DISEASES OF THE LIVER
AND BILIARY SYSTEM

Diseases of the Liver and Biliary System

SHEILA SHERLOCK

DBE, FRS
MD (Edin.), Hon. DSc (Edin., New York, Yale),
Hon. MD (Cambridge, Dublin, Leuven, Lisbon,
Mainz, Oslo, Padua, Toronto), Hon. LLD (Aberd.),
FRCP, FRCPE, FRACP, Hon. FRCCP,
Hon. FRCPI, Hon. FACP

Professor of Medicine,
Royal Free and University College Medical School
University College London,
London

JAMES DOOLEY

BSc, MD, FRCP

Reader and Honorary Consultant in Medicine,
Royal Free and University College Medical School,
University College London,
London

ELEVENTH EDITION

Blackwell
Science

© 1963, 1968, 1975, 1981, 1985, 1989, 1993, 1997, 2002 by
Blackwell Science Ltd a Blackwell Publishing Company
Editorial Offices:
Osney Mead, Oxford OX2 0EL, UK
    Tel: +44 (0)1865 206206
108 Cowley Road, Oxford OX4 1JF, UK
    Tel: +44 (0)1865 791100
Blackwell Publishing USA, 350 Main Street, Malden, MA 02148-5018, USA
    Tel: +1 781 388 8250
Iowa State Press, a Blackwell Publishing Company, 2121 State Avenue, Ames,
Iowa 50014-8300, USA
    Tel: + 515 292 0140
Blackwell Munksgaard, Nørre Søgade 35, PO Box 2148, Copenhagen, DK-1016, Denmark
    Tel: +45 77 33 33 33
Blackwell Publishing Asia, 54 University Street, Carlton, Victoria 3053, Australia
    Tel: +61 (0)3 9347 0300
Blackwell Verlag, Kurfurstendamm 57, 10707 Berlin, Germany
    Tel: +49 (0)30 32 79 060
Blackwell Publishing, 10 rue Casimir Delavigne, 75006 Paris, France
    Tel: +33 1 53 10 33 10

First published 1955   Fourth edition 1968   Eighth edition 1989
Reprinted 1956   Reprinted 1969, 1971   Reprinted 1991
Second edition 1958   Fifth edition 1975   Ninth edition 1993
Reprinted 1959, 1961   Sixth edition 1981   Reprinted 1993
Third edition 1963   Reprinted 1982, 1983   Tenth edition 1997
Reprinted 1965, 1966   Seventh edition 1985   Eleventh edition 2002
                            Reprinted 1986, 1987

Catalogue records for this title are available from the Library of Congress and the British
Library

ISBN 0-632-05582-0

Set in 8/10 pt Palatino by Best-set Typesetter Ltd, Hong Kong
Printed and bound in Italy, by Rotolito Lombarda, Milan

For further information on Blackwell Science, visit our website: www.blackwell-science.com

Contents

v

5 Ultrasound, Computed Tomography and Magnetic Resonance Imaging, 67

6 Hepato-cellular Failure, 81

7 Hepatic Encephalopathy, 93

8 Acute Liver Failure, 111

9 Ascites, 127

10   The Portal Venous System and Portal Hypertension, 147

11   The Hepatic Artery and Hepatic Veins: the Liver in Circulatory Failure, 187

x   *Contents*

Preface to the Eleventh Edition

The eleventh edition welcomes the new Millenium. Progress in basic and clinical hepatology remains exponential. Since 1997, the advances have been wide-ranging, with those in molecular and cellular biology, and in diagnosis and treatment, leading the way. In a world in which information technology gives all too ready access to individual publications, the eleventh edition sets the new within established knowledge and practice.

Viral hepatitis remains the worldwide hepatological challenge. This is reflected in a change in format with separate chapters on hepatitis B and C. Molecular virology continues to expose the inner workings of all the viruses. New therapeutic approaches are proving more effective against hepatitis C. Molecular and cellular biologists are showing us the importance of apoptosis and the intricate regulation of fibrosis. Mutation analysis for diagnosis of genetic haemochromatosis is routine, while the identification of the haemochromatosis gene has led to a surge of exploration in iron metabolism. Canalicular transporters have been cloned and linked to cholestatic syndromes, giving a new perspective to the bile plug seen under the microscope. Advances in imaging, particularly magnetic resonance, continue to reduce the need for invasive techniques. Patients needing transplantation benefit from improvements in immuno-suppression and surgical techniques, while there is steady progress in the management of complications of cirrhosis.

This edition contains more than 1000 new references and 100 new figures. Developments in publishing allow a more colourful format, but care has been taken to preserve clarity. Experience has shown that students, interns, postgraduate trainees as well as generalists and specialist clinicians have found previous editions useful. The goal of the book remains unchanged: a textbook of manageable size, critical and current.

We are indebted to many colleagues for their generous contributions to this edition including in particular Professor Peter Scheuer, Professor Amar Dhillon and Dr Susan Davies for histological material, and Dr Robert Dick, Dr Tony Watkinson and Dr Jon Tibballs for radiological images. We would also like to express our great thanks to Dr Leslie Berger, Dr Andrew Burroughs, Dr John Buscombe, Dr Martyn Caplin, Professor Geoffrey Dusheiko, Dr David Harry, Dr Andrew Hilson, Professor Humphrey Hodgson, Professor Neil McIntyre, Dr Kevin Moore, Dr Marsha Morgan, Dr Chris Kibbler and Dr David Patch for their help in the preparation of this edition.

Miss Aileen Duggan and Miss Karma Raines have assisted tirelessly with their meticulous secretarial support. The clarity and style of figures preserved from previous editions owes much to the artistry of Miss Janice Cox over many years.

We are grateful to Blackwell Publishing and, in particular, Rebecca Huxley for her tireless help with both manuscript and proofs, and for responding without a murmur to demands within a tight schedule. We also thank Jane Fallows who has reformatted and coloured all the previous line drawings as well as creating the many new and visually inviting figures for the eleventh edition.

The preface to the first edition which was published in 1955 refers to daughters Amanda and Auriole. Amanda is now an ordained Minister in the Baptist Church, and Auriole is working with Kent Police. Grandchildren have arrived, including Alice aged 9 and Emily aged 6.

On the 13th July 2001, the senior author was elected a Fellow of the Royal Society in its 341st year, a Society founded to improve natural knowledge. This honour was achieved because of the support of all the clinicians and scientists who have contributed to the Liver Unit and its associated departments at The Royal Free. The new Millenium is indeed an exciting time for all those working to solve the puzzles within hepato-biliary disease.

SHEILA SHERLOCK
JAMES DOOLEY
November 2001

Preface to the First Edition

My aim in writing this book has been to present a comprehensive and up-to-date account of diseases of the liver and biliary system, which I hope will be of value to physicians, surgeons and pathologists and also a reference book for the clinical student. The modern literature has been reviewed with special reference to articles of general interest. Many older more specialized classical contributions have therefore inevitably been excluded.

Disorders of the liver and biliary system may be classified under the traditional concept of individual diseases. Alternatively, as I have endeavoured in this book, they may be described by the functional and morphological changes which they produce. In the clinical management of a patient with liver disease, it is important to assess the degree of disturbance of four functional and morphological components of the liver—hepatic cells, vascular system (portal vein, hepatic artery and hepatic veins), bile ducts and reticulo-endothelial system. The typical reaction pattern is thus sought and recognized before attempting to diagnose the causative insult. Clinical and laboratory methods of assessing each of these components are therefore considered early in the book. Descriptions of individual diseases follow as illustrative examples. It will be seen that the features of hepatocellular failure and portal hypertension are described in general terms as a foundation for subsequent discussion of virus hepatitis, nutrition liver disease and the cirrhoses. Similarly blood diseases and infections of the liver are included with the reticulo-endothelial system, and disorders of the biliary tract follow descriptions of acute and chronic bile duct obstruction.

I would like to acknowledge my indebtedness to my teachers, the late Professor J. Henry Dible, the late Professor Sir James Learmonth and Professor Sir John McMichael, who stimulated my interest in hepatic disease, and to my colleagues at the Postgraduate Medical School and elsewhere who have generously invited me to see patients under their care. I am grateful to Dr A. G. Bearn for criticizing part of the typescript and to Dr A. Paton for his criticisms and careful proof reading. Miss D. F. Atkins gave much assistance with proof reading and with the bibliography. Mr Per Saugman and Mrs J. M. Green of Blackwell Scientific Publications have co-operated enthusiastically in the production of this book.

The photomicrographs were taken by Mr E. V. Willmott, FRPS, and Mr C. A. P. Graham from section prepared by Mr J. G. Griffin and the histology staff of the Postgraduate Medical School. Clinical photographs are the work of Mr C. R. Brecknell and his assistants. The black and white drawings were made by Mrs H. M. G. Wilson and Mr D. Simmonds. I am indebted to them all for their patience and skill.

The text includes part of unpublished material included in a thesis submitted in 1944 to the University of Edinburgh for the degree of MD, and part of an essay awarded the Buckston–Browne prize of the Harveian Society of London in 1953. Colleagues have allowed me to include published work of which they are jointly responsible. Dr Patricia P. Franklyn and Dr R. E. Steiner have kindly loaned me radiographs. Many authors have given me permission to reproduce illustrations and detailed acknowledgments are given in the text. I wish also to thank the editors of the following journals for permission to include illustrations: *American Journal of Medicine, Archives of Pathology, British Heart Journal, Circulation, Clinical Science, Edinburgh Medical Journal, Journal of Clinical Investigation, Journal of Laboratory and Clinical Investigation, Journal of Pathology and Bacteriology, Lancet, Postgraduate Medical Journal, Proceedings of the Staff Meetings of the Mayo Clinic, Quarterly Journal of Medicine, Thorax* and also the following publishers: Butterworth's Medical Publications, J. & A. Churchill Ltd, The Josiah Macy Junior Foundation and G. D. Searle & Co.

Finally I must thank my husband, Dr D. Geraint James, who, at considerable personal inconvenience, encouraged me to undertake the writing of this book and also criticized and rewrote most of it. He will not allow me to dedicate it to him.

SHEILA SHERLOCK

Chapter 1
Anatomy and Function

The liver, the largest organ in the body, weighs 1200–1500 g and comprises one-fiftieth of the total adult body weight. It is relatively larger in infancy, comprising one-eighteenth of the birth weight. This is mainly due to a large left lobe.

Sheltered by the ribs in the right upper quadrant, the upper border lies approximately at the level of the nipples. There are two anatomical lobes, the right being about six times the size of the left (figs 1.1–1.3). Lesser segments of the right lobe are the *caudate lobe* on the posterior surface and the *quadrate lobe* on the inferior surface. The right and left lobes are separated anteriorly by a fold of peritoneum called the falciform ligament,

posteriorly by the fissure for the ligamentum venosum and inferiorly by the fissure for the ligamentum teres.

The liver has a double blood supply. The *portal vein* brings venous blood from the intestines and spleen and the *hepatic artery*, coming from the coeliac axis, supplies the liver with arterial blood. These vessels enter the liver through a fissure, the *porta hepatis*, which lies far back on the inferior surface of the right lobe. Inside the porta, the portal vein and hepatic artery divide into branches to the right and left lobes, and the right and left hepatic bile ducts join to form the common hepatic duct. The *hepatic nerve plexus* contains fibres from the sympathetic ganglia

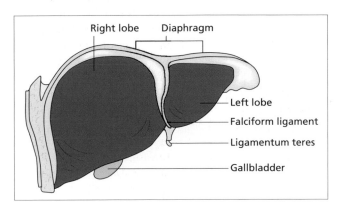

Fig. 1.1. Anterior view of the liver.

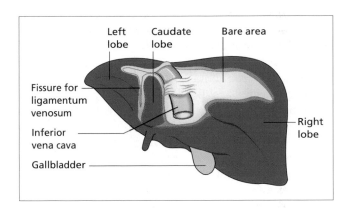

Fig. 1.2. Posterior view of the liver.

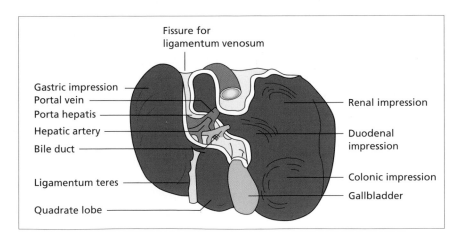

Fig. 1.3. Inferior view of the liver.

1

T7–T10, which synapse in the coeliac plexus, the right and left vagi and the right phrenic nerve. It accompanies the hepatic artery and bile ducts into their finest ramifications, even to the portal tracts and hepatic parenchyma [4].

The *ligamentum venosum*, a slender remnant of the ductus venosus of the fetus, arises from the left branch of the portal vein and fuses with the inferior vena cava at the entrance of the left hepatic vein. The *ligamentum teres*, a remnant of the umbilical vein of the fetus, runs in the free edge of the falciform ligament from the umbilicus to the inferior border of the liver and joins the left branch of the portal vein. Small veins accompanying it connect the portal vein with veins around the umbilicus. These become prominent when the portal venous system is obstructed inside the liver.

The venous drainage from the liver is into the *right* and *left hepatic veins* which emerge from the back of the liver and at once enter the inferior vena cava very near its point of entry into the right atrium.

Lymphatic vessels terminate in small groups of glands around the porta hepatis. Efferent vessels drain into glands around the coeliac axis. Some superficial hepatic lymphatics pass through the diaphragm in the falciform ligament and finally reach the mediastinal glands. Another group accompanies the inferior vena cava into the thorax and ends in a few small glands around the intrathoracic portion of the inferior vena cava.

The *inferior vena cava* makes a deep groove to the right of the caudate lobe about 2 cm from the mid-line.

The *gallbladder* lies in a fossa extending from the inferior border of the liver to the right end of the porta hepatis.

The liver is completely covered with peritoneum, except in three places. It comes into direct contact with the diaphragm through the bare area which lies to the right of the fossa for the inferior vena cava. The other areas without peritoneal covering are the fossae for the inferior vena cava and gallbladder.

The liver is kept in position by peritoneal ligaments and by the intra-abdominal pressure transmitted by the tone of the muscles of the abdominal wall.

Functional anatomy: sectors and segments

Based on the external appearances described above, the liver has a right and left lobe separated along the line of insertion of the falciform ligament. This separation, however, does not correlate with blood supply or biliary drainage. A *functional anatomy* is now recognized based upon studies of vascular and biliary casts made by injecting vinyl into the vessels and bile ducts. This classification correlates with that seen by imaging techniques.

The main portal vein divides into right and left branches and each of these supplies two further subunits (variously called sectors). The sectors on the right side are anterior and posterior and, in the left lobe, medial and lateral—giving a total of four sectors (fig. 1.4). Using this definition, the right and left side of the liver are divided not along the line of the falciform ligament, but along a slightly oblique line to the right of this, drawn from the inferior vena cava above to the gallbladder bed below. The right and left side are independent with regard to portal and arterial blood supply, and bile drainage. Three plains separate the four sectors and contain the three major hepatic vein branches.

Closer analysis of these four hepatic sectors produces a further subdivision into segments (fig. 1.5). The right anterior sector contains segments V and VIII; right posterior sector, VI and VII; left medial sector, IV; left lateral sector, segments II and III. There is no vascular anastomosis between the macroscopic vessels of the segments but communications exist at sinusoidal level. Segment I, the equivalent of the caudate lobe, is separate from the other segments and does not derive blood directly from the major portal branches or drain by any of the three major hepatic veins.

This functional anatomical classification allows interpretation of radiological data and is of importance to the

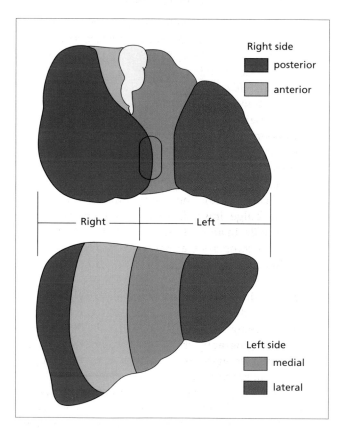

Fig. 1.4. The sectors of the human liver.

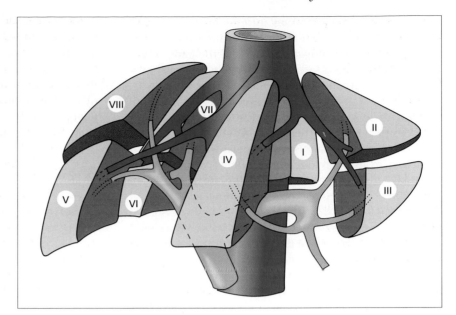

Fig. 1.5. Schematic representation of the functional anatomy of the liver. Three main hepatic veins (dark blue) divide the liver into four sectors, each of them receiving a portal pedicle; hepatic veins and portal veins are intertwined as the fingers of two hands [5].

surgeon planning a liver resection. There are wide variations in portal and hepatic vessel anatomy which can be demonstrated by spiral computed tomography (CT) and magnetic resonance imaging (MRI) reconstruction [41].

Anatomy of the biliary tract (fig. 1.6)

The *right* and *left hepatic ducts* emerge from the liver and unite in the porta hepatis to form the *common hepatic duct*. This is soon joined by the *cystic duct* from the gallbladder to form the common bile duct.

The *common bile duct* runs between the layers of the lesser omentum, lying anterior to the portal vein and to the right of the hepatic artery. Passing behind the first part of the duodenum in a groove on the back of the head of the pancreas, it enters the second part of the duodenum. The duct runs obliquely through the postero-medial wall, usually joining the main pancreatic duct to form the *ampulla of Vater* (1720). The ampulla makes the mucous membrane bulge inwards to form an eminence: the *duodenal papilla*. In about 10–15% of subjects the bile and pancreatic ducts open separately into the duodenum.

The dimensions of the common bile duct depend on the technique used. At operation it is about 0.5–1.5 cm in diameter. Using ultrasound the values are less, the common bile duct being 2–7 mm, with values greater than 7 mm being regarded as abnormal. Using endoscopic cholangiography, the duct diameter is usually less than 11 mm, although after cholecystectomy it may be more in the absence of obstruction.

The duodenal portion of the common bile duct is surrounded by a thickening of both longitudinal and circular muscle fibres derived from the intestine. This is called the *sphincter of Oddi* (1887).

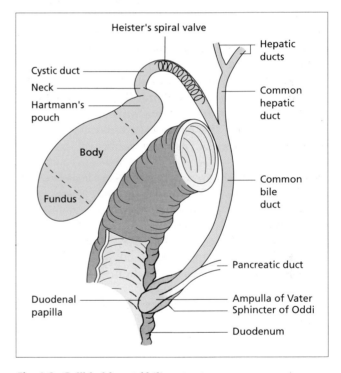

Fig. 1.6. Gallbladder and biliary tract.

The *gallbladder* is a pear-shaped bag 9 cm long with a capacity of about 50 ml. It always lies above the transverse colon, and is usually next to the duodenal cap overlying, but well anterior to, the right renal shadow.

Any decrease in concentrating power is accompanied by reduced distensibility. The fundus is the wider end and is directed anteriorly; this is the part palpated when the abdomen is examined. The body extends into a narrow neck which continues into the cystic duct. The *valves of Heister* are spiral folds of mucous membrane in the wall of the cystic duct and neck of the gallbladder. *Hartmann's pouch* is a sacculation at the neck of the gall-bladder; this is a common site for a gallstone to lodge.

The wall consists of a musculo-elastic network without definite layers, the muscle being particularly well developed in the neck and fundus. The mucous membrane is in delicate closely woven folds; instead of glands there are deep indentations of mucosa, the *crypts of Luschka*, which penetrate into the muscular layer. There is no submucosa or muscularis mucosae.

The *Rokitansky–Aschoff sinuses* are branching evaginations from the gallbladder lumen lined by mucosa reaching into the muscularis of the gallbladder. They play an important part in acute cholecystitis and gangrene of the gallbladder wall.

Blood supply. The gallbladder receives blood from the *cystic artery*. This branch of the hepatic artery is large, tortuous and variable in its anatomical relationships. Smaller blood vessels enter from the liver through the gallbladder fossa. The venous drainage is into the *cystic vein* and thence into the portal venous system.

The arterial blood supply to the supra-duodenal bile duct is generally by two main (axial) vessels which run beside the bile duct. These are supplied predominantly by the retro-duodenal artery from below, and the right hepatic artery from above, although many other vessels contribute. This pattern of arterial supply would explain why vascular damage results in bile duct stricturing [24].

Lymphatics. There are many lymphatic vessels in the submucous and subperitoneal layers. These drain through the cystic gland at the neck of the gallbladder to glands along the common bile duct, where they anastomose with lymphatics from the head of the pancreas.

Nerve supply. The gallbladder and bile ducts are liberally supplied with nerves, from both the parasympathetic and the sympathetic system.

Development of the liver and bile ducts

The liver begins as a hollow endodermal bud from the foregut (duodenum) during the third week of gestation. The bud separates into two parts—hepatic and biliary. The *hepatic* part contains bipotential progenitor cells that differentiate into hepatocytes or ductal cells, which form the early primitive bile duct structures (ductal plates). Differentiation is accompanied by changes in cytokeratin type within the cell [40]. Normally, this collection of rapidly proliferating cells penetrates adjacent mesodermal tissue (the septum transversum) and is met by ingrowing capillary plexuses from the vitelline and umbilical veins which will form the sinusoids. The connection between this proliferating mass of cells and the

foregut, the *biliary* part of the endodermal bud, will form the gallbladder and extra-hepatic bile ducts. Bile begins to flow at about the 12th week. Haemopoietic cells, Kupffer cells and connective tissue cells are derived from the mesoderm of the septum transversum. The fetal liver has a major haemopoietic function which subsides during the last 2 months of intra-uterine life so that only a few haemopoietic cells remain at birth.

Anatomical abnormalities of the liver

These are being increasingly diagnosed with more widespread use of CT and ultrasound scanning.

Accessory lobes. The livers of the pig, dog and camel are divided into distinct and separate lobes by strands of connective tissue. Occasionally, the human liver may show this reversion and up to 16 lobes have been reported. This abnormality is rare and without clinical significance. The lobes are small and usually on the under surface of the liver so that they are not detected clinically but are noted incidentally at scanning, operation or necropsy. Rarely they are intrathoracic. An accessory lobe may have its own mesentery containing hepatic artery, portal vein, bile duct and hepatic vein. This may twist and demand surgical intervention.

Riedel's lobe is fairly common and is a downward tongue-like projection of the right lobe of the liver. It is a simple anatomical variation; it is not a true accessory lobe. The condition is more frequent in women. It is detected as a mobile tumour on the right side of the abdomen which descends with the diaphragm on inspiration. It may come down as low as the right iliac region. It is easily mistaken for other tumours in this area, especially a visceroptotic right kidney. It does not cause symptoms and treatment is not required. Scanning may be used to identify Riedel's lobe and other anatomical abnormalities.

Cough furrows on the liver are parallel grooves on the convexity of the right lobe. They are one to six in number and run antero-posteriorly, being deeper posteriorly. They are said to be associated with a chronic cough.

Corset liver. This is a fibrotic furrow or pedicle on the anterior surface of both lobes of the liver just below the costal margin. The mechanism is unknown, but it affects elderly women who have worn corsets for many years. It presents as an abdominal mass in front of and below the liver and is isodense with the liver. It may be confused with a hepatic tumour.

Lobar atrophy. Interference with the portal supply or biliary drainage of a lobe may cause atrophy. There is usually hypertrophy of the opposite lobe. Left lobe atrophy found at post-mortem or during scanning is not uncommon and is probably related to reduced blood supply via the left branch of the portal vein. The lobe is decreased in size with thickening of the capsule, fibrosis and prominent biliary and vascular markings. The vascular problem may date from the time of birth.

Obstruction to the right or left hepatic bile duct by benign stricture or cholangiocarcinoma is now the most common cause of lobar atrophy [16]. The alkaline phosphatase is usually elevated. The bile duct may not be dilated within the atrophied lobe. Relief of obstruction may reverse the changes if cirrhosis has not developed. Distinction between a biliary and portal venous aetiology may be made using technetium-labelled iminodiacetic acid (IDA) and colloid scintiscans. A small lobe with normal uptake of IDA and colloid is compatible with a portal aetiology. Reduced or absent uptake of both isotopes favours biliary disease.

Agenesis of the right lobe [27]. This rare lesion may be an incidental finding associated, probably coincidentally, with biliary tract disease and also with other congenital abnormalities. It can cause pre-sinusoidal portal hypertension. The other liver segments undergo compensatory hypertrophy. It must be distinguished from lobar atrophy due to cirrhosis or hilar cholangiocarcinoma.

Anatomical abnormalities of the gallbladder and biliary tract are discussed in Chapter 33.

Surface marking (figs 1.7, 1.8)

Liver. The upper border of the right lobe is on a level with the 5th rib at a point 2 cm medial to the right mid-clavicular line (1 cm below the right nipple). The upper border of the left lobe corresponds to the upper border of the 6th rib at a point in the left mid-clavicular line (2 cm below the left nipple). Here only the diaphragm separates the liver from the apex of the heart.

The lower border passes obliquely upwards from the 9th right to the 8th left costal cartilage. In the right nipple line it lies between a point just under to 2 cm below the costal margin. It crosses the mid-line about mid-way between the base of the xiphoid and the umbilicus and the left lobe extends only 5 cm to the left of the sternum.

Gallbladder. Usually the fundus lies at the outer border of the right rectus abdominis muscle at its junction with the right costal margin (9th costal cartilage) (fig. 1.8). In an obese subject it may be difficult to identify the outer border of the rectus sheath and the gallbladder may then be located by the Grey–Turner method. A line is drawn from the left anterior superior iliac spine through the umbilicus; its intersection with the right costal margin indicates the position of the gallbladder. These guidelines depend upon the individual's build. The fundus may occasionally be found below the iliac crest.

Methods of examination

Liver. The lower edge should be determined by palpation just lateral to the right rectus muscle. This avoids mistaking the upper intersection of the rectus sheath for the liver edge.

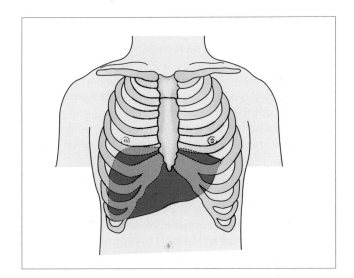

Fig. 1.7. The surface marking of the liver.

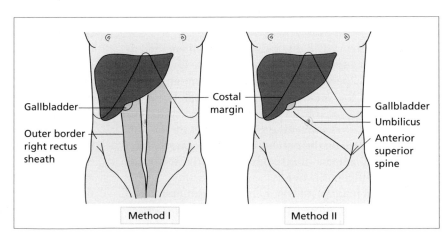

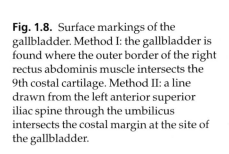

Fig. 1.8. Surface markings of the gallbladder. Method I: the gallbladder is found where the outer border of the right rectus abdominis muscle intersects the 9th costal cartilage. Method II: a line drawn from the left anterior superior iliac spine through the umbilicus intersects the costal margin at the site of the gallbladder.

Gallbladder

Outer border right rectus sheath

Costal margin

Gallbladder

Umbilicus

Anterior superior spine

Method I

Method II

The liver edge moves 1–3 cm downwards with deep inspiration. It is usually palpable in normal subjects inspiring deeply. The edge may be tender, regular or irregular, firm or soft, thickened or sharp. The lower edge may be displaced downwards by a low diaphragm, for instance in emphysema. Movements may be particularly great in athletes or singers. Some patients with practice become very efficient at 'pushing down' the liver. The normal spleen can become palpable in similar fashion. Common causes of a liver palpable below the umbilicus are malignant deposits, polycystic or Hodgkin's disease, amyloidosis, congestive cardiac failure and gross fatty change. Rapid change in liver size may occur when congestive cardiac failure is corrected, cholestatic jaundice relieved, or when severe diabetes is controlled. The surface can be palpated in the epigastrium and any irregularity or tenderness noted. An enlarged caudate lobe, as in the Budd–Chiari syndrome or with some cases of cirrhosis, may be palpated as an epigastric mass.

Pulsation of the liver, usually associated with tricuspid valvular incompetence, is felt by manual palpation with one hand behind the right lower ribs posteriorly and the other anteriorly on the abdominal wall.

The upper edge is determined by fairly heavy percussion passing downwards from the nipple line. The lower edge is recognized by very light percussion passing upwards from the umbilicus towards the costal margin. Percussion is a valuable method of determining liver size and is the only clinical method of determining a small liver.

The anterior liver span is obtained by measuring the vertical distance between the uppermost and lowermost points of hepatic dullness by percussion in the right mid-clavicular line. This is usually 12–15 cm. Direct percussion is as accurate as ultrasound in estimating liver span [33].

Friction may be palpable and audible, usually due to recent biopsy, tumour or peri-hepatitis. The venous hum of portal hypertension is audible between the umbilicus and the xiphisternum. An arterial murmur over the liver may indicate a primary liver cancer or acute alcoholic hepatitis.

The *gallbladder* is palpable only when it is distended. It is felt as a pear-shaped cystic mass usually about 7 cm long. In a thin person, the swelling can sometimes be seen through the anterior abdominal wall. It moves downwards on inspiration and is mobile laterally but not downwards. The swelling is dull to percussion and directly impinges on the parietal peritoneum, so that the colon is rarely in front of it. Gallbladder dullness is continuous with that of the liver.

Abdominal tenderness should be noted. Inflammation of the gallbladder causes a positive *Murphy's sign*. This is the inability to take a deep breath when the examining fingers are hooked up below the liver edge. The inflamed gallbladder is then driven against the fingers and the pain causes the patient to catch their breath.

The enlarged gallbladder must be distinguished from a *visceroptotic right kidney*. This, however, is more mobile, can be displaced towards the pelvis and has the resonant colon anteriorly. A *regenerative* or *malignant nodule* feels much firmer.

Imaging. A plain film of the abdomen, including the diaphragms, may be used to assess liver size and in particular to decide whether a palpable liver is due to actual enlargement or to downward displacement. On moderate inspiration the normal level of the diaphragm, on the right side, is opposite the 11th rib posteriorly and the 6th rib anteriorly.

Ultrasound, CT or MRI can also be used to study liver size, shape and content.

Hepatic morphology

Kiernan (1833) introduced the concept of hepatic lobules as the basic architecture. He described circumscribed pyramidal lobules consisting of a central tributary of the hepatic vein and at the periphery a portal tract containing the bile duct, portal vein radicle and hepatic artery branch. Columns of liver cells and blood-containing sinusoids extend between these two systems.

Stereoscopic reconstructions and scanning electron microscopy have shown the human liver as columns of liver cells radiating from a central vein, and interlaced in orderly fashion by sinusoids (fig. 1.9).

The liver tissue is pervaded by two systems of tunnels, the portal tracts and the hepatic central canals which dovetail in such a way that they never touch each other; the terminal tunnels of the two systems are separated by about 0.5 mm (fig. 1.10). As far as possible the two systems of tunnels run in planes perpendicular to each other. The sinusoids are irregularly disposed, normally in a direction perpendicular to the lines connecting the central veins. The terminal branches of the portal vein discharge their blood into the sinusoids and the direction of flow is determined by the higher pressure in the portal vein than in the central vein.

The *central hepatic canals* contain radicles of the hepatic vein and their adventitia. They are surrounded by a limiting plate of liver cells.

The *portal triads* (syn. portal tracts, Glisson's capsule) contain the portal vein radicle, the hepatic arteriole and bile duct with a few round cells and a little connective tissue (fig. 1.11). They are surrounded by a limiting plate of liver cells. Portal dyads are as frequent as triads, with the portal vein being the most frequently absent element. Within each linear centimetre of liver tissue obtained at

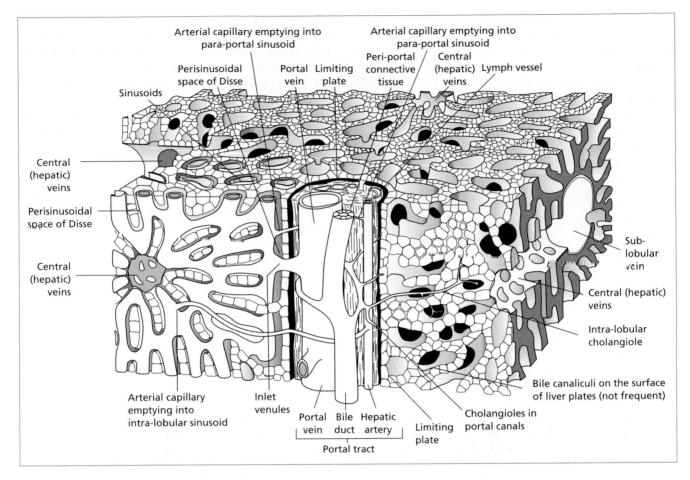

Fig. 1.9. The structure of the normal human liver.

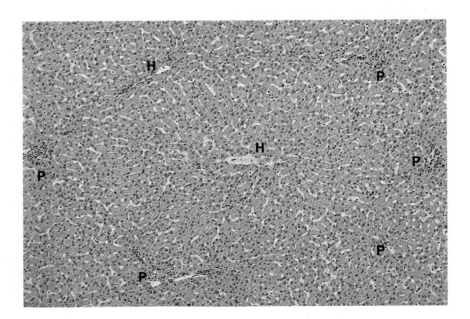

Fig. 1.10. Normal hepatic histology. H, terminal hepatic vein; P, portal tract. (H & E, ×60.)

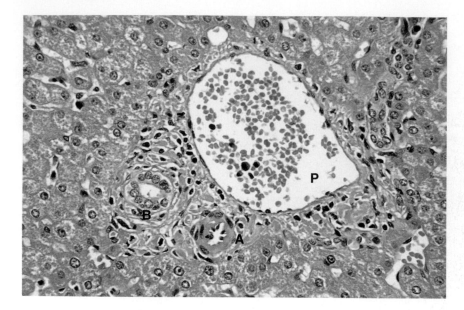

Fig. 1.11. Normal portal tract. A, hepatic artery; B, bile duct; P, portal vein. (H & E.)

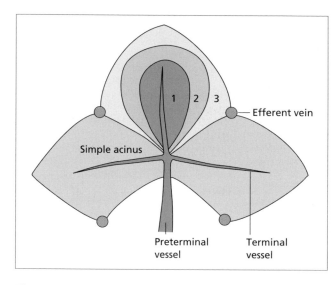

Fig. 1.12. The complex acinus according to Rappaport. Zone 1 is adjacent to the entry (portal venous) system. Zone 3 is adjacent to the exit (hepatic venous) system.

biopsy there are usually two interlobular bile ducts, two hepatic arteries and one portal vein per portal tract, with six full portal triads [8].

The liver has to be divided *functionally*. Traditionally, the unit is based on a central hepatic vein and its surrounding liver cells. However, Rappaport [28] envisages a series of functional acini, each centred on the portal triad with its terminal branch of portal vein, hepatic artery and bile duct (zone 1) (figs 1.12, 1.13). These interdigitate, mainly perpendicularly, with terminal hepatic veins of adjacent acini. The circulatory peripheries of acini (adjacent to terminal hepatic veins) (zone 3) suffer most from injury whether viral, toxic or anoxic. Bridging

necrosis is located in this area. The regions closer to the axis formed by afferent vessels and bile ducts survive longer and may later form the core from which regeneration will proceed. The contribution of each acinar zone to liver cell regeneration depends on the acinar location of damage [28].

The liver cells (*hepatocytes*) comprise about 60% of the liver. They are polygonal and approximately 30 μm in diameter. The nucleus is single or, less often, multiple and divides by mitosis. The lifespan of liver cells is about 150 days in experimental animals. The hepatocyte has three surfaces: one facing the sinusoid and space of Disse, the second facing the canaliculus and the third facing neighbouring hepatocytes (fig. 1.14). There is no basement membrane.

The sinusoids are lined by endothelial cells. Associated with the sinusoids are the phagocytic cells of the reticulo-endothelial system (Kupffer cells), and the hepatic stellate cells, which have also been called fat-storing cells, Ito cells and lipocytes.

There are approximately 202×10^3 cells in each milligram of normal human liver, of which 171×10^3 are parenchymal and 31×10^3 littoral (sinusoidal, including Kupffer cells).

The *space of Disse* is a tissue space between hepatocytes and sinusoidal endothelial cells. The *hepatic lymphatics* are found in the peri-portal connective tissue and are lined throughout by endothelium. Tissue fluid seeps through the endothelium into the lymph vessels.

The branch of the *hepatic arteriole* forms a plexus around the bile ducts and supplies the structures in the portal tracts. It empties into the sinusoidal network at different levels. There are no direct hepatic arteriolar–portal venous anastomoses.

The excretory system of the liver begins with the *bile*

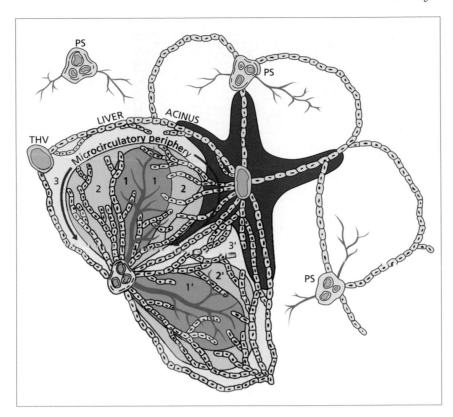

Fig. 1.13. Blood supply of the simple liver acinus, zonal arrangements of cells and the microcirculatory periphery. The acinus occupies adjacent sectors of the neighbouring hexagonal fields. Zones 1, 2 and 3, respectively, represent areas supplied with blood of first, second and third quality with regard to oxygen and nutrient content. These zones centre on the terminal afferent vascular branches, bile ductules, lymph vessels and nerves (PS) and extend into the triangular portal field from which these branches crop out. Zone 3 is the microcirculatory periphery of the acinus since its cells are as remote from their own afferent vessels as from those of adjacent acini. The *peri-venular* area is formed by the most peripheral portions of zone 3 of several adjacent acini. In injury progressing along this zone, the damaged area assumes the shape of a starfish (darker tint around a terminal hepatic venule, THV, in the centre). 1–3, microcirculatory zones; 1′–3′, zones of neighbouring acinus [28].

canaliculi (see figs 13.2, 13.3). These have no walls but are simply grooves on the contact surfaces of liver cells (see fig. 13.1). Their surfaces are covered by microvilli. The plasma membrane is reinforced by micro-filaments forming a supportive cytoskeleton (see fig. 13.2). The canalicular surface is sealed from the rest of the inter-cellular surface by junctional complexes including tight junctions, gap junctions and desmosomes. The intra-lobular canalicular network drains into thin-walled terminal bile ducts or ductules (cholangioles, canals of Hering) lined with cuboidal epithelium. These terminate in larger (interlobular) bile ducts in the portal canals. They are classified into small (less than 100 μm in diame-ter), medium (about 100 μm) and large (more than 100 μm).

Electron microscopy and hepato-cellular function (figs 1.14, 1.15)

The liver cell margin is straight except for a few anchor-ing pegs (desmosomes). From it, equally sized and spaced microvilli project into the lumen of the bile canaliculi. Along the sinusoidal border, irregularly sized and spaced microvilli project into the peri-sinusoidal tissue space. The microvillous structure indicates active secretion or absorption, mainly of fluid.

The *nucleus* has a double contour with pores allowing interchange with the surrounding cytoplasm. Human liver after puberty contains tetraploid nuclei and, at about age 20, in addition, octoploid nuclei are found. Increased polyploidy has been regarded as precancer-ous. In the chromatin network one or more nucleoli are embedded.

The *mitochondria* also have a double membrane, the inner being invaginated to form grooves or cristae. An enormous number of energy-providing processes take place within them, particularly those involving oxida-tive phosphorylation. They contain many enzymes, par-ticularly those of the citric acid cycle and those involved in β-oxidation of fatty acids. They can transform energy

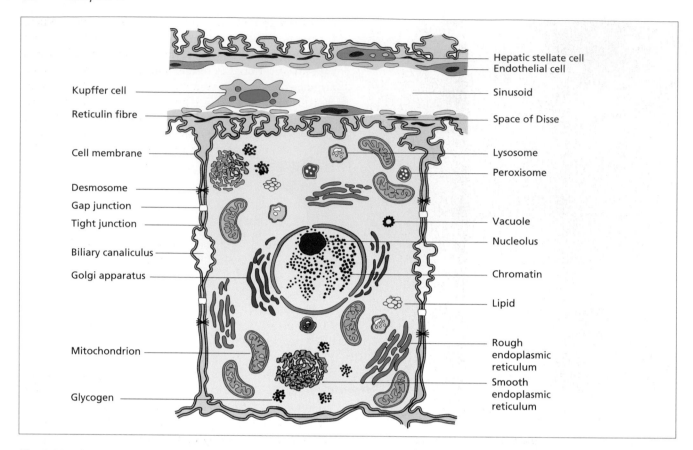

Fig. 1.14. The organelles of the liver cell.

so released into adenosine diphosphate (ADP). Haem synthesis occurs here.

The *rough endoplasmic reticulum* (RER) is seen as lamellar structures lined by ribosomes. These are responsible for basophilia under light microscopy. They synthesize specific proteins, particularly albumin, those used in blood coagulation and enzymes. They may adopt a helix arrangement, as polysomes, for co-ordination of this function. Glucose-6-phosphatase is synthesized. Triglycerides are synthesized from free fatty acids and complexed with protein to be secreted by exocytosis as lipoprotein. The RER may participate in glycogenesis.

The *smooth endoplasmic reticulum* (SER) forms tubules and vesicles. It contains the microsomes. It is the site of bilirubin conjugation and the detoxification of many drugs and other foreign compounds (P450 systems). Steroids are synthesized, including cholesterol and the primary bile acids, which are conjugated with the amino acids glycine and taurine. The SER is increased by enzyme inducers such as phenobarbital.

Peroxisomes are versatile organelles, which have complex catabolic and biosynthetic roles, and are distributed near the SER and glycogen granules. Peroxisomal enzymes include simple oxidases, β-oxidation cycles, the glyoxalate cycle, ether lipid synthesis, and cholesterol and dolichol biosynthesis. Several disorders of peroxisomal function are recognized of which Zellweger syndrome is one [14]. Endotoxin severely damages peroxisomes [7].

The *lysosomes* are dense bodies adjacent to the bile canaliculi. They contain many hydrolytic enzymes which, if released, could destroy the cell. They are probably intra-cellular scavengers which destroy organelles with shortened lifespans. They are the site of deposition of ferritin, lipofuscin, bile pigment and copper. Pinocytic vacuoles may be observed in them. Some pericanalicular dense bodies are termed *microbodies*.

The *Golgi apparatus* consists of a system of particles and vesicles again lying near the canaliculus. It may be regarded as a 'packaging' site before excretion into the bile. This entire group of lysosomes, microbodies and Golgi apparatus is a means of sequestering any material which is ingested and has to be excreted, secreted or stored for metabolic processes in the cytoplasm. The Golgi apparatus, lysosomes and canaliculi are concerned in cholestasis (Chapter 13).

The intervening cytoplasm contains granules of glycogen, lipid and fine fibrils.

The *cytoskeleton* supporting the hepatocyte consists

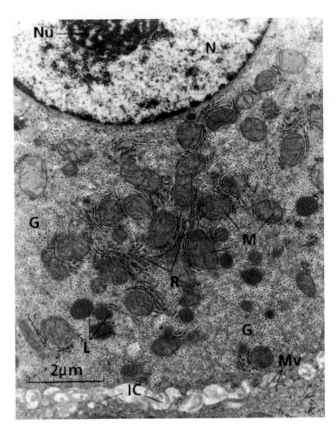

Fig. 1.15. Electron microscopic appearances of part of a normal human liver cell. G, glycogen granules; IC, intercellular space; L, lysosomes; M, mitochondria; Mv, microvilli in the intra-cellular space; N, nucleus; Nu, nucleolus; R, rough endoplasmic reticulum. (Courtesy of Ms J. Lewin.)

of microtubules, micro-filaments and intermediate filaments [12]. Microtubules contain tubulin and control subcellular mobility, vesicle movement and plasma protein secretion. Micro-filaments are made up of actin, are contractile and are important for the integrity and motility of the canaliculus and for bile flow. Intermediate filaments are elongated branched filaments comprising cytokeratins [40]. They extend from the plasma membrane to the peri-nuclear area and are fundamental for the stability and spatial organization of the hepatocyte.

Sinusoidal cells

The sinusoidal cells (endothelial cells, Kupffer cells, hepatic stellate cells and pit cells) form a functional and histological unit together with the sinusoidal aspect of the hepatocyte [34].

Endothelial cells line the sinusoids and have fenestrae which provide a graded barrier between the sinusoid and space of Disse (fig. 1.16). The Kupffer cells are attached to the endothelium.

The hepatic stellate cells lie in the space of Disse between the hepatocytes and the endothelial cells (fig. 1.17). *Disse's space* contains tissue fluid which flows outwards into lymphatics in the portal zones. When sinusoidal pressure rises, lymph production in Disse's space increases and this plays a part in ascites formation where there is hepatic venous outflow obstruction.

Endothelial cells. These cells form a continuous lining to the sinusoids. They differ from endothelial cells else-

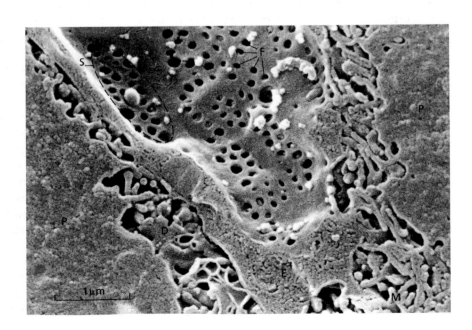

Fig. 1.16. Scanning electron micrograph of sinusoid showing fenestrae (F) grouped into sieve plates (S). D, space of Disse; E, endothelial cell; M, microvilli; P, parenchymal cell. (Courtesy of Professor E. Wisse.)

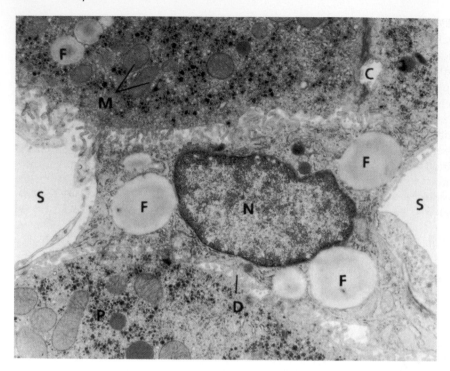

Fig. 1.17. Transmission electron micrograph of a hepatic stellate cell. Note the characteristic fat droplets (F). C, bile canaliculus; D, space of Disse; M, mitochondria; N, nucleus; P, parenchymal cell; S, lumen of sinusoid. (×12000.) (Courtesy of Professor E. Wisse.)

where in not having a regular basal lamina. The endothelial cells act as a sieve between the sinusoid and space of Disse, have specific and non-specific endocytotic activity and have a variety of receptors. Their capacity to act as a sieve is due to fenestrae, around 0.15 μm in diameter (fig. 1.16). These make up 6–8% of the total endothelial cell surface, and there are more in the centrilobular zone of the sinusoid than the peri-portal area. Extra-cellular matrix affects their function.

Fenestrae are clustered into sieve plates, and act as a biofilter between sinusoidal blood and the plasma within the space of Disse. They have a dynamic cytoskeleton [6]. This maintains and regulates their size, which can be changed by many influences including alcohol, nicotine, serotonin, endotoxin and partial hepatectomy. The fenestrae filter macro-molecules of differing size. Particles >0.2 μm diameter, which includes large triglyceride-rich parent chylomicrons, will not pass. Smaller triglyceride-depleted, cholesterol-rich and retinol-rich remnants can enter the space of Disse [15]. In this way the fenestrae have an important role in chylomicron and lipoprotein metabolism.

Endothelial cells have a high capacity for endocytosis (accounting for 45% of all pinocytotic vesicles in the liver) and are active in clearing macro-molecules and small particles from the circulation [35]. There is receptor-mediated endocytosis for several molecules including transferrin, caeruloplasmin, modified high density lipoprotein (HDL) and low density lipoprotein (LDL), hepatic lipase and very low density lipoprotein (VLDL). Hyaluronan (a major polysaccharide from con-

nective tissue) is taken up and this provides a method for assessing hepatic endothelial cell capacity. Endothelial cells can also clear small particles (<0.1 μm) from the circulation, as well as denatured collagen. Scanning electron microscopy has shown a striking reduction in the number of fenestrae, particularly in zone 3 in alcoholic patients, with formation of a basal lamina, which is also termed capillarization of the sinusoid [17].

Kupffer cells. These are highly mobile macrophages attached to the endothelial lining of the sinusoid, particularly in the peri-portal area. They stain with peroxidase. They have microvilli and intra-cytoplasmic-coated vesicles and dense bodies which make up the lysosomal apparatus. They proliferate locally but under certain circumstances macrophages can immigrate from an extra-hepatic site. They are responsible for removing old and damaged blood cells or cellular debris, also bacteria, viruses, parasites and tumour cells. They do this by endocytosis (phagocytosis, pinocytosis), including absorptive (receptor-mediated) and fluid phase (non-receptor-mediated) mechanisms [39]. Several processes aid this, including cell surface Fc and complement receptors. Coating of the particle with plasma fibronectin or opsonin also facilitates phagocytosis, since Kupffer cells have specific binding sites for fibronectin on the cell surface. These cells also take up and process oxidized LDL (thought to be atherogenic), and remove fibrin in disseminated intravascular coagulation. Alcohol reduces the phagocytic capacity.

Kupffer cells are activated by a wide range of agents, including endotoxin, sepsis, shock, interferon-γ, arachidonic acid and tumour necrosis factor (TNF). The result of activation is the production of an equally wide range of products: cytokines, hydrogen peroxide, nitric oxide, TNF, interleukin (IL) 1, IL6 and IL10, interferon-α and -β, transforming growth factor (TGF-β) and various prostanoids [34]. This whole array acts alone or in combination to stimulate other events in the cytokine cascade, but also increases discomfort and sickness. The Kupffer cell products may be toxic to parenchymal cells and endothelial cells. Kupffer cell-conditioned medium inhibits albumin synthesis in parenchymal cells, as do IL1, IL6 and TNF-α. The toxicity of endotoxin is caused by the secretory products of Kupffer cells since endotoxin itself is not directly toxic.

Hepatic stellate cells (fat-storing cells, lipocytes, Ito cells). These cells lie within the sub-endothelial space of Disse. They have long cytoplasmic extensions, some giving close contact with parenchymal cells, and others reaching several sinusoids, where they may regulate blood flow and hence influence portal hypertension [29]. In normal liver they are the major storage site of retinoids, giving the morphological characteristic of cytoplasmic lipid droplets. When empty of these droplets, they resemble fibroblasts. They contain actin and myosin and contract in response to endothelin-1 and substance P [30]. With hepatocyte injury, hepatic stellate cells lose their lipid droplets, proliferate, migrate to zone 3 of the acinus, change to a myofibroblast-like phenotype, and produce collagen type I, III and IV and laminin. Stellate cells also release matrix proteinases and inhibitory molecules of matrix proteinases (tissue inhibitor of metalloproteinases, TIMP) (Chapter 21) [3]. Collagenization of the space of Disse results in decreased access of protein-bound substrates to the hepatocyte.

Pit cells. These are highly mobile liver-specific natural killer lymphocytes attached to the sinusoidal surface of the endothelium [42]. They are short-lived cells and are renewed from circulating large granular lymphocytes which differentiate within the sinusoids. They have characteristic granules and rod-cored vesicles. Pit cells show spontaneous cytotoxicity against tumour- and virus-infected hepatocytes.

Sinusoidal cell interactions

There are complex interactions between Kupffer and endothelial cells, as well as sinusoidal cells and hepatocytes [31]. Kupffer cell activation by lipopolysaccharide suppresses hyaluronan uptake by endothelial cells, an effect probably mediated by leukotrienes [10]. Cytokines produced by sinusoidal cells can both stimulate and inhibit hepatocyte proliferation [22].

Hepatocyte death and regeneration
(fig. 1.18)

Normal liver structure and function depends upon a balance between cell death and regeneration [11, 20].

Cell death. Hepatocytes die as a result of either necrosis or apoptosis. The characteristic of *necrosis* is loss of plasma membrane integrity with release of the cellular contents locally which elicit an inflammatory response. This may potentiate the disease process and lead to further cell death.

Apoptosis is the mechanism by which cells, damaged, senescent or excess to requirement, self-destruct with the least production of inflammatory products [13, 26]. There is DNA fragmentation; organelles remain viable. Thus in comparison with necrotic cells, there is minimal release of injurious products, although there may still be a fibrotic reaction. Equilibrium within normal tissue depends upon the mitotic rate equalling the rate of apoptosis.

Pathological processes can alter the cellular mechanisms involved in apoptosis, leading to disease [25]. Increased apoptosis affecting cholangiocytes may lead to ductopenia. Experimentally, maximal stimulation of

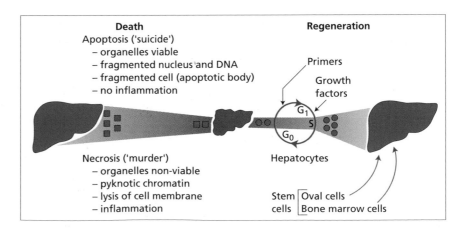

Fig. 1.18. Liver cell death and regeneration. Hepatocytes are lost either through apoptosis or necrosis. The liver normally regenerates through cellular replication. Priming is necessary for hepatocytes to respond to growth factors. If hepatocyte loss is massive or the toxic attack persists, cellular replication may not be possible. Liver cells may then be derived from stem cells either from within the liver (oval cells) or from the bone marrow.

hepato-cellular apoptosis leads to fulminant liver failure. Apoptosis is increased in alcoholic hepatitis [23]. If cells containing a mutation predisposing to malignant change do not undergo apoptosis, malignant transformation is enhanced.

The pathway to apoptopic cellular destruction is complex, and can be described in morphological and biochemical terms. Once the process is initiated a cascade of changes occurs, which may be irreversible after a particular stage is reached. There is great interest in the development of agents that interfere with the apoptotic process, since these may have a therapeutic place in diseases where apoptosis is increased or decreased.

Regeneration. When there is a need for additional hepatocytes, quiescent cells are stimulated by mediators (primers), including cytokines, to move into a primed state ($G_0 \rightarrow G_1$), when growth factors can stimulate DNA synthesis and cellular replication (fig. 1.18). Priming activates transcription factors including NFλB and STAT 3. Regeneration may be rapid, as seen after partial hepatectomy.

If hepatocytes are damaged so that this response is impaired, hepatocytes may be derived from cells associated with bile ductules, so-called oval cells. It is thought that these cells are derived from the cells of small bile ducts or canals of Hering and are related to embryonic ductal plate hepatocytes [32, 38].

Hepatocytes may also be derived from extra-hepatic stem cells, probably of bone marrow origin [9, 36]. Thus Y chromosome positive (male) hepatocytes and cholangiocytes are found in female livers transplanted into male recipients, and in the livers of female patients who have had a bone marrow transplant from a male donor [2, 37].

Extra-cellular matrix

This is obvious when there is liver disease, but also exists in a subtle form even in normal liver. In or around the space of Disse, all major constituents of a basement membrane can be found including type IV collagen, laminin, heparan sulphate, protoglycan and fibronectin. All cells impinging on the sinusoid can contribute to this matrix. The matrix within Disse's space influences hepato-cellular function [31], affecting expression of tissue-specific genes such as albumin as well as the number and porosity of sinusoidal fenestrations [21]. It may be important in liver regeneration.

Altered hepatic microcirculation and disease

In liver disease, particularly in the alcoholic, the liver microcirculation may be altered by collagenization of the space of Disse—formation of a basal lamina beneath the endothelium and modification of the endothelial fenestrations [17]. All these processes are maximal in zone 3. They contribute to deprivation of nutrients intended for the hepatocyte and to the development of portal hypertension.

Adhesion molecules

In hepatic inflammation lymphocytes are often the cells infiltrating the liver. There is an interaction between the receptor on the leucocyte surface, lymphocyte function-associated antigen (LFA-1) and an inter-cellular adhesion molecule (ICAM-1 or -2). ICAM-1 is expressed strongly on sinusoidal lining cells and weakly on portal and hepatic endothelium in normal liver. Induction of ICAM-1 on biliary epithelium, vascular endothelium and peri-venular hepatocytes is found in post-transplant rejection. Expression of this adhesion molecule on bile ducts has been found in primary biliary cirrhosis and primary sclerosing cholangitis [1].

Functional heterogeneity [18]

The relative functions of cells in the circulatory periphery of acini (zone 3) adjacent to terminal hepatic veins are different from those in the circulatory area adjacent to terminal hepatic arteries and portal veins (zone 1) (see figs 1.12, 1.13, table 1.1).

Krebs' cycle enzymes (urea synthesis and glutaminase) are found in the highest concentration in zone 1, whereas glutamine synthetase is peri-venous.

Oxygen supply is an obvious difference [18]; cells in zone 3 receive their oxygen supply last and are particularly prone to anoxic liver injury.

The drug-metabolizing P450 enzymes are present in greater amounts in zone 3. This is particularly so after enzyme induction, for instance with phenobarbital. Hepatocytes in zone 3 receive a higher concentration of any toxic product of drug metabolism. They also have a reduced glutathione concentration. This makes them particularly susceptible to hepatic drug reactions.

Hepatocytes in zone 1 receive blood with a high bile salt concentration and, therefore, are particularly important in bile-salt-dependent bile formation. Hepatocytes in zone 3 are important in non-bile-salt-dependent bile formation. There are also zonal differences in the hepatic transport rate of substances from the sinusoid to canaliculus.

The cause of the metabolic difference between the zones varies. For some functions (gluconeogenesis, glycolysis, ketogenesis) it appears to be dependent upon the direction of blood flow along the sinusoid. For others (cytochrome P450) the gene transcription rate differs between peri-venous and peri-portal hepatocytes. The

Table 1.1. Metabolism related to the zonal location of the hepatocyte whether acinar zone 1 ('peri-portal') or zone 3 ('central')

	Zone 1	Zone 3
Carbohydrates	Gluconeogenesis	Glycolysis
Proteins	Albumin } synthesis Fibrinogen	Albumin } synthesis Fibrinogen
Cytochrome P450	+	++
after phenobarbital	+	++++++++
Glutathione	++	−
Oxygen supply	+++	+
Bile formation		
bile-salt-dependent	++	−
non-bile-salt-dependent	−	++
Sinusoids	Small	Straight
	Highly anastomotic	Radial

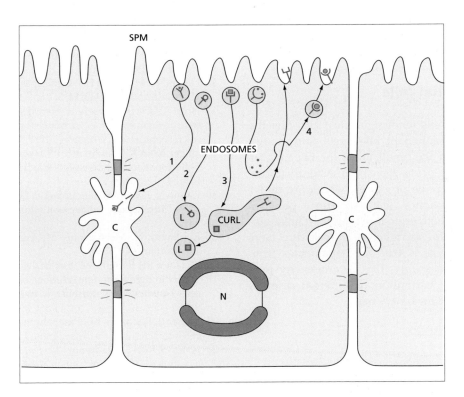

Fig. 1.19. Pathways of endocytosis from the sinusoidal plasma membrane (SPM). Receptors bound to ligand group together in a coated pit. There is endocytosis resulting in a coated vesicle which then loses its clatharin coat and fuses with other vesicles to form early endosomes (the site of sorting). Subsequent pathways include:

1 vesicular transport to the bile canaliculus (C) where the ligand and receptor are released (transcytosis) (e.g. polymeric IgA);

2 transfer of the ligand and receptor to a lysosome (L) where they are degraded;

3 the receptor and ligand are transferred to a compartment of uncoupling of receptor and ligand (CURL). The receptor and ligand separate. The receptor returns to sinusoidal plasma membrane and the ligand enters a lysosome and is degraded (e.g. LDL, asialoglycoprotein, insulin);

4 the ligand and receptor return to the plasma membrane (e.g. transferrin and its receptor after release of iron).

N, nucleus.

differential expression of glutamine synthetase across the acinus is already established in fetal liver.

Sinusoidal membrane traffic

The sinusoidal plasma membrane is a receptor-rich and metabolically dynamic domain which is separated from the bile canaliculus by a lateral domain which participates in cell–cell interactions (see fig. 1.14). Receptor-mediated endocytosis is responsible for the transfer of large molecules such as glycoproteins, growth factors and carrier proteins (transferrin). These ligands bind to receptors on the sinusoidal membrane, the occupied receptors cluster into a coated (clathrin) pit and endocytosis proceeds. The fate of the ligand within the cell varies according to the molecule involved, and the pathways are complex (fig. 1.19). Many ligands terminate in lysosomes where they are broken down while the receptor returns to the sinusoidal plasma membrane to perform again. Some ligands pass by vesicular transport across the cell to be discharged into the bile canaliculus.

Bile duct epithelial cells

Bile duct epithelial cells (cholangiocytes) [19] line the extra-hepatic and intra-hepatic bile ducts, and modify the bile derived from the canaliculi of the hepatocytes (Chapter 13). Cholangiocytes have both secretory (bicarbonate) and re-absorptive processes, which are under the control of hormones (e.g. secretin), peptides (endothelin-1) and cholinergic innervation. Cholangiocytes derived from different levels of the bile duct have different properties—as is true for hepatocytes from different areas of the acinus. This heterogeneity may explain in part the distribution of different diseases across specific areas of the biliary tree.

References

1 Adams DH, Hubscher SG, Shaw J *et al*. Increased expression of intercellular adhesion molecule 1 on bile ducts in primary biliary cirrhosis and primary sclerosing cholangitis. *Hepatology* 1991; **14**: 426.
2 Alison MR, Poulsom R, Jeffery R *et al*. Hepatocytes from non-hepatic adult stem cells. *Nature* 2000; 406: 257.
3 Arthur MJP, Mann DA, Iredale JP. Tissue inhibitors of metalloproteinases, hepatic stellate cells and liver fibrosis. *J. Gastroenterol. Hepatol.* 1998; **13**: S33.
4 Bioulac-Sage P, Lafon ME, Saric J *et al*. Nerves and perisinusoidal cells in human liver. *J. Hepatol.* 1990; **10**: 105.
5 Bismuth H. Surgical anatomy and anatomical surgery of the liver. *World J. Surg.* 1982; **6**: 3.
6 Braet F, De Zanger R, Baekeland M *et al*. Structure and dynamics of the fenestrae-associated cytoskeleton of rat liver sinusoidal endothelial cells. *Hepatology* 1995; **21**: 180.
7 Contreras MA, Khan M, Smith BT *et al*. Endotoxin induces structure–function alterations of rat liver peroxisomes: Kupffer cells released factors as possible modulators. *Hepatology* 2000; **31**: 446.
8 Crawford AR, Lin X-Z, Crawford JM. The normal adult human liver biopsy: a quantitative reference standard. *Hepatology* 1998; **28**: 323.
9 Crosbie OM, Reynolds M, McEntee G *et al. In vitro* evidence for the presence of haematopoietic stem cells in the adult human liver. *Hepatology* 1999; **29**: 1193.
10 Deaciuc IV, Bagby GJ, Niesman MR *et al*. Modulation of hepatic sinusoidal endothelial cell function by Kupffer cells: an example of intercellular communication in the liver. *Hepatology* 1994; **19**: 464.
11 Fausto N. Liver regeneration. *J. Hepatol.* 2000; **32** (suppl. 1): 19.
12 Feldmann G. The cytoskeleton of the hepatocyte. *J. Hepatol.* 1989; **8**: 380.
13 Feldmann G. Liver apoptosis. *J. Hepatol.* 1997; **26** (suppl. 2): 1.
14 FitzPatrick DR. Zellweger syndrome and associated phenotypes. *J. Med. Genet.* 1996; **33**: 863.
15 Fraser R, Dobbs BR, Rogers GWT. Lipoproteins and the liver sieve: the role of the fenestrated sinusoidal endothelium in lipoprotein metabolism, atherosclerosis, and cirrhosis. *Hepatology* 1995; **21**: 863.
16 Hadjis NS, Blumgart LH. Clinical aspects of liver atrophy. *J. Clin. Gastroenterol.* 1989; **11**: 3.
17 Horn T, Christoffersen P, Henriksen JH. Alcoholic liver injury: defenestration in noncirrhotic livers. A scanning microscopic study. *Hepatology* 1987; **7**: 77.
18 Jungermann K, Kietzmann T. Oxygen: modulator of metabolic zonation and disease of the liver. *Hepatology* 2000; **31**: 255.
19 Kanno N, LeSage G, Glaser S *et al*. Functional heterogeneity of the intrahepatic biliary epithelium. *Hepatology* 2000; **31**: 555.
20 Kaplowitz N. Mechanisms of liver cell injury. *J. Hepatol.* 2000; **32** (suppl. 1): 39.
21 McGuire RF, Bissell DM, Boyles J *et al*. Role of extracellular matrix in regulating fenestrations of sinusoidal endothelial cells isolated from normal rat liver. *Hepatology* 1992; **15**: 989.
22 Maher JJ, Friedman SL. Parenchymal and nonparenchymal cell interactions in the liver. *Semin. Liver Dis.* 1993; **13**: 13.
23 Natori S, Rust C, Stadheim LM *et al*. Hepatocyte apoptosis is a pathologic feature of human alcoholic hepatitis. *J. Hepatol.* 2001; 34: 248.
24 Northover JMA, Terblanche J. A new look at the arterial supply of the bile duct in man and its surgical implications. *Br. J. Surg.* 1979; **66**: 379.
25 Patel T, Roberts LR, Jones BA *et al*. Dysregulation of apoptosis as a mechanism of liver disease: an overview. *Semin. Liver Dis.* 1998; **18**: 105.
26 Patel T, Steer CJ, Gores GJ. Apoptosis and the liver: a mechanism of disease, growth regulation and carcinogenesis. *Hepatology* 1999; **30**: 811.
27 Radin DR, Colletti PM, Ralls PW *et al*. Agenesis of the right lobe of the liver. *Radiology* 1987; **164**: 639.
28 Rappaport AM. The microcirculatory acinar concept of normal and pathological hepatic structure. *Beitr. Path.* 1976; **157**: 215.
29 Rockey DC, Weisiger RA. Endothelin induced contractility of stellate cells from normal and cirrhotic rat liver: implica-

tions for regulation of portal pressure and resistance. *Hepatology* 1996; **24**: 233.

30 Sakamoto M, Ueno T, Kin M *et al*. Ito cell contraction in response to endothelin-1 and substance P. *Hepatology* 1993; **18**: 978.

31 Selden C, Khalil M, Hodgson HJF *et al*. What keeps hepatocytes on the straight and narrow? Maintaining differentiated function in the liver. *Gut* 1999; **44**: 443.

32 Sell S. Heterogeneity and plasticity of hepatocyte lineage cells. *Hepatology* 2001; 33: 738.

33 Skrainka B, Stahlhut J, Fullbeck CL *et al*. Measuring liver span. Bedside examination vs. ultrasound and scintiscan. *J. Clin. Gastroenterol*. 1986; **8**: 267.

34 Smedsrod B, De Bleser PJ, Braet F *et al*. Cell biology of liver endothelial and Kupffer cells. *Gut* 1994; **35**: 1509.

35 Smedsrod B, Pertoft H, Gustafson S *et al*. Scavenger functions of the liver endothelial cell. *Biochem. J*. 1990; **266**: 313.

36 Theise ND, Badve S, Saxena R *et al*. Derivation of hepato-cytes from bone marrow cells in mice after radiation-induced myeloablation. *Hepatology* 2000; **31**: 235.

37 Theise ND, Nimmakayalu M, Gardner R *et al*. Liver from bone marrow in humans. *Hepatology* 2000; 32: 11.

38 Theise ND, Saxena R, Portmann BC *et al*. The canals of Hering and hepatic stem cells in humans. *Hepatology* 1999; **30**: 1425.

39 Toth CA, Thomas P. Liver endocytosis and Kupffer cells. *Hepatology* 1992; **16**: 255.

40 van Eyken P, Desmet VJ. Cytokeratins and the liver. *Liver* 1993; **13**: 113.

41 van Leeuwen MS, Noordzij J, Fernandez MA *et al*. Portal venous and segmental anatomy of the right hemiliver: observations based on three-dimensional spiral CT renderings. *Am. J. Roentgenol*. 1994; **163**: 1395.

42 Wisse E, Luo D, Vermijlen D *et al*. On the function of pit cells, the liver-specific natural killer cells. *Semin. Liver Dis*. 1997; **17**: 265.

10 Pimstone NR, Stadalnik RC, Vera DR *et al.* Evaluation of hepatocellular function by way of receptor-mediated uptake of a technetium-99m labelled asialoglycoprotein analogue. *Hepatology* 1994; **20**: 917.

11 Reichel C, Nacke A, Sudhop T *et al.* The low-dose monoethylglycinexylidide test: assessment of liver function with fewer side-effects. *Hepatology* 1997; **25**: 1323.

12 Stremmel W, Wojdat R, Groteguth R *et al.* Liver function tests in a clinical comparison. *Gastroenterology* 1992; **30**: 784.

13 Tredger JM, Sherwood RA. The liver: new functional, prognostic and diagnostic tests. *Ann. Clin. Biochem.* 1997; **34**: 121.

14 Urbain D, Muls V, Thys O *et al.* Aminopyrine breath test improves long-term prognostic evaluation in patients with alcoholic cirrhosis in Child classes A and B. *J. Hepatol.* 1995; **22**: 179.

15 Virgolini I, Müller C, Höbart J *et al.* Liver function in acute viral hepatitis as determined by a hepatocyte-specific ligand: ^{99m}Tc-galactosyl-neoglycoalbumin. *Hepatology* 1992; **15**: 593.

16 Wahllander A, Mohr S, Paumgartner G. Assessment of hepatic function: comparison of caffeine clearance in serum and saliva during the day and at night. *J. Hepatol.* 1990; **10**: 129.

Lipid and lipoprotein metabolism

Lipids

The liver is central to lipid (cholesterol, phospholipid, triglyceride) and lipoprotein metabolism. Lipids are insoluble in water. Lipoproteins, hydrophobic within and hydrophilic on the outside, allow their transport in the plasma.

Cholesterol is found in cell membranes and is a precursor of bile acids and steroid hormones. It is synthesized in the liver, small intestine and in other tissues. Some is derived from intestinal absorption, reaching the liver in chylomicron remnants.

Cholesterol synthesis takes place mainly from acetyl coenzyme A (CoA) in the microsomal fraction and in cytosol (fig. 2.6). Hepatic synthesis is inhibited by cholesterol feeding and by fasting, and is increased by a biliary fistula or bile duct ligation and also by an intestinal lymph fistula. The rate-limiting step is the conversion of 3-hydroxy-3-methylglutaryl-CoA (HMG-CoA) to mevalonate by the enzyme HMG-CoA reductase. The mechanism controlling this process is uncertain. Cholesterol in membranes and in bile is present almost exclusively as free cholesterol. Bile provides the only significant route for cholesterol excretion. In plasma and in certain tissues such as liver, adrenal and skin, cholesterol esters (cholesterol esterified with long-chain fatty acids) are also found. Cholesterol esters are more non-polar than free cholesterol and therefore are even less soluble in water. Esterification is carried out in plasma by the enzyme lecithin cholesterol acyl transferase (LCAT) which is synthesized in the liver.

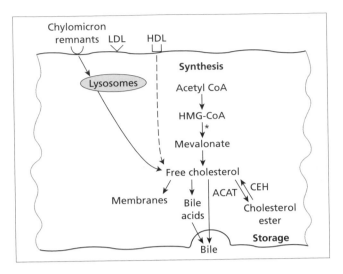

Fig. 2.6. Hepatic cholesterol balance. Free cholesterol is derived from intra-cellular synthesis, and from the uptake of chylomicron remnants and lipoproteins from the circulation. Storage is as cholesterol ester: ACAT (acyl CoA-cholesterol ester transferase, which esterifies free cholesterol to fatty acids) and CEH (cholesteryl ester hydrolase, which hydrolyses the ester linkage). Bile acids are synthesized from free cholesterol, and both are secreted into bile. 3-hydroxy-3-methylglutaryl coenzyme A (HMG-CoA) reductase is the rate-limiting step. HDL, high density lipoprotein; LDL, low density lipoprotein.

Phospholipids are a heterogeneous group of compounds. They contain one or more phosphoric acid groups and another polar group. This may be a heterogeneous base such as choline or ethanolamine. In addition there are one or more long-chain fatty acid residues. The phospholipids are much more complex in terms of chemical reactivity than cholesterol and cholesterol esters. They are important constituents of cell membranes and take part in a large number of chemical reactions. The most abundant phospholipid in plasma and most cellular membranes is phosphatidyl choline (lecithin).

Triglycerides are simpler compounds than the phospholipids. They have a backbone of glycerol, the hydroxy groups of which have been esterified with fatty acids. Naturally occurring triglycerides contain a variety of fatty acids; they act as a store of energy and also a method of transport of energy from the gut and liver to peripheral tissues.

Lipoproteins

These are essential for the circulation and metabolism of lipids. They are particles and are separated by their differing density on ultracentrifugation. This explains their nomenclature. Their surface comprises apolipoprotein, of several different types (table 2.3), free cholesterol and phospholipids. Inside there is cholesterol ester, triglycerides and fat-soluble vitamins.

Table 2.3. Properties of lipoproteins

Lipoproteins	Apolipoprotein	Source	Carries
Chylomicrons	B48, AI, C-II, E	Intestine	Dietary fat
VLDL	B100, C-II, E	Liver	Hepatic triglyceride and cholesterol
LDL	B100	From VLDL	Cholesterol
HDL	A-I, A-II	Peripheral tissue	Cholesterol ester

HDL, high density lipoprotein; LDL, low density lipoprotein; VLDL, very low density lipoprotein.

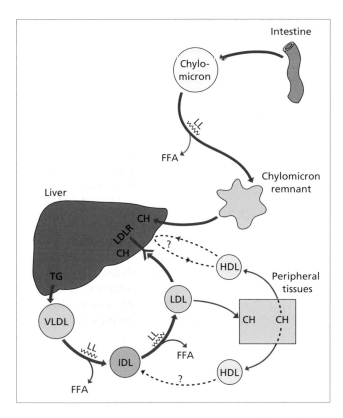

Fig. 2.7. The role of the liver in lipoprotein metabolism. CH, cholesterol; FFA, free fatty acid; LDLR, LDL receptor; LL, lipoprotein lipase; TG, triglyceride. (For lipoproteins see table 2.3.)

There are several metabolic cycles for lipoprotein, of which two are prominent: one is involved in fat absorbed from the intestine, and the other is responsible for the handling of endogenously synthesized lipid (fig. 2.7). There is overlap between the two.

Dietary fat is absorbed from the small intestine, and incorporated into chylomicrons. These enter the circulation (via the thoracic duct) where the triglyceride is removed by the action of lipoprotein lipases. The triglyceride is utilized or stored in tissue. The chylomicron remnant is taken up by the liver by the LDL receptor-related protein. The cholesterol enters metabolic pathways or plasma membranes, or is excreted in bile.

In the endogenous pathway, cholesterol and triglyceride leave the liver in VLDL. In the circulation the triglyceride is removed by the action of lipoprotein lipases. As a result VLDL particles become smaller, forming intermediate density lipoprotein (IDL), and then LDL, the major carrier for cholesterol. The predominant route for removal of LDL is by LDL receptors on the liver surface, but there are receptors on other cells which become important in the formation of atheromatous plaques.

HDL is the particle facilitating cholesterol removal from peripheral tissues. Cholesterol is transported out of the cell by the cholesterol-efflux regulatory protein, expressed from the adenosine triphosphate (ATP) binding cassette transporter 1 gene (ABC1) [2]. The HDL cholesterol is either taken up by the liver, or is incorporated into IDL resulting in the mature LDL. This removal of peripheral cholesterol is an important pathway, as reflected in the protective effect of a high HDL–cholesterol level against coronary artery disease. The metabolism of the HDL particle is still unclear.

Most apolipoproteins are made by the liver, some by the intestines. Apart from being components of lipoproteins, some have other functions: Apo A-1 activates plasma LCAT; C-11 activates lipoprotein lipase.

Changes in liver disease [1]

Cholestasis. Total and free cholesterol are increased. This is not due simply to the retention of cholesterol normally excreted in the bile. The mechanism is uncertain. Four factors have been implicated: regurgitation of biliary cholesterol into the circulation; increased hepatic synthesis of cholesterol; reduced plasma LCAT activity; and regurgitation of biliary lecithin, which produces a shift of cholesterol from pre-existing tissue cholesterol into the plasma. Whereas slight increases to 1.5–2 times normal are sometimes seen in acute cholestasis, very high values are found in chronic conditions, especially post-operative stricture and primary biliary cirrhosis. Values of over five times the upper limit of normal are associated with skin xanthomas. Malnutrition lowers the serum cholesterol so that values may be normal in carcinomatous biliary obstruction.

The level of cholesterol ester is decreased due to LCAT deficiency. Triglycerides tend to be increased. An abnormal lipoprotein, lipoprotein X, very rich in free cholesterol and lecithin is found which appears on electron microscopy as bilamellar discs. The red cell changes in cholestasis are related to abnormalities in cholesterol and lipoprotein.

Parenchymal injury. Triglyerides tend to be increased relating to an accumulation of triglyceride-rich LDL. Cholesterol ester is reduced due to a low LCAT. In cirrhosis total serum cholesterol values are usually normal.

Low results indicate malnutrition or decompensation. In the fatty liver due to alcohol, VLDL is increased, together with triglycerides. With drug toxicity, failure of apolipoprotein synthesis leads to difficulty in export of triglycerides as VLDL, and hence fatty liver.

Serum cholesterol esters, lipoproteins, LCAT and lipoprotein X are not estimated routinely. They are not of any established value in the diagnosis or assessment of liver function.

References

1 Harry DS, McIntyre N. Plasma lipids and lipoproteins. In Bircher J, Benhamou J-P, McIntyre N, Rizzetto M, Rodés J, eds. *Oxford Textbook of Clinical Hepatology*, 2nd edn. Oxford University Press, Oxford, 1999, p. 287.
2 Owen J. Role of ABC1 gene in cholesterol efflux and atheroprotection. *Lancet* 1999; **354**: 1402.

Bile acids

Bile acids [5] are synthesized in the liver and other tissues, 250–500 mg being produced and lost in the faeces daily. Synthesis is under negative feedback control. The primary bile acids, cholic acid and chenodeoxycholic acid, are formed from cholesterol (fig. 2.8). There are two different metabolic pathways for bile acid synthesis. The well-established pathway is 7α-hydroxylation of cholesterol in the liver. A more recently described alternate pathway begins with 27α-hydroxylation of cholesterol in various tissues. Both enzymes belong to the cytochrome P450 group but differ in their substrate specificity [12], subcellular localization and tissue distribution. The C-7α-hydroxylase is found in the endoplasmic reticulum while the C-27α-hydroxylating enzyme is

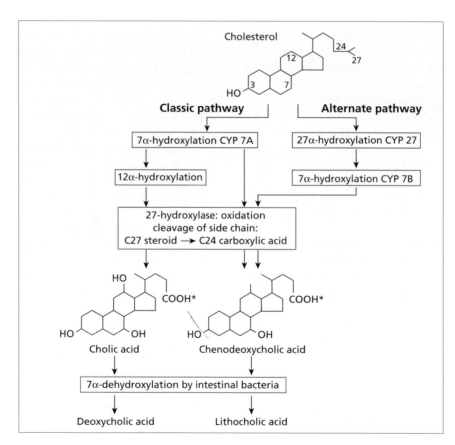

Fig. 2.8. Bile salt synthesis. There are two pathways: classic (neutral) and alternate (acidic).

Classic pathway: 7α-hydroxylation is the initial, rate-limiting step, converting cholesterol to 7α-hydroxycholesterol. The cytochrome P450 enzyme responsible (CYP 7A) is restricted to hepatic microsomes. After further modifications, including 12α-hydroxylation for precursors of cholic acid, the mitochondrial enzyme sterol 27-hydroxylase cleaves the side chain, with the formation of chenodeoxycholate or cholate. The asterisks (*) indicate the site of conjugation with glycine and taurine.

Alternate pathway: cholesterol is transported to mitochondria. CYP 27 catalyses 27-hydroxylation. This reaction can occur in many tissues. 7α-hydroxylation follows—by an oxysterol 7α-hydroxylase distinct from CYP 7A in the classic pathway. The alternate pathway leads to the predominant formation of chenodeoxycholic acid.

found in mitochondria. The interplay between these two synthetic pathways in maintaining bile salt pool size and cellular cholesterol levels is under study [2].

Hepatic synthesis is controlled by the amount of bile acid returning to the liver in the entero-hepatic circulation. When exposed to colonic bacteria the primary bile acids undergo 7α-dehydroxylation with the production of the secondary bile acids, deoxycholic and a very little lithocholic acid. Tertiary bile acids, largely ursodeoxycholic acid, are formed in the liver by epimerization of secondary bile acids. In human bile the amount of the trihydroxy acid (cholic acid) roughly equals the sum of the two dihydroxy acids (chenodeoxycholic and deoxycholic).

The bile acids are conjugated in the liver with the amino acids glycine or taurine. This prevents absorption in the biliary tree and small intestine but permits conservation by absorption in the terminal ileum. Sulphation and glucuronidation (as a detoxifying mechanism) may be increased with cirrhosis or cholestasis when these conjugates are found in excess in the urine and also in bile [9]. Bacteria can hydrolyse bile salts to bile acid and glycine or taurine.

Bile salts are excreted into the biliary canaliculus against an enormous concentration gradient between liver and bile. This depends in part on the intra-cellular negative potential of approximately $-35\,mV$, which provides potential-dependent facilitated diffusion, and also ATP-stimulated transporters (the major one being the canalicular bile salt export pump). The bile salts enter into micellar and vesicular association with cholesterol and phospholipids. In the upper small intestine the bile salt micelles are too large and too polar (hydrophilic) to be absorbed. They are intimately concerned with the digestion and absorption of lipids. When the terminal ileum and proximal colon are reached, absorption of bile acid takes place by an active transport process found only in the ileum. Non-ionic passive diffusion occurs throughout the whole intestine and is most efficient for unconjugated, dihydroxy bile acid. Oral administration of ursodeoxycholic acid interferes with the small intestinal absorption of both chenodeoxycholic and cholic acid [8].

The absorbed bile salts enter the portal venous system and reach the liver where they are taken up with great avidity by the hepatocytes. This depends upon a sodium-coupled co-transport system using the sodium gradient across the sinusoidal membrane as a driving force. Chloride ions may also be involved. The most hydrophobic bile acids (unconjugated mono- and dihydroxy bile acids) probably enter the hepatocyte by simple diffusion ('flip-flop') across the lipid membrane. The mechanism of bile acid passage across the liver cell from sinusoid to bile canaliculus is controversial.

Cytosolic bile acid-binding proteins, for example 3α-hydroxysteroid dehydrogenase, are involved [10]. The role of microtubules is uncertain. Vesicles seem to play a role but only at higher bile acid concentrations [3]. The bile acids are reconjugated and re-excreted into bile. Lithocholic acid is not re-excreted.

This entero-hepatic circulation of bile salts takes place 2–15 times daily (fig. 2.9). Because absorption efficiency varies among the individual bile acids they have different synthesis and fractional turnover rates.

In cholestasis bile acids are excreted in the urine by active transport and passive diffusion. They tend to be sulphated and these conjugates are actively secreted by the renal tubule [11].

Changes in disease

Bile salts increase the biliary excretion of water, lecithin, cholesterol and conjugated bilirubin. Ursodeoxycholic acid produces a much greater choleresis than chenodeoxycholic or cholic acid [6].

Altered biliary excretion of bile salts with defective biliary micelle formation is important in the pathogenesis of gallstones (Chapter 34). It also leads to the steatorrhoea of cholestasis.

Bile salts form a micellar solution with cholesterol and phospholipid, and in this way help to emulsify dietary fat and also play a part in the mucosal phase of absorption. Diminished secretion leads to steatorrhoea (fig. 2.10). They assist pancreatic lipolysis and release gastrointestinal hormones.

Disordered intra-hepatic metabolism of bile salts may be important in the pathogenesis of cholestasis (Chapter 13). They used to be thought to have a role in the pruritus of cholestasis but data now suggest that other substances are responsible (Chapter 13).

Bile salts may be responsible for target cells in the peripheral blood of jaundiced patients (Chapter 4) and for the secretion of conjugated bilirubin in urine. If bile acids are deconjugated by small intestinal bacteria, the resulting free bile acids are absorbed. Micelle formation and absorption of fat are then impaired. This may partly explain the malabsorption complicating diseases with bacterial overgrowth in the small intestine.

Removal of the terminal ileum interrupts the enterohepatic circulation and allows large amounts of primary bile acids to reach the colon and to be dehydroxylated by bacteria, thus reducing the body's bile salt pool. The altered bile salts in the colon excite a profound electrolyte and water loss with diarrhoea.

Lithocholic acid is mostly excreted in the faeces and only slightly absorbed. It is cirrhotogenic to experimental animals and can be used to produce experimental gallstones. Taurolithocholic acid can also cause intra-

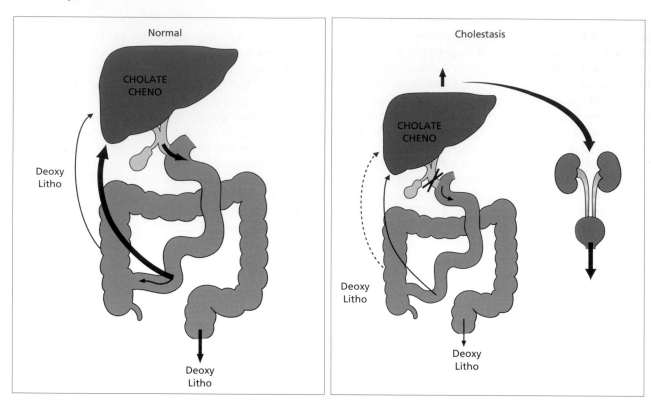

Fig. 2.9. The entero-hepatic circulation of bile acids in normal subjects and in cholestasis.

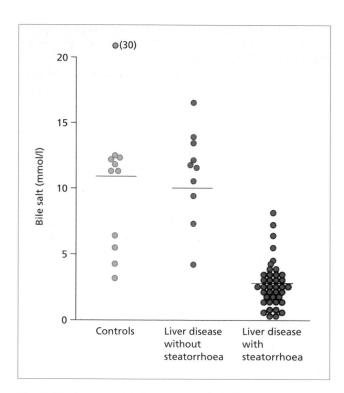

Fig. 2.10. Patients with chronic, non-alcoholic liver disease and steatorrhoea show a reduced bile salt concentration in their aspirated intestinal contents compared with control subjects and patients with chronic liver disease without steatorrhoea.

hepatic cholestasis, perhaps by interfering with the bile-salt-independent fraction of bile flow.

Serum bile acids

Gas–liquid chromatography allows individual bile acids to be distinguished, but the method is time consuming and the equipment expensive.

Enzymatic assays are based on the use of bacterial 3-hydroxysteroid dehydrogenase. The use of a bioluminescence assay has improved the sensitivity of this enzymatic technique up to that of radio-immunoassay. The method is simple and inexpensive if the equipment is available. Radio-immunoassay techniques can also measure individual bile acids.

The serum concentration of total bile acids reflects the extent to which bile acids reabsorbed from the intestine have escaped extraction on their first passage through the liver. The value reflects the instantaneous balance between intestinal absorption and hepatic uptake. Intestinal load is more important than hepatic extraction in regulating peripheral serum bile acid levels.

Raised levels of serum bile acids are specific for hepato-biliary disease. The sensitivity of serum bile acid estimations is less than originally thought for detecting hepato-cellular damage in viral hepatitis or chronic liver disease. The addition to the fasting serum bile acid value of a 2-h post-prandial level adds little in sensitivity [4]. The dual cholate clearance test (simultaneous ^{2}H-cholate orally and ^{13}C-cholate intravenously) has been used to measure intrinsic hepatic clearance as a reflection of liver function and the severity of liver disease [7].

Estimations of individual bile acids are not diagnostic. In cholestasis the ratio of serum trihydroxy to dihydroxy acid increases. Patients with hepato-cellular failure usually have a low ratio, the main bile acid being chenodeoxycholic acid. This is due to a reduction in the activity of the 12α-hydroxylase enzyme in the hepatocyte.

Amino acid conjugation is preserved even with severe hepato-cellular damage [1].

References

1 Arisaka M, Arisaka O, Nittono H *et al.* Conjugating ability of bile acids in hepatic failure. *Acta Paediatr. Scand.* 1986; **75**: 875.

2 Cooper AD. Bile salt biosynthesis: an alternate synthetic pathway joins the mainstream. *Gastroenterology* 1997; **113**: 2005.

3 Crawford JM, Gollan JL. Transcellular transport of organic anions in hepatocytes: still a long way to go. *Hepatology* 1991; **14**: 192.

4 Greenfield SM, Soloway RD, Carithers RL Jr *et al.* Evaluation of postprandial serum bile acid response as a test of hepatic function. *Dig. Dis. Sci.* 1986; **31**: 785.

5 Hofmann AF. The continuing importance of bile acids in liver and intestinal disease. *Arch. Intern. Med.* 1999; **159**: 2647.

6 Loria P, Carulli N, Medici G *et al.* Determinants of bile secretion: effect of bile salt structure on bile flow and biliary cation secretion. *Gastroenterology* 1989; **96**: 1142.

7 Shrestha R, McKinley C, Showalter R *et al.* Quantitative liver function tests define the functional severity of liver disease in early stage cirrhosis. *Liver Transplant Surg.* 1997; **3**: 166.

8 Stiehl A, Raedsch R, Rudolph G. Acute effects of ursodeoxycholic and chenodeoxycholic acid on the small intestinal absorption of bile acids. *Gastroenterology* 1990; **98**: 424.

9 Stiehl A, Raedsch R, Rudolph G *et al.* Biliary and urinary excretion of sulphated, glucuronidated and tetrahydroxylated bile acids in cirrhotic patients. *Hepatology* 1985; **5**: 492.

10 Stolz A, Takikawa H, Ookhtens M *et al.* The role of cytoplasmic proteins in hepatic bile acid transport. *Ann. Rev. Physiol.* 1989; **51**: 161.

11 Summerfield JA, Cullen J, Barnes S *et al.* Evidence for renal control of urinary excretion of bile acids and bile acid sulphates in the cholestatic syndrome. *Clin. Sci. Mol. Med.* 1977; **52**: 51.

12 Vlahcevic ZR, Pandak WM, Stravitz RT. Regulation of bile acid biosynthesis. *Gastroenterol. Clin. N. Am.* 1999; **28**: 1.

Amino acid metabolism

Amino acids derived from the diet and from tissue breakdown reach the liver for metabolism. Specific Na$^+$-independent and Na$^+$-dependent systems mediate the transport of free amino acids across the sinusoidal membrane of the hepatocyte [7]. Some are transaminated or deaminated to keto acids which are then metabolized by many pathways including the tricarboxylic acid cycle (Krebs–citric acid cycle). Others are metabolized to ammonia and urea (Krebs–Henseleit urea cycle).

The maximal rate of urea synthesis in chronic liver disease is markedly reduced. However, experimentally, at least 85% of liver must be removed before this mechanism fails significantly and before blood and urinary amino acid levels increase. A low blood urea concentration is an occasional feature of fulminant liver failure. A rise in blood ammonia level also represents a failure of the Krebs urea cycle and this increase has been related to hepatic encephalopathy.

Clinical significance

A generalized or selective amino aciduria is a feature of hepato-cellular disease. In patients with severe liver disease the usual picture is an increase in the plasma concentration of one or both of the aromatic amino acids, tyrosine and phenylalanine, together with methionine, and a reduction in the branched-chain amino acids valine, leucine and isoleucine (fig. 2.11) [6]. The changes are explained by impaired hepatic function, portosystemic shunting of blood, hyperinsulinaemia and hyperglucagonaemia. Patients with minimal liver disease also show changes, particularly a reduction in plasma proline, perhaps reflecting increased collagen

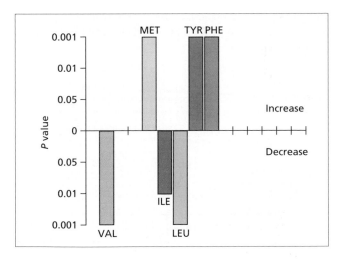

Fig. 2.11. The plasma amino acid pattern in cryptogenic cirrhosis (mean of 11 patients) compared with normal individuals. The aromatic amino acids and methionine are increased while the branched-chain amino acids are decreased. ILE, isoleucine; LEU, leucine; MET, methionine; PHE, phenylalanine; TYR, tyrosine; VAL, valine [6].

production. There is no difference in the ratio between branched-chain and aromatic amino acids whether or not the patients show hepatic encephalopathy.

In fulminant hepatitis there is marked generalized aminoaciduria involving particularly cystine and tyrosine and this carries a bad prognosis.

Plasma proteins

The plasma proteins produced by the hepatocyte are synthesized on polyribosomes bound to the rough endoplasmic reticulum, from which they are discharged into the plasma [9]. Falls in concentration usually reflect decreased hepatic synthesis although changes in plasma volume and losses, for instance into gut or urine, may contribute.

The hepatocyte makes albumin, fibrinogen, α_1-antitrypsin, haptoglobin, caeruloplasmin, transferrin and prothrombin (table 2.4). Some liver-produced proteins are acute phase reactors and rise in response to tissue injury such as inflammation (table 2.4). These include fibrinogen, haptoglobin, α_1-antitrypsin, C_3 component of complement and caeruloplasmin. An acute phase response may contribute to well-maintained or increased serum concentrations of these proteins, even with hepato-cellular disease.

The mechanism is complex but cytokines (interleukin (IL) 1, IL6, TNF-α) play a role [1, 8]. IL6 binds to the cell-surface receptor and this stimulates a message from the hepatocyte membrane to the nucleus where there is induction of specific nuclear factors which interact with promoter elements at the 5' end of several acute phase plasma protein genes. There are also post-transcriptional as well as transcriptional mechanisms. Cytokines not only stimulate production of acute phase proteins but also inhibit the synthesis of albumin, transferrin and a range of other proteins.

The *immunoglobulins* IgG, IgM and IgA are synthesized by the B cells of the lymphoid system.

Some 10 g of *albumin* is synthesized by the normal liver daily (figs 2.12, 2.13), whereas those with cirrhosis can only synthesize about 4 g (35 mg/kg/day in Child C cirrhosis) [2, 3]. The fractional synthetic rate of albumin is approximately 6% per day compared with 25% for total liver protein [3]. In liver disease, the fall in serum albumin concentration is slow, for the half-life of albumin is about 22 days. Thus a patient with fulminant liver failure may die with a virtually normal serum albumin value. A patient with decompensated cirrhosis would be expected to have a low level.

α_1-*Antitrypsin* deficiency is inherited (Chapter 25).

Haptoglobin is a glycoprotein composed of two types of polypeptide chains, α and β, which are covalently associated by disulphide bonds. Haptoglobin is largely synthesized by hepatocytes. Hereditary deficiencies are frequent in American black people. Low values are found in severe, chronic hepato-cellular disease and in haemolytic crises.

Caeruloplasmin is the major copper-containing protein in plasma and is responsible for the oxidase activity. A low concentration is found in 95% of those who are homozygous and about 10% of those heterozygous for Wilson's disease (Chapter 24). Caeruloplasmin increases to normal if a patient with Wilson's disease has a hepatic transplant. One must estimate caeruloplasmin in all patients with chronic hepatitis so that Wilson's disease, with its mandatory copper chelation therapy, may be diagnosed. However, low values are also found in very severe, decompensated cirrhosis which is not due to Wilson's disease. High values are found in preg-

Table 2.4. Serum (plasma) proteins synthesized by the liver

	Normal concentration
Albumin	40–50 g/l
α_1-antitrypsin*	2–4 g/l
α-fetoprotein	<10 KU/l
α_2-macroglobulin	2.2–3.8 g/l
Caeruloplasmin*	0.2–0.4 g/l
Complement components (C_3, C_6 and C_1)	
Fibrinogen*	2–6 g/l
Haemopexin	0.8–1.0 g/l
Prothrombin (factor II)†	
Transferrin	2–3 g/l

* Acute phase proteins.
† Vitamin K dependent; also factors VII and X.

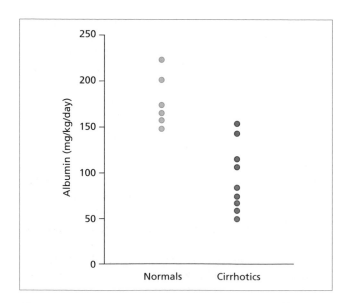

Fig. 2.12. The absolute synthesis of serum albumin (^{14}C carbonate method) in cirrhosis is reduced [10].

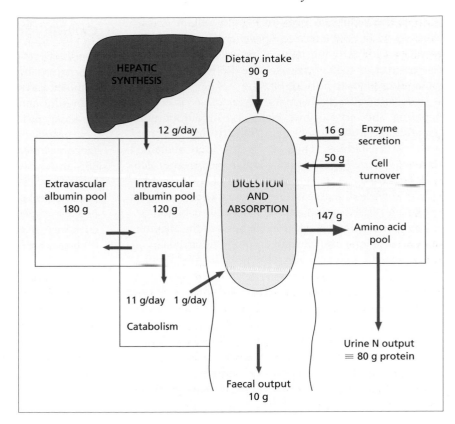

Fig. 2.13. The turnover of plasma albumin in a 70-kg adult seen in the context of the daily protein economy of the gastrointestinal tract and overall nitrogen balance. The total exchangeable albumin pool of about 300 g is distributed between the intravascular and extravascular compartments in a ratio of approximately 2:3. In this simplified schema the balance sheet is expressed in terms of grams of protein (6.25×grams of nitrogen). Losses do not include relatively minor routes, e.g. 2 g/day from the skin [9].

nancy, following oestrogen therapy and with large bile duct obstruction.

Transferrin is the iron transport protein. The plasma transferrin is more than 90% saturated with iron in patients with untreated idiopathic haemochromatosis. Reduced values may be found with cirrhosis.

The C_3 *component of complement* tends to be reduced in cirrhosis, normal in chronic hepatitis and increased in compensated primary biliary cirrhosis. Low values in fulminant hepatic failure and alcoholic cirrhosis with or without hepatitis reflect reduced hepatic synthesis and there is a correlation with prolonged prothrombin time and depression of serum albumin concentration [4]. There is also a contribution from increased consumption due to activation of the complement system. Transient reductions are found in the early 'immune complex' stage of acute hepatitis B.

Alpha-fetoprotein is a normal component of plasma protein in human fetuses older than 6 weeks, and reaches maximum concentration at between 12 and 16 weeks of fetal life. A few weeks after birth it disappears from the circulation but reappears in the blood of patients with primary liver cancer and can be shown in the tumour by indirect immunofluorescence. Raised values are also found with embryonic tumours of the ovary and testis and in embryonic hepatoblastoma. It may also be present with carcinomas of the gastrointesti-

nal tract with hepatic secondaries. Raised values are also found in active chronic hepatitis and during acute viral hepatitis, where they may indicate hepato-cellular regeneration. However, very high values are virtually confined to primary liver cancer. In a hepatitis B or C positive patient, rising values are of particular significance as an indicator of the development of hepato-cellular carcinoma (Chapter 31).

Electrophoretic pattern of serum proteins

Electrophoresis is used to determine the proportions of the various serum proteins. In cirrhosis, albumin is reduced.

The α_1-globulins contain glycoproteins and hormone-binding globulins. They tend to be low in hepato-cellular disease, falling in parallel with the serum albumin. An increase accompanies acute febrile illnesses and malignant disease. Ninety per cent of α_1-globulin consists of α_1-antitrypsin and an absent α_1-globulin may indicate α_1-antitrypsin deficiency.

The α_2- and β-globulins include lipoproteins. In cholestasis the increase in α_2- and β-globulin components correlates with the height of serum lipids.

The γ-globulins rise in hepatic cirrhosis due to increased production. The increased numbers of plasma cells in marrow, and even in the liver itself, may be the source. The γ-globulin peak in hepato-cellular disease shows a wide base (*polyclonal gammopathy*). *Monoclonal gammopathy* is rare and may be age-related rather than related to chronic liver disease. The dip between β- and γ-globulins tends to be bridged.

Immunoglobulins. IgG is markedly increased in chronic hepatitis and cryptogenic cirrhosis. In autoimmune hepatitis the raised level of IgG falls during treatment with corticosteroids. There is a slow and sustained increase in viral hepatitis and it is also increased in alcoholic cirrhosis.

IgM is markedly increased in primary biliary cirrhosis and to a lesser extent in viral hepatitis and cirrhosis.

IgA is markedly increased in cirrhosis of the alcoholic but also in primary biliary and cryptogenic cirrhosis.

The increase in serum secretory IgA, the predominant immunoglobulin in bile, may be related to communication of the bile canaliculus with the space of Disse and/or through the bile duct into the portal blood vessels [5].

In chronic hepatitis with active inflammation and cryptogenic cirrhosis the pattern is surprisingly similar, with increases in IgG, IgM and to a lesser extent IgA.

About 10% of patients with chronic cholestasis due to large bile duct obstruction show increases in all three main immunoglobulins.

Patterns are not diagnostic of any one disease but together with other data add support to considering a particular diagnosis.

References

1 Andus T, Bauer J, Gerok W. Effects of cytokines on the liver. *Hepatology* 1991; **13**: 364.
2 Ballmer PE, Reichen J, McNurlan MA *et al*. Albumin but not fibrinogen synthesis correlates with galactose elimination capacity in patients with cirrhosis of the liver. *Hepatology* 1996; **24**: 53.
3 Barle H, Nyberg B, Essen P *et al*. The synthesis rates of total liver protein and plasma albumin determined simultaneously *in vivo* in humans. *Hepatology* 1997; **25**: 154.
4 Ellison RT, Horsburgh CR Jr, Curd J. Complement levels in patients with hepatic dysfunction. *Dig. Dis. Sci.* 1990; **35**: 231.
5 Fukuda Y, Nagura H, Asai J *et al*. Possible mechanisms of elevation of serum secretory immunoglobulin A in liver disease. *Am. J. Gastroenterol.* 1986; **81**: 315.
6 Morgan MY, Marshall AW, Milsom JP *et al*. Plasma amino-acid patterns in liver disease. *Gut* 1982; **23**: 362.
7 Moseley RH. Hepatic amino acid transport. *Semin. Liver Dis.* 1996; **16**: 137.
8 Sehgal PB. Interleukin-6: a regulator of plasma protein gene expression in hepatic and nonhepatic tissues. *Mol. Biol. Med.* 1990; **7**: 117.
9 Tavill AS. The synthesis and degradation of liver-produced proteins. *Gut* 1972; **13**: 225.
10 Tavill AS, Craigie A, Rosenoer VM. The measurement of the synthetic rate of albumin in man. *Clin. Sci.* 1968; **34**: 1.

Carbohydrate metabolism

The liver occupies a key position in carbohydrate metabolism (see fig. 2.1) [2]. The changes in cirrhosis are complex and not fully understood.

In fulminant acute hepatic necrosis the blood glucose level may be low. This is rare in chronic liver disease.

In fasted patients with cirrhosis the contribution of carbohydrates to energy production is reduced (2 vs. 38% in normal controls) with the contribution from fat increasing (86 vs. 45%) [3]. This may be caused by impaired release of hepatic glucose or a reduced reserve of glycogen in the liver. After eating a meal, however, cirrhotics, like control subjects, make immediate use of dietary carbohydrate, indeed perhaps to a greater degree, because of a reduced ability to store and then mobilize energy as triglyceride [1].

The oral and intravenous glucose tolerance tests may show impairment in cirrhosis and there is relative insulin resistance (Chapter 25).

Galactose tolerance is also impaired in hepato-cellular disease and oral and intravenous tests have been devised. Results are independent of insulin secretion. Galactose removal by the liver has been used to measure hepatic blood flow.

References

1 Avgerinos A, Harry D, Bousboulas S *et al*. The effect of an eucaloric high carbohydrate diet on circulating levels of glucose, fructose and nonesterified fatty acids in patients with cirrhosis. *J. Hepatol.* 1992; **14**: 78.
2 Kruszynska YT. Carbohydrate metabolism. In Bircher J, Benhamou J-P, McIntyre N, Rizzetto M, Rodes J, eds. *Oxford Textbook of Clinical Hepatology*, 2nd edn. Oxford University Press, Oxford, 1999, p. 257.
3 Schneeweiss B, Graninger W, Ferenci P *et al*. Energy metabolism in patients with acute and chronic liver disease. *Hepatology* 1990; **11**: 387.

Effects of ageing on the liver [6]

Although there are many studies of hepatic function and ageing, results have been conflicting or unsubstantiated. Differences could be due to the study protocols used.

However, liver weight and volume decrease with age, and liver blood flow is reduced [8]. There is compensatory hypertrophy of hepatocytes.

In animals the rate of hepatic regeneration declines with increasing age but whether this is related to lower circulating levels of hepato-trophic factors is not clear. Somatic mutations, including gene rearrangements, increase with age and are more frequent in the liver than the brain in experimental models [1].

Structural changes in the hepatocyte include an

increase in secondary lysosomes and residual bodies, with a concomitant accumulation of lipofuscin. There are conflicting data on structural changes in mitochondria. However impaired mitochondrial enzyme activity and defects in the respiratory chain are reported [4, 5]. No consistent mitochondrial DNA mutations are seen.

In animals, protein synthesis by the liver falls with age. Since the total protein content of cells remains relatively constant it is thought that protein turnover is also reduced [6]. Hepatic nitrogen clearance (conversion of α-amino nitrogen into urea nitrogen) is impaired with advancing age [2].

First-pass metabolism of drugs is reduced and this may be due to reduced liver mass and hepatic blood flow rather than to alterations in the relevant enzyme systems. It has been suggested that increased hepatocyte volume extends the path length for oxygen diffusion (the 'oxygen diffusion barrier' hypothesis) which might affect cell function [3]. Hepatic microsomal mono-oxygenase enzyme activity does not appear to decline with age [7].

Fatal reactions to halothane and drugs such as benoxyprofen are more frequent in the elderly, but the overall increase in adverse reactions observed may be related to the multiplicity of drugs that these patients receive.

Cholesterol saturation of bile increases with age due to enhanced hepatic secretion of cholesterol and decreased bile acid synthesis. This may explain age as a risk factor for cholesterol gallstones.

References

1 Dolle ME, Giese H, Hopkins CL *et al*. Rapid accumulation of genome rearrangements in liver but not in brain of old mice. *Nature Genet.* 1997; **17**: 431.

2 Fabbri A, Marchesini G, Bianchi G *et al*. Kinetics of hepatic amino-nitrogen conversion in ageing man. *Liver* 1994; **14**: 288.

3 LeCouter DG, McLean AJ. The ageing liver. Drug clearance and an oxygen diffusion barrier hypothesis. *Clin. Pharmacokinet.* 1998; **34**: 359.

4 Muller Hocker J, Aust D, Rohrbach H *et al*. Defects of the respiratory chain in the normal human liver and in cirrhosis during ageing. *Hepatology* 1997; **26**: 709.

5 Sastre J, Pallardó FV, Plá R *et al*. Ageing of the liver: age-associated mitochondrial damage in intact hepatocytes. *Hepatology* 1996; **24**: 1199.

6 Schmucker DL. Ageing and the liver: an update. *J. Gerontol.* 1998; **53A**: B315.

7 Ward W, Richardson A. Effect of age on liver protein synthesis and degradation. *Hepatology* 1991; **14**: 935.

8 Wynne HA, Cope LH, Mutch E *et al*. The effect of age upon liver volume and apparent liver blood flow in healthy man. *Hepatology* 1989; **9**: 297.

Chapter 3
Biopsy of the Liver

A needle biopsy of the liver was said to have been first performed by Paul Ehrlich in 1883 (table 3.1) [13] in a study of the glycogen content of the diabetic liver, and later in 1895 by Lucatello in Italy, for the diagnosis of tropical liver abscess. The first published series was by Schüpfer (1907) [38] in France, where the technique was used for the diagnosis of cirrhosis and hepatic tumours. The method, however, never achieved early popularity until the 1930s when it was used for general purposes by Huard and co-workers [20] in France, and by Baron [3] in the USA. The Second World War saw a rapid increase in the use of liver biopsy, largely to investigate the many cases of non-fatal viral hepatitis which were affecting the armed forces of both sides [2, 21, 39].

The indications and techniques have changed, the complications are better recognized and the risks have decreased. Interpretation of the biopsy is an important part of a histopathologist's training.

Selection and preparation of the patient

The patient is usually admitted to hospital. Outpatients selected must not be jaundiced or show any sign of decompensation such as ascites or encephalopathy. Outpatient biopsy should be avoided in cirrhotic patients or in those with tumours [34]. Outpatient biopsies are usually indicated because of patient preference and reduction of cost. The American Gastroenterological Association recommends that clinicians should decide whether the biopsy is done as an inpatient or outpatient, and this should not be dictated by insurance coverage [22].

The one-stage prothrombin time should not be more than 3 s prolonged over control values after 10 mg vitamin K is given intramuscularly. The platelet count should exceed 50 000.

In thrombocytopenic patients the risk of haemorrhage depends on the function of the platelets rather than on their numbers. A patient with 'hypersplenism' and a platelet count of less than 50 000 is much less likely to bleed than one with leukaemia who has a similar platelet count. This distinction particularly arises in patients with haematological problems or after organ transplants where the effects on the liver of cytotoxic therapy,

viruses and other infective agents and of the graft-versus-host reaction have to be resolved. In such patients, if the platelet count can be raised to greater than 60 000 by platelet infusion, biopsy seems to be safe. Care should also be taken in recently imbibing alcoholic patients who may have reduced platelet counts and platelet dysfunction, especially if acetyl salicylic acid has been consumed. In such patients the platelet count may be 100 000 and the prothrombin time only 3 s prolonged over control values, yet the bleeding time may be 25 min.

The patient's blood group should be known and facilities for blood transfusion must always be available.

Clinically significant haemorrhage complicated 12.5% of 155 liver biopsies in haemophiliacs [1]. Liver biopsy should not be performed in haemophilia A unless there are very definite indications when the factor VIII level should be raised, and maintained, to about 50% for at least 48 h.

Techniques

The Menghini needle obtains a specimen by aspiration (fig. 3.1) [30]. The sheathed 'Trucut' is a cutting technique of particular value in cirrhotic patients [8]. Fragmentation of the biopsy is greater with the Menghini method, but the procedure is quicker, easier and has less complications [34]. The cost of the needle is less.

Menghini 'one second' needle biopsy (fig. 3.1). The 1.4-mm diameter needle is used routinely. A short needle is available for paediatric use. The tip of the needle is

Table 3.1. History of liver biopsies [40]

Author	Date	Country	Purpose
Ehrlich	1883	Germany	Glycogen
Lucatello	1895	Italy	Tropical
Schüpfer	1907	France	Cirrhosis
Huard *et al.*	1935	France	General
Baron	1939	USA	General
Iversen & Roholm	1939	Denmark	Hepatitis
Axenfeld & Brass	1942	Germany	Hepatitis
Dible *et al.*	1943	UK	Hepatitis

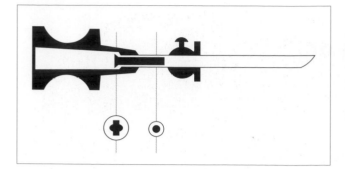

Fig. 3.1. Longitudinal section of the Menghini liver biopsy needle. Note the nail in the shaft of the needle [30].

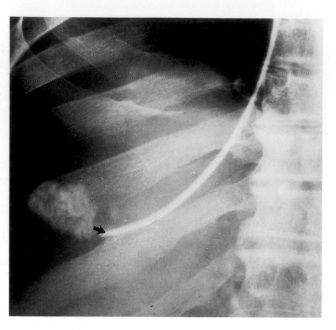

Fig. 3.2. Transvenous liver biopsy. The catheter is in the hepatic vein and contrast has been injected to show the wedged position. The Trucut needle is taking the liver biopsy (arrow).

Table 3.2. Indications for transjugular liver biopsy

Coagulation defects
Acute liver failure pre-transplant
Massive ascites
Small liver
Measurement of wedged hepatic venous pressure
Unco-operative patient

oblique and slightly convex towards the outside. The needle is fitted within its shaft with a blunt nail. This internal block prevents the biopsy from being fragmented or distorted by violent aspiration into the syringe.

Sterile solution (3 ml) is drawn into the syringe which is inserted through the anaesthetized track down to but not through the intercostal space. Two millilitres of solution are injected to clear the needle of any skin fragments. Aspiration is now commenced and maintained. This is the slow part of the procedure. With the patient holding his breath in expiration, the needle is rapidly introduced perpendicularly to the skin into the liver substance and extracted. This is the quick part of the procedure. The tip of the needle is now placed on sterile paper and some of the remaining saline flushed through the needle to deposit the biopsy gently onto the paper. The tissue is transferred into fixative.

Sedation is not given routinely before biopsy as it may interfere with the patient's co-operation. However, analgesia is sometimes needed after the procedure.

The *intercostal technique* is the most frequently used method [40]. It rarely fails, provided care is taken to assess liver size carefully by light percussion. A preliminary ultrasound or CT scan is useful. A small fibrotic liver is a contraindication. After adequate local anaesthesia, the needle is inserted in the 8th or 9th intercostal space in the mid-axillary line at the end of expiration with the patient breathing quietly. The direction is slightly posterior and cranial which helps to avoid the gallbladder. If an epigastric mass is present or imaging indicates left lobe disease, an anterior approach is made.

Transjugular (*transvenous liver biopsy*) [25]. A special Trucut needle is inserted through a catheter placed in the hepatic vein via the jugular vein. The needle is then introduced into the liver tissue by transfixing the hepatic venous wall (fig. 3.2). The correct position is confirmed by injecting contrast medium into the needle.

The technique is used in those who have a coagulation disorder, massive ascites, a small liver or who are unco-operative. It is useful in acute liver failure to determine prognosis and the need for liver transplantation [11]. In patients with advanced liver disease, it has the advantage of measuring wedged and free hepatic venous pressure and of opacifying the hepatic vein (table 3.2).

Biopsies are smaller than with the intercostal technique, but are adequate in two-thirds of patients with cirrhosis and extensive fibrosis, and in 99% of those without fibrosis and with normal architecture. Complications are between 0 and 20%. Mortality is very low, but perforation of the liver capsule can be fatal [26]. The disadvantage is the greater complexity. The cost is 10 times that of trans-capsular biopsy.

Directed (*guided biopsy*). The lesion is recognized under imaging, which is usually ultrasound, but may be CT. The Trucut biopsy needle is advanced into it (fig. 3.3). In patients with poor coagulation, a gel foam plug may be injected through the outer cannula of the Trucut needle after the inner cutting needle, with its contained speci-

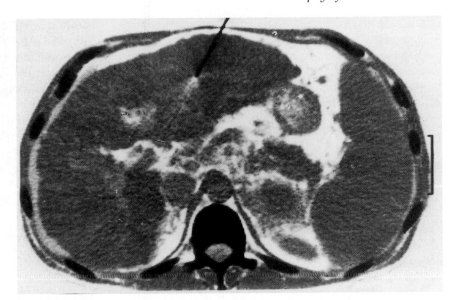

Fig. 3.3. CT scan of a 45-year-old male with hepatitis B positive cirrhosis. An irregular liver outline and splenomegaly are clearly seen. A directed biopsy of a suspected neoplasm of the left lobe of liver diagnosed hepato-cellular carcinoma.

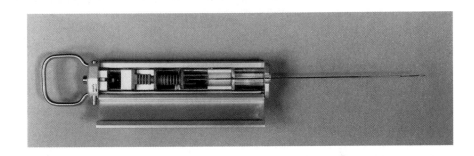

Fig. 3.4. The Biopty gun (Biopter).

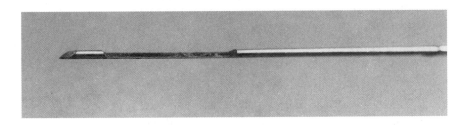

Fig. 3.5. The Trucut needle tip has an outer cannula and inner cutting needle. The inner needle is advanced and a liver biopsy is cored out.

men, has been removed [45]. This is effective in preventing major bleeding. Preliminary ultrasound may be used to assess liver size, the position of the gallbladder and any anatomical abnormality or focal lesion. The ultrasound may be performed in relation to the biopsy, preferably by the operator, and a portable ultrasound machine may be used. In diffuse disease, ultrasound decreases the incidence of major and minor complications such as pain, hypotension and bleeding [44].

Directed liver biopsy gives a higher percentage of positives than the trans-capsular technique. In chronic liver disease, the blind technique is approximately 81% accurate, but this can be raised to 95% if a directed form of liver biopsy is used [33]. Ultrasound-guided liver

biopsy increases the cost but new generation, portable ultrasound may be less expensive and reduction of major and minor complications is similarly cost-effective [27, 35].

The *Biopty gun* uses a modified 18- or 14-gauge Trucut needle and is operated with one hand (figs 3.4, 3.5). It is fired by a fast and powerful spring mechanism. It allows precise positioning of the needle and is less painful than the manual procedure. It is particularly useful for focal lesions [43].

Fine-needle-guided biopsy. Using a 22 swg (0.7 mm) needle adds to the safety. It is particularly useful for the diagnosis of focal lesions although diagnostic accuracy is variable [6]. Because of the size, fine-needle biopsy is not so useful in generalized disease such as chronic hepatitis or cirrhosis.

Cytological examination of the aspirate is useful for tumour typing [15].

After-care. Bleeding is most likely within the first 3–4h [23]. Pulse rate and blood pressure are charted every 15 min for the first hour and every 30 min for the next 2 h.

Inpatients continue to have their pulse rates charted for 24 h and routine visits are paid 4 and 8 h post-biopsy. A very careful watch must be kept on the patient. Rest in bed is essential for 24 h.

During the puncture the patient may complain of a drawing feeling across the epigastrium. Afterwards some patients have a slight ache in the right side for about 24 h and some complain of pain referred from the diaphragm to the right shoulder.

Outpatients are admitted to a supervised day ward at 9.00 a.m. The biopsy is never done later than 11.00 a.m. Pulse and blood pressure are monitored as for inpatients. The patient remains recumbent until 4.00 p.m., is seen at 4.30 p.m. by the physician and is allowed to go home at 5.00 p.m., accompanied and being driven. The patient should stay less than a 30-min drive from the hospital. The patient should not be alone and must have a telephone available. The transvenous biopsy technique is unsuitable for outpatients because of premedication and usually more severe liver disease and a higher rate of complications. The usual indication for outpatient biopsy is the diagnosis and management of chronic hepatitis, cirrhosis or alcoholic liver disease.

Difficulties

Failures arise in patients with cirrhosis, especially with ascites, for the tough liver is difficult to pierce and a few liver cells may be extracted, leaving the fibrous framework behind. Another difficulty may be pulmonary emphysema; the liver is then pushed downwards by the low diaphragm so that the trocar passes above it.

Failure is often due to the needle not being sharp enough to penetrate the capsule. Disposable needles are an advantage for they are sharp.

The percentage of successes increases with the diameter of the needle used, but so does the complication rate, and one must be weighed against the other. The 1-mm Menghini needle, for instance, which is extremely safe, often fails to procure adequate hepatic tissue for diagnosis. The Trucut needle causes more haemorrhages.

Liver biopsy in paediatrics

The Menghini technique may be employed. In infants a local anaesthetic, with 15–60 mg pentobarbital 30 min before the biopsy, is adequate. The child is restrained by adhesive strapping across the upper thighs and chest and the subcostal approach used. If the liver is small then the intercostal route is employed, the assistant compressing the chest at the end of expiration to arrest respiration.

Complications (4.5%) are more frequent in children than in adults and bleeding is particularly likely in those with cancer or having bone marrow transplants [7]. In older children, general anaesthesia is usually preferred, depending on the co-operation of the child.

Transjugular biopsy can be used in children [14].

Risks and complications

The mortality from various large combined series is about 0.01% (table 3.3). Complications are reported in 0.06–0.32% of patients [41].

In 17 years, some 8000 needle biopsies of the liver have been performed at the Royal Free Hospital with only two deaths, one in a haemophiliac and one in a patient with acute viral hepatitis [40]. In spite of the low mortality and complication rate, liver biopsy must only be performed when the patient can be expected to benefit from the information and where it cannot be obtained by less invasive means.

Pleurisy and peri-hepatitis

A friction rub caused by fibrinous peri-hepatitis or pleurisy may be heard on the next day. It is of little consequence and pain subsides with analgesics. A chest X-ray may show a small pneumothorax.

Haemorrhage

In a series of 9212 biopsies, there were 10 (0.11%) fatal

Table 3.3. Fatalities from needle liver biopsy

Source	Date	Reference	Biopsies	Mortality (%)
USA	1953	[1,2]	20016	0.17
Europe combined	1964	[3]	23382	0.01
Germany	1967	[4]	80000	0.015
Italy	1986	[5]	68276	0.009
USA	1990	[6]	9212	0.11

1 Zamcheck. *N. Engl. J. Med.* 1953; **249**: 1020.
2 Zamcheck. *N. Engl. J. Med.* 1953; **249**: 1062.
3 Thaler. *Wien. Klin. Wchschr.* 1964; **29**: 533.
4 Lindner. *Dtsch. Med. Wschr.* 1967; **92**: 1751.
5 Piccinino. *J. Hepatol.* 1986; **2**: 165 [34].
6 McGill. *Gastroenterology* 1990; **99**: 1396 [28].

and 22 (0.24%) non-fatal haemorrhages [28]. Malignancy, age, female sex and number of passes were the only predictable factors for bleeding. The complication rate is higher when referrals are from a haematology department than when predominantly hepatological problems are being investigated. Haemorrhage usually develops when least expected and when, at the time of biopsy, the risk seemed small. It might be related to factors other than peripheral clotting, for instance the concentration of clotting factors in hepatic parenchyma and the failure of mechanical compression of the needle tract by elastic tissue [12].

Bleeding from the puncture wound usually consists of a thin trickle lasting 10–60 s and the total blood loss is only 5–10 ml. Serious haemorrhage is usually intra-peritoneal but may be intrathoracic from an intercostal artery. The bleeding results from perforation of distended portal or hepatic veins or aberrant arteries. The occasional laceration of a major intra-hepatic vessel cannot be avoided. In some cases, a tear of the liver follows deep breathing during the intercostal procedure.

Perforation of the capsule with intra-peritoneal haemorrhage may follow transvenous biopsy.

Spontaneous recovery may ensue, otherwise angiography followed by transcatheter embolization is usually successful (figs 3.6, 3.7).

Severe haemothorax usually responds to blood transfusion and chest aspiration.

Haemorrhage is rare in the non-jaundiced.

Intra-hepatic haematomas

At 2–4 h post-biopsy, intra-hepatic haematomas are detected by ultrasound in only about 2% [18]. This is probably an underestimate as the haematomas remain isoechoic for the first 24–48 h and are not detected by ultrasound. The day after biopsy, haematomas, usually asymptomatic, are detected in 23% [31]. They can cause fever, rises in serum transaminases, a fall in haematocrit and, if large, right upper quadrant tenderness and an enlarging liver. They may be seen in the arterial phase of a dynamic CT scan as triangular hyper-dense segments. Sometimes a distal portal vein branch may be noted during the arterial phase. Occasionally, haematomas are followed by delayed haemorrhage.

Haemobilia

Haemobilia follows bleeding from a damaged hepatic vessel, artery or vein, into the bile duct (fig. 3.8). It is marked by biliary colic with enlargement and tenderness of the liver and sometimes the gallbladder. The diagnosis is confirmed by ultrasound, magnetic resonance (MR) cholangiography or endoscopic retrograde cholangiopancreatography (ERCP). It may be treated by hepatic arterial embolization; however, spontaneous recovery is usual.

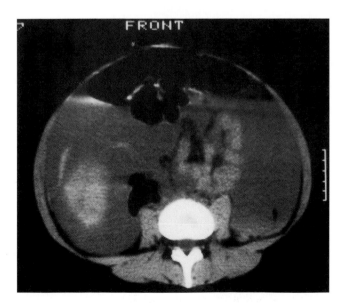

Fig. 3.6. CT scan taken 4 h post-biopsy in a patient with hepatic metastases and jaundice showing haemorrhage around and into the liver.

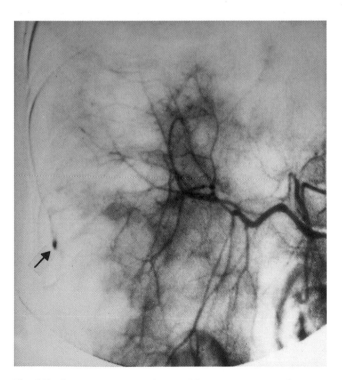

Fig. 3.7. Same patient as in fig. 3.6. Hepatic arteriography (DSA technique) shows blood beside the liver (arrow). The bleeding point was later successfully embolized via the hepatic artery.

Arteriovenous fistula

An arteriovenous fistula is shown by hepatic arteriography (figs 3.9, 3.10).

Histology shows marked phlebosclerosis of the portal vein tributaries [16]. The fistula may close spontaneously, otherwise it can be treated by direct hepatic arterial catheterization and embolization of the feeding artery.

Biliary peritonitis

This is the second commonest complication after haemorrhage. It was seen 49 times in 123 000 biopsies with 12 deaths. The bile usually comes from the gallbladder, which may be in an unusual position, or from dilated bile ducts. Biliary scintigraphy demonstrates the leak [42]. Surgical management is usually necessary although conservative measures with intravenous fluids, antibiotics and intensive care monitoring may be successful.

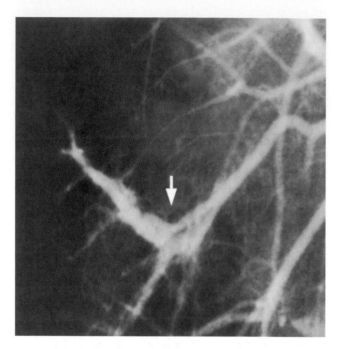

Fig. 3.9. Hepatic arteriography taken post liver biopsy shows an arteriovenous fistula (arrow).

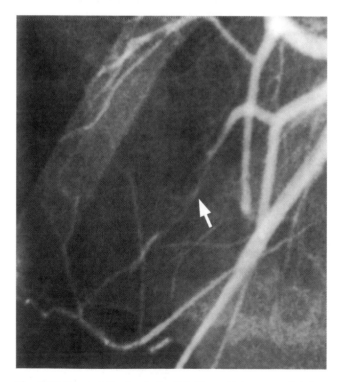

Fig. 3.10 Same patient as in fig. 3.9. The arteriovenous fistula has been successfully embolized (arrow).

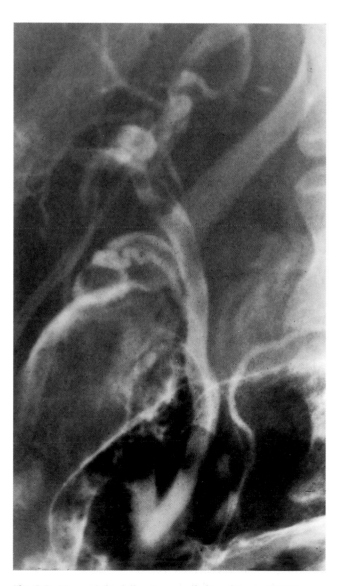

Fig. 3.8. Haemobilia following needle liver biopsy. ERCP shows linear filling defects in the common bile duct.

Puncture of other organs

Puncture of organs such as the kidney or colon is rarely clinically significant.

Infection

Transient bacteraemia is relatively common, particularly in patients with cholangitis. Septicaemia is rarer; blood cultures are usually positive for *Escherichia coli*.

Carcinoid crisis

This can follow percutaneous biopsy [4].

Sampling variability

It is surprising that such a small biopsy should so often be representative of changes in the whole liver. Cholestasis, steatosis, viral hepatitis and the reticuloses are fortunately diffuse. This is also true of most cirrhoses, although in macronodular cirrhosis it is possible to aspirate a large nodule and find normal architecture. There is sampling variability in the diagnosis of cirrhosis in the presence of acute hepatitis or chronic hepatitis. The focal granulomatous diseases such as sarcoidosis, tumour deposits and abscesses may be missed; this is infrequent if serial sections are cut.

Misdiagnosis is often due to smallness of the sample, especially failure to obtain portal zones, the focal nature of the disease process and particularly the inexperience of the interpreter.

The diagnostic yield may be improved if three consecutive samples are obtained by redirecting the biopsy needle through a single entry site [29].

Fibrous tissue is increased under the capsule in operative biopsies and this may give a false impression of the liver as a whole.

Operative biopsies may show artefactual changes such as patchy loss of glycogen, haemorrhages, polymorph infiltration and even focal necrosis. These are presumably related to the effects of trauma, circulatory changes and hypoxia.

Naked eye appearances

A satisfactory biopsy is 1–4 cm long and weighs 10–50 mg.

The cirrhotic liver tends to crumble into fragments of irregular contour. The fatty liver has a pale greasy look and floats in the formol–saline fixative. The liver containing malignant deposits is dull white in colour. The liver from a patient with Dubin–Johnson hyperbilirubinaemia is diffusely chocolate coloured (see fig. 12.12).

In cholestatic jaundice, the greenish central areas contrast with the less green periphery. The vascular centres of lobules in hepatic congestion may be obvious.

Preparation of the specimen

The biopsy is usually fixed in 10% formol–saline. The time taken to fix such a small piece is less than for a larger specimen. Routine stains include haematoxylin and eosin and a good stain for connective tissue. All specimens are stained for iron and by the diastase/PAS (periodic acid–schiff) method. Orcein staining is also useful. This shows hepatitis B surface antigen in the hepatocyte as a uniform, finely granular, brown material. It also stains copper-associated protein in lysosomes as black–brown granules, usually in the peri-portal area (zone 1). This is a useful indicator of cholestasis and is also sometimes found in Wilson's disease.

Adequate biopsies (3 mm in length) excised from paraffin blocks can be analysed retrospectively for iron and copper by atomic absorption spectrophotometry [32]. If iron overload is suspected, the specimen must not be fixed in saline as this leads to rapid loss of iron.

Frozen sections are needed to demonstrate lipids. These are stained with oil red O to show microvesicular fat.

Specimens for electron microscopy are fixed within seconds in glutaraldehyde and preserved at 4°C until processed. Electron microscopy is particularly valuable for diagnosis of tumours of uncertain origin and storage disorders, including Wilson's disease, Niemann–Pick disease and Dubin–Johnson syndrome.

Serial sections are important for the diagnosis of lesions such as granulomas which may be scattered through the liver.

Cytological preparations are made by smearing the aspirated tissue core on a slide.

Interpretation

The specimen should preferably be at least 2 cm in length with four portal zones if a reliable opinion is to be given. In the normal liver, zone 1 (portal) bears a regular relation to zone 3 (central). This orientation is an essential first step. Each portal zone consists of one or two bile ductules, a branch of the hepatic artery and of the portal vein, a few mononuclears and an occasional fibroblast. Using the 1.6-mm Menghini technique, a liver biopsy from a normal adult contains six full portal triads per linear centimetre of tissue [9]. Portal triads contain at least one of portal vein, hepatic artery and interlobular bile duct. Portal triads which do not contain one of these profiles (usually the portal vein) are almost as common as portal triads in normal liver.

The liver cell plates are one cell thick and contain abundant glycogen. Mitoses are not seen in the liver cells which are usually mononucleate and of regular size. The sinusoids are lined by Kupffer cells and can be seen converging upon zone 3.

Isolated sinusoidal dilatation prompts a search for a tumour or a disease associated with granulomas.

Liver biopsy appearances are described in individual chapters, and detailed histology can be found in the monographs of Klatskin and Conn [24] and Scheuer and Lefkowitch [37].

Indications (table 3.4) [40]

Numbers of liver biopsies are falling due to increasing use of cholangiography, imaging, virological and immunological diagnostic tools. Thus liver biopsies are rarely performed in patients with typical acute jaundice. Biopsy of patients with malignant tumours has to be related to the possibility of tumour seeding [8]. Focal lesions such as haemangioma or focal nodular hyperplasia are better diagnosed by imaging. Patients with typical primary biliary cirrhosis and positive serum mitochondrial antibodies, or those with fatty liver secondary to obesity, do not need a biopsy for diagnosis. Numbers are maintained by biopsies performed for the management of patients with chronic hepatitis or following hepatic transplantation.

Drug-related liver disease can be difficult to identify and the history is essential. Sometimes the distinction from acute viral hepatitis is impossible.

Chronic hepatitis remains a most important indication. Biopsy is needed for diagnosis and to follow the progress and the effects of treatment. A semiquantitative assessment can be made of inflammation (grading) and fibrosis (progression) (Knodell score) (Chapter 19) [10].

The diagnosis of *cirrhosis* demands connective tissue stains, particularly for reticulin.

Alcohol-related disease liver biopsy is used for diagnosis and prognosis but also as a deterrent to further consumption.

Table 3.4. Indications for liver biopsy

Drug-related hepatitis
Chronic hepatitis
Cirrhosis
Liver disease in the alcoholic
Intra-hepatic (ductopenic) cholestasis
Infective conditions
Storage diseases
Post-hepatic transplantation
Complications of renal transplantation
Space-occupying lesions
Unexplained hepatomegaly or enzyme elevations

Extra-hepatic cholestasis can usually be diagnosed by cholangiography with imaging and without the need for liver biopsy, but this is particularly useful in small duct disease (ductopenia) (Chapter 13).

Infections. These include tuberculosis, brucellosis, syphilis, histoplasmosis, coccidioidomycosis, pyogenic infection, leptospirosis, amoebiasis and opportunistic infections such as herpes, cytomegalovirus and cryptosporidosis. When indicated, the appropriate stains for the causative organism should be applied and a portion of the biopsy cultured.

Liver biopsy is useful in elucidating the cause of *fever* of unknown origin [19].

Storage diseases. These include amyloidosis and glycogen disease (Chapter 25). Haemochromatosis and Wilson's disease can be diagnosed and the effect of therapy is assessed by serial biopsies.

Orthotopic liver transplant. Liver biopsy is useful in the pre-transplant work-up. Post-transplant pathology includes rejection, infection and bile leaks. Liver biopsy is essential to unravel these complications. The protocol 5-day biopsy is particularly useful in diagnosing episodes of rejection [5].

Renal transplants. Liver biopsy is useful in evaluating the chronic liver disease in kidney recipients [36].

Space-occupying lesions are diagnosed by direct biopsy under imaging.

Other indications include obscure hepatomegaly or splenomegaly, and abnormal biochemical tests of uncertain cause, particularly where fatty liver is suspected.

Special methods [37]

Bile canaliculi may be shown by staining for adenosine triphosphatase (ATPase) and glucose-6-phosphatase. Electron microscopy may be combined with histochemistry. ATPase is localized to the microvilli of the canaliculi and 5-nucleotidase to the microvilli of the sinusoidal border. Acid phosphatase is found in Kupffer cells, degenerating foci and regenerating nodules; alkaline phosphatase defines cholangioles.

Immunohistochemical stains may be used to demonstrate antigens of viral hepatitis A, B, C, D and E, also herpes and adenovirus. Immunohistochemistry is also used to diagnose amyloid disease and α_1-antitrypsin deficiency.

Markers for bile duct epithelial cells such as cytokeratin 7 are useful in cholestatic disorders and especially for ductular reactions and ductopenia. Immunostaining for specific tumour markers may be useful in detecting the origin of tumour metastases and diagnosing hepatocellular carcinoma from cholangiocarcinoma. Studies on the expression of oncogenic products have not yet reached clinical application.

Factor VIII-related antigen is used to diagnose angiosarcoma and epithelioid haemangio-endothelioma.

In situ hybridization techniques, using complementary DNA or RNA sequences, are being increasingly used to assess viral replication, for instance cytomegalovirus, herpes and hepatitis B or C viruses (HBV or HCV).

Polymerase chain reaction (PCR) is useful in human immunodeficiency virus (HIV), HBV and HCV infections, but the whole biopsy is required for the analysis.

Mononuclear cells derived from liver biopsies may be studied by histochemistry using monoclonal antibodies specific for various surface antigens [17]. Flow cytometry is used to immunotype lymphocytes from fresh liver tissue.

Polarized light is useful for showing malarial and schistosomal pigment, crystals or amyloid after Congo red staining.

Ultraviolet light may help to identify porphyrins in fresh frozen sections from patients with porphyria cutanea tarda.

Quantitative analysis of liver biopsy specimens is plagued by sampling difficulties and by failure to find a suitable standard of reference. In the liver with normal structure, results are reasonably reliable. Difficulties arise particularly in biopsies from cirrhotic livers where the proportion of fibrous tissue is uncertain. DNA, which is confined to the nucleus, is probably the best reference base although this may be valueless where the proportion of cells of different types is variable. Alternatively, the substance being investigated may be referred to dry weight or to total nitrogen content of the biopsy.

References

1 Aledort LM, Levine PH, Hilgartner M *et al*. A study of liver biopsies and liver disease among haemophiliacs. *Blood* 1985; **66**: 367.

2 Axenfeld H, Brass K. Klinische und bioptische Untersuchungen über den sogenannten Icterus catarrhalis. *Frankfurt Z. Pathol*. 1942; **57**: 147.

3 Baron E. Aspiration for removal of biopsy material from the liver. *Arch. Intern. Med*. 1939; **63**: 276.

4 Bissonnette RT, Gibney RG, Berry BR *et al*. Fatal carcinoid crisis after percutaneous fine-needle biopsy of hepatic metastasis: case report and literature review. *Radiology* 1990; **174**: 751.

5 Brunt EM, Peters MG, Flye MW *et al*. Day-5 protocol liver allograft biopsies document early rejection episodes and are predictive of recurrent rejection. *Surgery* 1992; **111**: 511.

6 Buscarini L, Fornari F, Bolondi L *et al*. Ultrasound-guided fine-needle biopsy of focal liver lesions: techniques, diagnostic accuracy and complications. *J. Hepatol*. 1990; **11**: 344.

7 Cohen MB, A-Kader HH, Lambers D *et al*. Complications of percutaneous liver biopsy in children. *Gastroenterology* 1992; **102**: 629.

8 Colombo M, del Ninno E, de Franchis R *et al*. Ultrasound assisted percutaneous liver biopsy: superiority of the Trucut over the Menghini needle for diagnosis of cirrhosis. *Gastroenterology* 1988; **95**: 487.

9 Crawford AR, Lin X-Z, Crawford JM. The normal adult human liver biopsy: a quantitative reference standard. *Hepatology* 1998; **28**: 323.

10 Desmet VJ, Gerber M, Hoofnagle JH *et al*. Classification of chronic hepatitis: diagnosis, grading and staging. *Hepatology* 1994; **19**: 1513.

11 Donaldson BW, Gopinath R, Wanless IR *et al*. The role of transjugular liver biopsy in fulminant liver failure: relation to other prognostic indicators. *Hepatology* 1993; **18**: 1370.

12 Ewe K. Bleeding after liver biopsy does not correlate with indices of peripheral coagulation. *Dig. Dis. Sci*. 1981; **26**: 388.

13 Frerichs FT von. *Über den Diabetes*. Hirschwald, Berlin, 1884.

14 Furuya KN, Burrows PE, Phillips MJ *et al*. Transjugular liver biopsy in children. *Hepatology* 1992; **15**: 1036.

15 Glenthoj A, Sehested M, Torp-Pedersen S. Diagnostic reliability of histological and cytological fine needle biopsies from focal liver lesions. *Histopathology* 1989; **15**: 375.

16 Hashimoto E, Ludwig J, MacCarty RL *et al*. Hepatoportal arteriovenous fistula: morphologic features studied after orthotopic liver transplantation. *Hum. Pathol*. 1989; **20**: 707.

17 Hata K, Van Thiel DH, Herberman RB *et al*. Phenotypic and functional characteristics of lymphocytes isolated from liver biopsy specimens from patients with active liver disease. *Hepatology* 1992; **15**: 816.

18 Hederstrom E, Forsberg L, Floren C-H *et al*. Liver biopsy complications monitored by ultrasound. *J. Hepatol*. 1989; **8**: 94.

19 Holtz T, Moseley RH, Scheiman JM. Liver biopsy in fever of unknown origin: a reappraisal. *J. Clin. Gastroenterol*. 1993; **17**: 29.

20 Huard P, May JM, Joyeux B. La ponction biopsie du foie et son utilité dans le diagnostique des affections hépatiques. *Ann. Anat. Path. Anat. Norm. Méd-chir*. 1935; **12**: 1118.

21 Iversen P, Roholm K. On aspiration biopsy of the liver, with remarks on its diagnostic significance. *Acta. Med. Scand*. 1939; **102**: 1.

22 Jacobs WH, Goldberg SB and the Patient Care Committee of the American Gastroenterological Association. Statement on outpatient percutaneous liver biopsy. *Dig. Dis. Sci*. 1989; **34**: 322.

23 Janes CH, Lindor KD. Outcome of patients hospitalized for complications after outpatient liver biopsy. *Ann. Intern. Med*. 1993; **118**: 96.

24 Klatskin G, Conn HO. *Histopathology of the Liver*, vols 1 and 2. Oxford University Press, New York, 1993.

25 Lebrec D. Various approaches to obtaining liver tissue: choosing the biopsy technique. *J. Hepatol*. 1996; **25** (suppl. 1): 20.

26 Lebrec D, Goldfarb G, Degott C *et al*. Transvenous liver biopsy—an experience based on 1000 hepatic tissue samplings with this procedure. *Gastroenterology* 1982; **82**: 338.

27 Lindor KD, Bru C, Jorgensen RA *et al*. The role of ultrasonography and automatic-needle biopsy in outpatient percutaneous liver biopsy. *Hepatology* 1996; **23**: 1079.

28 McGill DB, Rakela J, Zinsmeister AR *et al*. A 21-year experience with major haemorrhage after percutaneous liver biopsy. *Gastroenterology* 1990; **99**: 1396.

29 Maharaj B, Maharaj RJ, Leary WP *et al.* Sampling variability and its influence on the diagnostic yield of percutaneous needle biopsy of the liver. *Lancet* 1986; **i**: 523.

30 Menghini G. One-second needle biopsy of the liver. *Gastroenterology* 1958; **35**: 190.

31 Minuk GY, Sutherland LR, Wiseman DA *et al.* Prospective study of the incidence of ultrasound-detected intrahepatic and subcapsular haematomas in patients randomized to 6 or 24h of bed rest after percutaneous liver biopsy. *Gastroenterology* 1987; **92**: 290.

32 Olynyk JK, O'Neill R, Britton RS *et al.* Determination of hepatic iron concentration in fresh and paraffin-embedded tissue: diagnostic implications. *Gastroenterology* 1994; **106**: 674.

33 Pagliaro L, Rinaldi F, Craxi A *et al.* Percutaneous blind biopsy vs. laparoscopy with guided biopsy in diagnosis of cirrhosis: a prospective, randomised trial. *Dig. Dis. Sci.* 1983; **28**: 39.

34 Piccinino F, Sagnelli E, Pasquale G *et al.* Complications following percutaneous liver biopsy. A multicentre retrospective study on 68276 biopsies. *J. Hepatol.* 1986; **2**: 165.

35 Pisha T, Gabriel S, Therneau T *et al.* Cost-effectiveness of ultrasound-guided liver biopsy. *Hepatology* 1998; **27**: 1220.

36 Rao KV, Anderson WR, Kasiske BL *et al.* Value of liver biopsy in the evaluation and management of chronic liver disease in renal transplant recipients. *Am. J. Med.* 1993; **94**: 241.

37 Scheuer PJ, Lefkowitch JH. *Liver Biopsy Interpretation*, 6th edn. WB Saunders, Philadelphia, 2000.

38 Schüpfer F. De la possibilité de faire 'intra vitam' un diagnostic histo-pathologique précis des maladies du foie et de la rate. *Sem. Méd.* 1907; **27**: 229.

39 Sherlock S. Aspiration liver biopsy, technique and diagnostic application. *Lancet* 1945; **ii**: 397.

40 Sherlock S, Dick R, van Leeuwen DJ. Liver biopsy today. The Royal Free Hospital experience. *J. Hepatol.* 1984; **1**: 75.

41 Tobkes AI, Nord HJ. Liver biopsy: review of methodology and complications. *Digestion* 1995; **13**: 267.

42 Veneri RJ, Gordon SC, Fink-Bennett D. Scintigraphic and culdoscopic diagnosis of bile peritonitis complicating liver biopsy. *J. Clin. Gastroenterol.* 1989; **11**: 571.

43 Whitmire LF, Galambos JT, Phillips VM *et al.* Imaging guided percutaneous hepatic biopsy: diagnostic accuracy and safety. *J. Clin. Gastroenterol.* 1985; **7**: 511.

44 Younossi ZM, Teran JC, Ganiats TG. Ultrasound-guided liver biopsy for parenchymal liver disease: an economic analysis. *Dig. Dis. Sci.* 1998; **43**: 46.

45 Zins M, Vilgrain V, Gayno S *et al.* US-guided percutaneous liver biopsy with plugging of the needle track: a prospective study in 72 high-risk patients. *Radiology* 1992; **184**: 841.

Chapter 4
The Haematology of Liver Disease

General features

Hepato-cellular failure, portal hypertension and jaundice may affect the blood picture. Chronic liver disease is usually accompanied by 'hypersplenism'. Diminished erythrocyte survival is frequent. In addition both parenchymal hepatic disease and cholestatic jaundice may produce blood coagulation defects. Dietary deficiencies, alcoholism, bleeding and difficulties in hepatic synthesis of proteins used in blood formation or coagulation add to the complexity of the problem.

Spontaneous bleeding, bruising and purpura, together with a history of bleeding after minimal trauma such as venepuncture, are more important indications of a bleeding tendency in patients with liver disease than laboratory tests.

Blood volume

Plasma volume is frequently increased in patients with cirrhosis, especially with ascites and also with long-standing obstructive jaundice or with hepatitis. This hypervolaemia may partially, and sometimes totally, account for a low peripheral haemoglobin or erythrocyte level. Total circulating haemoglobin is reduced in only about half the patients.

Erythrocyte changes

The red cells may be *hypochromic*. This is often due to gastrointestinal bleeding leading to iron deficiency. In portal hypertension anaemia follows gastro-oesophageal bleeding and is enhanced by thrombocytopenia and disturbed blood coagulation. In cholestasis or cirrhosis of the alcoholic, haemorrhage may be from an ulcer or gastritis. Epistaxis, bruising and bleeding gums add to the anaemia.

The erythrocytes are usually *normocytic*. This is a combination of the microcytosis of chronic blood loss and the macrocytosis inherent in patients with liver disease. Thus the red cell membrane cholesterol and phospholipid content and/or ratio is changed and this results in various morphological abnormalities including thin macrocytes and target cells.

Thin macrocytes are frequent and are associated with a macronormoblastic marrow. These resolve when liver function improves.

Target cells are also thin macrocytes. They are found in both hepato-cellular and cholestatic jaundice. They are flat, macrocytic and have an increased surface area and increased resistance to osmotic lysis. They are particularly prominent in cholestasis where a rise in bile acids may contribute by inhibiting lecithin cholesterol acyl transferase (LCAT) activity [12]. The red cell membrane LCAT is decreased, resulting in loading of the membrane with both cholesterol and lecithin. Membrane fluidity is unchanged.

Spur cells are cells with unusual thorny projections. They are also termed *acanthocytes* (fig. 4.1). They are associated with far advanced liver disease, usually in alcoholics. Severe anaemia and haemolysis are also found. Their appearance is a bad prognostic sign. They disappear after liver transplantation [11]. The mechanism of their formation is unclear but they may be derived from *echinocytes*, which are also called burr cells [28]. These spiculated cells are not usually seen on dry blood films but are present on wet films or scanning electron microscopy in many patients with liver disease. They form because of an interaction with the abnormal HDL found in liver disease [28]. There is excess accumulation of unesterified cholesterol compared with phospholipid, with resultant reduced membrane fluidity and the formation of thorny projections. Reticulo-endothelial cells in the spleen modify these rigid cells with removal of membrane.

Alcoholics show genuine *thick macrocytes* which are probably related to the toxic effect of alcohol on the bone marrow. Folic acid and B_{12} deficiency may contribute.

Bone marrow of chronic hepato-cellular failure is hyperplastic and macronormoblastic. In spite of this, erythrocyte volume is depressed and the marrow therefore does not seem able to compensate completely for the anaemia (*relative marrow failure*).

Folate and B_{12} metabolism

The liver stores folate and converts it to its active storage form, tetrahydrofolate. Folate deficiency may accom-

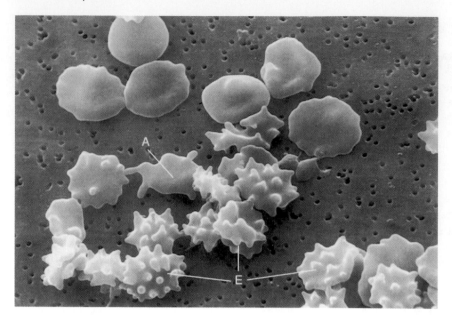

Fig. 4.1. Scanning electron micrograph of abnormal red cells from a patient with alcoholic hepatitis, showing echinocytes (E) at various stages of development, and an acanthocyte (A). (Courtesy of Dr J. Owen and Ms J. Lewin.)

pany chronic liver disease, usually in the alcoholic. This is largely due to dietary deficiency. Serum folate levels are low. Folate therapy is useful. The liver also stores vitamin B_{12} [27]. Hepatic levels are reduced in liver disease. When hepatocytes become necrotic the vitamin is released into the blood and high serum B_{12} levels are recorded. This is shown in hepatitis, active cirrhosis and with primary liver cancer. Values in cholestatic jaundice are normal.

Megaloblastic anaemia is rare with chronic liver disease and vitamin B_{12} therapy is rarely needed.

Erythrocyte survival and haemolytic anaemia

Increased red cell destruction is almost constant in hepato-cellular failure and jaundice of all types [35]. This is reflected in erythrocyte polychromasia and reticulocytosis.

The mechanism is extremely complex. The major factor is hypersplenism with destruction of red blood cells in the spleen. Also, spur cells have membrane defects, particularly decreased fluidity, and this, with the altered architecture, exacerbates splenic destruction. In some instances, however, the spleen is not the site of erythrocyte destruction. Splenectomy or corticosteroid therapy have little effect [35].

Haemolysis may occur in Wilson's disease (Chapter 24), and this diagnosis is likely in the young patient presenting with haemolysis and liver dysfunction.

Haemolysis may be acute in patients with alcoholic hepatitis who also have hypercholesterolaemia (*Zieve's syndrome*) [43].

Rarely, an autoimmune haemolytic anaemia with a positive Coombs' test is seen in chronic hepatitis, primary biliary cirrhosis and primary sclerosing cholangitis. Haemolytic anaemia may also follow liver transplantation due to 'passenger lymphocytes' in a mismatch donor organ [14] or a delayed transfusion reaction. A syndrome of haemolysis, elevated liver enzymes and a low platelet count (the HELLP syndrome) is a rare complication of the third trimester of pregnancy (Chapter 27) [34]. Haemolysis is a complication of ribavirin therapy due to oxidative damage to the red cell membrane with binding of specific IgG [13].

Aplastic anaemia is a rare complication of acute viral hepatitis, usually type non-A, non-B, non-C. It may be fatal but response to intensive immunosuppressive treatment is reported [7]. It may follow liver transplantation [16].

Changes in the leucocytes and platelets

Leucopenia and thrombocytopenia are commonly found in patients with cirrhosis, usually with a mild anaemia ('*hypersplenism*').

Leucocytes

The leucopenia is of the order of $1.5–3.0\times10^9/l$, with the depression mainly affecting polymorphs. Occasionally it may be more severe.

Leucocytosis accompanies cholangitis, fulminant hepatitis, alcoholic hepatitis, hepatic abscess and malignant disease. Atypical lymphocytes are found in the peripheral blood in viral infections such as infectious mononucleosis and viral hepatitis.

Platelets

Abnormalities in platelet count and function are common in patients with all forms of liver disease.

Platelet count. In patients with chronic liver disease and portal hypertension, a low platelet count is due in part to increased splenic sequestration and to low thrombopoietin levels. Thus, although platelet counts rise after the insertion of a transjugular intra-hepatic porto-systemic shunt, they do not return to normal [18]. Plasma concentrations of thrombopoietin, the key regulator of platelet function produced mainly by the liver, are reduced in patients with cirrhosis, correlate with platelet count, and rise after liver transplantation [17, 32, 38].

In chronic liver disease increased destruction of platelets is minimal and their half-life is normal, calling into question whether there is any biological effect of the IgG and IgM antibodies detected in patients with chronic hepatitis [20, 26]. Decreased production of platelets from the bone marrow follows alcohol excess, folic acid deficiency and viral hepatitis.

Platelet function, in particular aggregation, is impaired in patients with cirrhosis, particularly Child's grade C, due to an intrinsic defect and circulating serum factors [42]. There is reduced availability of arachidonic acid for prostaglandin production, and also a reduction in platelet adenosine triphosphate and 5-hydroxytryptamine [21]. Abnormal platelet aggregation due to disseminated intravascular coagulation may be an additional important factor in severe liver failure.

The thrombocytopenia of chronic liver disease (usually $60–90 \times 10^9/l$) is extremely frequent and is largely due to hypersplenism. It is very rarely of clinical significance. Unless the patient is actually suffering from the leucopenia or thrombocytopenia the spleen should not be removed; mere demonstration of a low platelet or leucocyte count is not sufficient. The circulating platelets and leucocytes, although in short supply, are functioning well, in contrast to those of leukaemia. Splenectomy is contraindicated. The mortality in patients with liver disease is high and the operation is liable to be followed by splenic and portal vein thrombosis which preclude later operations on the portal vein and may make hepatic transplantation more difficult.

The liver and blood coagulation [9, 24, 31]

Disturbed blood coagulation in patients with hepatobiliary disease is particularly complex. This is due to the many changes in pathways which lead to fibrin production occurring at the same time as changes in the fibrinolytic process (fig. 4.2, table 4.1). Changes in platelet number and function are discussed in the previous section. Despite the complexity of the changes, the end

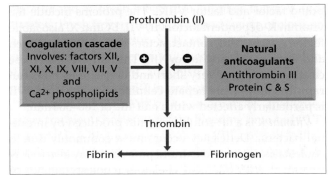

(a)

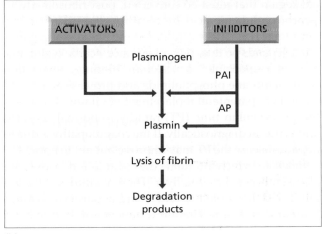

(b)

Fig. 4.2. Normal pathways of (a) coagulation and (b) fibrinolysis. Liver disease effects virtually all components. PAI, plasminogen activator inhibitor; AP, antiplasmin.

Table 4.1. Effect of liver disease on haemostasis

Reduced synthesis of clotting factors
  hepatic dysfunction *per se*
  vitamin K deficiency/malabsorption
Reduced synthesis of inhibitors of coagulation
Production of abnormal/dysfunctional proteins
Enhanced fibrolytic activity
  reduced clearance of activators of fibrinolysis
  reduced production of inhibitors of fibrinolysis
Reduced hepatic clearance of activated clotting factors
Disseminated intravascular coagulation
  multifactorial including endotoxaemia
Platelet abnormalities
  number
  function

result is reduced coagulation, which needs therapeutic intervention if there is bleeding or if a procedure is planned that risks haemorrhage.

The hepatocyte is the principal site of *synthesis* of all the *coagulation proteins* with the exception of von Wille-

Table 4.3. Hepato-biliary disease and bone marrow transplantation

Problem	Related to
Pre-existing	
Fungal	Granulocytopenia
Viral (hepatitis type B, C)	Blood products
Drug	Medication
Biliary	Stones
Post-transplantation	
Early neutropenic phase (up to 4 weeks)	
acute graft-versus-host disease	Donor marrow
veno-occlusive disease	Cytoreductive therapy
nodular regenerative hyperplasia	
drug induced	Including TPN
Extra-hepatic bacterial sepsis	Bacteria/endotoxin
fungal	
biliary disease	Sludge
Intermediate (4–15 weeks)*	
Viral	Cytomegalovirus
	Hepatitis type B, C
Late (>15 weeks)	
chronic graft-versus-host disease	Multi-organ disease
chronic viral infection	
fungal	Immunosuppression
tumour recurrence	

*As well as continuing early problems.

hepatic venous pressure to be measured [31]. Four histological abnormalities correlate with the clinical severity of disease: occluded hepatic venules, eccentric luminal narrowing/phlebosclerosis, hepatocyte necrosis and sinusoidal fibrosis [30]. These findings suggest that there is extensive injury to zone 3 structures by the cytoreductive therapy. Studies suggest that ursodeoxycholic acid [8], defibrotide [5] and tissue plasminogen activator [34] may be useful in the prevention or treatment of veno-occlusive disease.

Opportunistic *fungal* and *bacterial infections* occur during neutropenic periods and may cause abnormal liver function; *viral infections* occur later.

Helpful data to identify the cause of the hepatic abnormality include: (a) timing of the changes related to drugs, chemotherapy, radiation and bone marrow infusion; (b) the dose of cytoreductive (conditioning) therapy; (c) the source of donor marrow; (d) pretreatment viral serology; (e) the degree of immunosuppression; and (f) evidence of systemic disease. Bacteriological and virological data are important. Often more than one process is involved. In one series transvenous liver biopsy provided useful data for patient management in over 80% of cases [31].

After bone marrow transplantation, hepato-biliary scintiscanning and ultrasound commonly show abnormalities of questionable clinical significance. Doppler ultrasonography is not reliable for the diagnosis of veno-occlusive disease [28].

Lymphoma

Hepatic involvement occurs in about 70% of cases and immediately puts the patient into stage IV [14]. It may be seen as diffuse infiltrates, as focal tumour-like masses, as portal zone cellularity (fig. 4.4), as an epithelioid cell reaction or as lymphoid aggregates [14]. Rarely, lymphomatous infiltration presents as acute liver failure [40].

In *Hodgkin's disease*, typical tissue is seen spreading out from the portal tracts, with lymphocytes, large pale epithelioid cells, eosinophils, plasma cells and giant Reed–Sternberg cells (fig. 4.5). Later, fibroblasts are found in a supporting connective tissue reticulum.

In patients with known extra-hepatic Hodgkin's disease, but without obvious Reed–Sternberg cells in sections of the liver, hepatic involvement is suggested by portal infiltrates larger than 1 mm in diameter, changes of acute cholangitis, portal oedema and portal infiltrates with a predominance of atypical lymphocytes. These changes should stimulate a wider search for the diagnostic Reed–Sternberg cell in further sections [6].

In *non-Hodgkin's lymphoma*, the portal zones are usually involved. In small cell lymphocytic lymphoma, a dense, monotonous proliferation of normal-appearing lymphocytes is seen. The more aggressive lymphomas also involve portal zones and form tumour nodules. Large cell lymphoma may infiltrate sinusoids.

In *histiocytic medullary reticulosis*, large numbers of reticulum cells fill the sinusoids and portal tracts. Occasionally, the deposits may be single and large.

Liver granulomas with or without hepatic involvement are found with most lymphomas. Caseation without evidence of tuberculosis has been reported [15].

Paraproteinaemia and amyloidosis may be complications.

Diagnosis of hepatic involvement

Detection of hepatic involvement can be extremely difficult. It is unlikely if hepatomegaly is not found. Fever, jaundice and splenomegaly increase the likelihood. Increases in serum γ-GT and transaminase values are suggestive, although often non-specific.

Focal defects may be shown by ultrasound, CT and MRI scanning. Enlarged abdominal lymph nodes may also be seen.

Needle liver biopsy rarely reveals Hodgkin's tissue if the CT scan is normal. Ultrasound or CT-guided liver biopsy add to the chances of obtaining Hodgkin's tissue. Laparoscopy with liver biopsy may establish the diagnosis in the absence of positive CT scans [26]. Needle biopsy does not exclude hepatic involvement if only an

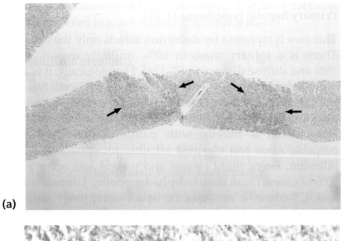

(a)

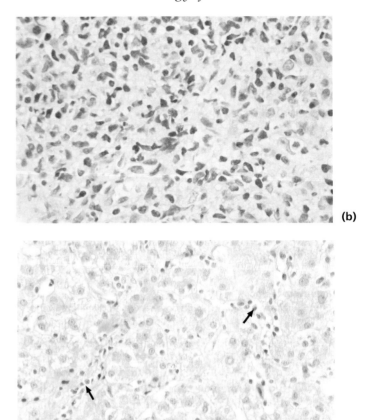

(b)

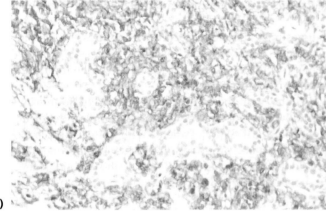

(c)

(d)

Fig. 4.4. Patterns of hepatic histology in lymphoma. (a) Low power showing dense portal cellular infiltrates (arrows) (H & E). (b) Higher power of portal area showing intermediate and large mononuclear cells. (c) Immunohistochemistry showing that the cells have a B cell phenotype (stained brown with antibody to CD20). Bile ducts are not stained. (d) Sinusoidal pattern of infiltration by lymphoma cells. Occasional atypical mononuclear cells are seen within the hepatic sinusoids (arrows).

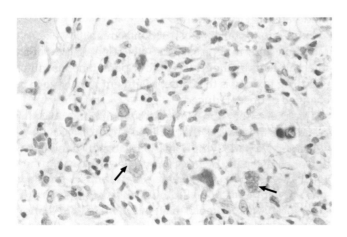

Fig. 4.5. Infiltration of portal zones by Hodgkin's cells including large Reed–Sternberg like cells (arrow) (H & E).

epithelioid histiocyte reaction is seen. Sinusoidal dilatation in zone 2 and 3 is found in 50% and may give a clue to the diagnosis [3].

Presentation as jaundice may provide great diagnostic difficulties (table 4.4). Lymphoma should always be considered in patients with jaundice, fever and weight loss.

Jaundice in lymphoma (table 4.4)

Hepatic infiltrates may be massive or present as space-occupying lesions. Large intra-hepatic deposits are the commonest cause of deep jaundice. Histological evidence is essential for diagnosis.

Biliary obstruction is more frequent with non-Hodgkin's lymphoma than with Hodgkin's disease [9]. It is usually due to hilar glands which are less mobile than those along the common bile duct which can be pushed aside. Occasionally the obstructing glands are peri-ampullary. Primary lymphoma of the bile duct itself is reported [20]. Investigations include endoscopic or percutaneous cholangiography and brush cytology. Known lymphoma elsewhere draws attention to this as a possible cause of bile duct obstruction. Differentiation from other causes of extra-hepatic biliary obstruction is difficult, and depends on the appearances on scanning

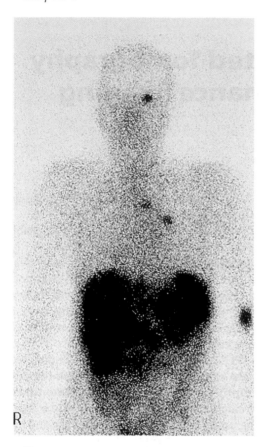

R

Fig. 5.1. ^{111}In-DTPA octreotide scan in a patient with carcinoid syndrome. Apart from the large intra-hepatic tumour, the scan shows metastases in the skull, mediastinum and left arm.

some diffuse hepatic abnormalities are shown. Residents who are not specialists in US can master the basic technique and apply it in the outpatient department or on the ward, for example to image liver and gallbladder before liver biopsy or to detect dilated bile ducts.

US has problems with hepato-biliary examination in the fat or gaseous patient, those with a high liver lying entirely covered by the rib margin and post-operative patients with dressings and painful scars.

A normal US shows the liver to have mixed echogenicity (fig. 5.2). Portal and hepatic veins, inferior vena cava and aorta are shown. The normal intra-hepatic bile ducts are thin and run parallel to large portal vein branches. The right and left hepatic ducts are 1–3 mm in diameter and the common duct 2–7 mm in diameter. US is the screening investigation of choice for patients with cholestasis (Chapter 13). The gallbladder is an ideal organ for sonography (Chapter 32).

The portal vein originates at the junction of the superior mesenteric and splenic veins. US can show a dilated portal vein and collaterals in portal hypertension, an obstructed or scarred portal vein due to tumour or thrombus, and the bunch of vessels of cavernomatous transformation in chronic portal vein thrombosis. Assessment of portal vein patency by real-time US, however, is not always accurate, particularly in patients with previous portal or biliary surgery. Doppler US has a greater sensitivity and specificity. In the absence of Doppler US, real-time US remains a useful first investigation in patients who have bled from oesophageal varices, to assess patency of the portal vein. The patency of portal systemic shunts can also be confirmed.

In heart failure, US shows dilated hepatic veins and inferior vena cava. In Budd–Chiari syndrome, hepatic veins may not be seen. Doppler US again adds diagnostic information over and above real-time US [2].

Focal hepatic lesions are better detected by US than diffuse disease. Lesions down to 1 cm in diameter can be seen. Simple cysts have smooth walls and echo-free contents with through transmission of the sound waves (fig. 33.4). The appearance is diagnostic and with small cysts more accurate than CT. Hydatid cysts produce a characteristic appearance with the contained daughter cysts. Cavernous haemangioma, the commonest liver neoplasm, is usually hyperechoic often with through transmission (fig. 5.3). Such a lesion less than 3 cm in diameter detected incidentally in a patient with normal liver function tests and defined by an experienced ultrasonographer generally needs no further investigation. Lesions more than 3 cm or where the appearances are not classic, or where metastases (especially hypervascular) are suspected, would need further confirmation by dynamic enhanced CT, red blood cell scintiscan or MRI.

Malignant masses (primary or secondary carcinoma) produce a range of appearances on US including a hyper- or hypoechoic pattern (fig. 5.4), well circumscribed or infiltrative. Appearances highly suggestive of metastases include the bull's eye appearance (a hyperechoic rim surrounding a hypoechoic centre). Necrotic tumours may mimic abscess or cyst. Clinical data are paramount—underlying cirrhosis, a proven primary tumour or raised tumour markers in the serum being important. Guided biopsy or aspiration will usually follow to establish the actual pathology.

Diffuse hepatic disease may be detected by US as may anatomical anomalies. In cirrhosis the edge of the liver may be irregular and/or small (fig. 5.5), the hepatic echo pattern coarse (i.e. increased irregular echogenicity) and there may be splenomegaly ascites [1].

A fatty liver may show bright echoes [19]. Accurate quantification of fat, however, is not possible, partly because of the normal variation in echo pattern between normal individuals.

US is the current first choice (together with α-fetoprotein) to screen for the development of hepatocellular carcinoma in patients with cirrhosis.

US is the first choice examination when a hepatic

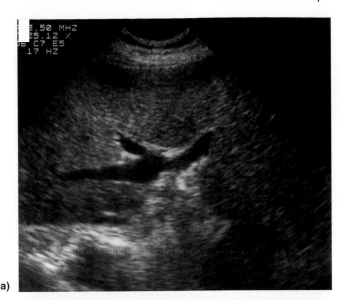

(a)

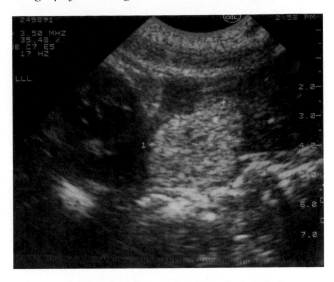

Fig. 5.3. Ultrasonography showing a 3-cm hyperechoic mass in the liver. This is characteristic of a cavernous haemangioma.

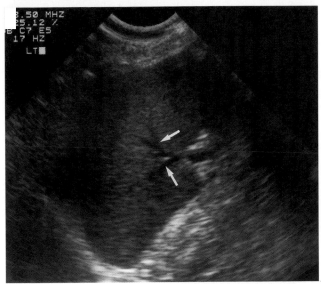

(b)

Fig. 5.2. Ultrasound appearance of normal liver. (a) Normal homogeneous echo pattern and the echo-free portal vein and its intra-hepatic branches. (b) Hepatic veins (arrowed) converge to enter the inferior vena cava.

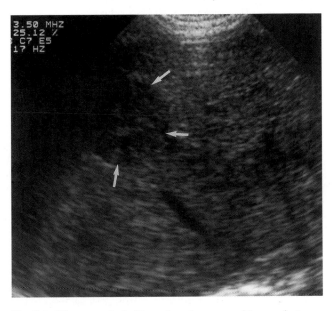

Fig. 5.4. Ultrasound of a liver showing a round hypoechoic mass (arrowed) with altered echo pattern—hepato-cellular carcinoma within a cirrhotic liver.

abscess is suspected. There is an area of reduced echogenicity with or without a surrounding capsule. Sometimes the pus has a similar echogenicity to liver and the abscess is not detected. Clinical features should draw attention to the possibility of a false negative result and CT ordered as a second option. US-guided aspiration for microbiology is necessary. Therapeutic aspiration or catheter drainage may follow.

Doppler ultrasound [12]

Doppler US depends upon the principle that the velocity and direction of flow in a vessel can be derived from

the difference between the frequency of the US signal emitted from the transducer and that reflected back (echo) from the vessel. The technique is difficult and needs an experienced sonographer. Hepatic veins, hepatic artery and portal vein (fig. 10.23) each have unique Doppler signals (Chapter 10). This technique may aid diagnosis in suspected hepatic vein block [2], hepatic artery thrombosis (after liver transplantation) and portal vein thrombosis. In portal hypertension the direction of portal flow and the patency of porto-

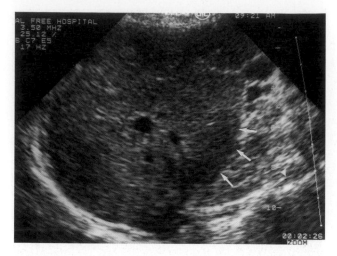

Fig. 5.5. Ultrasound scan in cirrhosis showing irregular edge of liver (arrowed) together with coarse echo pattern.

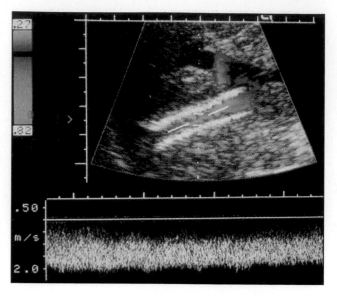

Fig. 5.6. Doppler US scan showing blood flow (blue) through a TIPS shunt.

systemic shunts can be seen. Flattening of the Doppler waveform from the hepatic veins suggests the presence of cirrhosis [4].

Monitoring of flow through transjugular intrahepatic portosystemic shunts (TIPS) by 2–3 monthly Doppler US is useful in detecting shunt dysfunction before clinical signs occur (fig. 5.6).

Endoscopic ultrasound

This technique can detect small peri-ampullary carcinomas and demonstrate the bile duct and gallbladder better than transcutaneous US (Chapter 32). Its use is restricted, however, by the availability of the equipment, and endoscopic and ultrasonic expertise.

Computed tomography [6, 25]

The liver is displayed as a series of adjacent cross-sectional slices. The hard copy scan is depicted as if seen from below. Typically 10–12 images are needed to examine the whole liver. Conventional CT has been replaced by spiral CT. In the conventional method, individual exposures are taken at 7–10-mm intervals through the area of interest. The breath must be held for each slice.

Spiral CT, where a continuous spiral exposure is made, can be completed during a single breath-hold, and thus more quickly (15–30 s). Images are still reconstructed as individual cross-sections. The great advantage of this method is that the scan can be completed while there is peak concentration of contrast medium in the blood vessels of interest. The detail is superior to conventional CT, particularly for small blood vessels. Tumour detection is improved. Computer reconstruction allows three-dimensional pictures which show the relationship of

blood vessels to tumours, and, with intravenous cholangiographic medium, the biliary tree.

The CT scan demonstrates detailed anatomy across the whole abdomen at the level of the slice (fig. 5.7). Oral contrast is usually given to help identify stomach and duodenum. Enhancement by intravenous contrast medium, given as a bolus, an infusion or by arterioportography, demonstrates blood vessels, followed by the hepatic parenchyma. There is renal excretion of contrast. Intravenous cholangiography as a source of contrast is very occasionally used to delineate the biliary system but is restricted to patients with normal liver function tests. CT gives good visualization of adjacent organs, particularly kidneys, pancreas, spleen and retroperitoneal lymph nodes.

CT demonstrates focal hepatic lesions and some diffuse conditions. Advantages over US are that it is less operator dependent and hard copy films can be more readily understood by the clinician. It is more reproducible and obese patients are well suited for CT. Gas-filled bowel may rarely produce some artefacts—solved by altering the patient's position. Pain, post-operative scars and dressings are no hindrance. CT-guided biopsy and aspiration are accurate.

Disadvantages are cost, the exposure to radiation and lack of portability—the patient must be brought to the scanner.

The liver appears homogeneous with an attenuation value (in Hounsfield units) similar to kidney and spleen. Portal vein branches are seen at the hilum. Intravenous enhancement is necessary to differentiate these from dilated bile ducts confidently. Hepatic veins are usually seen. Enhanced CT shows the portal vein and can be used to check patency. Invading tumour or obstructing

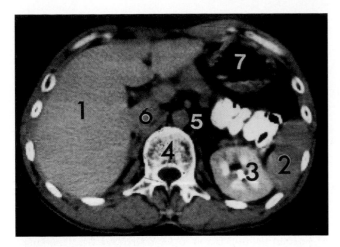

Fig. 5.7. CT scan (enhanced by contrast) showing the liver (1), spleen (2), kidney (3), vertebral body (4), aorta (5), head of the pancreas (6) and stomach (7).

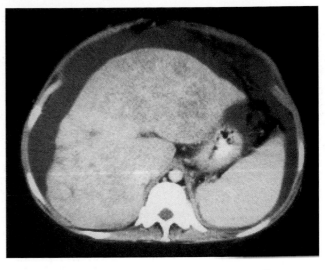

Fig. 5.8. Enhanced CT scan showing patchy areas of low attenuation in the liver (pseudo-tumour appearance) and ascites in a patient with Budd–Chiari syndrome.

thrombus may be seen. Cavernomatous transformation can be recognized with two or more enhancing vessels in place of the obstructed portal vein. Doppler US, however, remains the better technique to demonstrate abnormalities of the portal vein.

In Budd–Chiari syndrome there may be a patchy pattern of hepatic enhancement ('pseudo-tumour' appearance) (fig. 5.8) which may wrongly be interpreted as tumour within the liver. The caudate lobe is enlarged.

An enhanced CT demonstrates the splenic vein and in portal hypertension the collaterals around the spleen and retroperitoneum (fig. 5.9). Spontaneous and surgical shunts can be demonstrated.

Normal bile ducts, both intra- and extra-hepatic, are difficult to see. In the gallbladder, calcified stones are demonstrated and CT is used in the evaluation of patients for non-surgical therapy of gallbladder stones. US rather than CT, however, is the technique of choice to search for gallbladder stones.

The shape of the liver, any anatomical abnormalities or lobe atrophy are seen. Liver volume can be calculated from the slices taken but is a research tool.

CT demonstrates diffuse liver disease due to cirrhosis (fig. 5.10), fat (fig. 5.11) and iron (fig. 5.12). A nodular, uneven edge to the liver which may be shrunken suggests cirrhosis. Ascites and splenomegaly support this diagnosis. CT is of particular value in suspected cirrhosis when clotting deficiencies preclude routine percutaneous liver biopsy.

Fatty liver shows a lower attenuation value than normal (fig. 5.11). Even in an unenhanced scan the blood vessels stand out with a higher attenuation value than liver parenchyma. Thus fatty liver may be diagnosed without the need for liver biopsy. CT measurements correlate with histological steatosis. Single energy CT scan-

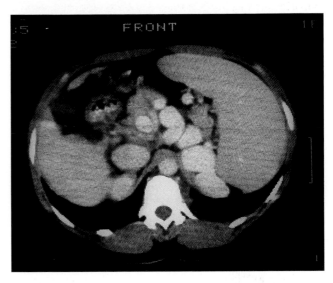

Fig. 5.9. Enhanced CT scan showing massive collaterals (white) around the large spleen due to portal hypertension.

ning is better than dual-energy CT which has a lower sensitivity, particularly when there is increased hepatic iron. However, overall, US is better than either CT method for diffuse steatosis [19].

In iron overload, hepatic density is increased on CT and the unenhanced liver is brighter than the spleen or kidney (fig. 5.12). Using dual-energy CT there is a correlation with liver iron but this is insufficient with moderate siderosis to make the method of practical value in the management of patients with haemochromatosis.

Liver with a high copper content usually has a normal attenuation value.

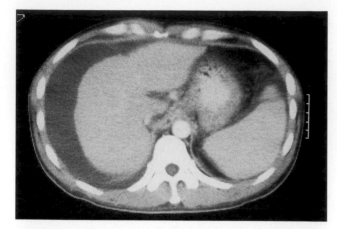

Fig. 5.10. Enhanced CT scan showing a shrunken liver with a nodular margin and ascites due to cirrhosis.

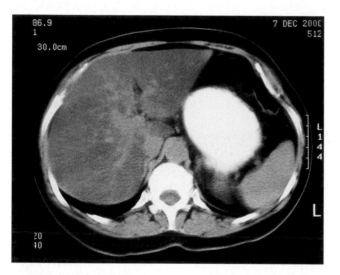

Fig. 5.11. Unenhanced CT scan in a patient with a fatty liver showing blood vessels outlined within the hepatic parenchyma which has a very low attenuation value.

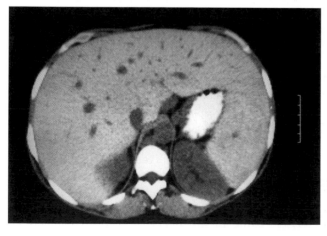

Fig. 5.12. Unenhanced CT scan of secondary iron overload in thalassaemia major. The liver shows increased density, greater than that of the kidney. Portal vein radicles are very prominent.

Space-occupying lesions of 1 cm and more in diameter can be detected by CT. Both unenhanced and enhanced scans should be done. Thus a filling defect on an unenhanced scan may be rendered isodense by intravenous contrast injection and missed. Conversely, an area isodense with normal liver on the unenhanced scan may only be seen after enhancement.

Benign lesions (often detected by chance) include simple cysts and cavernous haemangioma. Simple cysts can usually be confidently identified because of the low attenuation value of the centre, equivalent to water (fig. 33.5). Smaller cysts, however, may suffer from a partial volume effect (i.e. an artificially high attenuation value because of averaging with the surrounding block of normal tissue). US is necessary to confirm the small cyst.

Cavernous haemangioma appears as a low attenuation area on an unenhanced scan which subsequently fills in with contrast from the periphery (fig. 5.13). In the majority of cases the CT appearance is unequivocal. Where there is any question of the aetiology of the lesion, an MRI scan may be necessary.

CT scans can detect solid lesions greater than 1 cm in diameter due to primary or secondary malignant tumour (fig. 5.14). They usually have a lower attenuation value than normal liver that remains on enhancement. Calcification is present in some metastases such as from colon. Highly vascular metastases (kidney, choriocarcinoma, carcinoid) may fill in with enhancement. Most primary tumours do not. Whether confirmation by image-guided biopsy is necessary will depend upon the clinical situation and the results of tumour markers, α-fetoprotein and carcino-embryonic antigen (CEA). The sensitivity of CT in showing hepato-cellular carcinoma is 87%, compared with 80% for US and 90% for hepatic angiography [23]. The sensitivity for satellite lesions is lower at 59% for CT and angiography, and 17% for US. Injection of iodized oil (lipiodol) into the hepatic artery followed by CT 2 weeks later (fig. 31.12) may be used to detect small lesions [20], but many still escape detection—the sensitivity in a study of lesions 9–40 mm in diameter being only 53% [29].

CT scanning after injection of contrast into the splenic or superior mesenteric artery (CT arterio-portography) is the most sensitive method for detecting hepatic metastases (fig. 5.15) and also shows benign and malignant primary hepatic tumours [28]. Because it is invasive it is generally reserved for candidates for surgical resection. CT portography detects 75% of hepato-cellular carcinomas less than 2 cm in diameter [8] and 88% of primary and secondary hepatic malignant lesions [9].

Adenomas and focal nodular hyperplasia usually give negative defects but can be missed both by CT and US because they have characteristics close to that of normal liver tissue. Focal nodular hyperplasia classically has

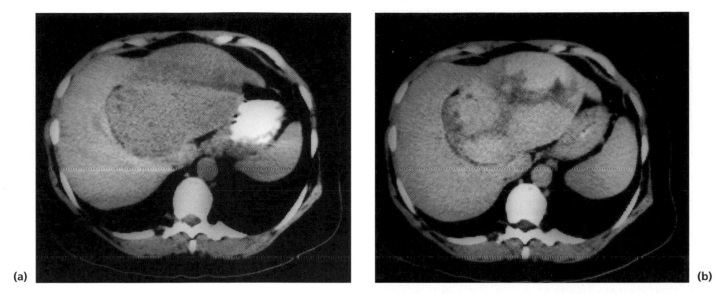

Fig. 5.13. (a) An unenhanced CT scan showing a large, low attenuation lesion in the left lobe of the liver. (b) Following enhancement, dynamic scanning shows gradual infilling of the lesion which eventually became isodense with the remainder of the liver. These are the characteristic appearances of a cavernous haemangioma.

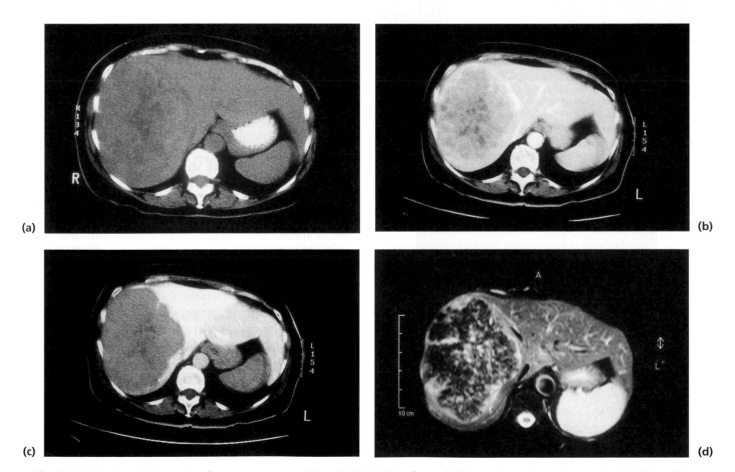

Fig. 5.14. Hepato-cellular carcinoma appearances on CT and MRI. (a) Unenhanced CT scan. Low attenuation area in right lobe. (b) Contrast enhanced CT scan. (c) CT portogram. (d) MRI scan (T_2-weighted) showing a predominantly low intensity lesion.

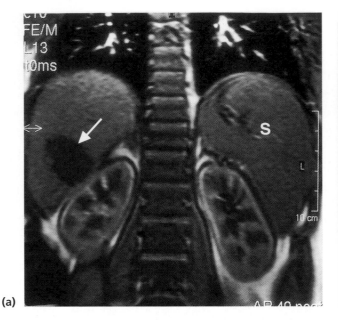

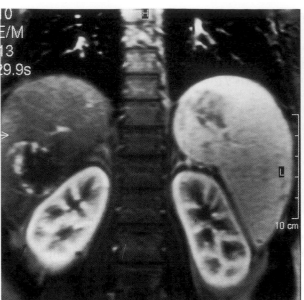

(a)

(b)

Fig. 5.19. MRI of hepatic haemangioma. (a) T_1-weighted scan showing a typical low intensity lesion in the right lobe (arrow). (b) There is bright high intensity infilling at the periphery after gadolinium enhancement. Note incidental splenomegaly (S).

Several approaches can be used to quantify the iron concentration by, for example, comparing the signal from liver with that of muscle on specific sequences [13]. Accurate quantification is likely only to be possible in units with a specific interest, and MRI is not currently widely used in the management of patients with haemochromatosis.

MR cholangiopancreatography (MRCP) has emerged as a valuable technique for showing pathology in the intra- and extra-hepatic biliary tree (fig. 5.21) (Chapter 32) [17, 24]. No contrast is required. The peripheral radicals of the intra-hepatic bile ducts are usually more fully demonstrated than on contrast cholangiography (percutaneous transhepatic cholangiography, endoscopic retrograde cholangiopancreatography). MR angiography allows non-invasive investigation of arterial and venous anatomy, and pathology (Figs 5.22, 5.23).

MRI techniques are advancing rapidly. Developments will include optimizing the spin–echo sequence, using fast imaging sequences and applying new contrast media such as gadolinium and manganese derivatives and ferrite [22]. At present the results for MRI of the liver are comparable to CT. MRI promises much for the future but its use may well be limited geographically by cost, availability and expertise.

CT remains the better choice if scanning of the chest or bones is needed to evaluate malignant hepatic disease, or if guided biopsy is necessary.

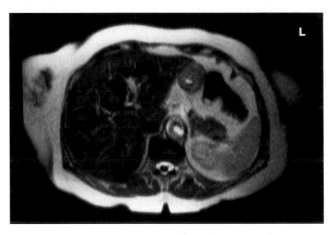

Fig. 5.20. MRI scan (T_2-weighted) showing black low intensity liver due to iron in a patient with haemochromatosis.

MR spectroscopy

MR spectroscopy allows non-invasive evaluation of biochemical changes in tissue *in vivo*. Changes in molecules involved in selected areas of cellular metabolism can be detected. The technique currently remains experimental, but has been applied to patients with liver disease [30]. Phosphorus-31 spectroscopy shows an increase in phospholipid membrane precursors (phosphomonoester or PME peak) and a decrease in phospholipid membrane degradation products and endoplasmic reticulum (phosphodiester or PDE peak). These changes correlate with severity of liver disease and may reflect increased turnover of cell membranes as the liver regenerates. Clinical application of the technique remains elusive but

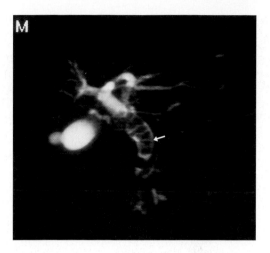

Fig. 5.21. MRCP showing the bile duct packed full of stones (arrow).

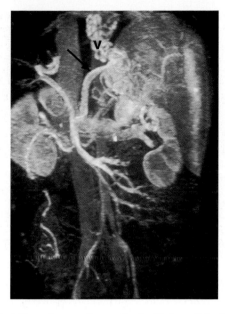

Fig. 5.23. MR angiogram in a patient with hepatitis C cirrhosis, showing a large collateral vein (arrow) feeding a leash of varices (v).

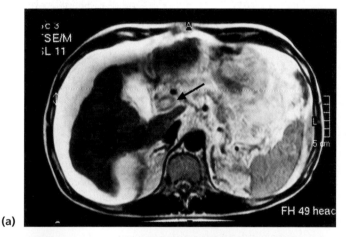

(a)

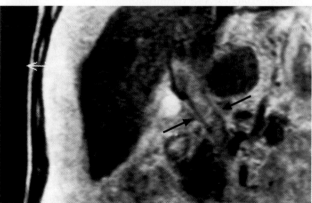

(b)

Fig. 5.22. MR angiography. T_1-weighted scan. (a) Cross-section in a patient with cirrhosis and ascites, showing thrombus in the portal vein (arrow). (b) Coronal scan, showing thrombus between a rim of blood (arrows) in a partially patent portal vein.

a role in acute liver failure and assessment of donor liver tissue is possible.

Conclusions and choice

The choice of technique for hepato-biliary imaging depends upon the problem that has to be solved and the availability of the appropriate apparatus, operator and interpreter (table 5.1). Strict diagnostic algorithms cannot be formulated that will service *all units*. Radio-isotope scanning has been superseded by US, CT and MRI which are better in detecting lesions and character-izing them. With an experienced ultrasonographer, this technique is the initial examination of choice for the majority of problems. Equivocal results can be further studied by CT or MRI as necessary.

CT and MRI characterize most lesions better than US but are more costly and less widely available. In some centres CT replaces US as the primary procedure, often more out of availability and convenience (for the clinician) than need.

For the diagnosis of jaundice, US is the preferred screening investigation. If necessary this may be fol-lowed by MRI and/or MRCP scanning to help in the diagnosis and to show the extent of disease.

For the diagnosis of gallbladder stones, US is the primary method of choice.

Tc-IDA scanning provides an alternative non-invasive method to US for diagnosing acute cholestasis, and is used to demonstrate post-operative biliary patency and

Table 5.1. Non-invasive imaging for hepato-biliary disease

Question	Choice		
	First	Second	Third
Mass in liver	US	CT/MRI	
Hepatic metastases	US	CT/MRI	
Screen cirrhotic for HCC	US	CT	
Tumour resectable	CT*	MRI	
Haemangioma	US	MRI	
Abscess	US/CT		
Hydatid cyst	US	MRI/CT	
Portal vein patent	USDop	US/CT/MRI	
Portal hypertension	USDop	US	CT
Budd–Chiari	USDop	US	CT/MRI
Shunt patent	USDop	US/CT/MRI	
Assessment of trauma	US/CT		
Cirrhosis	US	CT	
Fatty liver	US	CT/MRI	
Iron	CT	MRI	
Gallbladder stone	US		
Acute cholecystitis	US/IDA		
Dilated bile ducts	US	MRCP	
Duct stone	US†	MRCP	
Bile leak	IDA		
Pancreatic tumour	US/CT	EUS	

*CT portography.
†Only of value if positive.
CT, computed tomography; EUS, endoscopic ultrasound; HCC, hepato-cellular carcinoma; IDA, scintiscan with iminodiacetic acid derivative; MRCP, magnetic resonance cholangiopancreatography; MRI, magnetic resonance imaging; US, ultrasound; USDop, Doppler ultrasound.

leaks. It is also used in infants in the diagnostic work-up of possible biliary atresia (see fig. 32.9).

References

1 Aubé C, Oberti F, Korali N et al. Ultrasonographic diagnosis of hepatic fibrosis or cirrhosis. *J. Hepatol.* 1999; **30**: 472.

2 Bolondi L, Gaiani S, Li Bassi S et al. Diagnosis of Budd–Chiari syndrome by pulsed Doppler ultrasound. *Gastroenterology* 1991; **100**: 1324.

3 Caplin ME, Buscombe JR, Hilson AJ et al. Carcinoid tumour. *Lancet* 1998; **352**: 799.

4 Colli A, Cocciolo M, Riva C et al. Abnormalities of Doppler waveform of hepatic veins in patients with chronic liver disease: correlation with histological findings. *Am. J. Roentgenol.* 1994; **162**: 833.

5 de Beeck BO, Luypaert R, Dujardin M et al. Benign liver lesions: differentiation by magnetic resonance. *Eur. J. Radiol.* 1999; **32**: 52.

6 El Sherif A, McPherson SJ, Dixon AK. Spiral CT of the abdomen: increased diagnostic potential. *Eur. J. Radiol.* 1999; **31**: 43.

7 Huebner RH, Park KC, Shepherd JE et al. A meta-analysis of the literature for whole-body FDG PET detection of recurrent colorectal cancer. *J. Nucl. Med.* 2000; **41**: 1177.

8 Ikeda K, Saitoh S, Koida I et al. Imaging diagnosis of small hepatocellular carcinoma. *Hepatology* 1994; **20**: 82.

9 Irie T, Takeshita K, Wada Y et al. CT evaluation of hepatic tumours: comparison of CT with arterial portography, CT with infusion hepatic arteriography, and simultaneous use of both techniques. *Am J. Roentgenol.* 1995; **164**: 1407.

10 Ito K, Mitchell DG, Matsunaga N. MR imaging of the liver: techniques and clinical applications. *Eur. J. Radiol.* 1999; **32**: 2.

11 Khan MA, Combs CS, Brunt EM et al. Positron emission tomography in the evaluation of hepatocellular carcinoma. *J. Hepatol.* 2000; **32**: 792.

12 Killi RM. Doppler sonography of the native liver. *Eur. J. Radiol.* 1999; **32**: 21.

13 Kreeftenberg HG, Mooyaart EL, Huizenga JR et al. Quantification of liver iron concentration with magnetic resonance imaging by combining T1-, T2-weighted spin echo sequences and a gradient echo sequence. *Neth. J. Med.* 2000; **56**: 133.

14 Krinsky GA, Lee VS, Theise ND et al. Hepatocellular carcinoma and dysplastic nodules in patients with cirrhosis: prospective diagnosis with MR imaging and explantation correlation. *Radiology* 2001; **219**: 445.

15 Li KC, Chan F. New approaches to the investigation of focal hepatic lesions. *Bailliéres Best Pract. Res. Clin. Gastroenterol.* 1999; **13**: 529.

16 Macdonald GA, Peduto AJ. Magnetic resonance imaging (MRI) and diseases of the liver and biliary tract. Part 1. Basic principles, MRI in the assessment of diffuse and focal hepatic disease. *J. Gastroenterol. Hepatol.* 2000; **15**: 980.

17 Macdonald GA, Peduto AJ. Magnetic resonanace imaging and diseases of the liver and biliary tract. Part 2. Magnetic resonance cholangiography and angiography and conclusions. *J. Gastroenterol. Hepatol.* 2000; **15**: 992.

18 Matsui O, Kadoya M, Kameyama T et al. Adenomatous hyperplastic nodules in the cirrhotic liver: differentiation from hepatocellular carcinoma with MR imaging. *Radiology* 1989; **173**: 123.

19 Mendler M-H, Bouillet P, Le Sidaner A et al. Dual energy CT in the diagnosis and quantification of fatty liver: limited clinical value in comparison to ultrasound scan and single-energy CT, with special reference to iron overload. *J. Hepatol.* 1998; **28**: 785.

20 Palma LD. Diagnostic imaging and interventional therapy of hepatocellular carcinoma. *Br. J. Radiol.* 1998; **71**: 808.

21 Poletti PA, Mirvis SE, Shanmuganathan K et al. CT criteria for management of blunt liver trauma: correlation with angiographic and surgical findings. *Radiology* 2000; **216**: 418.

22 Reimer P, Jähnke N, Fiebich M et al. Hepatic lesion detection and characterization: value of nonenhanced MR imaging, superparamagnetic iron oxide-enhanced MR imaging, and spiral CT-ROC analysis. *Radiology* 2000; **217**: 152.

23 Rizzi PM, Kane PA, Ryder SD et al. Accuracy of radiology in detection of hepatocellular carcinoma before liver transplantation. *Gastroenterology* 1994; **107**: 1425.

24 Sackmann M, Beuers U, Helmberger T. Biliary imaging: magnetic resonance cholangiography vs. endoscopic retrograde cholangiography. *J. Hepatol.* 1999; **30**: 334.

25 Savci G. The changing role of radiology in imaging liver tumours: an overview. *Eur. J. Radiol.* 1999; **32**: 36.

26 Shi W, Johnston CF, Buchanan KD *et al.* Localization of neuroendocrine tumours with ^{111}In DTPA-octreotide scintigraphy (Octreoscan): a comparative study with CT and MR imaging. *Q. J. Med.* 1998; **91**: 295.

27 Sica GT, Ji H, Ros PR. CT and MR imaging of hepatic metastases. *Am. J. Roentgenol.* 2000; **174**: 691.

28 Soyer P, Bluemke DA, Fishman EK. CT during arterial portography for the preoperative evaluation of hepatic tumours: how, when, and why? *Am. J. Roentgenol.* 1994; **163**: 1325.

29 Taourel PG, Pageaux GP, Coste V *et al.* Small hepatocellular carcinoma in patients undergoing liver transplantation: detection with CT after injection of iodized oil. *Radiology* 1995; **197**: 377.

30 Taylor-Robinson SD. Applications of magnetic resonance spectroscopy to chronic liver disease. *Clin. Med.* 2001; **1**: 54.

Chapter 6
Hepato-cellular Failure

Hepato-cellular failure can complicate almost all forms of liver disease. It may follow virus hepatitis, or the cirrhoses, fatty liver of pregnancy, hepatitis due to drugs, overdose with drugs such as acetaminophen (paracetamol), ligation of the hepatic artery near the liver, or occlusion of the hepatic veins. The syndrome does not complicate portal venous occlusion alone. Circulatory failure, with hypotension, may precipitate liver failure.

It may be terminal in chronic cholestasis, such as primary biliary cirrhosis or cholestatic jaundice associated with malignant replacement of liver tissue or acute cholangitis. It should be diagnosed cautiously in a patient suffering from acute biliary obstruction.

Although the clinical features may differ, the overall picture and treatment are similar, irrespective of the aetiology. Acute liver failure poses special problems (Chapter 8).

There is no constant hepatic pathology and in particular necrosis is not always seen. The syndrome is therefore functional rather than anatomical. It comprises some or all of the following features.

- General failure of health.
- Jaundice.
- Hyperdynamic circulation and cyanosis.
- Fever and septicaemias.
- Neurological changes (hepatic encephalopathy).
- Ascites (Chapter 9).
- Changes in nitrogen metabolism.
- Skin and endocrine changes.
- Disordered blood coagulation (Chapter 4).

General failure of health

The most conspicuous feature is easy fatiguability. Wasting can be related to difficulty in synthesizing tissue proteins. Anorexia and poor dietary habits add to the malnutrition.

Jaundice

Jaundice is largely due to failure of the liver cells to metabolize bilirubin, so it is some guide to the severity of liver cell failure.

In acute failure, due to such causes as virus hepatitis,

jaundice parallels the extent of liver cell damage. This is not so evident in cirrhosis, where jaundice may be absent or mild. When present it represents active hepato-cellular disease and indicates a bad prognosis. Diminished erythrocyte survival adds a haemolytic component to the jaundice.

Vasodilatation and hyperdynamic circulation

This is associated with all forms of hepato-cellular failure, but especially with decompensated cirrhosis [33]. It is shown by flushed extremities, bounding pulses and capillary pulsations. Peripheral blood flow is increased. Arterial blood flow is increased in the lower limbs. Portal blood flow is increased. Renal blood flow, and particularly cortical perfusion, is reduced. Cardiac output is raised [11, 24] and evidenced by tachycardia, an active precordial impulse and frequently an ejection systolic murmur (figs 6.1, 6.2). These circulatory changes only rarely result in heart failure.

The blood pressure is low and, in the terminal phase, further reduces kidney function. At this stage the impaired liver blood flow contributes to hepatic failure and the fall in cerebral blood flow adds to the mental changes [8]. Such hypotension is ominous and attempts at elevation by raising circulatory volume by blood

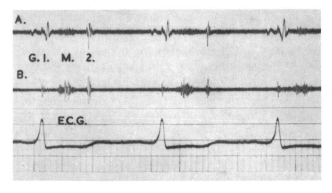

Fig. 6.1. Cirrhosis. Phonocardiogram at apex (A) and base (B) shows ejection-type systolic murmur (M) and an auricular sound (pre-systolic gallop) (G) [19].

81

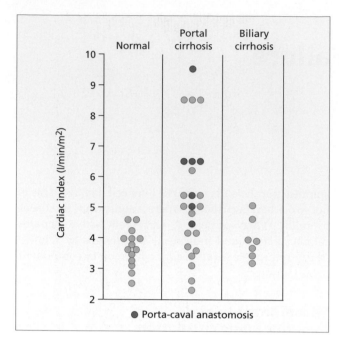

Fig. 6.2. The cardiac output is raised in many patients with hepatic cirrhosis but within normal limits in biliary cirrhosis. Mean normal cardiac index is $3.68\pm0.601/min/m^2$. Mean in hepatic cirrhosis is $5.36\pm1.981/min/m^2$ [24].

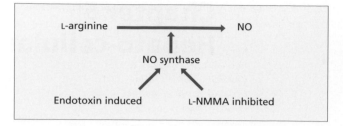

Fig. 6.3. Nitric oxide (NO) is a general vasodilator. It is produced from L-arginine, NO synthase being the responsible enzyme. This is induced by endotoxin and inhibited by L-NMMA.

transfusion or by such drugs as dopamine are of only temporary benefit.

Systemic vascular peripheral resistance is reduced as is the arteriovenous oxygen difference. In patients with cirrhosis, whole body oxygen consumption is decreased and tissue oxidation is abnormal. This has been related to the hyperdynamic circulation and to arteriovenous shunting. Thus, the vasodilator state of liver failure may contribute to general tissue hypoxia.

Vasomotor tone is decreased as shown by reduced vasoconstriction in response to mental exercise, the Valsalva manoeuvre and tilting from horizontal to vertical [19, 20]. Autonomic neuropathy is a poor prognostic indicator [6]. Large numbers of normally present, but functionally inactive, arteriovenous anastomoses may have opened under the influence of a vasodilator substance. The effective arterial blood volume falls as a consequence of the enlargement of the arterial vascular compartment induced by arterial vasodilatation. This activates the sympathetic and renin–angiotensin systems and is important in sodium and water retention and ascites formation (Chapter 9). The hyperdynamic splanchnic circulation is related to portal hypertension (Chapter 10).

The nature of the vasodilators concerned remains speculative. They are likely to be multiple. The substances might be formed by the sick hepatocyte, fail to be inactivated by it or bypass it through intra- or extra-hepatic portal-systemic shunts. The vasodilators are

likely to be of intestinal origin. In cirrhosis, increased permeability of the intestinal mucosa and porto-systemic shunting allow endotoxin and cytokines to reach the systemic circulation and these could be responsible (see fig. 6.9) [17, 18].

Nitric oxide (NO). This endothelium-derived potent vasodilator may be involved in the hyperdynamic circulation [26]. It is released from L-arginine by a family of NO synthase enzymes encoded by different genes (fig. 6.3). The endothelial constituent, NO synthase (NO S3), plays an important part in regulating normal vasoconstrictor tone [3].

L-arginine analogues such as NG-monomethyl-L-arginine (L-NMMA) inhibit NO release. They have been shown to reverse many of the vasodilator effects of NO. Inhibitors have been shown to reverse the hyperdynamic circulation in portal-hypertensive rats [16]. Cirrhotic rats show increased sensitivity to the pressor effect of NO inhibition and portal pressure rises [25]. NO synthase is inducible after stimulation with bacterial endotoxin or cytokines. NO is important in ascites formation and the hepato-renal syndrome (Chapter 9), and in portal hypertension (Chapter 10) [36].

Various gastrointestinal peptides, such as vaso-active intestinal polypeptide (VIP) type II, have little effect on the portal circulation. Glucagon is unlikely to be the sole vasodilator responsible.

Prostaglandins (E_1, E_2 and E_{12}) have vasodilatory actions and prostanoids are released into the portal vein in patients with chronic liver disease [38]. They may play a part in vasodilatation.

The cirrhotic shows arterial hyporeactivity to endogenous vasoconstrictors [23].

After hepatic transplantation, portal pressure becomes normal, and the cardiac index and splanchnic flow remain high due to the persistence of portal-systemic collateral flow [9].

Hepato-pulmonary syndrome

About a third of patients with decompensated cirrhosis

Table 6.1. Pulmonary changes complicating chronic hepato-cellular disease

Hypoxia
Intra-pulmonary shunting
Ventilation–perfusion mismatch
Reduced transfer factor
Pleural effusion
Raised diaphragms
Basal atelectasis
Primary pulmonary hypertension
Porto-pulmonary shunting
Chest X-ray mottling

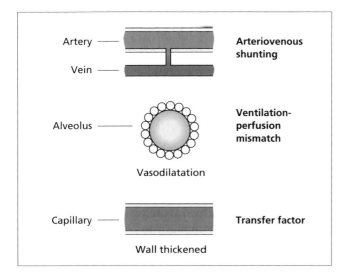

Fig. 6.4. Pulmonary changes in liver failure.

Table 6.2. Hepato-pulmonary syndrome

Advanced chronic liver disease
Arterial hypoxaemia
Intra-pulmonary vascular dilatation
No primary cardiopulmonary disease

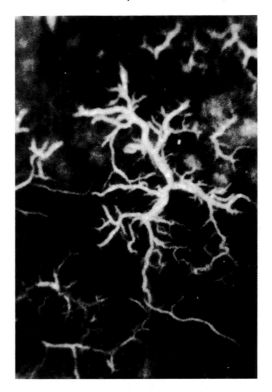

Fig. 6.5. Cirrhosis. Macroscopic appearances of the pleura showing dilated pleural vessels resembling a spider naevus [1].

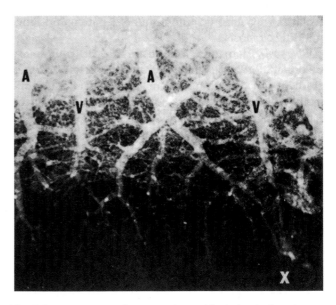

Fig. 6.6. Arteriogram from a patient with cirrhosis showing a slice of the basal region of the left lung. Arteries (A) and veins (V) alternate: X is the site of the arteriovenous shunting, into which a large arterial branch can be directly traced. The injection medium was barium suspension [1].

have reduced arterial oxygen saturation and are sometimes cyanosed (table 6.1, fig. 6.4) [29]. Causes include the hepato-pulmonary syndrome (table 6.2) [32]. This is defined as a clinical disorder associated with advanced liver disease and with disturbed pulmonary gas exchange leading to hypoxaemia and with widespread intra-pulmonary vascular dilatations in the absence of detectable primary cardio-pulmonary disease [13, 30, 32]. The alveolar–arterial oxygen gradient (AaPo_2) exceeds 15 mmHg (breathing room air). The intra-pulmonary shunting is through microscopic arteriovenous fistulae. The peripheral branches of the pulmonary artery are markedly dilated in the lungs and in the pleura where spider naevi may sometimes be seen (fig. 6.5) [1]. Arterial right-to-left large shunts causing cyanosis are rare (fig. 6.6) [1].

Reduction of diffusing capacity is present without a restrictive ventilatory defect [35]. This is likely to be due

atic porto systemic shunt improves oxygenation in hepato-pulmonary syndrome. *Gastroenterology* 1998; **109**: 987.

29 Rodman T, Sobel M, Close HP. Arterial oxygen unsaturation and the ventilation perfusion defect of Laennec's cirrhosis. *N. Engl. J. Med.* 1960; **263**: 73.

30 Rodriguez-Roisin R, Agusti AGN, Roca J. The hepato-pulmonary syndrome: new name, old complexities. *Thorax* 1992; **47**: 897.

31 Ruff F, Hughes JMB, Stanley N *et al.* Regional lung function in patients with hepatic cirrhosis. *J. Clin. Invest.* 1971; **50**: 2403.

32 Sherlock S. The liver–lung interface. *Semin. Resp. Med.* 1988; **9**: 247.

33 Sherlock S. Vasodilatation associated with hepatocellular disease: relation to functional organ failure. *Gut* 1990; **31**: 365.

34 Stanley NN, Williams AJ, Dewar CA *et al.* Hypoxia and hydrothoraces in a case of liver cirrhosis: correlation of physiological, radiographic, scintigraphic and pathological findings. *Thorax* 1977; **32**: 457.

35 Stanley NN, Woodgate DJ. Mottled chest radiograph and gas transfer defect in chronic liver disease. *Thorax* 1972; **27**: 315.

36 Stark ME, Szurszewski JH. Role of nitric oxide in gastrointestinal and hepatic function and disease. *Gastroenterology* 1992; **103**: 1928.

37 Stoller JK, Moodie D, Schiavone WA *et al.* Reduction of intrapulmonary shunt and resolution of digital clubbing associated with primary biliary cirrhosis after liver transplantation. *Hepatology* 1990; **11**: 54.

38 Wernze H, Tittor W, Goerig M. Release of prostanoids into the portal and hepatic vein in patients with chronic liver disease. *Hepatology* 1986; **6**: 911.

39 Willett IR, Sutherland RC, O'Rourke MF *et al.* Pulmonary hypertension complicating hepato-cellular carcinoma. *Gastroenterology* 1984; **87**: 1180.

40 Wong J, Vanderford PA, Fineman JR *et al.* Endothelin-1 produces pulmonary vasodilation in the intact unborn lamb. *Am. J. Physiol.* 1993; **265**: H1318.

Fever and septicaemia

About one-third of patients with decompensated cirrhosis show a continuous low-grade fever which rarely exceeds 38°C. This is unaffected by antibiotics or by altering dietary protein. It seems to be related to the liver disease. Cytokines such as tumour necrosis factor may be responsible, at least in alcoholics (fig. 6.9) [8]. Cytokines released as part of the inflammatory response have undesirable effects, particularly vasodilatation, endothelial activation and multi-organ failure.

The human liver is bacteriologically sterile and the portal venous blood only rarely contains organisms. However, in the cirrhotic, bacteria, particularly intestinal, could reach the general circulation either by passing through a faulty hepatic filter or through porto-systemic collaterals [2].

Septicaemia is frequent in terminal hepato-cellular failure. Multiple factors contribute. Kupffer cell and polymorphonuclear function are impaired [3, 5]. Serum

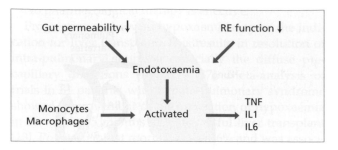

Fig. 6.9. Anorexia, fever, weight loss and a fatty liver in patients with hepato-cellular failure may be related to endotoxaemia with production of cytokines: tumour necrosis factor (TNF), interleukin-1 (IL1) and IL6. RE, reticulo-endothelial.

shows a reduction in factors such as fibronectin, opsonins and chemo-attractants, including members of the complement cascade. Systemic toxaemia of intestinal origin results in deterioration of the scavenger functions of the reticulo-endothelial system and also to renal damage (fig. 6.9) [6]. These factors contribute to blood culture positive episodes. They are particularly important in spontaneous bacterial peritonitis which affects 75% of cirrhotic patients with ascites (Chapter 9).

Urinary tract infections are particularly common in cirrhotic patients and are usually Gram-negative. Indwelling urinary catheters play a part.

Pneumonia especially affects alcoholics. Other infections include lymphangitis and endocarditis [4]. Of patients with acute liver failure, 50% show infections, often arising from soft tissues, the respiratory or urinary tract or central venous cannulas [7]. Clinical features may be atypical with inconspicuous fever, no rigors and only slight leucocytosis.

In both acute and chronic liver failure, about two-thirds of the infections are Gram-positive, often staphylococcal, and Gram-negative in one-third [1, 7]. Grade C cirrhotics are usually affected. The hospital mortality is 38%. Bad prognostic features are an absence of fever, elevated serum creatinine and marked leucocytosis [1]. Recurrent infections are ominous and sufferers should be considered for liver transplant.

Patients with liver failure should receive prophylactic antibiotics during invasive practical procedures and after gastrointestinal bleeding. Parenteral broad-spectrum antibiotics should be commenced when infection is suspected.

References

1 Barnes PF, Arevalo C, Chan LS *et al.* A prospective evaluation of bacteremic patients with chronic liver disease. *Hepatology* 1988; **8**: 1099.

2 Caroli J, Platteborse R. Septicémie porto-cave. Cirrhosis du foie et septicémie à colibacille. *Sem. Hôp. Paris* 1958; **34**: 472.

3 Imawari M, Hughes RD, Gove CD *et al*. Fibronectin and Kupffer cell function in fulminant hepatic failure. *Dig. Dis. Sci.* 1985; **30**: 1028.

4 McCashland TM, Sorrell MF, Zetterman RK. Bacterial endocarditis in patients with chronic liver disease. *Am. J. Gastroenterol.* 1994; **89**: 924.

5 Rajkovic IA, Williams R. Abnormalities of neutrophil phagocytosis, intracellular killing, and metabolic activity in alcoholic cirrhosis and hepatitis. *Hepatology* 1986; **6**: 252.

6 Rimola A, Soto R, Bory F *et al*. Reticuloendothelial system phagocytic activity in cirrhosis and its relation to bacterial infections and prognosis. *Hepatology* 1984; **4**: 53.

7 Rolando N, Harvey F, Brahm J *et al*. Prospective study of bacterial infection in acute liver failure: an analysis of 50 patients. *Hepatology* 1990; **11**: 49.

8 Yoshioka K, Kakumu S, Arao M *et al*. Tumor necrosis factor α production by peripheral blood mononuclear cells of patients with chronic liver disease. *Hepatology* 1989; **10**: 769.

Fetor hepaticus

This is a sweetish, slightly faecal smell of the breath which has been likened to that of a freshly opened corpse, or mice. It complicates severe hepato-cellular disease especially with an extensive collateral circulation. It is presumably of intestinal origin, for it becomes less intense after defaecation or when the gut flora is changed by wide-spectrum antibiotics. Methyl mercaptan has been found in the urine of a patient with hepatic coma who exhibited fetor hepaticus [1]. This substance can be exhaled in the breath and might be derived from methionine, the normal demethylating processes being inhibited by liver damage.

In patients with acute liver disease, fetor hepaticus, particularly if so extreme that it pervades the room, is a bad omen and often precedes coma. It is very frequent in patients with an extensive portal-collateral circulation, when it is not such a grave sign. Fetor may be a useful diagnostic sign in patients seen for the first time in coma.

Reference

1 Challenger F, Walshe JM. Fœtor hepaticus. *Lancet* 1995; **i**: 1239.

Changes in nitrogen metabolism

Ammonia metabolism (Chapter 7). The failing liver is unable to convert ammonia to urea.

Urea production is impaired, but the reserve powers of synthesis are so great that the blood urea concentration in hepato-cellular failure is usually normal. Low values may be found in fulminant hepatitis. Maximal rate of urea synthesis is a good measure of hepato-cellular function, but is too complicated for routine use [2].

Amino acid metabolism. An excess of amino acid in the urine is usual [3]. In both acute and chronic liver disease a common pattern of plasma amino acids is found. The aromatic amino acids, tyrosine and phenylalanine, are raised together with methionine. The concentration of the three branched-chain amino acids, valine, isoleucine and leucine, is reduced [1]. This results in a lowering of the ratio of branched-chain to aromatic amino acids and this is irrespective of the presence or absence of hepatic encephalopathy.

Serum albumin level falls in proportion to the degree of hepato-cellular failure and its duration. Protein is absorbed and retained, but is not used for serum protein manufacture. The low serum protein values may also reflect an increased plasma volume.

Plasma prothrombin falls with the serum protein level. The consequent prolonged prothrombin time is not restored to normal by vitamin K therapy. Other proteins concerned in blood clotting may be deficient. In terminal liver failure the bleeding diathesis may be so profound that the patient is exsanguinated by such simple procedures as a paracentesis abdominis (Chapter 4).

References

1 Morgan MY, Milsom JP, Sherlock S. Plasma amino acid patterns in liver disease. *Gut* 1982; **23**: 362.

2 Rudman D, Di Fulco TJ, Galambos JT *et al*. Maximal rates of excretion and synthesis of urea in normal and cirrhotic subjects. *J. Clin. Invest.* 1973; **52**: 2241.

3 Walshe JM. Disturbances of amino-acid metabolism following liver injury. *Q. J. Med.* 1953; **22**: 483.

Skin changes

> An older Miss Muffett
> Decided to rough it
> And lived upon whisky and gin.
> Red hands and a spider
> Developed outside her—
> Such are the wages of sin. [1]

Vascular spiders [1, 3, 5]

Synonyms: *arterial spider, spider naevi spider telangiectasis, spider angioma*

Arterial spiders are found in the vascular territory of the superior vena cava and very rarely below a line joining the nipples. Common sites are the necklace area, the face, forearms and dorsum of the hand (fig. 6.10). They fade after death.

An arterial spider consists of a central arteriole, radiating from which are numerous small vessels resembling a spider's legs (fig. 6.11). It ranges in size from a pinhead to 0.5 cm in diameter. When sufficiently large it can be seen

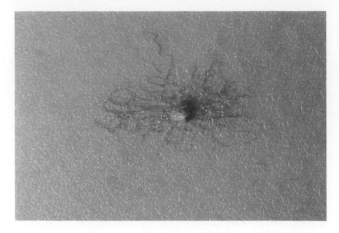

Fig. 6.10. A vascular spider. Note the elevated centre and radiating branches.

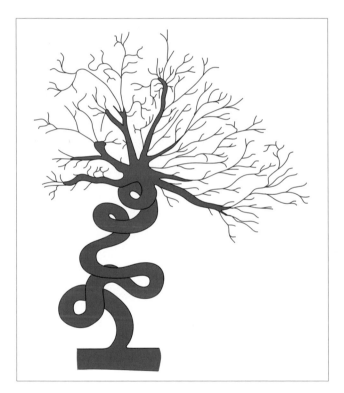

Fig. 6.11. Schematic diagram of an arterial spider [3].

or felt to pulsate, and this effect is enhanced by pressing on it with a glass slide. Pressure on the central prominence with a pinhead causes blanching of the whole lesion, as would be expected from an arterial lesion.

Arterial spiders may disappear with improving hepatic function, whereas the appearance of fresh spiders is suggestive of progression. The spider may also disappear if the blood pressure falls. Spiders can bleed profusely.

In association with vascular spiders, and having a similar distribution, numerous small vessels may be scattered in random fashion through the skin, usually on the upper arms. These resemble the silk threads in American dollar bills and the condition is called *paper money skin*.

A further association is the appearance of *white spots* on the arms and buttocks on cooling the skin [3]. Examination with a lens shows that the centre of each spot represents the beginnings of a spider.

Vascular spiders are most frequently associated with cirrhosis, especially of the alcoholic. They may appear transiently with viral hepatitis. Rarely they are found in normal persons, especially children. During pregnancy, they appear between the second and fifth months, disappearing within 2 months of delivery. A few spiders are not sufficient to diagnose liver disease, but many new ones, with increasing size of old ones, should arouse suspicion.

Differential diagnosis

Hereditary haemorrhagic telangiectasis. The lesions are usually on the upper body. Mucosal ones are common inside the nose, on the tongue, lips and palate, and in the pharynx, oesophagus and stomach. The nail beds, palmar surfaces and fingers are frequently involved. Visceral angiography usually shows lesions elsewhere.

The telangiectasis is punctiform, flat or a little elevated, with sharp margins. It is connected with a single vessel, or with several, which makes it resemble the vascular spider. Pulsation is difficult to demonstrate.

The lesion is a thinning of the telangiectatic vessel but the veins show muscular hypertrophy [4].

Telangiectasia may be associated with cirrhosis. Calcinosis, Raynaud's phenomenon, sclerodactyly and telangiectasia (*CRST syndrome*) may be found in patients with primary biliary cirrhosis.

Campbell de Morgan's spots are very common, increasing in size and number with age. They are bright red, flat or slightly elevated and occur especially on the front of the chest and the abdomen.

The venous star is found with elevation of venous pressure. It usually overlies the main tributary to a vein of large size. It is 2–3 cm in diameter and is not obliterated by pressure. Venous stars are seen on the dorsum of the foot, legs, back and on the lower border of the ribs.

Palmar erythema (liver palms)

The hands are warm and the palms bright red in colour, especially the hypothenar and thenar eminences and pulps of the fingers (fig. 6.12). Islets of erythema may be found at the bases of the fingers. The soles of the feet may be similarly affected. The mottling blanches on pressure and the colour rapidly returns. When a glass slide is pressed on the palm it flushes synchronously with the

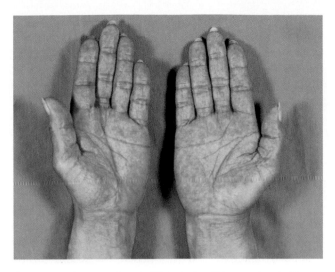

Fig. 6.12. Palmar erythema ('liver palms') in a patient with hepatic cirrhosis.

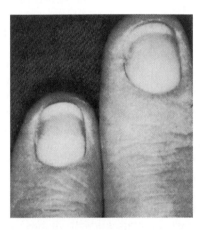

Fig. 6.13. White nails in a patient with hepatic cirrhosis.

pulse rate. The patient may complain of throbbing, tingling palms.

Palmar erythema is not so frequently seen in cirrhosis as are vascular spiders. Although both may be present, they may appear independently, making it difficult to define a common aetiology.

Many normal people have *familial* palmar flushing, unassociated with liver disease. A similar appearance may be seen in prolonged rheumatoid arthritis, in pregnancy, with chronic febrile diseases, leukaemia and thyrotoxicosis.

White nails

White nails, due to opacity of the nail bed, were found in 82 of 100 patients with cirrhosis and occasionally in certain other conditions (fig. 6.13) [2]. A pink zone is seen at the tip of the nail and in a severe example the lunula cannot be distinguished. The lesions are bilateral, with the thumb and index finger being especially involved.

Mechanism of skin changes

The selective distribution of vascular spiders is not understood. Exposure of upper parts of the body to the elements may damage the skin so that it becomes susceptible to the development of spiders when the appropriate internal stimulus exists. Children may develop spiders on the knees and one nudist with cirrhosis was said to be covered with vascular spiders. The number of spiders does not correlate with the hyperdynamic circulation, although when the cardiac output is very high the spiders pulsate particularly vigorously.

The vascular spiders and palmar erythema have been traditionally attributed to oestrogen excess. They are also seen in pregnancy when circulating oestrogens are increased. Oestrogens have an enlarging, dilating effect on the spiral arterioles of the endometrium, and such a mechanism may explain the closely similar cutaneous spiders [1]. Oestrogens have induced cutaneous spiders in men [1], although this is not usual when such therapy is given for prostatic carcinoma. The liver certainly inactivates oestrogens, although oestradiol levels in cirrhosis are often normal. The ratio between oestrogens and androgens may be more important. In male cirrhotics, although the serum oestradiol was normal, free serum testosterone was reduced. The oestradiol/free testosterone ratio was highest in male cirrhotics with spiders [5].

The aetiology of the other skin lesions remains unknown.

References

1 Bean WB. *Vascular Spiders and Related Lesions of the Skin.* Blackwell Scientific Publications, Oxford, 1959.
2 Lloyd CW, Williams RH. Endocrine changes associated with Laennec's cirrhosis of the liver. *Am. J. Med.* 1948; **4**: 315.
3 Martini GA. Über Gefässveränderungen der Haut bei Leberkranken. *Z. Klin. Med.* 1955; **150**: 470.
4 Martini GA, Straubesand J. Zur Morphologie der Gefässpinnen ('vascular spiders') in der Haut Leberkranker. *Virchows Arch.* 1953; **324**: 147.
5 Pirovino M, Linder R, Boss C *et al.* Cutaneous spider nevi in liver cirrhosis: capillary microscopical and hormonal investigations. *Klin. Wochenschr.* 1988; **66**: 298.

Endocrine changes

Endocrine changes may be found in association with cirrhosis. They are more common in cirrhosis of the alcoholic and if the patient is in the active, reproductive phase of life. In the male, the changes are towards feminization. In the female, the changes are less and are towards gonadal atrophy.

Hypogonadism

Diminished libido and potency are frequent in men with active cirrhosis and a large number are sterile. The impotence and its severity are greater if the cirrhotic patient is alcoholic [7]. Patients with well-compensated disease may have large families.

The testes are soft and small. Seminal fluid is abnormal in some cases. Secondary sexual hair is lost and men shave less often. Prostatic hypertrophy has a lower incidence in men with cirrhosis [5].

Other signs include female body habitus and a female escutcheon. Gynaecomastia is particularly common in alcoholics.

The female has ovulatory failure. The pre-menopausal patient loses feminine characteristics, particularly breast and pelvic fat. She is usually infertile; menstruation is erratic, diminished or absent, but rarely excessive. Any breast or uterine atrophy is of little significance in the post-menopausal woman.

In women with non-alcoholic liver disease, sexual behaviour, desire, frequency and performance are not impaired [1].

Gynaecomastia, sometimes unilateral, is rare, and the incidence in cirrhotics may not differ from that of controls [6] (fig. 6.14). Total oestrogen/free testosterone and oestradial/free testosterone ratios are higher in cirrhotic patients, but cannot be correlated with the presence of gynaecomastia.

The breasts may be tender. Enlargement is caused by hyperplasia of the glandular elements [5]. Young men with chronic autoimmune hepatitis may develop gynaecomastia but alcoholic liver disease is the commonest association.

Spironolactone therapy is the commonest cause of gynaecomastia in cirrhotic patients. This decreases serum testosterone levels and reduces hepatic androgen-receptor activity [10].

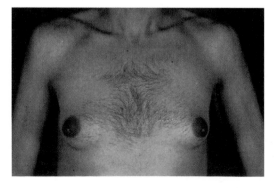

Fig. 6.14. Gynaecomastia in a patient with cirrhosis.

Relation to alcohol

It is difficult to disentangle the hypothalamic–pituitary–gonadal dysfunction in patients with chronic liver disease from the aetiology of the liver disease and particularly from the effects of alcohol.

Feminization is more frequent with alcoholic cirrhosis than with other types. Acute administration of alcohol to normal men increases the hepatic metabolism of testosterone.

The hepatic uptake of sex steroids depends on liver function. Chronic administration of alcohol raises sex hormone binding globulin (SHBG) so reducing the free fraction of plasma testosterone and the amount presented to the liver [11]. However, low dehydroepiandrosterone with raised oestradiol and androstenedione are found in patients with non-alcoholic liver disease [3]. The direct effect of alcohol on the testes may add to the general effects of liver disease. Acutely, alcohol also raises plasma gonadotrophins. Impotence is greater if the cirrhotic patient is alcoholic [7].

Mechanism

The three principal unconjugated oestrogens (oestrone, oestradiol and oestriol) are found in the plasma of normal men. They are produced by the testes and adrenals and also from peripheral conversion of the major circulating androgens. Oestradiol is the most biologically potent oestrogen. It is bound to SHBG and to albumin. The biologically active unbound form is marginally raised in patients with cirrhosis and the total only minimally increased. The changes in plasma oestrogens are insufficient to account for the degree of feminization.

The human liver has both androgen and oestrogen receptors which render it sensitive to androgens and oestrogens [9, 15]. Reduced oestrogen receptor concentrations in patients with chronic liver disease reflect the degree of liver dysfunction and not the specific type of liver disease [4]. In cirrhosis, the end organ sensitivities to sex hormones may be changed. Hepatic androgen receptors fall and hepatic oestrogen receptor concentrations increase [15].

Feminization may be related to hepatic regeneration [16]. Partial hepatic resection or liver transplantation are associated with increases in serum oestrogens and reductions in testosterone, while oestrogen receptors increase [13].

Primary liver cancer occasionally presents with feminization [14]. Serum oestrone levels are high and can return to normal when the tumour is removed. The tumour can be shown to function as trophoblastic tissue.

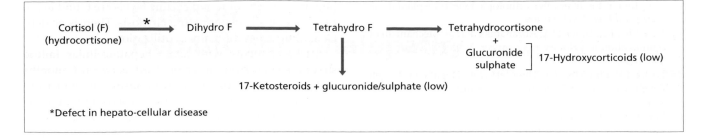

Fig. 6.15. The metabolism of cortisol by the liver. In hepato-cellular disease there is difficulty in reducing the 4–3 ketonic group but not in conjugation. Urinary 17-ketosteroids and 17-hydroxycorticoids are therefore reduced.

Hypothalamic–pituitary function

Plasma gonadotrophins are usually normal although a minority of cirrhotic patients have high values. These normal levels, in spite of testicular failure, suggest either a primary testicular defect or a failure of the pituitary–hypothalamus. Impaired release of luteinizing hormone suggests a possible hypothalamic defect, at least in those with alcoholic liver disease [2].

Hypothalamic–pituitary dysfunction in some women with non-alcoholic liver disease may lead to amenorrhoea and oestrogen deficiency and also to osteoporosis [8].

Metabolism of hormones [12]

A reduced rate of hormonal metabolism might be related to a decrease in hepatic blood flow, to shunting of blood through or around the liver or to an increase in SHBG which would reduce the free diffusible fraction of circulating hormone [11].

Steroid hormones are conjugated in the liver. Derivatives of oestrogens, cortisol and testosterone are conjugated as a glucuronide or sulphate and so excreted in the bile or urine. There seems to be little difficulty in the process even in the presence of hepato-cellular disease. The conjugated hormones excreted in the bile undergo an entero-hepatic circulation. In cholestasis the biliary excretion of oestrogens, and especially of polar conjugates, is greatly reduced. There are changes in the urinary pattern of excretion. Any failure of hormone metabolism results in a rise in blood hormone levels. This alters the normal homeostatic balance between secretion rates of hormones and their utilization. These feedback mechanisms between plasma hormone levels and hormone secretion prevent any but temporary rises in circulating levels. This may explain some of the difficulty in relating plasma hormone levels to clinical features.

Testosterone is converted to a more potent metabolite —dihydrotestosterone. It is degraded in the liver and conjugated for urinary excretion as 17-oxysteroids.

Oestrogens are metabolized and conjugated for excretion in urine or bile.

Cortisol is degraded primarily in the liver by a ring reduction to tetrahydrocortisone and subsequently conjugated with glucuronic acid (fig. 6.15).

Prednisone is converted to prednisolone.

References

1 Bach N, Schaffner F, Kapelman B. Sexual behaviour in women with nonalcoholic liver disease. *Hepatology* 1989; **9**: 698.

2 Bannister P, Handley T, Chapman C *et al.* Hypogonadism in chronic liver disease: impaired release of luteinizing hormone. *Br. Med. J.* 1986; **293**: 1191.

3 Bannister P, Oakes J, Sheridan P *et al.* Sex hormone changes in chronic liver disease: a matched study of alcoholic vs. nonalcoholic liver disease. *Q. J. Med.* 1987; **63**: 305.

4 Becker U, Andersen J, Poulsen HS *et al.* Variation in hepatic oestrogen receptor concentrations in patients with liver disease. A multivariate analysis. *Scand. J. Gastroenterol.* 1992; **27**: 355.

5 Bennett HS, Baggenstoss AH, Butt HR. The testis, breast and prostate of men who die of cirrhosis of the liver. *Am. J. Clin. Pathol.* 1950; **20**: 814.

6 Cavanaugh J, Niewoehner CB, Nuttall FQ. Gynecomastia and cirrhosis of the liver. *Arch. Intern. Med.* 1990; **150**: 563.

7 Cornely CM, Schade RR, Van Thiel DH *et al.* Chronic advanced liver disease and impotence: cause and effect? *Hepatology* 1984; **4**: 1227.

8 Cundy TF, Butler J, Pope RM *et al.* Amenorrhoea in women with nonalcoholic chronic liver disease. *Gut* 1991; **32**: 202.

9 Eagon PK, Elm MS, Stafford EA *et al.* Androgen receptor in human liver: characterization and quantification in normal and diseased liver. *Hepatology* 1994; **19**: 92.

10 Francavilla A, Di Leo A, Eagon PK *et al.* Effect of spironolactone and potassium canrenoate on cytosolic and nuclear androgen and oestrogen receptors of rat liver. *Gastroenterology* 1987; **93**: 681.

11 Guechot J, Vaubourdolle M, Ballet F *et al.* Hepatic uptake of sex steroids in men with alcoholic cirrhosis. *Gastroenterology* 1987; **92**: 203.

12 Johnson PJ. Sex hormones and the liver. *Clin. Sci.* 1984; **66**: 369.

13 Kahn D, Makowka L, Zeng P *et al.* Estrogen and androgen

ration, particularly when sudden, the clinician should be on guard for the occasional patient with intracranial haemorrhage, trauma, infection or tumour with the associated neurological signs, as well as a drug-induced or other metabolic cause.

With hepatic encephalopathy, differences in clinical history and examination are usual, particularly in the more chronic cases. The picture depends on the nature and severity of aetiological and precipitating factors. Children may show a particularly acute reaction, often with mania.

For descriptive purposes, features of encephalopathy can be separated into changes in consciousness, personality, intellect and speech.

Disturbed consciousness with disorder of sleep is usual. Hypersomnia appears early and progresses to reversal of the normal sleep pattern. Reduction of spontaneous movement, a fixed stare, apathy, and slowness and brevity of response are early signs. Further deterioration results in reaction only to intense or noxious stimuli. Coma at first resembles normal sleep, but progresses to complete unresponsiveness. Deterioration may be arrested at any level. Rapid changes in the level of consciousness are accompanied by delirium.

Personality changes are most conspicuous with chronic liver disease. These include childishness, irritability and loss of concern for family. Even in remission the patient may present similar personality features suggesting frontal lobe involvement. They are usually co-operative, pleasant people with an ease in social relationships and frequently a jocular, euphoric mood.

Intellectual deterioration varies from slight impairment of organic mental function to gross confusion. Isolated abnormalities appearing in a setting of clear consciousness relate to disturbances in visual spatial gnosis. These

are most easily elicited as constructional apraxia, shown by an inability to reproduce simple designs with blocks or matches (fig. 7.1). Number connection tests (fig. 7.2) may be used serially to assess progress but to be most informative should be compared with normal values for the same age group [66, 86].

Writing is oblivious of ruled lines and a daily writing chart is a good check of progress (fig. 7.1). Failure to distinguish objects of similar size, shape, function and position may lead to symptoms such as micturating and defaecating in inappropriate places. Insight into such anomalies of behaviour is frequently preserved.

Speech is slow and slurred and the voice is monotonous. In deep stupor, dysphasia becomes marked and is always combined with perseveration.

Some patients have *fetor hepaticus*. This is a sour, faecal smell in the breath, due to volatile substances normally formed in the stool by bacteria. These mercaptans if not removed by the liver are excreted through the lungs and appear in the breath. Fetor hepaticus does not correlate with the degree or duration of encephalopathy and its absence does not exclude hepatic encephalopathy.

The most characteristic neurological abnormality is the 'flapping' tremor (*asterixis*). This is due to impaired inflow of joint and other afferent information to the brainstem reticular formation resulting in lapses in posture. It is demonstrated with the patient's arms outstretched and fingers separated or by hyperextending the wrists with the forearm fixed (fig. 7.3). The rapid flexion–extension movements at the metacarpophalangeal and wrist joints are often accompanied by lateral movements of the digits. Sometimes arms, neck, jaw, protruded tongue, retracted mouth and tightly closed eyelids are involved and the gait is ataxic. Absent at rest, less marked on movement and maximum on sustained

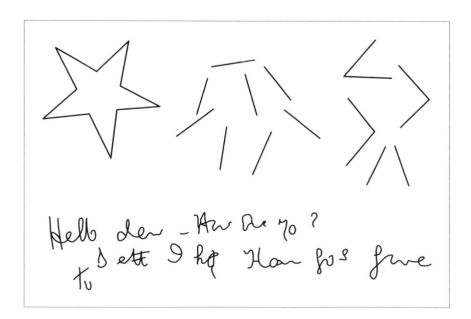

Fig. 7.1. Focal disorders in chronic portal-systemic encephalopathy elicited in patients with full consciousness and minimal intellectual defect, in the absence of gross tremor or visual disorder. Above: constructional apraxia. Below: writing difficulty. 'Hello dear. How are you? Better I hope. That goes for me too'.

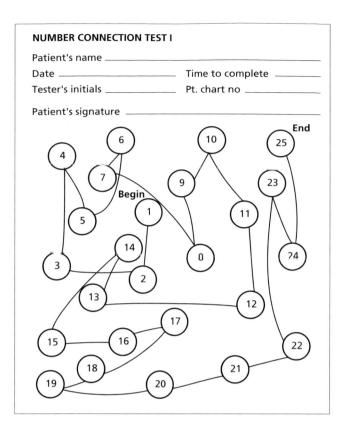

NUMBER CONNECTION TEST I

Patient's name _____

Date _____   Time to complete _____

Tester's initials _____   Pt. chart no _____

Patient's signature _____

Fig. 7.2. The Reitan number connection test.

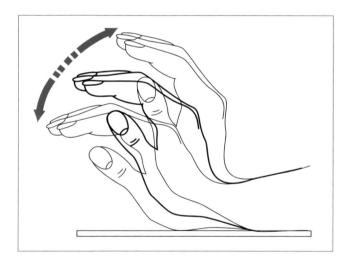

Fig. 7.3. 'Flapping' tremor elicited by attempted dorsiflexion of the wrist with the forearm fixed.

posture, the tremor is usually bilateral, although not bilaterally synchronous, and one side may be affected more than the other. It may be appreciated by gentle elevation of a limb or by the patient gripping the doctor's hand. In coma the tremor disappears. A 'flapping' tremor is not specific for hepatic pre-coma. It can also be observed in uraemia, in respiratory failure and in severe heart failure.

Table 7.2. The clinical grades of hepatic encephalopathy

I	Mild confusion, euphoria, anxiety or depression
	Shortened attention span
	Slowing of ability to perform mental tasks (addition/subtraction)
	Reversal of sleep rhythm
II	Drowsiness, lethargy, gross deficits in ability to perform mental tasks
	Obvious personality changes
	Inappropriate behaviour
	Intermittent disorientation of time (and place)
	Lack of sphincter control
III	Somnolent but rousable
	Persistent disorientation of time and place
	Pronounced confusion
	Unable to perform mental tasks
IV	Coma with (IVa) or without (IVb) response to painful stimuli

Deep tendon reflexes are usually exaggerated. Increased muscle tone is present at some stage and sustained ankle clonus is often associated with rigidity. During coma patients become flaccid and lose their reflexes.

The plantar responses are usually flexor becoming extensor in deep stupor or coma. Hyperventilation and hyperpyrexia may be terminal. The diffuse nature of the cerebral disturbance is further shown by excessive appetite, muscle twitchings, grasping and sucking reflexes. Disorders of vision include reversible cortical blindness [45].

The clinical course fluctuates, and frequent observation of the patient is necessary. Clinical grading should be used as a part of the clinical record of neuropsychiatric signs (table 7.2).

Investigations

Cerebrospinal fluid

This is usually clear and under normal pressure. Patients in hepatic coma may show an increased CSF protein concentration, but the cell count is normal. Glutamic acid and also glutamine may be increased.

Electroencephalogram

There is a bilateral synchronous slowing of the wave frequency (with an increase in wave amplitude) from the normal α-rhythm of 8–13 cycles per second (Hz) down to the δ range of below 4 cycles per second (fig. 7.4). This is best graded using frequency analysis. Alerting stimuli, such as opening the eyes, fail to reduce the background rhythmic activity. The change starts in the frontal or central region and progresses posteriorly.

holic hepatitis. *Opiates, benzodiazepines* and *barbiturates* depress cerebral function and have a prolonged action when hepatic detoxication is delayed.

Infections, especially with bacteraemia and including 'spontaneous' bacterial peritonitis, may be the precipitant.

Coma may occasionally be initiated by a large *protein meal* or *severe constipation*.

Transjugular intrahepatic portal-systemic shunts (TIPS) precipitate or worsen hepatic encephalopathy in about 20–30% of cases. This incidence varies depending on the patient population and selection [31, 72]. As with surgical shunts, the wider the diameter of TIPS inserted, the more likely is encephalopathy. Independent predictors of post-TIPS hepatic encephalopathy are the presence of encephalopathy before the procedure and reduced liver function [59]. There is a decline in the frequency of hepatic encephalopathy 3 months after TIPS despite a sustained increase in arterial ammonia. This is not totally explained by a reduction in shunt flow or alteration in liver function. Cerebral adaptation to the effect of toxins has been suggested [59].

Chronic type

This relates to extensive portal-systemic shunting, which may consist simply of the myriad of small anastomotic vessels developing in the cirrhotic patient or, more often, one major collateral channel, such as the spleno-renal, gastro-renal, umbilical or inferior mesenteric vein.

Fluctuations in encephalopathy are related to dietary protein and diagnosis can be confirmed by noting the effect clinically and on the EEG of a precipitant such as a high-protein diet or by demonstrating improvement by protein withdrawal. Clinical and biochemical evidence of liver disease may be equivocal or absent, and the neuropsychiatric disorder may dominate the picture.

The intermittent neuropsychiatric disturbance may continue for many years and the diagnosis is very likely to fall between various specialist interests. The psychiatrist is interested in the non-specific organic reaction and may not consider underlying liver disease. The neurologist focuses attention on the neurological features, while the hepatologist, recognizing the cirrhosis, fails to elicit the neurological signs or assumes that the patient is just 'odd' or an alcoholic. The patient may be seen for the first time in coma or in remission, adding to the diagnostic difficulty.

The *acute psychiatric states* often present shortly (2 weeks to 8 months) after porta-caval anastomosis as a paranoid–schizophrenic picture or as hypomania. 'Classic' portal-systemic encephalopathy, with EEG slowing, is usually present in addition. Formal psychiatric treatment may be required as well as treatment of the hepatic encephalopathy.

Hepato-cerebral degeneration: myelopathy

More persistent neuropsychiatric syndromes are probably related to organic changes in the central nervous system, not only in the brain but also in the spinal cord. Progressive *paraplegia* may commence insidiously in those with a large portal-systemic collateral circulation. The encephalopathy is not severe. The spinal cord shows demyelination. The paraplegia is progressive and the usual treatment for portal-systemic encephalopathy is ineffective.

Chronic cerebellar and *basal ganglia* signs with parkinsonism, the tremor being unaffected by intention, may develop after some years of chronic hepatic encephalopathy. Permanent cerebral damage is probably present, for treatment has little effect on the tremor.

Focal cerebral symptoms, epileptic attacks and dementia have also been noted.

Differential diagnosis

A *low sodium state* can develop in cirrhotic patients on a restricted sodium diet and having diuretics and abdominal paracenteses. This is shown by apathy, headache, nausea and hypotension. The diagnosis is confirmed by finding low serum sodium levels with a rise in blood urea concentration. The condition may be combined with impending hepatic coma.

Acute alcoholism provides a particularly difficult problem especially as the two syndromes may coexist (Chapter 22). Many symptoms attributed to alcoholism may be due to portal-systemic encephalopathy. Delirium tremens is distinguished by continuous motor and autonomic over-activity, total insomnia, terrifying hallucinations and a finer, more rapid tremor. The patient is flushed, agitated, inattentive and perfunctory in his replies. Tremor, absent at rest, becomes coarse and irregular on activity. Profound anorexia, often with retching and vomiting, is common.

Portal-systemic encephalopathy in an alcoholic has similar features to that in the non-alcoholic except for the frequent absence of rigidity, hyper-reflexia and ankle clonus due to concomitant peripheral neuritis. An EEG is helpful, as is the observation of a favourable response to dietary protein withdrawal and lactulose.

Wernicke's encephalopathy is common with profound malnutrition and with alcoholism.

Hepato-lenticular degeneration (*Wilson's disease*) is found in young people, often with a family history. The symptoms do not fluctuate, the tremor is choreo-athetoid rather than 'flapping', the Kayser–Fleischer corneal ring is seen and disturbances in copper metabolism can usually be demonstrated.

Latent *functional psychoses*, such as depression or paranoia, are frequently released by impending hepatic coma. The type of reaction is related to the previous personality, and to intensification of personality traits. The psychiatric importance of the syndrome is emphasized by such patients often being admitted to mental hospitals. Conversely, a chronic psychiatric state in patients with known liver disease may not be related to the liver dysfunction. In such patients investigations are designed to demonstrate the chronic syndrome and in particular a large collateral circulation by arterio-portography or by CT scanning after intravenous contrast enhancement. Clinical and EEG changes induced by high and low protein feeding may also be useful.

Prognosis

Prognosis depends on the extent of liver cell failure. The chronic group with relatively good liver function but with an extensive collateral circulation combined with increased intestinal nitrogen have the best prognosis and the acute hepatitis group the worst. In cirrhosis, the outlook is poor if the patient has ascites, jaundice and a low serum albumin level—all indicative of liver failure. The survival probability in cirrhotic patients after the first episode of acute hepatic encephalopathy is 42% at 1 year and 23% at 3 years [12].

Assessment of therapy is made difficult by fluctuations in the clinical course. The value of any new method can only be assessed after large numbers of patients have been treated by controlled regimes. Results in patients with chronic encephalopathy (largely related to porto-systemic shunting) with recovery as the rule, must be separated from acute hepato-cellular failure in which recovery is rare.

Older patients have the added disadvantage of cerebral vascular disease. Children with portal vein obstruction having a portal-systemic shunt develop no intellectual or psychological side-effects [1].

Pathogenetic mechanisms [28, 33]

The essentially reversible nature of the syndrome with such widespread cerebral changes suggests a metabolic mechanism. However, no single metabolic derangement accounts for hepatic encephalopathy. The basic processes are failure of hepatic clearance of gut-derived substances, either through hepato-cellular failure or shunting, and altered amino acid metabolism, both of which result in changes in cerebral neurotransmission. Several neuroactive toxins, in particular ammonia, and neurotransmitter systems (table 7.4) are thought to be involved and inter-relate. Reduced cerebral metabolic rates for oxygen and glucose found in hepatic encephalopathy are thought to be due to the reduced neuronal activity.

Table 7.4. Neurotransmitters implicated in hepatic encephalopathy

Neurotransmitter system	Normal action	Hepatic encephalopathy
Glutamate	Neuro-excitation	Dysfunction ↓ receptors interference by NH_4^+
GABA/BZ	Neuro-inhibitor	Increased endogenous BZs ?GABA
Dopamine Noradrenaline	Motor/cognitive	Inhibition false neurotransmitters (aromatic amino acids)
Serotonin	Arousal	?Dysfunction synaptic deficit? ↑serotonin turnover

BZ, benzodiazepine; GABA, γ-aminobutyric acid.

Portal-systemic encephalopathy

Every patient with hepatic pre-coma or coma has a circulatory pathway through which portal blood may enter the systemic veins and reach the brain without being metabolized by the liver.

In patients with poor hepato-cellular function, such as acute hepatitis, the shunt is through the liver itself. The damaged cells are unable to metabolize the contents of the portal venous blood completely so that they pass unaltered into the hepatic veins (fig. 7.5).

In patients with more chronic forms of liver disease, such as cirrhosis, the portal blood bypasses the liver through enlarged natural 'collaterals'. The portal–hepatic vein anastomoses, developing around the nodules in a cirrhotic liver, may also act as internal shunts. The picture is a common complication of porta-caval anastomosis and TIPS. The condition is analogous to the neuropsychiatric disturbance developing in a dog with an Eck fistula (porta-caval shunt) if it is fed meat.

Encephalopathy is unusual if liver function is adequate. In hepatic schistosomiasis, where the collateral circulation is great and liver function good, coma is rare. If shunting is sufficiently great, however, encephalopathy may develop in the absence of obvious liver disease, for instance in extra-hepatic portal hypertension and congenital shunts [82].

Patients going into hepatic coma are suffering from cerebral intoxication by intestinal contents which have not been metabolized by the liver (*portal-systemic encephalopathy*). The nature of the cerebral intoxicant is nitrogenous. A picture indistinguishable from impending hepatic coma can be induced in some patients with

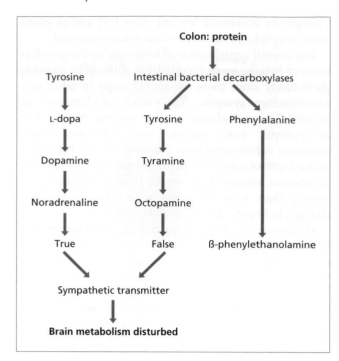

Fig. 7.8. The possible role of false sympathetic neuro-transmitters in the disturbed cerebral metabolism in liver disease.

abnormal blood–brain barrier. There may also be reduced efflux of aromatic amino acids from the brain [36]. An increase in phenylalanine level in the brain leads to inhibition of dopa production and the formation of false neurotransmitters such as phenylethanolamine and octopamine.

A change in this neurotransmitter system in hepatic encephalopathy has some support from the improvement after L-dopa and bromocriptine treatment, but the number of patients who improve is limited and the results are equivocal. Serum and urinary octopamine levels are increased in hepatic encephalopathy. However, intraventricular infusion of enormous quantities of octopamine, with resulting depression of brain dopamine and adrenaline, failed to cause coma in normal rats. Moreover, when brain catecholamines were measured post-mortem in cirrhotic patients with encephalopathy, no reduction was found compared with cirrhotics who were not encephalopathic at the time of death [17].

Serotonin

The neurotransmitter serotonin (5-hydroxytryptamine or 5-HT) is involved in the control of cortical arousal and thus the conscious state and the sleep/wake cycle. The precursor tryptophan is one of the aromatic amino acids increased in the plasma in liver disease. It is also increased in the CSF and brain of patients with hepatic

coma and therefore has the potential to increase brain serotonin synthesis. In hepatic encephalopathy there are also other changes in serotonin metabolism including related enzymes (monoamine oxidase, MAO), receptors and metabolites (5-hydroxyindole acetic acid, 5-HIAA). There is increased expression of the neuronal isoform of the monoamine-metabolizing enzyme MAO-A [55]. These changes, together with the appearance of encephalopathy in patients with chronic liver disease treated with ketanserin (a 5-HT blocker) for portal hypertension [81], implicate the serotonin system in hepatic encephalopathy. Where the dysfunction in this system primarily lies awaits further study.

γ-Aminobutyric acid (GABA) and endogenous benzodiazepines

GABA is the principal inhibitory neurotransmitter in the brain [7]. It is usually synthesized from glutamate by glutamate dehydrogenase in presynaptic nerves and stored in vesicles. It binds to a specific GABA receptor in the postsynaptic membrane. This receptor is part of a larger receptor complex which also has binding sites for benzodiazepines and barbiturates (fig. 7.9). The binding of any of these ligands opens a chloride channel and after the influx of chloride there is hyperpolarization of the postsynaptic membrane, and neuroinhibition.

GABA is synthesized by gut bacteria, and that entering the portal vein is metabolized by the liver. In the presence of liver failure or portal-systemic shunting it enters the systemic circulation. There are increased GABA levels in the plasma of patients with liver disease and hepatic encephalopathy [41]. Suggestions that GABA might be involved in hepatic encephalopathy came mainly from experimental models of acute liver failure, but in subsequent studies in autopsied brain tissue from cirrhotic patients with encephalopathy, GABA *per se* does not seem to be involved.

However, the focus on the GABA–benzodiazepine receptor complex led to data suggesting that endogenous benzodiazepines are present in patients with hepatic encephalopathy and that these may interact with the receptor complex and cause neuroinhibition. Benzodiazepine-like compounds have been detected in the plasma and CSF of patients with hepatic encephalopathy due to cirrhosis [57] and in the plasma in fulminant hepatic failure [6]. Cirrhotics with hepatic encephalopathy who had taken no synthetic benzodiazepines for at least 3 months showed significantly higher values for benzodiazepine-like activity than controls without liver disease, using a radio-receptor assay [57]. Stool from cirrhotic patients contains five times the benzodiazepine-like activity as stool from controls [3]. The relationship between plasma endogenous benzodiazepines and encephalopathy is controversial.

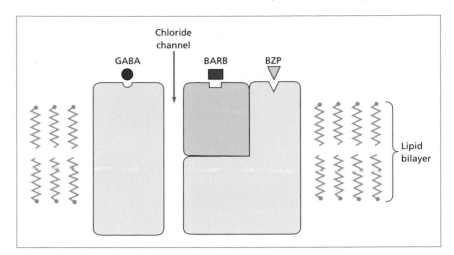

Fig. 7.9. Simplified model of the GABA-receptor/ionophore complex embedded in a postsynaptic neural membrane. Binding of any of the depicted ligands, γ-aminobutyric acid (GABA), barbiturates (BARB) or benzodiazepines (BZP), to its specific binding site increases chloride-ion conductance through the membrane with resultant hyperpolarization and neuroinhibition [73].

Some studies show a correlation [57] while others do not [4]. However, both central benzodiazepine receptors (coupled GABA-A receptors) and peripheral type benzodiazepine receptors are increased in the brain in chronic liver failure [13, 32].

It remains unclear whether the changes in the benzodiazepine receptor or endogenous ligands are significant pathogenetically or are simply associated phenomena. Nevertheless involvement of this neurotransmitter system is consistent with the increased sensitivity to benzodiazepines of cirrhotic patients [8]. Also the benzodiazepine antagonist flumazemil reverses encephalopathy temporarily (the drug has a short half-life) in some patients. [5]

Other metabolic abnormalities

Neuronal nitric oxide synthase may be increased in hepatic encephalopathy and make a contribution to the altered cerebral perfusion in chronic liver disease [67].

These patients are often alkalotic. This may result from toxic stimulation of the respiratory centre by ammonium, from administration of alkalis such as citrate in transfusions or with potassium supplements, or from hypokalaemia. Urea synthesis consumes bicarbonate. Progressive loss of urea cycle capacity is associated with increased plasma bicarbonate levels (and metabolic alkalosis) and ammonia excretion by the kidney increases. [27]

Hypoxia increases cerebral sensitivity to ammonia. The stimulation of the respiratory centre results in increase in depth and rate of respiration. Hypocapnia follows and this reduces cerebral blood flow. The increase in the blood organic acids (lactate and pyruvate) is correlated with the reduction in CO_2 tension.

Any potent diuretic can precipitate hepatic coma. This may be related to hypokalaemia [15] and to readier penetration of ammonium ions through the blood-brain barrier in the presence of alkalosis. In addition to hypokalaemia, other electrolyte disturbances or a profound diuresis seem to initiate encephalopathy.

Changes in carbohydrate metabolism

The hepatectomized dog dies in hypoglycaemic coma. Hypoglycaemic episodes are rare in chronic liver disease but may complicate fulminant hepatitis (Chapter 8).

α-Ketoglutaric and pyruvic acids are transported from the periphery to the metabolic pool in the liver, and blood levels increase as the neurological state deteriorates. These levels probably reflect severe liver damage. The fall in blood ketones also reflects severity of hepatic dysfunction. There is progressive impairment of intermediate carbohydrate metabolism as the liver fails.

Astrocyte swelling

Studies using MR spectroscopy show a depletion of myoinositol and an increase in glutamine/glutamate ('osmolytes'). It has been suggested that an associated increase in astrocyte hydration may be a major pathogenetic event in the development of hepatic encephalopathy [26].

Conclusions

No unifying mechanism explains hepatic encephalopathy. The brain controls neuropsychiatric behaviour through multiple inhibitory and stimulatory receptor-mediated pathways. Although neurotransmitters are produced locally they depend upon substrates and influences from further afield (fig. 7.10). When the liver fails or there is portal-systemic shunting there is a complex pattern of changes which influence multiple neurotransmitter systems.

Of the systems discussed, the effects of ammonia

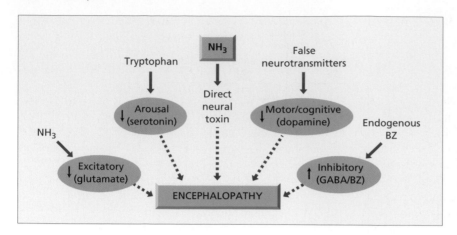

Fig. 7.10. Multifactorial mechanism of hepatic encephalopathy. The altered neurotransmitter state leaves the brain more sensitive to other insults including narcotics, sepsis, hypoxia and hypotension. BZ, benzodiazepines; GABA, γ-aminobutyric acid.

appear central to hepatic encephalopathy, with changes in glutamate, serotonin and endogenous benzodiazepine-mediated neurotransmission awaiting further study. The place of false neurotransmitters and GABA appears less persuasive than initially thought.

Cerebral metabolism is undoubtedly abnormal in liver disease. This is thought to be an effect rather than the cause of neurotransmitter-mediated changes. In the chronic case, actual structural changes in the brain can be demonstrated. The end result is a brain with abnormal neurotransmitter function, which is unduly sensitive to insults (opiates, electrolyte imbalance, sepsis, hypotension, hypoxia) that would be without effect in the normal patient.

Treatment of hepatic encephalopathy [16]

Treatment broadly divides into three areas.
1 Identification and treatment of the precipitating cause.
2 Intervention to reduce the production and absorption of gut-derived ammonia and other toxins. This involves reduction and modification of dietary protein, alteration of enteric bacteria and the colonic environment (antibiotics, lactulose/lactilol), and stimulation of colonic emptying (enemas, lactulose/lactilol).
3 Prescription of agents to modify neurotransmitter balance directly (bromocriptine, flumazemil), or indirectly (branched-chain amino acids). These are of limited clinical value at present.

The choice of treatment (table 7.6) depends on the clinical picture: subclinical, acute or persistent chronic encephalopathy.

Diet [46, 62]

In the acute attack dietary protein is reduced to 20 g/day. Calorie intake is maintained at 2000 cal/day or above, orally or intravenously. During recovery, protein is added in 10 g increments on alternate days. Any relapse

Table 7.6. Treatment of hepatic pre-coma and coma

Acute
Identify precipitating factor
Empty bowels of nitrogen-containing materials
   stop haemorrhage
   phosphate enema
Protein-restricted diet; raise dietary protein slowly with recovery
Lactulose or lactilol
Neomycin 1 g four times a day by mouth for 1 week
Maintain calorie, fluid and electrolyte balance
Stop diuretics, check serum electrolyte levels

Chronic
Avoid nitrogen-containing drugs
Protein, largely vegetarian intake, at limit of tolerance
Ensure at least two free bowel movements daily
Lactulose or lactilol
If symptoms worsen adopt the regime for acute coma

is treated by a return to the previous level. In patients after an acute episode of coma, a normal protein intake is soon achieved.

It is important in cirrhotic patients to avoid protein restriction for any longer than is necessary since these patients have a higher than normal protein requirement (1.2 g/kg/day) to remain in positive balance. Guidelines recommend that the daily protein intake in patients with liver disease should if possible be around 1.0–1.5 g/kg depending upon the degree of hepatic decompensation [46, 62]. In the acute case, a short period of protein deprivation may not be harmful but prolonged restriction of protein in the cirrhotic patient without encephalopathy is inappropriate [75].

If animal protein is not well tolerated, vegetable protein may be used. The latter is less ammoniagenic and contains small amounts of methionine and aromatic amino acids. It is also more laxative and increases the intake of dietary fibre so that there is increased incorporation and elimination of nitrogen contained in faecal bacteria [84]. It may be difficult to take because of flatulence, diarrhoea and bulk.

Antibiotics

Neomycin, given orally, is very effective in decreasing gastrointestinal ammonium formation. Little neomycin is absorbed from the gut although blood levels have been detected and impaired hearing or deafness may follow its long-term use. Thus it should only be used for the acute case for 5–7 days (4–6 g/day in divided doses). Neomycin should be used with particular caution in patients with renal insufficiency. In acute hepatic coma, lactulose is given, and neomycin added if the response is slow or partial. Surprisingly the two drugs seem to act synergistically [85], perhaps because of action on different bacterial populations.

Metronidazole (200 mg four times per day orally) seems to be as effective as neomycin [53]. Because of dose-related central nervous system toxicity, it should not be used long term.

Rifaximin, a non-absorbed derivative of rifamycin, is effective for grade 1–3 hepatic encephalopathy at a dose of 1200 mg/day [87].

Lactulose and lactilol

The human intestinal mucosa does not have an enzyme to split these synthetic disaccharides. When given by mouth *lactulose* reaches the caecum where it is broken down by bacteria predominantly to lactic acid (fig. 7.11). The osmotic volume of the colon is increased. The faecal pH drops. The growth of lactose-fermenting organisms is favoured and organisms such as bacteroides, which are ammonia formers, are suppressed. It may be of particular value in hepatic encephalopathy induced by bleeding. The colonic fermentative bacteria prefer lactulose to blood when both are present [54]. It may 'detoxify' short-chain fatty acids produced in the presence of blood and proteins.

The mode of action is uncertain. Faecal acidity would reduce the ionization and hence absorption of ammonia (also amines and other toxic nitrogenous compounds); faecal ammonia is not increased. Lactulose more than doubles the colonic output of bacterial mass and 'soluble' nitrogen [84] which is then no longer available for absorption as ammonia.

The aim of treatment with lactulose is to produce acid stools without diarrhoea. The dose is 10–30 ml three times a day and is adjusted to produce two semi-soft stools daily.

Side-effects include flatulence, diarrhoea and intestinal pain. Diarrhoea can be so profound that serum sodium increases to over 145 mmol/l, serum potassium falls and alkalosis develops. The blood volume falls and

may impair renal function. These side-effects are particularly likely if the daily dose exceeds 100 ml. Some of the side-effects may be related to contamination of lactulose syrup with other sugars. Crystalline lactulose may be less toxic.

Lactilol (β-galactoside sorbitol) is a second-generation disaccharide easily produced in chemically pure crystalline form, which can be dispensed as a powder. It is not broken down or absorbed in the small intestine, but is metabolized by colonic bacteria [61].

Lactilol seemed to be as effective as lactulose in chronic and acute portal-systemic encephalopathy [51]. Patients responded more quickly to lactilol than lactulose, and there was less diarrhoea and flatulence (table 7.7) [10, 51].

However, lactitol is no longer routinely available on prescription, but can be obtained from the manufactuer under special circumstances for patients intolerant of lactulose.

Lactilol and lactulose have been used for the treatment of subclinical hepatic encephalopathy [50]. Psycho-

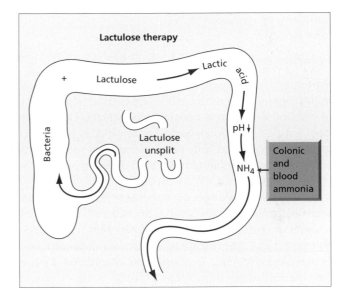

Fig. 7.11. Lactulose reaches the colon unsplit. It is then converted by bacteria to organic acids and an acid stool results. This may also affect the ionization of ammonia in the colon and reduce its absorption.

Table 7.7. The effects of lactilol compared with lactulose

Colonic effects similar
As effective in encephalopathy
Quicker action
More convenient (powder)
Less sweet
Less diarrhoea and flatulence

metric performance improved. A dose of lactitol of 0.3–0.5 g/kg/day was well tolerated and effective [71].

Purgation. Hepatic encephalopathy follows constipation and remissions are associated with return to a normal bowel action. The value of enemas and purgation with magnesium sulphate in patients with hepatic coma must be emphasized. Lactulose or lactose enemas may be used and are superior to water [80]. All enemas must be neutral or acid to reduce ammonium absorption. Magnesium sulphate enemas can cause dangerous hypermagnesaemia [14]. Phosphate enemas are safe.

Sodium benzoate and L-ornithine -L-aspartate

Sodium benzoate promotes urinary excretion of ammonia and is as effective as lactulose and is less expensive.

L-ornithine-L-aspartate treatment promotes hepatic removal of ammonia by stimulating residual hepatic urea cycle activity and promoting glutamine synthesis, particularly in skeletal muscle [70]. Control studies show that both oral and intravenous administration reduce ammonia levels and improve encephalopathy in patients with cirrhosis [35, 76].

Levodopa and bromocriptine

If portal-systemic encephalopathy is related to a defect in dopaminergic neurotransmission then replenishment of cerebral dopamines should be beneficial. Dopamine does not pass the blood–brain barrier, but its precursor, levodopa, does and can cause temporary arousal in acute hepatic encephalopathy [44]. However, only a few patients benefit.

Bromocriptine is a specific dopamine receptor agonist with a prolonged action. As an adjunct to protein restriction and lactulose it has given clinical, psychometric and EEG improvement in chronic portal-systemic encephalopathy [52]. It should be considered in the rare patient with intractable chronic portal-systemic encephalopathy and good, stable liver function resistant to dietary protein restriction and lactulose.

Flumazenil

This is a benzodiazepine-receptor antagonist which can induce transient, variable but distinct improvement in some patients with hepatic encephalopathy associated with fulminant liver failure or cirrhosis. A randomized, double-blind study of flumazenil was only beneficial in a subgroup of cirrhotic patients with severe hepatic encephalopathy [5]. Overall results showed improvement in neurological score in 15% of treated patients

compared with 3% on placebo. EEG improved in 25% of treated patients compared with 4% on placebo. The place of this group of compounds in the clinical situation has yet to be established.

Branched-chain amino acids

In cirrhotic patients the serum branched chain amino acids valine, leucine and isoleucine are low, and aromatic amino acid levels are increased. The reduced ratio of branched-chain to aromatic amino acids has been related to the development of hepatic encephalopathy through increased supply of precursors of neurotransmitters. Infusions of solutions containing a high concentration of branched-chain amino acids have been used to treat acute and chronic hepatic encephalopathy. Results have been extremely conflicting, perhaps related to differences in the nature of amino acid solutions, the ways of administration and the patients studied. Analysis of controlled trials shows that there is no consensus that intravenous branched-chain amino acids control hepatic encephalopathy [47].

Despite individual studies showing benefit of oral branched-chain amino acid treatment the benefit of this expensive treatment also remains controversial [19, 49].

Other precipitating factors

Patients are extremely sensitive to sedatives and whenever possible these are avoided. If an overdose is suspected, the appropriate antagonist should be given. If the patient is uncontrollable and some sedation is necessary, a small dose of temazepam or oxazepam is given; morphine and paraldehyde are absolutely contraindicated. Chlordiazepoxide and heminevrin used with caution are valuable in the alcoholic with impending hepatic coma. Drugs known to induce hepatic coma such as oral amino acids and diuretics are disallowed.

Potassium deficiency can be treated by fruit juices or by effervescent or slow-release potassium chloride. If it is urgent, potassium chloride may be added to an intravenous infusion.

Zinc deficiency in patients with cirrhosis should be treated with supplementation. Theoretically deficiency may reduce metabolism of ammonia to urea because of the dependency on zinc of some of the enzymes involved, but studies of zinc therapy in hepatic encephalopathy have not established benefit [68].

Shunt occlusion

Surgical shunt occlusion can reverse the severe portal-systemic encephalopathy following a porta-caval anastomosis. Alternatively the shunt may be occluded by invasive radiology with the insertion of a balloon or a steel coil. This may also be done for a spontaneous gastro-spleno-renal shunt [34, 39].

Temporary hepatic support

Complicated methods of temporary hepatic support are not applicable to hepatic coma in the cirrhotic. Such a patient is either terminal or can be expected to come out of coma without them.

Hepatic transplantation

This may be the ultimate answer to the problem of chronic hepatic encephalopathy. One patient with a history of 3 years showed marked improvement lasting 9 months following transplantation [60]. Another patient with chronic hepato-cerebral degeneration and spastic paraparesis showed remarkable improvement after orthotopic liver transplantation [65].

References

1 Alagille D, Carlier J-C, Chiva M *et al.* Long-term neuropsychological outcome in children undergoing portal-systemic shunts for portal vein obstruction without liver disease. *J. Pediatr. Gastroenterol. Nutr.* 1986; **5**: 861.

2 Amodio P, Del Piccolo F, Marchetti P *et al.* Clinical features and survival of cirrhotic patients with subclinical cognitive alterations detected by the number connection test and computerized psychometric tests. *Hepatology* 1999; **29**: 1662.

3 Aronson L, Gacad RC, Kaminsky-Russ K *et al.* Evidence of gut production of 'endogenous' benzodiazepines: implications for hepatic encephalopathy. *Gastroenterology* 1996; **110**: A1144.

4 Avallone R, Zeneroli ML, Venturini I *et al.* Endogenous benzodiazepine-like compounds and diazepam binding inhibitor in serum of patients with liver cirrhosis with and without overt encephalopathy. *Gut* 1998; **42**: 861.

5 Barbaro G, Di Lorenzo G, Soldini M *et al.* Flumazenil for hepatic encephalopathy grade III and IVa in patients with cirrhosis: an Italian multicentre double-blind, placebo-controlled, cross-over study. *Hepatology* 1998; **28**: 374.

6 Basile AS, Harrison PM, Hughes RD *et al.* Relationship between plasma benzodiazepine receptor ligand concentrations and severity of hepatic encephalopathy. *Hepatology* 1994; **19**: 112.

7 Basile AS, Jones EA. Ammonia and GABA-ergic neurotransmission: interrelated factors in the pathogenesis of hepatic encephalopathy. *Hepatology* 1997; **25**: 1303.

8 Batki G, Fisch HU, Karlaganis G *et al.* Mechanism of the excessive sedative response of cirrhotics to benzodiazepines. Model experiments with triazolam. *Hepatology* 1987; **7**: 629.

9 Bernthal P, Hays A, Tarter RE *et al.* Cerebral CT scan abnormalities in cholestatic and hepato-cellular disease and their relationship to neuro-psychologic test performance. *Hepatology* 1987; **7**: 107.

10 Blanc P, Daures J-P, Rouillon J-M *et al.* Lactitol or lactulose in the treatment of chronic hepatic encephalopathy: results of a meta-analysis. *Hepatology* 1992; **15**: 222.

11 Blei AT. *Helicobacter pylori*, harmful to the brain? *Gut* 2001; **48**: 590.

12 Bustamante J, Rimola A, Ventura P-J *et al.* Prognostic significance of hepatic encephalopathy in patients with cirrhosis. *J. Hepatol.* 1999; **30**: 890.

13 Butterworth RF. Complications of cirrhosis III. Hepatic encephalopathy. *J. Hepatol.* 2000; **32** (Suppl. 1): 171.

14 Collinson PO, Burroughs AK. Severe hypermagnesaemia due to magnesium sulphate enemas in patients with hepatic coma. *Br. Med. J.* 1986; **293**: 1013.

15 Conn HO. Effects of high–normal and low–normal serum potassium levels on hepatic encephalopathy: facts, half-facts or artifacts? *Hepatology* 1994; **20**: 1637.

16 Cordoba J, Blei AT. Treatment of hepatic encephalopathy. *Am. J. Gastroenterol.* 1997; **92**: 1429.

17 Cuilleret G, Pomier-Layrargues G, Pons F *et al.* Changes in brain catecholamine levels in human cirrhotic hepatic encephalopathy. *Gut* 1981; **21**: 565.

18 Das A, Dhiman RK, Saraswat VA *et al.* Prevalence and natural history of subclinical hepatic encephalopathy in cirrhosis. *J. Gastroenterol. Hepatol.* 2001; **16**: 531.

19 Fabbri A, Magrini N, Bianchi G *et al.* Overview of randomized clinical trials of oral branched-chain amino acid treatment in chronic hepatic encephalopathy. *J. Parenter. Enterol. Nutr.* 1996; **20**: 159.

20 Fischer JE, Baldessarini RJ. False neurotransmitters and hepatic failure. *Lancet* 1971; **2**: 75.

21 Frerichs FT. *A Clinical Treatise on Diseases of the Liver*, Vol. I. Translated by C Murchison. New Sydenham Society, London, 1960, p. 241.

22 Gitlin N, Lewis DC, Hinkley L. The diagnosis and prevalence of subclinical hepatic encephalopathy in apparently healthy, ambulant nonshunted patients with cirrhosis. *J. Hepatol.* 1986; **3**: 75.

23 Groeneweg M, Moerland W, Quero JC *et al.* Screening of subclinical hepatic encephalopathy. *J. Hepatol.* 2000; **32**: 748.

24 Groeneweg M, Quero JC, Bruijn ID *et al.* Subclinical hepatic encephalopathy impairs daily functioning. *Hepatology* 1998; **28**: 45.

25 Haseler LJ, Sibbitt WL Jr, Mojtahedzadeh HN *et al.* Proton MR spectroscopic measurement of neurometabolities in hepatic encephalopathy during oral lactulose therapy. *Am. J. Neuroradiol.* 1998; **19**: 1681.

26 Haussinger D, Kircheis G, Fischer R *et al.* Hepatic encephalopathy in chronic liver disease: a clinical manifestation of astrocyte swelling and low-grade cerebral oedema? *J. Hepatol.* 2000; **32**: 1035.

27 Haussinger D, Steeb R, Gerok W. Ammonium and bicarbonate homeostasis in chronic liver disease. *Klin. Wochenschr.* 1990; **68**: 75.

28 Hazell AS, Butterworth RF. Hepatic encephalopathy: an update of pathophysiologic mechanisms. *Proc. Soc. Exp. Biol. Med.* 1999; **222**: 99.

29 Hermengildo C, Monfort P, Felipo V. Activation of N-methyl-D-aspartate receptors in rat brain *in vivo* following acute ammonia intoxication: characterization by *in vivo* brain microdialysis. *Hepatology* 2000; **31**: 709.

30 Horsmans Y, Solbreux PM, Daenens C *et al.* Lactulose

Chapter 8
Acute Liver Failure

Acute liver failure describes the clinical syndrome of severe impairment of liver function (encephalopathy, coagulopathy and jaundice) within 6 months of the onset of symptoms. Although usually due to an acute insult (most frequently virus or drug) in a previously healthy person, acute liver failure may be the presenting feature of chronic liver disease in particular Wilson's disease, autoimmune chronic hepatitis or delta superinfection in a patient with chronic hepatitis B.

Acute liver failure developing within a few days or weeks after the acute insult has a high incidence of cerebral oedema and a risk of dying from brainstem herniation ('coning'). Other complications that may lead to death include bacterial and fungal infections, circulatory instability, renal and pulmonary failure, acid–base and electrolyte disturbances and coagulopathy. These make intensive care, referral to a specialist unit, the availability of liver transplantation and temporary hepatic support vitally important. The survival of patients has improved with such facilities, rising from about 20% in the early 1970s to 50% in the 1990s [90].

The key to optimizing treatment is early recognition of acute liver failure and transfer of the patient to a liver unit with facilities for liver transplantation. In a recent study of patients with acetaminophen (paracetamol) induced acute liver failure, 56 of the 124 patients who met the criteria for transplantation were not listed because of the rapid development of contraindications (multi-organ failure, cerebral oedema). Of those 68 patients listed for transplantation 24 developed contraindications while awaiting transplant [9]. This outcome highlights the need for rapid referral of patients with acute liver failure to a transplant centre to maximize the chance of survival.

Definition

The original definition of fulminant hepatic failure by Trey and Davidson in 1970 stipulated an onset of hepatic encephalopathy within 8 weeks of the first symptoms of illness, in patients without pre-existing liver disease. The recognition that different clinical patterns of acute liver failure relate to aetiology and prognosis, and that patients may have underlying chronic liver disease, has led to revision of this definition and the development of several classifications [10, 60].

One widely used classification broadly separates acute liver failure into hyper-acute, acute and sub-acute, based on the time interval between the development of jaundice and encephalopathy (table 8.1) [60]. An alternative classification [12] is fulminant and sub-fulminant liver failure (time from jaundice to encephalopathy less or more than 2 weeks). Late onset liver failure describes encephalopathy developing more than 8 weeks (but less than 24 weeks) after the first symptoms [32]. Classification of the patient into a particular subgroup has value in the assessment of prognosis and the urgency with which intervention is needed. In rapidly developing liver failure (hyper-acute) the chance of survival without transplantation is more than in acute liver failure. Classifications also have an important role in the interpretation of data from different units and countries and in the planning of trials.

Causes (tables 8.2, 8.3)

The most common cause of acute liver failure worldwide is viral hepatitis. The exception to this pattern is in the UK where acetaminophen self-poisoning has been the most frequent cause of acute liver failure.

Table 8.1. Classification of acute liver failure [60]

	Interval: jaundice to encephalopathy	Cerebral oedema	Prognosis	Leading causes
Hyper-acute	<7 days	Common	Moderate	Virus A, B; acetaminophen
Acute	8–28 days	Common	Poor	Non-A/B/C; drugs
Sub-acute	29 days to 12 weeks	Poor	Poor	Non-A/B/C; drugs

Table 8.2. Causes of acute liver failure

Infective
Hepatitis virus A, B, C, D, E, transfusion-transmitted virus (TTV)
Herpes simplex

Drug reactions and toxins
Acetaminophen (paracetamol) overdose
Antidepressants
Halothane
Isoniazid–rifampicin
Non-steroidal anti-inflammatory drugs
Mushroom poisoning
Herbal remedies
Ecstasy

Ischaemic
Ischaemic hepatitis
Surgical 'shock'
Acute Budd–Chiari syndrome

Metabolic
Wilson's disease
Fatty liver of pregnancy
Reye's syndrome

Miscellaneous (rare)
Massive malignant infiltration
Severe bacterial infection
Heat stroke

Table 8.3. Causes of acute liver failure: geographical variation

Cause	USA [77] 1994–1996 n = 295 (%)	India [1, 2] 1987–1993 n = 423 (%)	UK [8] 1991–1997 n = 989 (%)
Acetaminophen (paracetamol)	20	–	71
Viral (A, B, E*)	17	80	5
Non-A/B/C/E	15	12	7
Drug	12	5	5
Other	36	–	12

* Hepatitis E is rare in the USA and UK.

The hepatitis virus responsible varies from one geographical location to another. In the United States 30% of acute liver failure is due to virus, half being from hepatitis A and B and the remainder non-A/B/C/E [77]. The latter have typical prodromal symptoms and biochemical profiles, but no viral agent can be identified. In India, virtually all acute liver failure is viral with 40% being due to hepatitis E and 25–30% to hepatitis B [1, 2]. In Greece, the high carrier rate of hepatitis B is reflected in a greater proportion of patients having hepatitis B-related acute liver failure [61].

If appropriate testing is not done hepatitis B may not be diagnosed since one-third to one-half of patients with acute liver failure due to this virus become seronegative for hepatitis B surface antigen (HBsAg) after a few days

[76]. Hepatitis B virus (HBV) core mutants may complicate the picture further because of defective production of the normal viral antigens. They are an important aetiology in cases of acute hepatitis B related acute liver failure in India [2]. In about 50% of hepatitis B patients the acute liver failure is precipitated by another factor, usually acute infection or superinfection with delta virus [76]. Reactivation of viral replication in carriers of hepatitis B or C may lead to liver failure [36, 85] after antitumour chemotherapy or following cessation of immunosuppressive therapy.

The contribution of hepatitis C varies geographically being low (0–10%) in the USA and Europe and higher (around 20%) in Taiwan [19]. Patients with superinfection of chronic hepatitis C with acute hepatitis A may be at risk of acute liver failure [86]. This risk is the basis for offering hepatitis vaccination to patients with chronic liver disease, although the cost-effectiveness of this strategy has been questioned [56].

Hepatitis E causes epidemics of acute hepatitis not only in India but also in central Asia, Mexico and China. Pregnant women are particularly at risk of acute liver failure. In Western countries acute liver failure due to hepatitis E has been reported in individuals with links to endemic areas [49].

Hepatitis G infection does not appear to be responsible for fulminant hepatic failure [78]. Transfusion-transmitted virus (TTV) has been implicated in 25% of cases of idiopathic acute liver failure [17].

Other viruses can cause a fatal hepatic necrosis especially in immunocompromised individuals. These include herpes simplex, cytomegalovirus, adenoviruses, Epstein–Barr and parvovirus B19 [46].

Acetaminophen is predictably hepato-toxic in overdose and has been the most common suicidal agent taken in the UK (Chapter 20). Since 1998 there has been a reduction in the frequency of severe acetaminophen-related hepato-toxicity [64, 83] due the sale of acetaminophen in blister packs rather than bottles, and a restriction in the number of tablets obtainable without prescription.

Acetaminophen may be hepato-toxic when taken in therapeutic doses in patients concurrently drinking excess alcohol. The characteristic picture is of very high serum aspartate transaminase levels (reported up to 48 000 iu/l) usually accompanied by a lower level of alanine transaminase [93]. Alcohol-enhanced acetaminophen hepato-toxicity, however, appears to be a less frequent clinical event in the UK [51].

Idiosyncratic drug reactions may cause acute liver failure. The most frequent culprits are anti-tuberculosis medication [1, 8], non-steroidal agents [6], anaesthetic agents and antidepressants. Acute liver failure is also reported with the recreational drug 'ecstasy' (3,4-methylene dioxymetamphetamine) [4]. Herbal remedies have been associated with hepato-cellular damage and acute liver failure [81]. Carbon tetrachloride poisoning usually causes more renal than hepatic damage. This is true of most industrial poisons although acute liver failure can follow occupational exposure to the solvent 2-nitropropane [39].

Mushroom poisoning is common in France and in areas where unusual fungi are gathered and eaten. Hepatic failure is preceded by muscarinic effects, such as profuse sweating, vomiting and diarrhoea. Early recognition is important to optimize supportive measures and to be alerted to the possibility of liver failure [45].

Pregnant women may develop hepatic necrosis due to eclampsia or fatty liver (Chapter 27).

Vascular causes of ischaemic hepatitis include low cardiac output in a patient with underlying cardiac disease, acute Budd–Chiari syndrome, and surgical shock with or without Gram-negative septicaemia.

Massive infiltration of the liver with tumour such as in lymphoma [74] can lead to acute liver failure. Such a cause should be considered in the differential diagnosis since liver transplantation is contraindicated, and specific therapy may be life saving.

Acute Wilson's disease must always be excluded in any patient who is less than 35 years old, particularly if haemolysis is associated. In these patients acute liver failure may result from a superimposed acute viral hepatitis [75].

Autoimmune hepatitis may rarely present as subfulminant hepatic failure [40].

Clinical features

The patient, previously having been well, typically develops non-specific symptoms such as nausea and malaise. Jaundice follows and then features of hepatic encephalopathy. Coma may develop rapidly within a few days. Transfer of the patient to a specialist liver centre with a transplantation service needs to be done earlier rather than later. It must be realized that a patient with acute liver disease and prolonged coagulation can deteriorate and die. Advice from a liver centre should be sought. If on admission there is encephalopathy, immediate transfer should be discussed.

In the early stages, jaundice bears little relation to neuropsychiatric changes which may even develop before jaundice. Later, jaundice is deep. Liver size is usually small.

Vomiting is common but abdominal pain rare. Tachycardia, hypotension, hyperventilation and fever are later features. The clinician must be alert to the delay between acetaminophen overdose and liver damage which may present after a period of 2–3 days or apparent clinical recovery.

Focal neurological signs, high fever or a slow response to conventional treatment should prompt a search for alternative causes for encephalopathy.

Patients with a more gradual onset of hepatic insuffi-

ciency (over weeks rather than days, and variously called sub-fulminant, sub-acute or late onset) infrequently develop cerebral oedema. Ascites and renal failure appear, and the prognosis is worse than in those patients with a more rapid course.

Common complications of acute liver failure include infections, haemodynamic disturbances and cerebral oedema. These complications together with hepatic encephalopathy and other related problems are discussed below.

The overall mortality of an attack of acute hepatitis is about 1%, with the risk for non-A, non-B (1.5–2.5%) being greater than that for hepatitis B (1%) or A (0.2–0.4%) [41]. The short-term prognosis for acute liver failure is much worse than for liver failure associated with chronic liver disease, but in acute liver failure the hepatic lesion is potentially reversible, and survivors usually recover completely.

Late onset hepatic failure. This term refers to a group of patients in whom encephalopathy develops after an illness of more than 8 weeks but less than 24 weeks from the first symptoms, in the absence of pre-existing liver disease. In most patients, the cause cannot be found [31]. Nausea, malaise and abdominal discomfort are followed by ascites, encephalopathy and renal impairment. Survival was about 20% without transplantation. A 1-year survival of 55% has been reported after transplantation [31].

Distinction from chronic liver disease

A note should be made of any history of liver disease, the duration of symptoms and the presence of a hard liver, marked splenomegaly and vascular spiders on the skin (table 8.4). A problem arises in the alcoholic where recent heavy drinking adds acute hepatitis to underlying chronic liver disease. In these circumstances the liver is large. Potential reversibility of acute alcoholic hepatitis merits more supportive effort than could be given to the usual end-stage cirrhosis where the liver would not be expected to regenerate.

Investigations (table 8.5)

Blood is taken to identify problems needing immediate

Table 8.4. Liver failure: distinction between acute and acute-on-chronic types

	Acute	Acute-on-chronic
History	Short	Long
Nutrition	Good	Poor
Liver	±	+ hard
Spleen	±	+
Spiders	o	++

Table 8.5. Investigations of acute liver failure

Haematology
Haemoglobin, platelets, WBC, prothrombin, blood group

Biochemical
Blood glucose, serum bilirubin, aspartate transaminase, alkaline
    phosphatase, albumin, globulin, immunoglobulins
Serum urea, sodium, potassium, bicarbonate, chloride, calcium,
    phosphate
Serum amylase
Store 8 ml serum for later use

Microbiology, virology
Hepatitis B antigen and IgM anticore
Hepatitis A (IgM) antibody
Hepatitis C antibody
Hepatitis E antibody
Serum anti-delta
Blood culture, aerobic and anaerobic
Sputum, urine, stool (culture and microscopy)
Store serum for virological studies

Other essential
Chest X-ray, electrocardiogram, fluid intake and output, blood
    gases

Additional (not always necessary)
Blood alcohol or other drug level
Urine electrolyte concentration
Plasma fibrin degradation products
Hepatic scan

attention, to establish a baseline for hepatic and renal function, to establish the cause and to check criteria for survival/transplantation.

Haematology

The prothrombin time (together with the degree of encephalopathy) is central to the assessment of the severity of the clinical situation, and its progress. Haemoglobin and white count are obtained. A falling platelet count may reflect disseminated intravascular coagulation.

Biochemistry

Blood glucose, blood urea, electrolytes and creatinine are measured. Bilirubin, albumin, transaminase, alkaline phosphatase and amylase are routinely done. Serum bilirubin is important prognostically for non-acetaminophen patients. Serum albumin is usually initially normal, but later a low albumin reflects a poor prognosis. The transaminases are of little prognostic value. Levels tend to fall as the patient's condition worsens. Blood gas analysis for pH is important in the prognostic evaluation of acetaminophen-related liver failure.

Virological markers

Acute hepatitis A should be diagnosed by a serum IgM anti-A antibody. Serum HBsAg is checked, but the IgM core antibody is necessary for certain diagnosis. HBsAg may have been cleared and hepatitis B surface antibody (HBsAb) will not have appeared. Serum HBV DNA is then usually negative. Such rapid viral clearance indicates a favourable prognosis, perhaps because it implies a good immune response to the HBV. In those positive for HBV, serum anti-delta should be sought. Anti-hepatitis C virus (anti-HCV) should be performed, but is likely to be negative this early in the disease (Chapter 18). PCR for HCV RNA is required for diagnosis of HCV-related acute hepatic failure.

Hepatitis E serology should be done if geographically appropriate.

Electroencephalogram (EEG)

This has been used to assess the clinical state and determine prognosis (fig. 8.1). However, the guidelines now used for decisions on clinical management, and in particular liver transplantation, no longer depend on the EEG. Repeated measurement may, however, be necessary when clinical and laboratory features do not move in the same direction.

Continuous EEG recording, however, has shown 50% of patients with acute liver failure to have sub-clinical seizure/epileptiform activity. This is not recognized clinically without EEG because the patient is paralysed and ventilated. EEG monitoring has been recommended for patients reaching stage 3 or 4 encephalopathy [32].

Scanning and liver biopsy

Scanning will show a reduction in liver size. However, correlation of liver size with survival is imprecise. Liver histology shows considerable variability of necrosis from area to area which may be prognostically misleading [38].

In a retrospective study a liver volume of less than 1000 ml and/or hepatic parenchymal necrosis of greater than 50% indicated a poor prognosis, but findings above these two thresholds did not necessarily indicate a good outcome [79]. Hepatic regenerative changes on histology (associated with less than 50% parenchymal necrosis) were present in the good prognostic group. However, both CT scanning and transjugular liver biopsy are done in the radiology department and transfer of the patient can worsen haemodynamic instability and intercranial hypertension. From the practical point of view clinical and laboratory data rather than scanning and biopsy are used for decision making.

CT of the brain is unreliable in detecting early cerebral

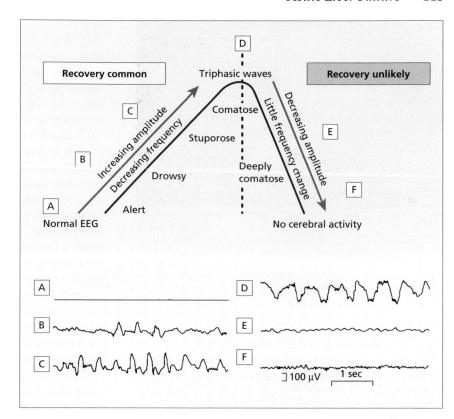

Fig. 8.1. Evolution of the EEG in liver failure. The progression from grade A to D is marked by increasing amplitude, decreasing frequency and increasing drowsiness. At D, triphasic waves appear and the interrupted line indicates the limit beyond which recovery is unlikely. From E to F amplitude decreases with little frequency change and at F there is no cerebral activity.

oedema, and the movement of the patient to the radiology unit carries the risk of deterioration.

Associations

Hepatic encephalopathy

The neurological sequelae of acute liver failure are hepatic encephalopathy and cerebral oedema with raised intracranial pressure (ICP). Clinically they overlap (fig. 8.2). Early in the clinical course encephalopathy usually develops without evidence of increased ICP. Once stupor to deep coma with or without decerebrate posturing (grade 3–4 encephalopathy) develops, the patient is at high risk of developing cerebral oedema.

The pathogenesis of hepatic encephalopathy is multifactorial (Chapter 7) and centres on failure of the liver to remove toxic, mainly nitrogenous, substances from the circulation. In contrast to the coma of cirrhotic patients, portal-systemic encephalopathy due to shunting of blood past the liver is of minor importance. Blood ammonia (and presumably amine) levels are increased but do not correlate with the depth of coma or the prognosis. Measurement of blood ammonia is not necessary for management.

The onset of encephalopathy is often sudden. It may precede jaundice. The features are unlike those seen in chronic liver disease with agitation, changes in personality, delusions and restlessness. The patient may show

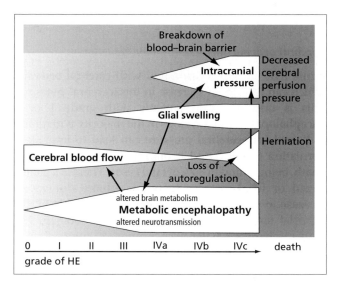

Fig. 8.2. Brain dysfunction in acute liver failure. Proposed interrelation of metabolic encephalopathy, ICP and changes in cerebral blood flow during the progression of the disease. HE, hepatic encephalopathy. (From [33] with permission.)

antisocial behaviour or character disturbance. Nightmares, headaches and dizziness are other inaugural, non-specific symptoms. Delirium, mania and fits indicate stimulation of the reticular system. Unco-operative behaviour often continues while consciousness is clouded. The delirium is of the noisy, restless variety and

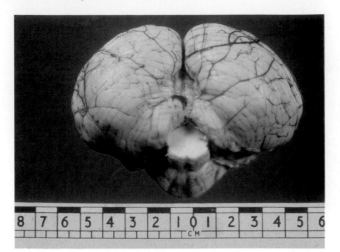

Fig. 8.3. Cerebral oedema in a patient who died in hepatic coma. Note the indented cerebellum.

attacks of screaming are spontaneous or induced by minor stimuli. Violent behaviour is common. 'Flapping' tremor may be transient and overlooked. Fetor hepaticus is usually present.

The prognosis for patients with grade 1 or 2 encephalopathy (confused or drowsy) is good. For grade 3 or 4 it is much poorer.

Cerebral oedema (intracranial hypertension)

Acute liver failure is associated with cerebral oedema, which can lead to an increase in intracerebral pressure. This is uncommon in patients with grade 1 or 2 encephalopathy, but develops in the majority with grade 4. Raised intracerebral pressure can lead to brainstem herniation (fig. 8.3) and is the most common cause of death, being found in 80% of fatal cases. There is a generalized or focal increase in brain volume due to an increase in water content. The cause is probably multifactorial and currently not fully understood [15, 48]. Two mechanisms have been proposed: cytotoxic and vasogenic.

The *cytotoxic* hypothesis depends on the accumulation of osmolytes such as glutamine, particularly in astrocytes, with subsequent osmotic uptake of water into the cells. In the brain astrocytes are the site of ammonia metabolism by amidation of glutamate to glutamine. In acute liver failure cerebral glutamine concentrations rise. Brain-stem herniation correlates with arterial ammonia concentration [20].

The *vasogenic* hypothesis depends on changes in cerebral blood flow and the blood–brain barrier. Cerebral blood flow has a wide variation between individuals with acute liver failure and it is not clear whether this is related to systemic changes or is locally induced. Cere-

bral vasodilatation is associated with a poor prognosis. Hypoxia and prostaglandins may be involved. It is possible that the changes in cerebral blood flow may also be related to glutamine through the production of nitric oxide. Surges of intracranial hypertension may result from vascular engorgement secondary to inappropriate vasodilatation.

Disruption of the blood–brain barrier with leakage of plasma into the cerebrospinal fluid has been proposed as a mechanism for cerebral oedema but this hypothesis has not been substantiated.

The net blood supply to the brain depends on the balance between carotid arterial pressure and intracerebral pressure. Cerebral blood flow appears to be inadequate in most patients with grade 4 encephalopathy resulting in cerebral hypoxia [89], and these changes may be related to the development of cerebral oedema. Cerebral blood flow autoregulation (maintained blood flow despite falling or rising blood pressure) is lost in patients with fulminant hepatic failure [47]. Loss of this protective mechanism could exacerbate cerebral changes due to systemic hypotension (giving cerebral ischaemia) and cerebral hyperperfusion (increasing cerebral blood volume and interstitial water) [48].

Clinically, raised intracerebral pressure is suggested by systolic hypertension (sustained or intermittent), increased muscle tone and myoclonus which progress to extension and hyperpronation of the arms and extension of the legs (decerebrate posturing). Dysconjugate eye movements and skewed positions of the eyes may be seen. If not controlled by treatment, this clinical picture progresses to loss of pupillary reflexes and respiratory arrest from brainstem herniation.

Coagulopathy

The liver synthesizes all the coagulation factors (except factor VIII), inhibitors of coagulation and proteins involved in the fibrinolytic system (Chapter 4). It is also involved in the clearance of activated clotting factors. The coagulopathy of fulminant hepatic failure is thus complex and due not only to factor deficiency, but also to enhanced fibrinolytic activity most likely caused by intravascular coagulation [63]. The platelet count may fall due to increased consumption or reduced production, and platelet function is also abnormal in fulminant hepatic failure.

The resulting coagulopathy predisposes to bleeding. This is a potential cause of death; it may be spontaneous, from the mucous membranes, from the gastrointestinal tract or into the brain.

The prothrombin time is the most widely used test to assess coagulation. It is a guide to prognosis and is one of the criteria used in deciding whether transplantation should be done (see table 8.7) [58].

Hypoglycaemia, hypokalaemia, metabolic changes

Hypoglycaemia is found in 40% of patients with acute liver failure. It may be persistent and intractable. Plasma insulin levels are high due to reduced hepatic uptake; gluconeogenesis is reduced in the failing liver. Hypoglycaemia can cause rapid neurological deterioration and death and is one aspect of the condition which can be treated satisfactorily.

Hypokalaemia is common and due in part to urinary losses with inadequate replacement, and administration of glucose. Serum sodium levels tend to be low, falling markedly in the terminal stages. Other electrolyte changes include hypophosphataemia, hypocalcaemia and hypomagnesaemia.

Acid–base changes are common. Respiratory alkalosis is due to hyperventilation, probably related to direct stimulation of the respiratory centre by unknown toxic substances. Respiratory acidosis can be caused by elevated ICP and respiratory depression, or pulmonary complications. Lactic acidosis develops in about half of the patients reaching grade 3 coma. It is related to inadequate tissue perfusion due to hypotension and hypoxaemia. A metabolic acidosis is more frequent in acetaminophen-induced acute liver failure; the fall in pH is one of the criteria used in transplant decisions (see table 8.7).

Infection [70]

Ninety per cent of patients with acute liver failure and grade 2 or more encephalopathy have clinical or bacteriological evidence of infection (fig. 8.4) [68]. Twenty-five per cent have associated bacteraemia. The majority of infections are respiratory. The high rate of infection can be related to poor host defences with impaired Kupffer cell and polymorph function and to the reduction of factors such as fibronectin, opsonins and chemoattractants, including components of the complement system. Poor respiratory effort and cough reflex, and the presence of endotracheal tubes, venous lines and urinary catheters place the patient at increased risk.

Infections in the blood, respiratory tract and urine are usually detected within 3 days of admission. In some cases the source of infection may never be found, but tips of intravenous catheters should be cultured after removal, and are often incriminated. The typical manifestations of sepsis, such as fever and leucocytosis, may be absent (fig. 8.4). More than two-thirds of infections are due to Gram-positive organisms, usually staphylococci, but streptococci and Gram-negative bacilli are also found.

Fungal infections are found in about one-third of patients, often unrecognized and ominous [69]. These patients share particular clinical features (table 8.6).

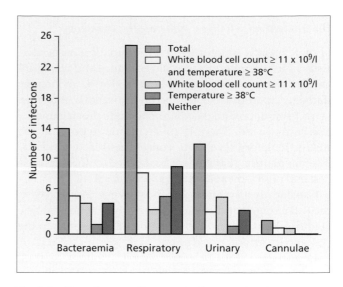

Fig. 8.4. Clinical signs of bacterial infection related to significant microbiological cultures in 50 patients with acute liver failure. Raised temperature and white cell count were poor indicators of bacterial infection. (From [68] with permission.)

Table 8.6. Features of systemic fungal infection [69]

Deterioration in coma grade after initial improvement
Pyrexia unresponsive to antibiotics
Established renal failure
Markedly elevated white cell count

Fungal resistance to short-term prophylaxis with fluconizole is unlikely [35].

Overall, infections make a major contribution to clinical deterioration and death. The severity of the systemic inflammatory response relates to prognosis [72].

Renal

Due to decreased urea synthesis by the liver, the blood urea concentration may not be a good indicator of kidney function, and the serum creatinine is preferred. Renal failure, which develops in about 55% of patients, may be related to liver cell failure itself (hepato-renal syndrome), to acute tubular necrosis secondary to complications of acute liver failure (sepsis, endotoxaemia, bleeding, hypotension), or direct nephrotoxicity of the drug or other insult responsible for the hepatic damage (e.g. acetaminophen overdose). The hepato-renal syndrome (Chapter 9) results from a combination of factors including a hyperdynamic circulation with lowered renal perfusion pressure, activation of the sympathetic nervous system, and increased synthesis of vasoactive mediators which decrease glomerular capillary ultrafiltration [54].

Haemodynamic changes: systemic hypotension

Hypotension is a feature of liver failure. It is associated with a low peripheral vascular resistance and increased cardiac output which relate to the degree of hepatic damage. Apart from sepsis and endotoxaemia, the cause is unclear but possible mediators include prostaglandins and nitric oxide. There is covert tissue hypoxia at the microcirculatory level with conse-quent lactic acidosis. The circulatory changes are associated with decreased cerebral perfusion and renal vasoconstriction.

Cardiac dysrhythmias of most types are noted in the later stages and relate to electrolyte abnormalities, acidosis, hypoxia and the insertion of catheters into the pulmonary artery.

Depression of brainstem function due to cerebral oedema and herniation eventually leads to circulatory failure.

Pulmonary complications

These include aspiration of gastric contents or blood, atelectasis, infection and respiratory depression due to brainstem compression. Intrapulmonary arteriovenous shunting adds to the hypoxia. There may be pulmonary oedema. Adult respiratory distress syndome (ARDS) is usually refractory to treatment and fatal.

Chest X-rays show abnormalities in over half of patients. These include lobar collapse, patchy consolidation, aspiration pneumonia and, in one-quarter, noncardiogenic pulmonary oedema.

Acute pancreatitis

Acute haemorrhagic and necrotizing pancreatitis is frequent in patients dying with acute liver failure. It is difficult to recognize in the comatose patient but, rarely, it may be the cause of death. Serum amylase levels are raised in about one-third of patients and should be monitored.

Aetiological factors include haemorrhage into and around the pancreas, the causative virus, corticosteroid therapy and shock.

Prognosis

The overall survival for those reaching grade 3 or 4 encephalopathy is 20% without transplantation. If only grade 1 or 2 coma is reached, survival is around 65%. Those who survive do not develop cirrhosis.

The advent of successful liver transplantation for acute liver failure has made prediction of survival particularly important. Indications, whether clinical or laboratory, that spontaneous recovery is unlikely are therefore of vital importance. Prognosis is worse in older patients, although under 10 year olds are also at particu-

lar risk [58]. Coexistence of other disease worsens the prognosis.

Aetiology is important. In one series, 12.5% of halothane-related patients survived without transplantation compared with 66% for hepatitis A, 38.9% for hepatitis B and 50% for acetaminophen overdose [59].

If any precipitant of encephalopathy can be identified, particularly the administration of sedatives, the prognosis is better. The patient improves as the drug is eliminated.

Unfavourable clinical signs include a small liver and ascites. Decerebrate rigidity, with loss of the oculovestibular reflex and respiratory failure are particularly ominous. Such patients, if they survive, may rarely be left with residual brainstem and cerebral cortical injury [57].

Prothrombin time is the best indicator of survival [58]. The association of a clotting factor V concentration of less than 15% with coma is also ominous [11]. At this level survival is only 10% for all aetiologies except hepatitis A and acetaminophen overdose where the outlook is better. Hypoglycaemia is another bad sign.

Liver biopsy is rarely indicated but, if necessary, can be performed by the transjugular route. The extent of hepato-cellular necrosis and interlobular confluent necrosis is related to outcome. Hepatic parenchymal necrosis of more than 50% is associated with a reduced survival [79].

An important univariate and multivariate analysis was made of predictive factors in 586 patients with acute liver failure managed medically (table 8.7) [58]. In patients with viral hepatitis and drug reactions, three static variables—aetiology (non-A–E hepatitis or drug), age (less than 10 years and more than 40 years) and duration of jaundice before encephalopathy (greater than 7 days)—and two dynamic variables, a serum bilirubin exceeding 18 mg (300 μmol/l) and a prothrombin time exceeding 50 s, indicated a poor prognosis. In acetaminophen overdose, survival correlated with arterial blood pH, peak prothrombin time and serum creatinine.

These criteria have been validated by other centres and some have found a slightly lower predictive accuracy (71 and 68% for acetaminophen-induced and non-acetaminophen-induced acute liver failure) [3]. Acute Physiology and Chronic Health Evaluation scores (APACHE II and III) may improve decision making and the defining of patients in clinical trials [9, 52].

Another commonly applied set of criteria uses the concurrent presence of confusion or coma and an age-corrected factor V between 20 or 30% of normal [14].

These criteria use clinical and laboratory data that are straightforward to collect and there is currently no other generally accepted system in use. The King's College criteria are most widely used.

Assessment of hepatocyte necrosis on liver biopsy, or reduced liver volume on CT scanning, are used in some

Table 8.7. King's College Hospital criteria for liver transplantation in acute liver failure [58]

Acetaminophen (paracetamol)

pH < 7.30 (irrespective of grade of encephalopathy)

or

Prothrombin time >100 s (INR > 7) and serum creatinine >300 µmol/l in patients with grade III or IV encephalopathy

Non-acetaminophen patients

Prothrombin time >100 s (INR > 7) (irrespective of grade of encephalopathy)

or

Any three of the following variables (irrespective of grade of encephalopathy)
 age <10 or >40 years
 aetiology: non-A–E hepatitis, 'viral' hepatitis no agent identified, halothane hepatitis, idiosyncratic drug reaction
 duration of jaundice before onset of encephalopathy >7 days
 prothrombin time >50 s (INR > 3.5)
 serum bilirubin >300 µmol/l

Table 8.8. Management of acute liver failure

Problem	Treatment
Hepatic encephalopathy	Reduce protein by mouth
	Phosphate enema twice daily
	No sedation
	Lactulose 30 ml dose
Cerebral oedema	Intravenous mannitol
	Avoid hyperthermia
	Monitor ICP
Hypoglycaemia	100 ml 50% glucose if blood glucose falls below 3 mmol/l
	Check blood glucose hourly
	Infusion 10–50% dextrose
	Check hypokalaemia
Hypocalcaemia	10 ml 10% calcium gluconate i.v. daily
Renal failure	Haemofiltration
Respiratory failure	Intubation
	Ventilation
	Oxygen
	Maintain normal blood gases
Hypotension	Albumin
	Vaso-constrictors
Infection	Frequent cultures
	Prophylactic antibiotics (see text)
	Specific antibiotics later
Bleeding	No arterial puncture
	H₂ blocker
	Sulcralfate
	Fresh frozen plasma and platelets

ICP, intracranial pressure.

centres, and in the case of biopsy may alter the diagnosis in 17% of cases [27]. However, debate as to their discriminant value and practical problems in arranging them safely, at the appropriate time, have limited their use.

The causes of death are: cerebral oedema, infection, bleeding, respiratory and circulatory failure, renal failure, hypoglycaemia and pancreatitis.

Survival depends on the capacity of the liver to regenerate and this is almost impossible to predict. It is probably under humoral control and a hepatocyte growth factor has been identified. Human hepatocyte growth factor is increased in the blood in patients with acute liver failure, but is not a useful prognostic measure.

No criteria are ever likely to predict the outcome of acute liver failure with certainty. However, prediction of a low chance of survival, for example 20%, is clinically useful in directing a decision to transplant with a 60–80% chance of survival.

Treatment [8]

Over the years survival of patients with acute liver failure has improved due to meticulous attention to the detail of good supportive care combined with better knowledge of the most important functions lost when the liver cell fails. These patients are mercifully rare, and should be treated in a special unit with experience in the management of acute liver failure and facilities for liver transplantation. The complex problems associated with multiple organ failure require close monitoring and prompt treatment (table 8.8). The clinical state of the patient may change rapidly. Frequent review is essential. Such patients should be managed in a high dependency or intensive care area by an appropriately trained team of nurses.

The measures described below apply predominantly to patients in grade 3 and 4 coma and must be modified for those in the lower grades.

The patient is barrier nursed. Attendants should wear gloves, gowns and masks and should have been vaccinated against hepatitis B. The grade of encepalopathy (Chapter 7) must be charted hourly.

Temperature, pulse and blood pressure should be recorded at least hourly and preferably continuously. A strict fluid balance chart recording input and output is imperative. Care should be taken to avoid fluid overload.

A naso-gastric tube is passed. An H₂-antagonist or proton pump inhibitor is given to reduce the risk of gastroduodenal erosions and bleeding. Lack of acid may increase gastric bacteria. Prophylaxis using sulcralfate is an alternative. Enteral nutrition should be given containing calories appropriate to the individual patient. Earlier in the course of the illness oral supplements should be given.

To detect early evidence of complications, such as renal and respiratory failure, monitoring using invasive methods is necessary so that preventative measures can be taken. A urinary catheter, central venous catheter and arterial line should be placed, the last two after clotting factor and if necessary platelet infusion.

Hypoglycaemia is frequent, and on arrival the blood sugar is estimated; 100 ml of 50% glucose is given intravenously if the blood glucose is less than 60 mg/dl (3.5 mmol/l). A continuous infusion of dextrose 5 or 10% is given, the volume according to fluid needs. If enteral nutrition is given hypoglycaemia is less likely.

The blood sugar is checked every hour and further 50% glucose given if hypoglycaemia recurs. If it is necessary to move a patient from one centre to another, a 20% dextrose infusion should be given during the journey.

Hypomagnesaemia is a frequent finding often associated with hypokalaemia.

Respiratory status is monitored using pulse oximetry. Oxygen by mask is given. Mechanical ventilation is necessary if respiratory failure is shown by a rise in arterial P_{CO_2} (>6.5 kPa) or fall in P_{O_2} (<10 kPa), although this is a rare indication. More often endotracheal intubation is necessary for the comatose patient to prevent aspiration or when sedation is becoming necessary because of agitation.

Infections occur in up to 90% of patients with acute liver failure [68]. Particular risk factors are a high maximum INR and intubation of the trachea [67].

To pre-empt *septic complications*, sputum and urine should be sent for culture daily. Venous and arterial line sites should be inspected regularly; cannulas should be replaced if inflamed, or if fever develops, or otherwise routinely every 3–5 days. The tip of the catheter is sent for culture.

Studies of prophylactic selective systemic antibiotics and intestinal decontamination have shown benefit both individually and in combination. Their use is, however, controversial. Prophylactic intravenous antibiotics reduce infection by 80% but do not improve outcome or reduce the length of stay. Selective enteric decontamination adds no benefits to parenteral antibiotics (fig. 8.5) [71]. In this study multi-resistant bacteria were found and were thought to be related to the third-generation cephalosporin used. The most appropriate antibiotic regimen will depend on the incidence, type and sensitivity of bacteria on the individual liver unit. Regular microbiological surveillance is essential. Blanket use of broad-spectrum antibiotics should be narrowed down to a specific choice once positive cultures are available.

Without prophylaxis fungal infections are found in about 30% of patients [69]. Trials in which oral amphotericin B have been used have reduced the rate of fungal infection below 5% (fig. 8.5) [71]. Treatment of systemic fungal infection is with amphotericin B and flucytosine.

Hypotension is extremely difficult, if not impossible to control. When crystalloid or albumin infusions do not correct the fall in blood pressure, a vaso-constrictor agent such as noradrenaline (norepinephrine) may be given although combinations of vaso-active drugs may be more useful [8].

When *renal failure* develops, monitoring of fluid balance becomes even more critical. Dopamine infusion may slow or reverse the change in renal function although its use is questionable in critically ill patients [8, 54]. Continuous arteriovenous haemofiltration [22] is indicated when the serum creatinine rises above about 400 μmol/l (4.5 mg/dl), and to correct fluid overload, acidosis and hyperkalaemia. Haemodialysis on an intermittent basis causes haemodynamic instability. It may increase ICP.

Coagulopathy is managed by routine intravenous vitamin K. Fresh frozen plasma and platelets are given if there is bleeding or for invasive procedures such as insertion of an arterial line or extradural pressure transducer.

Hepatic encephalopathy is treated by the usual routine (Chapter 7) with no protein by mouth, and phosphate enemas. Lactulose is given via the naso-gastric tube (initially 15–30 ml). Exacerbating factors, such as sepsis, electrolyte imbalance and haemorrhage, should be treated. Sedation must be avoided if at all possible. If absolutely necessary, if the patient is violent, a small dose of a short-acting benzodiazepine (e.g. midazolam) may be given. Neomycin is avoided because of possible nephrotoxicity. Antibiotics given to prevent or treat infection will also serve to treat the encephalopathy. Flumazemil is a benzodiazepine-receptor antagonist which can produce variable, short-lived but distinct improvement in some patients with hepatic encephalopathy. This drug at present, however, has no defined role in the management of encephalopathy.

Cerebral oedema is an important cause of death. *ICP monitoring* with an epidural pressure transducer is used in specialist units [16, 43, 50] allowing detection of subclinical episodes of intracranial hypertension. Control of cerebral oedema may prolong survival giving a greater chance of the patient reaching transplantation [43]. Complications of transducer insertion, including intracranial bleeding and sepsis, occur in about 4%, with fatal haemorrhage in 1% [16]. The type of transducer chosen depends on local expertise, although the complication rate with epidural placement is less than with sub-dural bolts and parenchymal monitors [16]. A platelet count of less than 50×10^9/litre is regarded as a contraindication because of the risk of bleeding [43]. Increases of ICP to 25–30 mmHg sustained for more than 5 min are treated with mannitol 1 g/kg body weight (up to 100 g given in a 20% solution as an intravenous bolus). Urine output must be monitored to confirm a diuresis. In patients with renal failure, mannitol should only be used in combination with ultrafiltration, to avoid hyperosmolarity and fluid overload.

ICP monitoring allows the cerebral perfusion pressure (mean arterial pressure minus ICP) to be calculated. A pressure of less than 50 mmHg has been considered a contraindication to transplantation because of a poor neurological outcome. However, patients with a lower perfusion pressure and prolonged intracranial hypertension (greater than 35 mmHg for 24–38 h) have survived with complete neurological recovery [23].

Monitoring of the *jugular bulb venous oxygen saturation* may be used but this approach is not widespread. The jugular vein is catheterized retrogradely until the catheter tip sits in the jugular bulb. Samples of blood are taken; oxygen saturations of less than 55% indicate cerebral ischaemia. This is managed either by increasing blood flow, decreasing ICP or using agents to reduce the metabolic demands of the brain. Oxygen saturations of greater than 85% may reflect a hyperaemic cerebral circulation which similarly needs correcting [48].

It is important to nurse the patient with the upper trunk and head elevated between 20 and 30° above the horizontal since this lowers ICP. Further elevation may raise ICP and lower mean arterial pressure [21]. Corticosteroids are not effective. Hyperventilation, to induce cerebral vasoconstriction and reduce cerebral blood volume, has an effect which is not sustained [29]. Thiopental infusion by decreasing the cerebral metabolic rate, is effective in some patients where mannitol and haemofiltration have failed [37] but because of possible haemodynamic effects should be done with ICP monitoring.

Hypothermia prevents brain oedema experimentally either by reducing blood–brain transfer of ammonia and/or by reducing extra-cellular brain glutamate concentrations [73]. Preliminary studies in patients with acute liver failure also show a reduction in ICP. Further studies are needed to optimize this approach and determine whether it can be used to stabilize patients until a donor liver is available [42]. These results emphasize however, that hyperthermia should be avoided.

When ICP monitoring cannot be done, the clinical team should be alert for signs of raised ICP (see above), and administer mannitol if this is suspected.

Epileptiform activity detected by EEG should be treated with phenytoin, to reduce the increase in cerebral oxygen consumption that occurs [32].

N-acetylcysteine, initially introduced and validated for the acute treatment (12–15 h) of acetaminophen self-poisoning, has been shown to be of value in patients with acetaminophen-induced acute liver failure when continued for longer than the first 16 h [44]. Survival is increased, and cerebral oedema, hypotension and renal failure reduced. A previous study suggesting that N-acetylcysteine improves blood flow and oxygen

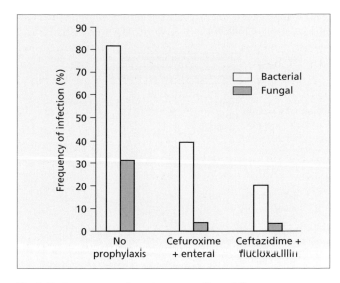

Fig. 8.5. Prevention of sepsis in acute liver failure: comparison of results from studies at King's College Hospital. Prophylactic parenteral antibiotics reduced infections. Enteral decontamination had no additional benefit. Oral amphotericin B (antifungal) was given with both antimicrobial regimens. (Data from [67, 68, 70, 71] courtesy of Dr N. Rolando.)

delivery and extraction in acute liver failure has not been substantiated [87].

Corticosteroids. Large doses of corticosteroids are of no benefit in acute liver failure. They may even be of negative value. The complications include infections and gastric erosions.

Artificial and bio-artificial liver support

The aim is to provide support until the native liver recovers its function spontaneously, or until a donor liver is available. Much research has focused on the use of columns or membranes that would allow removal of toxic metabolites. Charcoal haemoperfusion, despite early promise, has not shown benefit in controlled trials [59]. More recent *artificial liver support* systems (Bio-Logic-DT™ and the Molecular Absorbent Recirculating System [MARS]) [65] use systems which attempt to remove tightly protein-bound toxins by perfusion over resins or albumin. The MARS system uses an albumin-impregnated dialysis membrane and a dialysate containing 5% human albumin. The dialysate is perfused over charcoal and resin adsorbents and finally dialysed to remove water-soluble toxins including ammonia. Preliminary experience with both of these artificial liver support systems have shown some benefit but controlled studies in the setting of acute liver failure are awaited.

Bio-artificial liver support systems use bio-reactors containing viable hepatocytes in culture. Three systems have reached an advanced stage of clinical assessment:

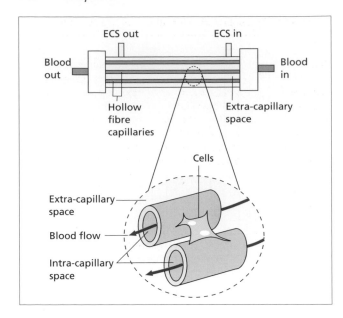

Fig. 8.6. Bio-artificial liver support. Diagram of hollow fibre cartridge device. Cells are cultured on the extra-capillary side of the semipermeable fibres while blood or medium flows through the lumen. ECS, extra-capillary space. (From [82] with permission.)

the 'Bio-artificial Liver' (BAL), the 'Extra-corporeal Liver Assist Device' (ELAD) [30] and the 'Berlin Extra-corporeal Liver support System' (BELS) [28, 65]. The BAL and BELS systems use primary porcine hepatocytes, while the ELAD system uses a hepatoblastoma cell line. Anticoagulated plasma or whole blood is passed through a device allowing metabolic transfer between cells and perfusate (fig. 8.6). Protocols differ as to whether the plasma or blood is first passed over a charcoal column or other device. None of the systems use primary human hepatocytes. Whether the use of a mixture of parenchymal and non-parenchymal cells is more effective is not yet known.

The function of such bio-artificial liver devices has been shown experimentally. Preliminary results in patients with acute liver failure have been encouraging with a reduction in encephalopathy, serum ammonia and ICP, an increase in cerebral perfusion and an improvement in prothrombin time, factor 5 level and galactose elimination capacity. A pilot controlled study of the ELAD system showed no statistically significant benefit. In patients with acute liver failure treated with the BAL system, 18 showed statistically significant improvement in level of consciousness, a reduction in intracranial hypertension and an increase in cerebral perfusion pressure [88]. A randomized control trial is in progress. These techniques hold promise for the future but whether the results will ever regularly lead to a recovery of the native liver rather than bridge the gap to successful transplantation remains to be seen.

Liver transplantation

Hepatic transplantation has to be considered for patients reaching grade 3 and 4 coma due to fulminant hepatic failure. The survival rate for these patients without transplantation is usually less than 20%. Survival rates with transplantation are 60–80%. However, it is frequently difficult to judge both the right time and the necessity for transplant. If too early, the operation may be unnecessary and the patient will be committed to lifetime immunosuppression; if too late, the chances of successful transplantation are reduced.

Indications [92]. The decision to select ('list') an individual for potential transplant is based on validated criteria (see prognosis section above). These include pH, age, aetiology, time between onset of jaundice and encephalopathy, prothrombin time and serum bilirubin level [58], or a plasma factor V level of less than 20% of normal [11]. In the original studies, use of these criteria identified about 95% of fatal cases. The predictive accuracy of these criteria in subsequent studies is in some cases above and in others below the original report, but the criteria remain central to the assessment of the patient admitted with acute liver failure [3, 62, 80].

However, there is a delay on average of about 2 days in obtaining an acceptable donor liver after putting out the request. Although the majority will have survived and still require a transplant, and some will have improved and not need a transplant, some will have died (table 8.9) or developed problems that make them inappropriate to transplant. The prognostic criteria have a lower predictive value (around 50%; range 17–82%) in identifying which patients will not need a transplant [66]. This has led to the suggestion that all patients with hyper-acute and acute (fulminant and sub-fulminant) liver failure should be listed for transplantation on admission to hospital, or when they reach grade 3 encephalopathy [62], and that the decision as to whether or not transplantation is necessary should be reviewed when the donor liver becomes available.

These prognostic uncertainties emphasize the need for early dialogue and transfer of patients with acute liver failure to a specialist liver unit with the facilities for transplantation (table 8.10). Children in particular

Table 8.9. Hepatic transplantation for acute liver failure (Paris experience) [7]

Number of patients	112
Died waiting	18%
Transplanted	92
Alive	71%

Table 8.10. Checklist of information when referring patient with fulminant hepatic failure to liver unit

Patient details

Probable cause of liver failure

Risk factors

Drug overdose, when taken, blood levels, treatment

Past medical history

Previous surgery

Previous psychiatric history

Cardiorespiratory status

Current grade of encephalopathy

Assessment of renal and septic status

Obvious Kayser–Fleischer rings

Weight and height

Investigations

Full blood count, platelets

Prothrombin time (fibrin degradation products)

Urea, sodium, potassium, bicarbonate, creatinine, blood glucose, amylase

Bilirubin, transaminase, alkaline phosphatase, albumin

Blood gases

Urine output

Positive bacteriological culture

Viral serology (HAV IgM, HBsAg, HB core IgM)

Chest X-ray

Central venous pressure

Current medication/fluid regime

Scanning data: liver, brain

Electroencephalogram

Table 8.11. Transplantation for fulminant hepatic failure

Centre	References	Date	Number	Survival (%)
London/ Cambridge	Williams and O'Grady [91]	1990	56	58
Paris	Devictor et al. [24]	1992	19	68
San Francisco	Ascher et al. [5]	1995	35	92
Pittsburgh	Dodson et al. [26]	1994	115	60
Paris	Bismuth et al. [14]	1995	116	68
USA (12 centres)	Schiødt et al. [77]	1999	121	76
European Registry	Fischer et al. [34]	1999	2205	61

should be transferred before the development of hepatic encephalopathy.

Contraindications. Absolute contraindications are active ongoing infection; ARDS and inspired oxygen of greater than 60%; fixed dilated pupils for prolonged periods of time (1 h or more); and cerebral perfusion pressure <40 mmHg or ICP >35 mmHg for longer than 1–2 h [92]. Relative contraindications are a rapidly increasing requirement for vasopressor support, infection under treatment and a history of psychiatric problems [55].

Results. Technically the operation is less difficult than that for chronic liver disease as portal venous collaterals and adhesions are not present. Coagulation defects can be controlled with plasma derivatives and platelets.

Published results worldwide show a survival between 60 and 90% (table 8.11), the variation probably reflecting the severity of illness at the time of transplantation and the criteria for proceeding with transplantation. Survival is less than that seen overall when transplantation is done for liver cirrhosis [34]. The results in acute liver failure compare with an estimated 20% survival of patients reaching this stage of disease who are not

transplanted. Donor livers are hard to find at short notice, and livers that are not ideal, e.g. with an incompatible blood group or steatosis, may be used. This worsens the results [14].

Analysis of the influence of pre-transplantation status on outcome in acute liver failure has shown that in non-acetaminophen-induced liver failure, survival is related to aetiology and serum creatinine [25]. At the time of transplant indices of the severity of systemic illness (organ system failure and APACHE III score) and serum creatinine discriminated survivors from non-survivors. In the acetaminophen group, time from ingestion to transplantation was significantly shorter in the survivors than non-survivors (4 ± 1 vs. 6 ± 1 days). At the time of transplantation serum bilirubin and APACHE III score correlated with survival [25].

Liver transplantation has been performed in patients with fulminant hepatitis A, B and presumed non-A–E. Results in patients with hepatitis B are particularly satisfactory as the disease does not usually recur in the transplanted liver.

Auxiliary liver transplantation

The native liver is left in place, and the donor liver graft either placed in the right upper quadrant alongside the native liver (heterotopic), or part of the native liver is resected and replaced with a reduced size graft (orthotopic). The intention is to provide viable liver function from the graft, giving the native liver time to recover and regenerate. The advantage over conventional transplantation is the temporary need for immunosuppression.

Analysis of 47 patients transplanted in 12 European centres showed no difference in 1-year patient survival between those having a conventional orthotopic liver transplant (61% survival) compared with auxiliary liver transplantation (62%) [84]. Of patients surviving 1 year after auxiliary liver transplantation, 65% were free of immunosuppressive treatment. These results suggest that auxiliary liver transplantation (particularly partial orthotopic) may have an advantage over conventional orthotopic liver transplantation in acute liver failure because with a similar 1-year survival there is a chance of life free of immunosuppression. Reliable criteria to indicate which patients are most likely to benefit from this technique are needed. Factors associated with a high likelihood of complete liver regeneration include an age less than 40 years, liver failure due to acetaminophen or hepatitis A or B infection, and a delay between the onset of jaundice and encephalopathy of less than 7 days [18]. The problem with these criteria, however, is that they have been recognized as indicating favourable outcome even in patients with conservative management [34].

Living related liver transplantation

This is a well-established procedure of liver transplantation for children using a left or left lateral lobe from a living donor. It has been used in patients with fulminant/sub-fulminant hepatic failure [53] with a 90% 1-year survival in 14 recipients. The post-operative course in all donors was uneventful. Concerns with this approach for acute liver failure include issues of informed consent under the pressure of an emergency situation which may interfere with a potential donor's ability to make a well-considered decision. Additionally there are issues as to whether the hepatocyte mass from a left or left lateral hepatic lobe is always able to sustain recovery in such patients [34].

Hepatocyte transplantation

In experimental animals with acute liver failure hepatocyte transplantation may improve survival. Only a small number of cells is necessary, between 0.5 and 3% of the normal hepatocyte mass. A limited number of studies have been done in patients with acute liver failure who were not candidates for liver transplantation [13, 65]. There was an improvement in encephalopathy score, arterial ammonia, prothrombin time, and aminopyrine and caffeine clearances. No clinical improvement was seen in the first 24h after hepatocyte transplantation. None of the patients survived. Immunosuppression is necessary for the survival of the transplanted cells. Complications include hypoxaemia and infiltrates on chest X-ray after intraportal hepatocyte transplantation. No randomized, controlled data are available. Developments are needed in the method of delivery of hepatocytes, the prophylaxis of infections and strategies for preventing rejection without the need for immunosuppressive drugs.

Conclusion

Liver transplantation cannot be accepted as the perfect and ideal treatment for fulminant hepatic failure, but it gives survival to many patients who otherwise would have died. Early referral of patients to a specialist centre must be emphasized. This will increase the chance of the patient being fit enough for transfer. Delayed action loses the window of opportunity for safe transfer and greater success of transplantation. There are still considerable selection difficulties. Some patients will clearly be candidates for transplant, some will obviously be unsuitable. The doubt lies in the intermediate cases and how many in this category will recover with conservative treatment alone. The initial selection of potential candidates for transplantation is separate from the final decision to proceed. The success and role of artificial liver support systems and of auxiliary and living related liver transplantation await further evaluation.

References

1 Acharya SK, Dasarathy S, Kumer TL *et al.* Fulminant hepatitis in a tropical population: clinical course, and early predictors of outcome. *Hepatology* 1996; **23**: 1448.

2 Acharya SK, Panda SK, Saxena A *et al.* Acute hepatic failure in India: a perspective from the East. *J. Gastroenterol. Hepatol.* 2000; **15**: 473.

3 Anand AC, Nightingale P, Neuberger JM. Early indicators of prognosis in fulminant hepatic failure: an assessment of the King's criteria. *J. Hepatol.* 1997; **26**: 62.

4 Andreu V, Mas A, Bruguera M *et al.* Ecstasy: a common cause of severe acute hepatotoxicity. *J. Hepatol.* 1998; **29**: 394.

5 Ascher NL, Lake JR, Emond JC *et al.* Liver transplantation for fulminant hepatic failure. *Arch. Surg.* 1995; **128**: 677.

6 Banks AT, Zimmerman HJ, Ishak KG *et al.* Diclofenac-associated hepatotoxicity: analysis of 180 cases reported to the Food and Drug Administration as adverse reactions. *Hepatology* 1995; **22**: 820.

7 Benhamou JP. *Fulminant Hepatic Failure.* American Association for the Study of the Liver Disease Course Syllabus, 1990.

8 Bernal W, Wendon J. Acute liver failure; clinical features and management. *Eur. J. Gastroenterol. Hepatol.* 1999; **11**: 977.

9 Bernal W, Wendon J, Rela M *et al.* Use and outcome of liver transplantation in acetaminophen-induced acute liver failure. *Hepatology* 1998; **27**: 1050.

10 Bernuau J, Benhamou JP. Classifying acute liver failure. *Lancet* 1993; **342**: 252.

11 Bernuau J, Goudeau A, Poynard T *et al.* Multivariate analysis of prognostic factors in fulminant hepatitis B. *Hepatology* 1986; **6**: 648.

12 Bernuau J, Rueff B, Benhamou JP. Fulminant and subfulminant liver failure: definitions and causes. *Semin. Liver Dis.* 1986; **6**: 97.

13 Bilir BM, Guinette D, Karrer F *et al.* Hepatocyte transplantation in acute liver failure. *Liver Transplant.* 2000; **6**: 32.

14 Bismuth H, Samuel D, Castaing D *et al.* Orthotopic liver transplantation in fulminant and subfulminant hepatitis. The Paul Brousse experience. *Ann. Surg.* 1995; **222**: 109.

15 Blei AT, Larsen FS. Pathophysiology of cerebral oedema in fulminant hepatic failure. *J. Hepatol.* 1999; **31**: 771.

16 Blei AT, Olafsson S, Webster S *et al.* Complications of intracranial pressure monitoring in fulminant hepatic failure. *Lancet* 1993; **341**: 157.

17 Charlton M, Adjei P, Poterucha J *et al*. TT-virus infection in North American blood donors, patients with fulminant hepatic failure, and cryptogenic cirrhosis. *Hepatology* 1998; **28**: 839.

18 Chenard-Neu MP, Boudjema K, Bernuau J *et al*. Auxiliary liver transplantation: regeneration of the native liver and outcome in 30 patients with fulminant hepatic failure—a multicentre European study. *Hepatology* 1996; **23**: 1119.

19 Chu C-M, Sheen I-S, Liaw Y-F. The role of hepatitis C virus in fulminant viral hepatitis in an area with endemic hepatitis A and B. *Gastroenterology* 1994; **107**: 189.

20 Clemmesen JO, Larsen FS, Kondrup J *et al*. Cerebral herniation in patients with acute liver failure is correlated with arterial ammonia concentration. *Hepatology* 1999; **29**: 648.

21 Davenport A, Will EJ, Davison AM. Effect of posture on intracranial pressure and cerebral perfusion pressure in patients with fulminant hepatic and renal failure after acetaminophen self-poisoning. *Crit. Care Med*. 1990; **18**: 286.

22 Davenport A, Will EJ, Losowsky MS *et al*. Continuous arteriovenous haemofiltration in patients with hepatic encephalopathy and renal failure. *Br. Med. J*. 1987; **295**: 1028.

23 Davies M, Mutimer D, Lowes J *et al*. Recovery despite impaired cerebral perfusion in fulminant hepatic failure. *Lancet* 1994; **343**: 1329.

24 Devictor D, Desplanques L, Debray D *et al*. Emergency liver transplantation for fulminant liver failure in infants and children. *Hepatology* 1992; **16**: 1156.

25 Devlin J, Wendon J, Heaton N *et al*. Pretransplantation clinical status and outcome of emergency transplantation for acute liver failure. *Hepatology* 1995; **21**: 1018.

26 Dodson SF, Dehara K, Iwatsuki S. Liver transplantation for fulminant hepatic failure. *ASAIO J*. 1994; **40**: 86.

27 Donaldson BW, Gopinath R, Wanless IR *et al*. The role of transjugular liver biopsy in fulminant liver failure: relation to other prognostic indicators. *Hepatology* 1993; **18**: 1370.

28 Dowling DJ, Mutimer DJ. Artificial liver support in acute liver failure. *Eur. J. Gastroenterol. Hepatol*. 1999; **11**: 991.

29 Ede RJ, Gimson AES, Bihari D *et al*. Controlled hyperventilation in the prevention of cerebral oedema in fulminant hepatic failure. *J. Hepatol*. 1986; **2**: 43.

30 Ellis AJ, Hughes RD, Wendon JA *et al*. Pilot controlled trial of the extracorporeal liver assist device in acute liver failure. *Hepatology* 1996; **24**: 1446.

31 Ellis AJ, Saleh M, Smith H *et al*. Late-onset hepatic failure: clinical features, serology and outcome following transplantation. *J. Hepatol*. 1995; **23**: 363.

32 Ellis AJ, Wendon JA, Williams R. Subclinical seizure activity and prophylactic phenytoin infusion in acute liver failure: a controlled clinical trial. *Hepatology* 2000; **32**: 536.

33 Ferenci P. Brain dysfunction in fulminant hepatic failure. *J. Hepatol*. 1994; **21**: 487.

34 Fischer L, Sterneck M, Rogiers X. Liver transplantation for acute liver failure. *Eur. J. Gastroenterol. Hepatol*. 1999; **11**: 985.

35 Fisher NC, Cooper MA, Hastings JGM *et al*. Fungal colonization and fluconazole therapy in acute liver disease. *Liver* 1998; **18**: 320.

36 Flowers MA, Heathcote J, Wanless IR *et al*. Fulminant hepatitis as a consequence of reactivation of hepatitis B virus infection after discontinuation of low-dose methotrexate therapy. *Ann. Intern. Med*. 1990; **112**: 381.

37 Forbes A, Alexander GJM, O'Grady JG *et al*. Thiopental infusion in the treatment of intracranial hypertension complicating fulminant hepatic failure. *Hepatology* 1989; **10**: 306.

38 Hanau C, Munoz SJ, Rubin R. Histopathological heterogeneity in fulminant hepatic failure. *Hepatology* 1995; **21**: 345.

39 Harrison R, Letz G, Pasternak G *et al*. Fulminant hepatic failure after occupational exposure to 2-nitropropane. *Ann. Intern. Med*. 1987; **107**: 466.

40 Herzog D, Rasquin-Weber A-M, Debray D *et al*. Subfulminant hepatic failure in autoimmune hepatitis type 1: an unusual form of presentation. *J. Hepatol*. 1997; **27**: 578.

41 Hoofnagle JH, Carithers RL, Shapiro C *et al*. Fulminant hepatic failure: summary of a workshop. *Hepatology* 1995; **21**: 240.

42 Jalan R, Damink SWMO, Deutz NEP *et al*. Moderate hypothermia for uncontrolled intracranial hypertension in acute liver failure. *Lancet* 1999; **354**: 1164.

43 Keays RT, Alexander GJM, Williams R. The safety and value of extradural intracranial pressure monitors in fulminant hepatic failure. *J. Hepatol*. 1993; **18**: 205.

44 Keays R, Harrison PM, Wendon JA *et al*. Intravenous acetylcysteine in paracetamol induced fulminant hepatic failure: a prospective controlled trial. *Br. Med. J*. 1991; **303**: 1026.

45 Klein AS, Hart J, Brems JJ *et al*. Amanita poisoning: treatment and the role of liver transplantation. *Am. J. Med*. 1989; **86**: 187.

46 Langnas AN, Markin RS, Cattral MS *et al*. Parvovirus B19 as a possible causative agent of fulminant liver failure and associated aplastic anaemia. *Hepatology* 1995; **22**: 1661.

47 Larsen FS, Ejlersen E, Clemmesen JO *et al*. Preservation of cerebral oxidative metabolism in fulminant hepatic failure: an autoregulation study. *Liver Transplant. Surg*. 1996; **2**: 348.

48 Larsen FS, Knudsen GM, Hansen BA. Pathophysiological changes in cerebral circulation, oxidative metabolism and blood–brain barrier in patients with acute liver failure. *J. Hepatol*. 1997; **27**: 231.

49 Lau JYN, Sallie R, Fang JWS *et al*. Detection of hepatitis E virus genome and gene products in two patients with fulminant hepatitis E. *J. Hepatol*. 1995; **22**: 605.

50 Lidofsky SD, Bass NM, Prager MC *et al*. Intracranial pressure monitoring and liver transplantation for fulminant liver failure. *Hepatology* 1992; **16**: 1.

51 Makin A, Williams R. Paracetamol hepatoxicity and alcohol consumption in deliberate and accidental overdose. *Q. J. Med*. 2000; **93**: 341.

52 Mitchell I, Bihari D, Chang R *et al*. Earlier identification of patients at risk from acetaminophen-induced acute liver failure. *Crit. Care Med*. 1998; **26**: 279.

53 Miwa S, Hashikura Y, Mita A *et al*. Living-related liver transplantation for patients with fulminant and subfulminant hepatic failure. *Hepatology* 1999; **30**: 1521.

54 Moore K. Renal failure in acute liver failure. *Eur. J. Gastroenterol. Hepatol*. 1999; **11**: 967.

55 Mutimer DJ, Ayres RCS, Neuberger JM *et al*. Serious paracetamol poisoning and the results of liver transplantation. *Gut* 1994; **35**: 809.

56 Myers RP, Gregor JC, Marotta PJ. The cost-effectiveness of hepatitis A vaccination in patients with chronic hepatitis C. *Hepatology* 2000; **31**: 834.

57 O'Brien CJ, Wise RJS, O'Grady JG *et al*. Neurological sequelae in patients recovered from fulminant hepatic failure. *Gut* 1987; **28**: 93.

58 O'Grady JG, Alexander GJM, Hayllar KM *et al*. Early indicators of prognosis in fulminant hepatic failure. *Gastroenterology* 1989; **97**: 439.

59 O'Grady JG, Gimson AES, O'Brien CJ *et al.* Controlled trials of charcoal haemoperfusion and prognostic factors in fulminant hepatic failure. *Gastroenterology* 1988; **94**: 1186.

60 O'Grady JG, Schalm SW, Williams R. Acute liver failure: redefining the syndromes. *Lancet* 1993; **342**: 273.

61 Papaevangelou G, Tassopoulos N, Roumeliotou-Karayannis A *et al.* Etiology of fulminant viral hepatitis in Greece. *Hepatology* 1984; **4**: 369.

62 Pauwels A, Mostefa-Kara N, Florent C *et al.* Emergency liver transplantation for acute liver failure: evaluation of London and Clichy criteria. *J. Hepatol.* 1993; **17**: 124.

63 Pernambuco JR, Langley PG, Hughes RD *et al.* Activation of the fibrinolytic system in patients with fulminant liver failure. *Hepatology* 1993; **18**: 1350.

64 Prince MI, Thomas SHL, James OFW *et al.* Reduction in incidence of severe paracetamol poisoning. *Lancet* 2000; **355**: 2047.

65 Riordan SM, Williams R. Acute liver failure: targeted artificial and hepatocyte-based support of liver regeneration and reversal of multiorgan failure. *J. Hepatol.* 2000; **32** (Suppl. 1): 63.

66 Riordan SM, Williams R. Use and validation of selection criteria for liver transplantation in acute liver failure. *Liver Transplant.* 2000; **6**: 170.

67 Rolando N, Gimson A, Wade J *et al.* Prospective controlled trial of selective parenteral and enteral antimicrobial regimen in fulminant hepatic failure. *Hepatology* 1993; **17**: 196.

68 Rolando N, Harvey F, Brahm J *et al.* Prospective study of bacterial infection in acute liver failure: an analysis of 50 patients. *Hepatology* 1990; **11**: 49.

69 Rolando N, Harvey F, Brahm J *et al.* Fungal infection: a common, unrecognized complication of acute liver failure. *J. Hepatol.* 1991; **12**: 1.

70 Rolando N, Philpott HJ, Williams R. Bacterial and fungal infection in acute liver failure. *Semin. Liver Dis.* 1996; **16**: 389.

71 Rolando N, Wade JJ, Stangou A *et al.* Prospective study comparing the efficacy of prophylactic parenteral antimicrobials, with or without enteral decontamination, in patients with acute liver failure. *Liver Transplant. Surg.* 1996; **2**: 8.

72 Rolando N, Wade J, Davalos M *et al.* The systemic inflammatory response syndrome in acute liver failure. *Hepatology* 2000; **32**: 734.

73 Rose C, Michalak A, Pannunzio M *et al.* Mild hypothermia delays the onset of coma and prevents brain oedema and extracellular brain glutamate accumulation in rats with acute liver failure. *Hepatology* 2000; **31**: 872.

74 Rowbotham D, Wendon J, Williams R. Acute liver failure secondary to hepatic infiltration: a single centre experience of 18 cases. *Gut* 1998; **42**: 576.

75 Sallie R, Chiyende J, Tan KC *et al.* Fulminant hepatic failure resulting from coexistent Wilson's disease and hepatitis E. *Gut* 1994; **35**: 849.

76 Saracco G, Macagno S, Rosina F *et al.* Serologic markers with fulminant hepatitis in persons positive for hepatitis B surface antigen. A worldwide epidemiologic and clinical survey. *Ann. Intern. Med.* 1988; **108**: 380.

77 Schiødt FV, Atillasoy E, Shakil AO *et al.* Etiology and outcome for 295 patients with acute liver failure in the United States. *Liver Transplant. Surg.* 1999; **5**: 29.

78 Sergi C, Jundt K, Seipp S *et al.* The distribution of HBV, HCV and HGV among livers with fulminant hepatic failure of different aetiology. *J. Hepatol.* 1998; **29**: 861.

79 Shakil AO, Jones BC, Lee RG *et al.* Prognostic value of abdominal CT scanning and hepatic histopathology in patients with acute liver failure. *Dig. Dis. Sci.* 2000; **45**: 334.

80 Shakil AO, Kramer D, Mazariegos GV *et al.* Acute liver failure: clinical features, outcome analysis, and applicability of prognostic criteria. *Liver Transplant.* 2000; **6**: 163.

81 Sheikh NM, Philen RM, Love LA. Chaparral-associated hepatotoxicity. *Arch. Intern. Med.* 1997; **157**: 913.

82 Sussman NL, Chong MG, Koussayer T *et al.* Reversal of fulminant hepatic failure using an extracorporeal liver assist device. *Hepatology* 1992; **16**: 60.

83 Turvill JL, Burroughs AK, Moore KP. Change in occurrence of paracetamol overdose in UK after introduction of blister packets. *Lancet* 2000; **355**: 2048.

84 van Hoek B, de Boer J, Boudjema K *et al.* Auxiliary vs. orthotopic liver transplantation for acute liver failure. *J. Hepatol.* 1999; **30**: 699.

85 Vento S, Cainelli F, Mirandola F *et al.* Fulminant hepatitis on withdrawal of chemotherapy in carriers of hepatitis C virus. *Lancet* 1996; **347**: 92.

86 Vento S, Garofano T, Renzini C *et al.* Fulminant hepatitis associated with hepatitis A virus superinfection in patients with chronic hepatitis C. *N. Engl. J. Med.* 1998; **338**: 286.

87 Walsh TS, Hopton P, Philips BJ *et al.* The effect of *N*-acetylcysteine on oxygen transport and uptake in patients with fulminant hepatic failure. *Hepatology* 1998; **27**: 1332.

88 Watanabe FD, Mullon CJ-P, Hewitt WR *et al.* Clinical experience with a bioartificial liver in the treatment of severe liver failure. *Ann. Surg.* 1997; **225**: 484.

89 Wendon JA, Harrison PM, Keays R *et al.* Cerebral blood flow and metabolism in fulminant liver failure. *Hepatology* 1994; **19**: 1407.

90 Williams R. New directions in acute liver failure. *J. R. Coll. Physicians Lond.* 1994; **28**: 552.

91 Williams R, O'Grady JG. Liver transplantation: results, advances and problems. *J. Gastroenterol. Hepatol.* 1990; **5** (Suppl. 1): 110.

92 Williams R, Wendon J. Indications for orthotopic liver transplantation in fulminant liver failure. *Hepatology* 1994; **20**: 5S.

93 Zimmerman HJ, Maddrey WC. Acetaminophen (paracetamol) hepatotoxicity with regular intake of alcohol: analysis of instances of therapeutic misadventure. *Hepatology* 1995; **22**: 767.

Chapter 9
Ascites

Ascites is free fluid within the peritoneal cavity. It forms because of conditions directly involving the peritoneum (infection, malignancy), or diseases remote from the peritoneum (liver disease, heart failure, hypoproteinaemia). Cirrhosis is the commonest cause in the Western world, with malignancy, and less frequently cardiac failure and tuberculous peritonitis, being responsible for most other cases.

The pathophysiology underlying the formation of ascites in cirrhosis is complex. This is reflected in the number of theories put forward. There are many neurohormonal, renal and systemic vascular abnormalities. Theories have evolved as new observations are made to piece together the jigsaw of interactions leading to ascites.

The abnormalities associated with the formation of ascites in patients with cirrhosis are:
- portal hypertension
- renal retention of sodium
- splanchnic arterial vasodilatation
- systemic vascular changes
- increased splanchnic and hepatic lymph formation
- hypoalbuminaemia.

Portal hypertension and renal retention of sodium are universal. At their most extreme the abnormalities related to cirrhosis and ascites lead to the *hepato-renal syndrome*.

New avenues of treatment being explored have followed advances in knowledge, such as the use of splanchnic vasoconstrictors for hepato-renal syndrome. Drugs to increase water loss (aquaretics) are under investigation.

Liver transplantation is the ultimate therapy for ascites and hepato-renal syndrome. Replacement of the liver reverses the renal changes. However, this approach is only practical for the relatively stable patient. It is impracticable for rapidly progressing hepato-renal syndrome. New therapeutic strategies are needed to buy time before a donor liver becomes available.

Mechanism of ascites formation [27]

All proposed mechanisms involve inappropriate renal sodium and water retention, either secondary to vascular changes (*underfill and peripheral arterial vasodilatation hypotheses*) or as a primary event (*overfill theory*) (table 9.1). Liver disease and portal hypertenion are central to the process. Increased lymph production from the liver and splanchnic capillaries leads to ascites. Changes in the peritoneal membrane and its permeability may contribute.

Underfill and peripheral vasodilatation hypotheses

Vascular changes

Many circulatory changes are found in patients with cirrhosis, particularly as disease advances and there is decompensation (table 9.2). Theories of ascites formation based on vascular changes depend upon stimulation of the renin–angiotensin–aldosterone system (RAAS) as a result of a reduced effective circulating volume—that is, the compartment interacting with volume and baroreceptors.

The traditional *underfill theory* proposed sequestration of blood in the splanchnic venous bed, which with peripheral vasodilatation associated with arteriovenous shunting led to a reduction in the central vascular compartment.

The current modification of this theory is based upon *peripheral arterial vasodilatation* (fig. 9.1). Splanchnic arterial vasodilatation is found in some patients with cirrhosis and portal hypertension. Nitric oxide is thought to play a central role. This leads to net arterial vasodilatation, reduced arterial vascular resistance, increased cardiac output and reduced filling of the central pressure monitoring compartment. RAAS and sympathetic activity are increased. Splanchnic arterial vasodilatation is accompanied systemically by vasoconstriction in the renal, cerebral and muscle vascular beds.

Table 9.1. Sequence of events for the hypotheses of ascites formation

	Underfill/peripheral arterial vasodilatation	Overfill
Primary event	Vascular	Renal
Secondary event	Renal	Vascular

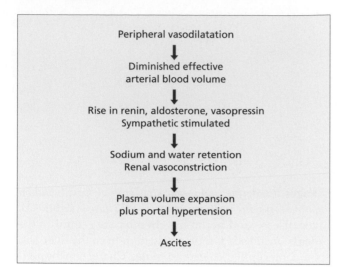

Fig. 9.1. The peripheral arterial vasodilatation hypothesis for ascites formation in cirrhosis [70].

Table 9.2. Circulatory changes in patients with cirrhosis

Increased	Plasma/total blood volume
	Non-central blood volume
	Cardiac output
	Portal pressure and flow
Reduced	Central blood volume
	Arterial blood pressure
	Splanchnic vascular resistance
	Systemic vascular resistance
	Renal blood flow

Vasodilators (table 9.3)

The factors responsible for splanchnic and peripheral arterial vasodilatation are not clearly understood. Some vasodilators may be of intestinal origin. Endothelial cells may respond to changes in shear stress, endotoxin or cytokines with the production of vasodilators such as nitric oxide. Nitric oxide synthesis is increased in cirrhotic patients. There is increased plasma nitric oxide and its metabolites, and increased nitric oxide in exhaled air [50]. Plasma concentrations of nitric oxide are higher in portal venous than peripheral venous blood, suggesting increased splanchnic production. In an experimental model of cirrhosis, inhibition of nitric oxide synthase significantly reduces plasma renin, aldosterone and vasopressin levels, and increases renal sodium and water excretion [51].

Another new potent vasodilator peptide, adrenomedullin, may also play a role. Plasma levels are increased in cirrhotic patients with ascites [31].

Table 9.3. Vasodilators implicated in vascular changes of cirrhosis and vasoconstrictors

	Vasodilators	Vasoconstrictors
Renal	Prostaglandin E_2	Endothelin-1
	Nitric oxide	Thromboxane A_2
	Kallikrein–kinin system	Angiotensin II
	Prostacyclin	Leukotrienes
		Adenosine
Systemic	Nitric oxide	Angiotensin II
	Atrial natriuretic peptide	Noradrenaline
	Adrenomedullin	Antidiuretic hormone
	Calcitonin gene-related peptide	Neuropeptide Y

Renal changes

Total body sodium and water balance depends upon the control of sodium and water reabsorption in the distal tubule and collecting duct. This is regulated by the RAAS and anti-diuretic hormone (ADH, vasopressin).

Renin is produced by the kidney in response to stretching of the afferent glomerular arterioles, and to renal baroreceptor and β-adrenergic stimulation. Under the influence of renin, angiotensinogen (produced by the liver) is converted to angiotensin I (a decapeptide), which in turn is converted to angiotensin II (an octapeptide) by angiotensin-converting enzyme (ACE). Angiotensin II is the main stimulant to the synthesis and secretion of aldosterone, a mineralocorticoid, from the glomerular cells of the adrenal cortex.

Aldosterone acts on cells in the collecting duct(ule), and through a cytoplasmic interaction increases both luminal uptake and basolateral passage of sodium.

Other factors affecting renin release are angiotensin II, nitric oxide, atrial natriuretic peptide (ANP), vasopressin (ADH), and adenosine (inhibitory), and prostaglandins, kallikrein, calcitonin and TNF-α (stimulatory). Angiotensin II also stimulates sodium and water retention in the proximal tubule.

In patients with cirrhosis and ascites, the normal regulation of sodium balance is lost. Sodium is retained avidly, urinary sodium excretion often being less than 5 mmol/day.

There is increased activity of the RAAS (fig. 9.2). Plasma levels of these hormones are increased because of stimulation of volume receptors in the central circulation. This is due to a reduction in 'effective circulating blood volume', which also activates the sympathetic system (raised circulating noradrenaline).

Naturesis after spironolactone therapy (an aldosterone antagonist) supports hyperaldosteronism as having an active part in sodium retention of the cirrhotic.

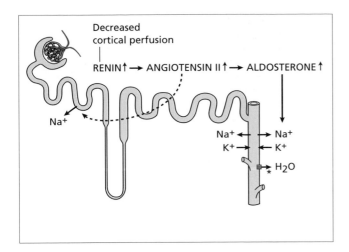

Fig. 9.2. Mechanisms of increased sodium and water reabsorption in cirrhosis. * Increased ADH-stimulated water reabsorption in collecting ducts.

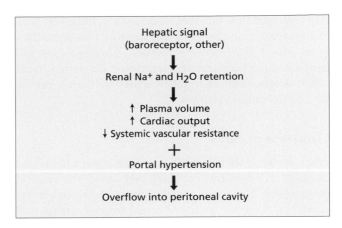

Fig. 9.3. Overfill hypothesis.

Overfill hypothesis (fig. 9.3)

A large proportion (30–60%) of cirrhotic patients do not have a measurable increase in the components of the RAAS. However, some of these patients have a defect of sodium handling even in the absence of ascites. Thus they do not excrete a sodium challenge appropriately and there is a tendency to sodium retention. This finding questions whether sodium and water retention in cirrhotics is truly related to prior systemic vascular changes followed by RAAS activation. An alternative proposal is that there is a primary renal change—responding to a hepatic signal—that leads to sodium retention (*overfill theory*) (fig. 9.3). Several signals have been suggested. Reduced hepatic synthesis of a natriuretic agent, reduced hepatic clearance of a sodium-retaining hormone, or a 'hepato-renal reflex' of unknown aetiology could be responsible. The hypothesis proposes that sodium and water retention lead to expansion of the plasma volume, an increase in cardiac output and a fall in systemic vascular resistance. The combination of portal hypertension and circulatory hypervolaemia lead to ascites. Central to the argument between this *overfill hypothesis* and the theories based on vascular abnormalities is whether or not changes in cardiovascular haemodynamics and in RAAS are present before the first evidence of renal sodium retention. Early involvement of angiotensin II in sodium retention is supported by data showing correction of the subtle renal sodium retention in pre-ascitic cirrhotic patients, with *low* systemic angiotensin II levels, by losartan, an angiotensin II receptor antagonist [28].

Other renal factors

Atrial natriuretic factor (ANF)

This is a potent vaso-relaxant natriuretic peptide released from the cardiac atria, probably in response to intravascular volume expansion. In early compensated cirrhosis, ANF may maintain sodium homeostasis despite the presence of mild anti-natriuretic factors. In the later stages renal resistance to ANF develops, rendering it ineffective. ANF probably has no primary role in the sodium retention of cirrhosis.

Prostaglandins

Several prostaglandins are synthesized in the kidney and although they are not primary regulators they modulate the effects of other factors and hormones locally.

Prostaglandin (PG) I_2 and E_2 are vasodilators, and also increase sodium excretion through vasodilatation and a direct effect on the loop of Henle. They stimulate renin production and inhibit cyclic adenosine monophostate (cAMP) synthesis, thereby interfering with the action of vasopressin (ADH).

Thromboxane A_2 is a vasoconstrictor, reducing renal blood flow, glomerular filtration and perfusion pressure.

$PGI_{2\alpha}$ is synthesized in the tubules and increases sodium and water excretion.

Prostaglandins therefore have a significant role in sodium and water homeostasis. In conditions where there is a reduced circulating volume, which includes cirrhosis, there is increased prostaglandin synthesis. This counterbalances renal vasoconstriction by antagonizing the local effects of renin, angiotensin II, endothelin 1, vasopressin and catecholamines.

The importance of this role is demonstrated clinically by the renal dysfunction seen in cirrhotics when non-steroidal anti-inflammatory agents are given [82]. Without the vasodilatatory influence of prostaglandins renal blood flow and glomerular filtration rate fall because of unopposed vasoconstriction due to renin and other factors. Such an imbalance may be the trigger for the hepato-renal syndrome.

Circulation of ascites

Once formed, ascitic fluid can exchange with blood through an enormous capillary bed under the visceral peritoneum. This plays a vital, dynamic role, sometimes actively facilitating transfer of fluid into the ascites and sometimes retarding it. Ascitic fluid is continuously circulating, with about half entering and leaving the peritoneal cavity every hour, there being a rapid transit in both directions. The constituents of the fluid are in dynamic equilibrium with those of the plasma.

Summary (fig. 9.4)

The *peripheral arterial dilatation hypothesis* of ascites formation proposes that renal sodium and water retention is due to reduced effective blood volume secondary to peripheral arterial vasodilatation particularly in the splanchnic bed. The renal changes are mediated by stimulation of the RAAS, an increase in sympathetic function, and other systemic and local peptide and hormone disturbances.

The *overfill* view suggests that renal retention of sodium is primary with secondary vascular changes and accumulation of ascites and oedema.

The increase in intra-sinusoidal pressure found in cirrhosis and hepatic venous obstruction in Budd–Chiari syndrome stimulates hepatic lymph formation and this adds to the ascites. An active role of the peritoneal capillary membrane in controlling the passage of fluid is possible.

Thus several changes occurring in sequence are responsible for the clinical features. Different disturbances are emphasized according to the stage of liver disease. At the extreme end of the spectrum of renal and vascular changes, hepato-renal syndrome develops.

Clinical features

Onset

Ascites may appear suddenly or develop insidiously over the course of months with accompanying flatulent abdominal distension.

Ascites may develop suddenly when hepato-cellular function is reduced, for instance by haemorrhage, 'shock', infection or an alcoholic debauch. This might be related to the fall in serum albumin values and/or to

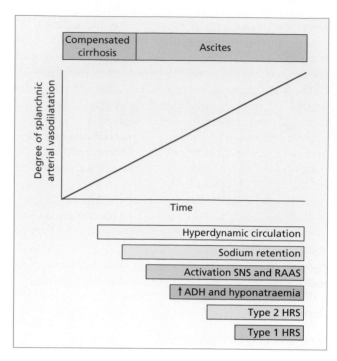

Fig. 9.4. Time course of circulatory, neurohormonal and renal function abnormalities in cirrhosis (in sequence of peripheral arterial vasodilation theory). ADH, antidiuretic hormone; HRS, hepato-renal syndrome; RAAS, renin–angiotensin–aldosterone system; SNS, sympathetic nervous system. (From [9] with permission.)

intravascular fluid depletion. Occlusion of the portal vein may precipitate ascites in a patient with a low serum albumin level.

The insidious onset proclaims a worse prognosis, possibly because it is not associated with any rectifiable factor.

There is gradually increasing abdominal distension and the patient may present with dyspnoea.

Examination

The patient is sallow and dehydrated. Sweating is diminished. Muscle wasting is profound. The thin limbs with the protuberant belly lead to the description of the patient as a 'spider man'. The ascites may be classified into mild, moderate or tense.

The abdomen is distended not only with fluid but also by air in the dilated intestines. The fullness is particularly conspicuous in the flanks. The umbilicus is everted and the distance between the symphysis pubis and umbilicus seems diminished.

The increased intra-abdominal pressure favours the protrusion of hernias in the umbilical, femoral or inguinal regions or through old abdominal incisions. Scrotal oedema is frequent.

Distended abdominal wall veins may represent porto-systemic collateral channels which radiate from the umbilicus and persist after control of the ascites. Inferior vena caval collaterals result from a secondary, functional block of the inferior vena cava due to pressure of the peritoneal fluid. They commonly run from the groin to the costal margin or flanks and disappear when the ascites is controlled and intra-abdominal pressure is reduced. Abdominal striae may develop.

Dullness on percussion in the flanks is the earliest sign and can be detected when about 2 litres are present. The distribution of the dullness differs from that due to enlargement of the bladder, an ovarian tumour or a pregnant uterus when the flanks are resonant to percussion. With tense ascites it is difficult to palpate the abdominal viscera, but with moderate amounts of fluid the liver or spleen may be ballotted.

A fluid thrill means much free fluid; it is a very late sign of fluid under tension.

The lung bases may be dull to percussion due to elevation of the diaphragm.

Secondary effects

A *pleural effusion* is found in about 5–10% of cirrhotics and in 85% of these it is right-sided [40]. It is due to defects in the diaphragm allowing ascites to pass into the pleural cavity (fig. 9.5). This can be shown by introducing ^{131}I albumin or air into the ascites and examining the pleural space afterwards. However, this technique only has a sensitivity of around 70%. Similarly, examination of pleural and ascitic fluid is not reliable to differentiate an effusion due to local pleural disease from that due to ascites [2].

Right hydrothorax may be seen in the absence of ascites due to the negative intra-thoracic pressure during breathing, drawing the peritoneal fluid through the diaphragmatic defects into the pleural cavity [37].

The pleural fluid is in equilibrium with the peritoneal fluid and control depends on medical treatment of the ascites. Aspiration is followed by rapid filling up of the pleural space by ascitic fluid. Transjugular intrahepatic portosystemic shunts (TIPS) have been successful [75].

Spontaneous bacterial empyema may be a complication [83].

Oedema usually follows the ascites and is related to hypoproteinaemia. A functional inferior vena caval block due to pressure of the abdominal fluid is an additional factor.

The *cardiac apex beat* is displaced up and out by the raised diaphragm.

The *neck veins* are distended. This is secondary to the increase in right atrial pressure and intra-pleural pressure which follows tense ascites and a raised diaphragm. A persisting increase in jugular venous pressure after ascites is controlled implies a cardiac cause for the fluid retention.

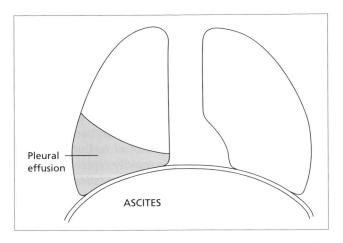

Fig. 9.5. A right-sided pleural effusion may accompany ascites and is related to defects in the diaphragm.

Ascitic fluid

Diagnostic paracentesis (of about 30 ml) is always performed, however obvious the cause of the ascites. Complications, including bowel perforation and haemorrhage can develop rarely after paracentesis in patients with cirrhosis.

Protein concentration rarely exceeds 1–2 g/100 ml. Higher values suggest infection. Obstruction to the hepatic veins (Budd–Chiari syndrome) is usually, but not always, associated with a very high ascitic fluid protein. Pancreatic ascites also has a high protein concentration.

If the serum albumin minus ascites albumin *gradient* is greater than 1.1 g/dl, the patient has portal hypertension.

Electrolyte concentrations are those of other extracellular fluids.

Ascitic fluid protein and white cell count, but not polymorph concentration, increase during a diuresis.

Fluid appears clear, green, straw-coloured or bile-stained. The volume is variable and up to 70 litre have been recorded. A blood-stained fluid indicates malignant disease or a recent paracentesis or an invasive investigation, such as liver biopsy or trans-hepatic cholangiography.

The *protein content* and *white cell count* should be measured and a *film* examined for organisms. Aerobic and anaerobic *cultures* should be performed.

The percentage of positive cultures can be markedly increased if ascitic fluid is inoculated directly into blood culture bottles at the bedside [62].

Cytology. The normal endothelial cells in the peritoneum can resemble malignant cells, so leading to an over-diagnosis of cancer.

The *rate of accumulation of fluid* is variable and depends on the dietary intake of sodium and the ability of the

cefotaxime [61]. This study used intravenous amoxycillin-clavulanic acid followed by oral therapy. Intravenous ciprofloxacin followed by oral treatment is also effective [76].

These regimens are for the initial empirical therapy of spontaneous bacterial peritonitis but the antibiotic choice should be reviewed once results of ascitic culture and sensitivity of the bacterial isolates are known. Because of renal toxicity, aminoglycosides should be avoided.

In a randomized study the administration of intravenous albumin to patients with spontaneous bacterial peritonitis treated with cefotaxime significantly reduced the incidence of renal impairment (10 vs. 33%) and hospital mortality (10 vs. 29%) [73]. The use of albumin was expensive. This study provides the lowest reported hospital mortality for spontaneous bacterial peritonitis. Further trials with lower doses of albumin or synthetic plasma expanders are awaited.

Diuretic therapy increases the total protein and ascitic opsonic activity. Paracentesis does not seem to increase the early and long-term risk of spontaneous bacterial peritonitis [72].

Because of reduced survival, spontaneous bacterial peritonitis is an indication to consider hepatic transplantation, particularly if recurrent.

Prophylaxis

The risk of spontaneous bacterial peritonitis is particularly high in cirrhotic patients with upper gastrointestinal haemorrhage. Oral administration of norfloxacin (400 mg/12h for a minimum of 7 days) is currently recommended for this group [62]. Spontaneous bacterial peritonitis and other infections should be ruled out before starting prophylaxis. The incidence of bacterial infections in patients with gastrointestinal haemorrhage is also reduced by combinations of ofloxacin with amoxycillin-clavulanic acid, ciprofloxacin with amoxycillin-clavulanic acid and oral ciprofloxacin alone [62].

In patients with a previous episode of spontaneous bacterial peritonitis the risk of recurrence during the subsequent year is 40–70%. Oral administration of norfloxacin (400 mg/day) is recommended in such patients who should then be evaluated for liver transplantation [62]. Trimethoprim-sulfamethoxazole is a less costly but effective alternative [71].

There is currently insufficient evidence to recommend prophylaxis for patients with a low ascitic fluid protein (< 1 g/dl) who have an increased risk of spontaneous bacterial peritonitis. There is a concern that long-term prophylaxis will lead to the emergence of resistant bacteria [57]. In patients with a high ascitic fluid protein (> 1 g/dl) without a past history of spontaneous bacterial peritonitis, prophylaxis is not thought necessary.

Treatment of cirrhotic ascites [7, 19, 65]

Therapy of ascites, whether by diuretics or paracentesis, reduces clinical symptoms and the patients is grateful. However, although the initial clinical response may be excellent, if fluid loss is excessive the result may be a patient in renal failure or with encephalopathy. Treatment must therefore be appropriate to the clinical state and the response properly monitored. The approach must be tailored to the patient. The spectrum of therapeutic intervention ranges from sodium restriction alone (rarely used), to diuretic use, therapeutic paracentesis, and for the most severe groups, TIPS and eventually liver transplantation.

Indications for treatment include the following:

Symptomatic ascites. Abdominal swelling sufficient to produce clinical symptoms, for example increasing girth or physical effort, requires treatment, most often with sodium restriction and diuretics. The presence of stable ascites *per se*, for example on scanning, without clinical symptoms, may not require active treatment, although to prevent deterioration advice on a reduction in sodium intake is wise. Inappropriate introduction of excessive treatment for ascites may lead to dizziness, muscle cramps, dehydration, hypotension and renal dysfunction.

Uncertain diagnosis. Control of ascites may allow such procedures as scanning and liver biopsy to be done. The urgency of the situation and degree of ascites will direct whether sodium restriction and diuretic is used, or paracentesis.

Gross ascites, causing abdominal pain and/or dyspnoea most often demands paracentesis.

Tense ascites with pain may lead to eversion and ulceration of an umbilical hernia, which is near to rupture. This complication has a very high mortality, due to shock, renal failure and sepsis, and urgent paracentesis is indicated.

Monitoring during treatment is mandatory. The patient is weighed daily. Fluid input as well as output is monitored. Urine volume and body weight provide a satisfactory guide to progress. Urinary electrolyte (sodium/potassium) determinations are helpful but not essential in determining therapy and monitoring the response. Serum electrolytes are measured two to three times per week while the patient is in hospital.

Treatment regimens include dietary sodium restriction, diuretics and abdominal paracentesis (table 9.5). Where liver disease is due to alcohol, the patient should be encouraged to abstain. The mild case is managed as an outpatient by diet and diuretics, but if admitted to hospital, paracentesis is usually a first procedure. In a survey of European hepatologists, 50% used paracentesis initially, to be followed by diuretics [7]. Fifty per cent regarded complete control of the ascites as desirable,

Table 9.5. General management of ascites

Bed rest. 70–90 mmol sodium diet. Check serum and urinary
electrolytes. Weigh daily. Measure urinary volume. Sample ascites
Spironolactone 100–200 mg daily
If tense ascites consider paracentesis (see table 9.8)
After 4 days consider adding frusemide (furosemide) 40 mg daily.
Check serum electrolytes
Stop diuretics if pre-coma ('flap'), hypokalaemia, azotaemia or
alkalosis
Continue to monitor weight. Increase diuretics as necessary

---

whereas the other half were satisfied with symptomatic relief without removing all the ascites. Thus consensus on standardized treatment regimes is difficult to reach because of the clinical spectrum of ascites, the clinical success of the different regimens and the lack of evidence-based studies comparing individual approaches.

Bed rest used to be a feature of initial therapy. Evidence for benefit is sparse but as part of an overall strategy it has been found to be beneficial [20]. This may be related to increased renal perfusion and portal venous blood flow during recumbency. However, modern clinical medicine does not allow the luxury of observing clinical responses to bed rest and sodium restriction alone over even a few days of hospital stay because of cost, and the clinical effectiveness and relative safety of more active therapies.

Sodium restriction/diet

The cirrhotic patient who is accumulating ascites on an unrestricted sodium intake excretes less than 10 mmol (approximately 0.2 g) sodium daily in the urine. Extra-renal loss is about 0.5 g. Sodium taken in excess of 0.75 g will result in ascites, every gram retaining 200 ml of fluid. Historically, such patients were recommended a diet containing 22–40 mmol/day. Current opinion, however, supports a 'no added salt' diet (approximately 70–90 mmol) combined with diuretic to increase urinary sodium excretion (table 9.4). The diets restricting sodium to 22–40 mmol were unpalatable and also compromised protein and calorie intake, which in patients with cirrhosis is critical for proper nutrition. Occasionally restrictions between 40 and 70 mmol/day may be necessary.

The average daily intake of sodium is about 150–250 mmol. To reduce intake to 70–90 mmol/day (approximately 1600–2000 mg) salt should not be used at the table or when cooking. Also various foods containing sodium should be restricted or avoided (table 9.6). Many low-sodium foods are now available including soups, ketchups and crackers.

A few ascitic patients may respond to this regimen

Table 9.6. Advice for 'no added salt diet' (70–90 mmol/day)

Omit

Anything containing baking powder or baking soda (contains
sodium bicarbonate): pastry, biscuits, crackers, cakes, self-raising
flour and ordinary bread (see restriction below)
All commercially prepared foods (unless designated low salt—check
packet)
Dry breakfast cereals except Shreaded Wheat, Puffed Wheat or
Sugar Puffs
Tinned/bottled savouries: pickles, olives, chutney, salad cream,
bottled sauces
Tinned meats/fish: ham, bacon, corned beef, tongue, oyster,
shellfish
Meat and fish pastes; meat and yeast extracts
Tinned/bottled vegetables, soups, tomato juice
Sausages, kippers
Cheese, ice cream
Candy, pastilles, milk chocolate
Salted nuts, potato crisps, savoury snacks
Drinks: especially Lucozade, soda water, mineral waters according
to sodium content (essential to check sodium content of mineral
waters, varies from 5 to 1000 mg/l)

Restrict

Milk (300 ml = half pint/day)
Bread (two slices/day)

Free use

Fresh and home-cooked fruit and vegetables of all kinds
Meat/poultry/fish (100 g/day) and one egg. Egg may be used to
substitute 50 g meat (2 oz)
Unsalted butter or margarine, cooking oils, double cream
Boiled rice, pasta (without salt), semolina
Seasonings help make restricted salt meal more palatable: include
lemon juice, onion, garlic, pepper, sage, parsley, thyme,
marjoram, bay leaves
Fresh fruit juice, coffee, tea
Mineral water (check sodium content)
Marmalade, jam
Dark chocolate, boiled sweets, peppermints, chewing gum
Salt substitutes (not potassium chloride)
Salt-free bread, crispbread, crackers or matzos

---

alone but usually the first line of treatment for ascites includes diuretics. Patients prefer the combination of diuretics and a modest restriction of sodium to severe sodium restriction alone. Very occasionally if there is a good response, diuretics may be withdrawn and the patient maintained on dietary sodium restriction alone.

Good responders are liable to be those:
• with ascites and oedema presenting for the first time in an otherwise stable patient—'virgin ascites'
• with a normal creatinine clearance (glomerular filtration rate)
• with an underlying reversible component of liver disease such as fatty liver of the alcoholic
• in whom the ascites has developed acutely in response to a treatable complication such as infection or bleeding, or after a non-hepatic operation

Prevention

The risk of hepato-renal syndrome is reduced by careful use and monitoring of diuretic therapy, and the early recognition of any complication such as electrolyte imbalance, haemorrhage or infection. Nephrotoxic drugs are avoided. The risk of renal deterioration after large volume paracentesis is reduced by the administration of salt-poor albumin. The risk of further episodes of spontaneous bacterial peritonitis in patients already having had one episode is reduced by prophylactic antibiotic. When spontaneous bacterial peritonitis is treated with antibiotics, the administration of albumin reduces the frequency of renal dysfunction [73].

Treatment

General measures

Since renal dysfunction may be related to hypovolaemia, measurement of the central venous pressure is important. An intravenous fluid challenge is appropriate with up to 1.5 litre of saline or, if available, colloid such as human albumin solution (HAS). Monitoring the patient for fluid overload is necessary although this is not usually a problem because advanced cirrhotics have increased venous compliance [34].

Potentially nephrotoxic drugs are stopped. A search for sepsis is made. Ascites is tapped for white cell count, Gram stain and culture. Blood, urine and cannula tips are cultured. A broad-spectrum antibiotic is started irrespective of proof of infection.

Tense ascites may be drained to improve renal haemo-dynamics by decreasing inferior vena caval and renal vein pressure.

Haemodialysis, although not formally studied in control trials, is not considered effective. Complications occur including arterial hypotension, coagulopathy, sepsis and gastrointestinal haemorrhage, and most patients die during treatment. Continuous arteriove-nous and venovenous haemofiltration have been used but not formally evaluated. Liver transplantation needs to be available rapidly for such therapy to be appropri-ate, but this is rarely the case in type 1 hepato-renal syndome. The promise of new pharmacological treat-ments provides a potentially new therapeutic approach which may avoid the need to consider renal support.

Liver transplantation

The survival of patients with type I hepato-renal syn-drome is short, from days to a few weeks, and this currently virtually removes liver transplantation as a therapeutic choice. New pharmacological approaches

reversing or stabilizing renal dysfunction may allow elective transplantation.

In patients with type 2 hepato-renal syndrome, liver transplantation results in return of acceptable renal func-tion in 90%, and the overall survival rates are similar to those without hepato-renal syndrome [29]. Patients with hepato-renal syndrome have a longer stay in the inten-sive care unit (21 vs. 4.5 days) and haemodialysis was required more often post-operatively (35 vs. 5%). Since cyclosporin A may contribute to renal deterioration, it has been suggested that azathioprine and steroids be given until a diuresis has started—usually by 48–72 h [29].

These results emphasize the need to identify patients at risk of hepato-renal syndrome and plan transplanta-tion as early as possible.

Pharmacological treatment [13, 16]

Vasodilators. These have been used in an attempt to reverse renal vasoconstriction. Dopamine at renal support doses has a renal vasodilatory effect. Although widely used clinically there is no clear evidence of efficacy. Prostaglandin administration is not associated with significant improvement in renal function.

Vasoconstrictors. The rationale for use of these agents is to reverse the intense splanchnic vasodilatation, which is considered an important factor in ascites formation and hepato-renal syndrome. Renal vasoconstriction reflects systemic and local responses to the reduced effective circulating volume.

Several regimens show promise using agonists of vasopressin V1 receptors. Initially, short-term intra-venous ornipressin was shown to improve circulatory dysfunction, suppress the renin–angiotensin–aldos-terone and sympathetic nervous system activity, and increase creatinine clearance [42]. With longer term treat-ment using ornipressin and albumin, renal function improved in four of eight patients with hepato-renal syndrome, but treatment had to be withdrawn in the remainder because of side-effects, including ischaemic events related to ornipressin [30]. Terlipressin (gly-pressin) is slowly converted into vasopressin *in vivo* and has a longer biological half-life. It has fewer side-effects than ornipressin. Terlipressin given to patients with hepato-renal syndrome type 1 for 2 days improved glomerular filtration rate [33]. Reversal of hepato-renal syndrome has been reported in seven of nine patients treated with terlipressin and intravenous albumin (5–15 days) without side-effects [80].

An alternative pharmacological approach has used long-term midrodine (an α-adrenergic agonist) com-bined with octreotide (an inhibitor of the release of glucagon) and intravenous albumin [6]. In all eight patients with type 1 hepato-renal syndrome, treated in this way renal function improved with no side-effects. Survival was long enough in four of the eight to allow successful liver transplantation.

A further study has shown benefit from prolonged (up to 27 days) intravenous ornipressin and dopamine in seven patients with type 1 hepato-renal syndrome which was reversed in four patients [32]. One patient had an ischaemic complication.

These studies represent a major advance in the management of hepato-renal syndrome. Based upon the 'peripheral arterial vasodilatation hypothesis', they suggest that vasoconstrictor drugs can be effective in the treatment of hepato-renal syndrome. Which agent and dose is best and whether albumin infusion is necessary needs randomized studies.

Antioxidant therapy

A preliminary uncontrolled study has suggested improvement in renal function after intravenous *n*-acetylcysteine [35]. Seven of 12 patients survived for 3 months including two patients who underwent successful liver transplantation.

Transjugular intrahepatic portosystemic shunt (TIPS)

Uncontrolled studies have shown that TIPS may improve renal perfusion and reduce the activity of the RAAS. In a prospective study of 31 non-transplantable patients approximately 75% had improvement in renal function after TIPS [12]. The 1-year survival was significantly better in type 2 than type 1 patients (70 vs. 20%). This study excluded patients with a Pugh score > 12, serum bilirubin > 15 mg/dl (250 μmol/l), and severe spontaneous encephalopathy. Controlled trials against other developing modalities would be useful to choose the optimal approach and select appropriate patients.

Extracorporeal albumin dialysis

A small randomized trial of MARS, the molecular absorbent recirculating system, has shown benefit for patients with type 1 hepato-renal syndrome [53]. This modified dialysis method uses an albumin-containing dialysate. Studies are underway to establish whether it has a role in such patients as a bridge to transplantation.

Summary

New approaches offer hope that hepato-renal syndrome, which previously had a dismal outlook, may be improved or reversed. The approaches remain investiga-

tional. The optimal approach may become clearer as randomized studies are achieved.

Hyponatraemia [26]

Hyponatraemia is common in cirrhotic patients with ascites, being found in around one-third. The cause is excess body water because of the inability of these patients to adjust the amount of water excreted in urine to that taken in. Serum sodium concentrations of less than 130 mmol/l are treated by fluid restriction, to avoid further falls. Advances in the understanding of the pathogenesis are leading to pharmacological approaches to treatment.

Mechanism

Eighty per cent of the water in the glomerular filtrate is reabsorbed in the proximal tubule and descending limb of Henle. The ascending limb of Henle and distal tubule are impermeable to water. Control of the volume of water passed in urine is dependent on the amount of water reabsorbed in the collecting tubule and collecting duct. This is under the control of vasopressin, which interacts with V2 receptors on the cells of the renal collecting ducts (see fig. 9.2). Vasopressin receptor activation stimulates the translocation of the water channel aquaporin 2 from a cytoplasmic vesicular compartment to the apical membrane. This mechanism may be effected by prostaglandins which inhibit vasopressin-stimulated water reabsorption.

Vasopressin is produced in the hypothalamus. Production is controlled in two ways: by osmoreceptors in the anterior hypothalamus under the influence of plasma osmolarity, and by parasympathetic stimulation as a result of activation of baroreceptors in the atria, ventricles, aortic arch and carotid sinus.

Water retention in cirrhotic patients with ascites is due to excess vasopressin as a result of baroreceptor stimulation. This is thought to be related to the reduced effective circulating volume as a result of splanchnic and other arterial vasodilatation—the same circulatory abnormality which leads to activation of the renin–angiotensin–aldosterone axis and the sympathetic nervous system and sodium retention. However, alterations in sodium and water handling are not synchronous, that for sodium occurring first (see fig. 9.4).

Data show that vasopressin levels are not grossly elevated in cirrhotic patients. The normal inhibition of vasopressin by a water load, however, is blunted or absent. Although there is reduced hepatic metabolism of vasopressin in patients with cirrhosis, related to the severity of disease, this is not thought to be the primary reason for water retention.

Pharmacological treatment

With greater understanding of the mechanisms involved several approaches are being studied to increase free water clearance. These are: (i) blocking secretion of vasopressin by the hypothalamus, or V2 receptors in the collecting ducts; or (ii) perturbing cAMP formation, which acts as the signal between vasopressin and aquaporin in collecting duct cells.

κ-Opioid receptor agonists inhibit vasopressin release. Experimentally and in human studies they increase urine volume [18]. However, because there is no significant decrease in circulating vasopressin levels with the agonist used (niravoline) the mechanism remains unclear [18].

In an experimental model of cirrhosis, the *V2 receptor antagonist*, OPC31260, induced a four-fold increase in water excretion [79].

Demeclocycline, a tetracycline, interferes with the generation and action of cAMP in collecting ducts, and in cirrhotics increases free water clearance and serum sodium. However, in patients with cirrhosis its use is associated with renal impairment.

Summary

Although advances are being made in pharmacological approaches to correct water retention and the associated hyponatraemia, these are not yet clinically applicable. The mainstay of treatment is fluid restriction. Intravenous albumin infusion may be effective in the short term [52]. Whichever approach is used, it should be recognized that hyponatraemia is a predictor of reduced survival in cirrhotic patients with ascites and is a risk factor for the hepato-renal syndrome [21].

References

1 Aalami OO, Allen DB, Organ CH. Chylous ascites; a collective review. *Surgery* 2000; **128**: 761.
2 Ackerman Z, Reynolds TB. Evaluation of pleural fluid in patients with cirrhosis. *J. Clin. Gastroenterol.* 1997; **25**: 619.
3 Albillos A, Cuervas-Mons V, Millan I *et al.* Ascitic fluid polymorphonuclear cell count and serum to ascites albumin gradient in the diagnosis of bacterial peritonitis. *Gastroenterology* 1990; **98**: 134.
4 Andreu M, Sola R, Sitges-Serra A *et al.* Risk factors for spontaneous bacterial peritonitis in cirrhotic patients with ascites. *Gastroenterology* 1993; **104**: 1133.
5 Angeli P, Albino G, Carraro P *et al.* Cirrhosis and muscle cramps: evidence of a causal relationship. *Hepatology* 1996; **23**: 264.
6 Angeli P, Volpin R, Gerunda G *et al.* Reversal of type 1 hepatorenal syndrome with the administration of midodrine and octreotide. *Hepatology* 1999; **29**: 1690.
7 Arroyo V, Ginès A, Saló J. A European survey on the treatment of ascites in cirrhosis. *J. Hepatol.* 1994; **21**: 667.
8 Arroyo V, Ginès P, Gerbes AL *et al.* Definition and diagnostic criteria of refractory ascites and hepatorenal syndrome in cirrhosis. *Hepatology* 1996; **23**: 164.
9 Arroyo V, Jimenèz W. Complications of cirrhosis. II. Renal and circulatory dysfunction. Lights and shadows in an important clinical problem. *J. Hepatol.* 2000; **32** (Suppl. 1): 157.
10 Blaise M, Pateron D, Trinchet J-C *et al.* Systemic antibiotic therapy prevents bacterial infection in cirrhotic patients with gastrointestinal haemorrhage. *Hepatology* 1994; **20**: 34.
11 Bories PN, Campillo B, Azaou L *et al.* Long-lasting NO overproduction in cirrhotic patients with spontaneous bacterial peritonitis. *Hepatology* 1997; **25**: 1328.
12 Brensing KA, Textor J, Perz J *et al.* Long-term outcome after transjugular intrahepatic portosystemic stent-shunt in non-transplant cirrhotics with hepatorenal syndrome: a phase II study. *Gut* 2000; **47**: 288.
13 Cárdenas A, Uriz J, Ginès P *et al.* Hepatorenal syndrome. *Liver Transplant.* 2000; **6**: S63.
14 Casafont F, Sanchez E, Martin L *et al.* Influence of malnutrition on the prevalence of bacterial translocation and spontaneous bacterial peritonitis in experimental cirrhosis in rats. *Hepatology* 1997; **25**: 1334.
15 Chang C-S, Chen G-H, Lien H-C *et al.* Small intestine dysmotility and bacterial overgrowth in cirrhotic patients with spontaneous bacterial peritonitis. *Hepatology* 1998; **28**: 1187.
16 Dagher L, Patch D, Marley R *et al.* Review article: pharmacological treatment of the hepatorenal syndrome in cirrhotic patients. *Aliment. Pharmacol. Ther.* 2000; **14**: 515.
17 Fernández-Esparrach G, Sánchez-Fueyo A, Ginès P *et al.* A prognostic model for predicting survival in cirrhosis with ascites. *J. Hepatol.* 2001; **34**: 46.
18 Gadano A, Moreau R, Pessione F *et al.* Aquaretic effects of niravoline, a kappa-opioid agonist, in patients with cirrhosis. *J. Hepatol.* 2000; **32**: 38.
19 Garcia-Tsao G. Current management of the complications of cirrhosis and portal hypertension: variceal haemorrhage, ascites, and spontaneous bacterial peritonitis. *Gastroenterology* 2001; **120**: 726.
20 Gentilini P, Casini-Raggi V, Di Fiore G *et al.* Albumin improves the response to diuretics in patients with cirrhosis and ascites: results of a randomized, controlled trial. *J. Hepatol.* 1999; **30**: 639.
21 Ginès A, Escorsell A, Ginès P *et al.* Incidence, predictive factors, and prognosis of the hepatorenal syndrome in cirrhosis with ascites. *Gastroenterology* 1993; **105**: 229.
22 Ginès A, Fernàndez-Esparrach G, Monescillo A *et al.* Randomised trial comparing albumin, dextran 70, and polygeline in cirrhotic patients with ascites treated by paracentesis. *Gastroenterology* 1996; **111**: 1002.
23 Ginès A, Planas R, Angeli P *et al.* Treatment of patients with cirrhosis and refractory ascites by Le Veen shunt with titanium tip: comparison with therapeutic paracentesis. *Hepatology* 1995; **22**: 124.
24 Ginès P, Arroyo V, Quintero E *et al.* Comparison of paracentesis and diuretics in the treatment of cirrhotics with tense ascites. Results of a randomized study. *Gastroenterology* 1987; **93**: 234.
25 Ginès P, Arroyo V, Vargas V *et al.* Paracentesis with intravenous infusion of albumin as compared with peritoneovenous shunting in cirrhosis with refractory ascites. *N. Engl. J. Med.* 1991; **325**: 829.

26 Ginès P, Berl T, Bernardi M *et al*. Hyponatraemia in cirrhosis: from pathogenesis to treatment. *Hepatology* 1998; **28**: 851.

27 Ginès P, Schrier RW. The arterial vasodilation hypothesis of ascites formation in cirrhosis. In Arroyo V, Ginès P, Rodés J, Schrier RW, eds. *Ascites and Renal Dysfunction in Liver Disease. Pathology, Diagnosis and Treatment*. Blackwell Science, Oxford, 1999, p. 411.

28 Girgrah N, Liu P, Collier J, Blendis L, Wong F. Haemodynamic, renal sodium handling, and neurohormonal effects of acute administration of low dose losartan, an angiotensin II receptor antagonist, in preascitic cirrhosis. *Gut* 2000; **46**: 114.

29 Gonwa TA, Morris CA, Goldstein RM *et al*. Long-term survival and renal function following liver transplantation in patients with and without hepatorenal syndrome—experience in 300 patients. *Transplantation* 1991; **51**: 428.

30 Guevara M, Ginès P, Fernández-Esparrach G *et al*. Reversibility of hepatorenal syndrome by prolonged administration of ornipressin and plasma volume expansion. *Hepatology* 1998; **27**: 35–41.

31 Guevara M, Ginès P, Jiménez W *et al*. Increased adrenomedullin levels in cirrhosis: relationship with haemodynamic abnormalities and vasoconstrictor systems. *Gastroenterology* 1998; **114**: 336.

32 Gülberg V, Bilzer M, Gerbes AL. Long-term therapy and retreatment of hepatorenal syndrome type 1 with ornipressin and dopamine. *Hepatology* 1999; **30**: 870.

33 Hadengue A, Gadano A, Moreau R *et al*. Beneficial effects of the 2-day administration of terlipressin in patients with cirrhosis and hepatorenal syndrome. *J. Hepatol.* 1998; **29**: 565.

34 Hadengue A, Moreau R, Gaudin C *et al*. Total effective vascular compliance in patients with cirrhosis: a study of the response to acute blood volume expansion. *Hepatology* 1992; **15**: 809.

35 Holt S, Goodier D, Marley R *et al*. Improvement in renal function in hepatorenal syndrome with *N*-acetylcysteine. *Lancet* 1999; **353**: 294.

36 Jacobson ED, Pawlik WW. Adenosine regulation of mesenteric vasodilation. *Gastroenterology* 1994; **107**: 1168.

37 Kakizaki S, Katakai K, Yoshinaga T *et al*. Hepatic hydrothorax in the absence of ascites. *Liver* 1998; **18**: 216.

38 Kao HW, Rakov HE, Savage E *et al*. The effect of large volume paracentesis on plasma volume—a cause of hypovolemia? *Hepatology* 1985; **5**: 403.

39 Kravetz D, Romero G, Argonz J *et al*. Total volume paracentesis decreases variceal pressure, size, and variceal wall tension in cirrhotic patients. *Hepatology* 1997; **25**: 59.

40 Lazaridis KN, Frank JW, Krowka MJ *et al*. Hepatic hydrothorax: pathogenesis, diagnosis, and management. *Am. J. Med.* 1999; **107**: 262.

41 Lebrec K, Giuily N, Hadengue A *et al*. Transjugular intrahepatic portosystemic shunts: comparison with paracentesis in patients with cirrhosis and refractory ascites: a randomised trial. *J. Hepatol.* 1996; **25**: 135.

42 Lenz K, Hörnargl H, Druml W *et al*. Ornipressin in the treatment of functional renal failure in decompensated liver cirrhosis. *Gastroenterology* 1991; **101**: 1060.

43 Llach J, Ginès P, Arroyo V *et al*. Effect of dipyridamole on kidney function in cirrhosis. *Hepatology* 1993; **17**: 59.

44 Llovet JM, Bartoli R, March F *et al*. Translocated intestinal bacteria cause spontaneous bacterial peritonitis in cirrhotic rats: molecular epidemiologic evidence. *J. Hepatol.* 1998; **28**: 307.

45 Llovet JM, Bartoli R, Planas R *et al*. Selective intestinal decontamination with norfloxacin reduces bacterial translocation in ascitic cirrhotic rats exposed to haemorrhagic shock. *Hepatology* 1996; **23**: 781.

46 Llovet JM, Moitinho E, Sala M *et al*. Prevalence and prognostic value of hepatocellular carcinoma in cirrhotic patients presenting with spontaneous bacterial peritonitis. *J. Hepatol.* 2000; **33**: 423.

47 Llovet JM, Planas R, Morillas R *et al*. Short-term prognosis of cirrhosis with spontaneous bacterial peritonitis: multivariate study. *Am. J. Gastroenterol.* 1993; **88**: 388.

48 Malinchoc M, Kamath PS, Gordon FD *et al*. A model to predict poor survival in patients undergoing transjugular intrahepatic portosystemic shunts. *Hepatology* 2000; **31**: 864.

49 Maroto A, Ginès A, Saló J *et al*. Diagnosis of functional kidney failure of cirrhosis with Doppler sonography: prognostic value of resistive index. *Hepatology* 1994; **20**: 839.

50 Martin P-Y, Ginès P, Schrier RW. Nitric oxide as a mediator of haemodynamic abnormalities and sodium and water retention in cirrhosis. *N. Engl. J. Med.* 1998; **339**: 533.

51 Martin P-Y, Ohara M, Ginès P *et al*. Nitric oxide synthase (NOS) inhibition for one week improves renal sodium and water excretion in cirrhotic rats with ascites. *J. Clin. Invest.* 1998; **101**: 235.

52 McCormick PA, Mistry P, Kaye G *et al*. Intravenous albumin infusion is an effective therapy for hyponatraemia in cirrhotic patients with ascites. *Gut* 1990; **31**: 204.

53 Mitzner SR, Stange J, Klammt S *et al*. Improvement of hepatorenal syndrome with extracorporeal albumin dialysis MARS: results of a prospective, randomised, controlled clinical trial. *Liver Transplant.* 2000; **6**: 277.

54 Moore K, Wendon J, Frazer M *et al*. Plasma endothelin immunoreactivity in liver disease and the hepatorenal syndrome. *N. Engl. J. Med.* 1992; **327**: 1774.

55 Moskovitz M. The peritoneovenous shunt: expectations and reality. *Am. J. Gastroenterol.* 1990; **85**: 917.

56 Navasa M, Follo A, Filella X *et al*. Tumor necrosis factor and interleukin-6 in spontaneous bacterial peritonitis in cirrhosis: relationship with the development of renal impairment and mortality. *Hepatology* 1998; **27**: 1227.

57 Novella M, Sola R, Soriano G *et al*. Continuous vs. inpatient prophylaxis of the first episode of spontaneous bacterial peritonitis with norfloxacin. *Hepatology* 1997; **25**: 532.

58 Perez-Ayuso RM, Arroyo V, Planas R *et al*. Randomised comparative study of efficacy of frusemide vs. spironolactone in nonazotaemic cirrhosis with ascites. *Gastroenterology* 1983; **84**: 961.

59 Platt JF, Ellis JH, Rubin JM *et al*. Renal duplex Doppler ultrasonography: a noninvasive predictor of kidney dysfunction and hepatorenal failure in liver disease. *Hepatology* 1994; **20**: 362.

60 Pockros PJ, Reynolds TB. Rapid diuresis in patients with ascites from chronic liver disease: the importance of peripheral oedema. *Gastroenterology* 1986; **90**: 1827.

61 Ricart E, Soriano G, Novella MT *et al*. Amoxicillin-clavulanic acid vs. cefotaxime in the therapy of bacterial infections in cirrhotic patients. *J. Hepatol.* 2000; **32**: 596.

62 Rimola A, Garcia-Tsao G, Navasa M *et al*. Diagnosis, treatment and prophylaxis of spontaneous bacterial peritonitis: a consensus document. *J. Hepatol.* 2000; **32**: 142.

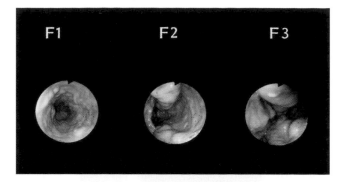

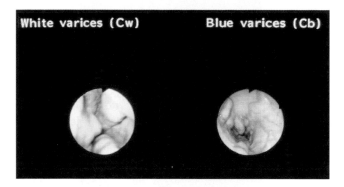

Fig. 10.17. The form (F) of the oesophageal varices (from [97]).

Fig. 10.18. Variceal colour through the endoscope (from [97]).

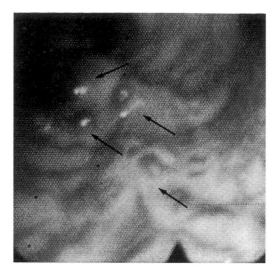

Fig. 10.19. Endoscopic view of cherry-red spots on oesophageal varices (arrows).

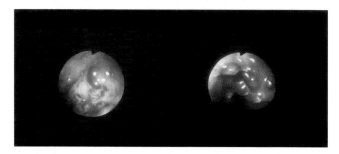

Fig. 10.20. Haemocystic spots on oesophageal varices (from [97]).

as raised cherry-red spots (fig. 10.19) and red wheal markings (longitudinal dilated veins resembling whip marks). They lie on top of large sub-epithelial vessels. The haemocystic spot is approximately 4 mm in diameter (fig. 10.20). It represents blood coming from the deeper extrinsic veins of the oesophagus straight out towards the lumen through a communicating vein into the more superficial submucosal veins. Red colour is usually associated with larger varices. All these colour changes, and particularly the red colour sign, predict variceal bleeding. Intra-observer error may depend on the skill and experience of the endoscopist. On the whole, agreement is good for size and red signs [22].

Portal hypertensive gastropathy is seen largely in the fundus, but can extend throughout the stomach (fig. 10.21). It is shown as a mosaic-like pattern with small polygonal areas, surrounded by a whitish-yellow depressed border [140]. Red point lesions and cherry-red spots predict a high risk of bleeding. Black–brown spots are due to intra-mucosal haemorrhage. Sclerotherapy increases the gastropathy [29].

Variceal (azygos) blood flow can be assessed during diagnostic endoscopy by a Doppler US probe passed down the biopsy channel of the standard gastroscope.

Portal hypertensive colopathy is seen in about half the patients with portal hypertension, usually in those with

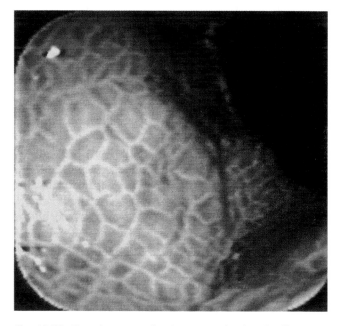

Fig. 10.21. Portal gastropathy. A mosaic of red and yellow is seen together with petechial haemorrhages.

gastropathy. Colonoscopy may be needed to diagnose lower gastrointestinal bleeding in cirrhotic patients [45].

Imaging the portal venous system

Ultrasound

Longitudinal scans at the sub-costal margins and transverse scans at the epigastrium are essential (fig. 10.22). The portal and superior mesenteric veins can always be seen. The normal splenic vein may be more difficult.

A large portal vein suggests portal hypertension, but this is not diagnostic. If collaterals are seen, this confirms portal hypertension. Portal vein thrombosis is accurately diagnosed and echogenic areas can sometimes be seen within the lumen.

Doppler ultrasound

Doppler US demonstrates the anatomy of the portal veins and hepatic artery (table 10.2). Satisfactory results depend on technical expertise. Small cirrhotic livers are difficult to see as are those of the obese. Colour-coded Doppler improves visualization (fig. 10.23). Portal venous obstruction is demonstrated by Doppler US as accurately as by angiography provided the Doppler is technically optimal.

Doppler US shows spontaneous hepato-fugal flow in portal, splenic and superior mesenteric veins in 8.3% of patients with cirrhosis [44]. Its presence correlates with severity of cirrhosis and with encephalopathy. Variceal bleeding is more likely if the flow is hepato-petal.

Table 10.2. Clinical uses of Doppler ultrasound

Portal vein
Patency
Hepato-fugal flow
Anatomical abnormalities
Portal-systemic shunt patency
Acute flow changes

Hepatic artery
Patency (post-transplant)
Anatomical abnormalities

Hepatic veins
Screening Budd–Chiari syndrome

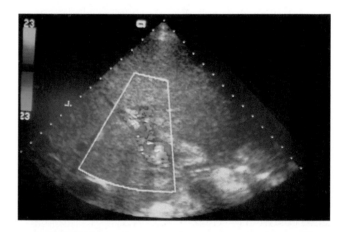

Fig. 10.23. Colour Doppler US of the porta hepatis shows the hepatic artery in red and portal vein in blue.

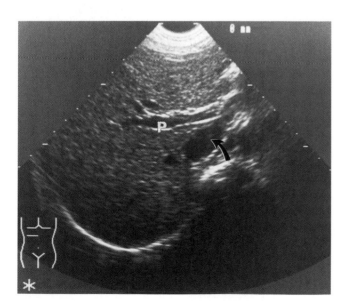

Fig. 10.22. Transverse US shows a patent portal vein (P); the arrow indicates the inferior vena cava.

Abnormalities of the intra-hepatic portal veins can be shown. These are important if surgery is contemplated.

Colour Doppler is a good way of demonstrating portal-systemic shunts and the direction of flow in them. These include surgical shunts but also transjugular intra-hepatic portosystemic shunts (TIPS). Intra-hepatic portal-systemic shunts may be visualized [72].

Colour Doppler screening is useful for patients suspected of the Budd–Chiari syndrome.

The hepatic artery is more difficult than the hepatic vein to locate because of its small size and direction. Nevertheless, duplex Doppler is the primary screening procedure to show a patent hepatic artery after liver transplantation.

Duplex Doppler has been used to measure portal blood flow. The average velocity of blood flowing in the portal vein is multiplied by the cross-sectional area of the vessel (fig. 10.24). There are observer errors in measurement, particularly of velocity. The method is most useful in measuring rapid, large, acute changes in flow

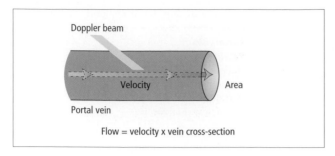

Fig. 10.24. The Doppler real-time US method of measuring portal venous flow.

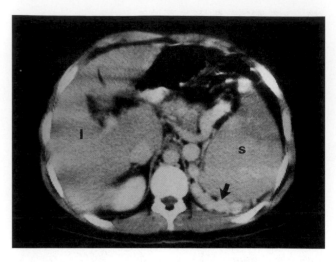

Fig. 10.25. Contrast-enhanced CT scan in a patient with cirrhosis and a large retroperitoneal retrosplenic collateral circulation (arrow). l, liver; s, spleen.

rather than monitoring chronic changes in portal haemodynamics.

Portal blood flow velocity correlates with the presence and size of oesophageal varices. In cirrhosis, the portal vein velocity tends to fall and when less than 16 cm/s portal hypertension is likely.

CT scan

After contrast, portal vein patency can be established and retroperitoneal, perivisceral and para-oesophageal varices may be visualized (fig. 10.25). Oesophageal varices may be shown as intraluminal protusions enhancing after contrast. The umbilical vein can be seen. Gastric varices show as rounded structures, indistinguishable from the gastric wall.

CT arterio-portography is done by rapid CT scanning (preferably helical) during selective injection of contrast into the superior mesenteric vein via a catheter [116]. It is particularly useful in showing focal lesions, the collateral circulation and arteriovenous shunts [141].

Magnetic resonance angiography

Magnetic resonance angiography gives excellent depiction of blood vessels as regions of absent signal (figs 10.26–10.28). Portal patency, morphology and flow of velocity may be demonstrated. Magnetic resonance angiography is more reliable than Doppler [43].

Venography

If the portal vein is patent by scanning, confirmation by venography is not necessary unless portal surgery or hepatic transplantation is being considered.

Patency of the portal vein is important particularly in the diagnosis of splenomegaly in childhood and in excluding invasion by a hepato-cellular carcinoma in a patient with cirrhosis.

Anatomy of the portal venous system must be known before such operations as portal-systemic shunt, hepatic resection or hepatic transplantation. The patency of a surgical shunt may be confirmed.

The demonstration of a large portal collateral circulation is essential for the diagnosis of chronic hepatic encephalopathy (figs 10.25, 10.29).

A filling defect in the portal vein or in the liver due to a space-occupying lesion may be demonstrated.

Venographic appearances

When the portal circulation is normal, the splenic and portal veins are filled but no other vessels are outlined. A filling defect may be seen at the junction of the splenic and superior mesenteric veins due to mixing with non-opacified blood. The size and direction of the splenic and portal veins are very variable. The intra-hepatic branches of the portal vein show a gradual branching and reduction in calibre. Later the liver becomes opaque due to sinusoidal filling. The hepatic veins may rarely be seen in later films.

In cirrhosis, the venogram varies widely. It may be completely normal or may show filling of large numbers of collateral vessels with gross distortion of the intra-hepatic pattern ('tree in winter' appearance) (fig. 10.30).

In extra-hepatic portal or splenic vein obstruction, large numbers of vessels run from the spleen and splenic vein to the diaphragm, thoracic cage and abdominal wall. Intra-hepatic branches are not usually seen, although, if the portal vein block is localized, para-portal vessels may short circuit the lesion (fig. 10.27) and produce a delayed but definite filling of the vein beyond.

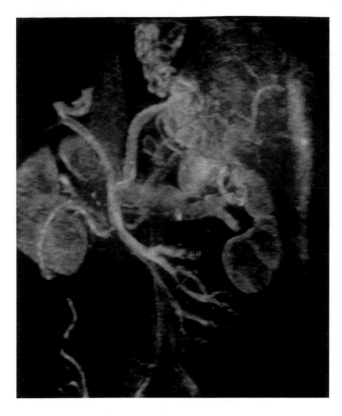 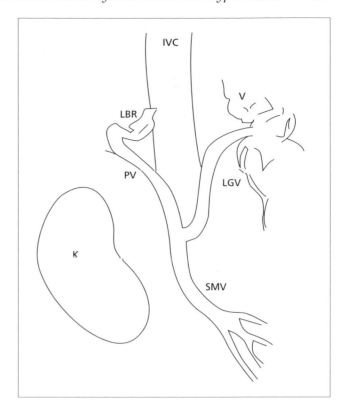

Fig. 10.26. Magnetic resonance angiography of a patient with cirrhosis showing the right kidney (K), superior mesenteric vein (SMV), portal vein (PV), left gastric vein (LGV), left branch of portal vein (LBR), gastro-oesophageal collateral veins (V) and the inferior vena cava (IVC).

Visceral angiography

Safety has increased with the use of smaller (French 5) arterial catheters. New contrast materials are less toxic to kidneys and other tissues and hypersensitivity reactions are rare.

The coeliac axis is catheterized via the femoral artery and contrast is injected. The material that flows into the splenic artery returns through the splenic and portal veins and produces a splenic and portal venogram. Similarly, a bolus of contrast introduced into the superior mesenteric artery returns through the superior mesenteric and portal veins which can be seen in radiographs exposed at the appropriate intervals (figs 10.31, 10.32).

Visceral angiography demonstrates the hepatic arterial system, so allowing space-filling lesions in the liver to be identified. A tumour circulation may diagnose hepato-cellular cancer or another tumour.

Knowledge of splenic and hepatic arterial anatomy is useful if surgery is contemplated. Haemangiomas, other space-occupying lesions and aneurysms may be identified.

The portal vein may not opacify if flow in it is hepatofugal or if there is 'steal' by the spleen or by large collateral channels. A superior mesenteric angiogram will confirm that the portal vein is in fact patent.

Digital subtraction angiography

The contrast is given by selective arterial injection with immediate subtraction of images. The portal system is very well visualized free of other confusing images (fig. 10.33). Spatial resolution is poorer than with conventional film-based angiography. The technique is particularly valuable for the parenchymal phase of hepatic angiography and for the diagnosis of vascular lesions such as haemangiomas or arteriovenous malformations.

Splenic venography

Contrast material, injected into the pulp of the spleen, flows into the portal venous system with sufficient rapidity to outline splenic and portal veins (fig. 10.30). The collateral circulation is particularly well visualized [2]. Splenic venography has now been replaced by less invasive procedures.

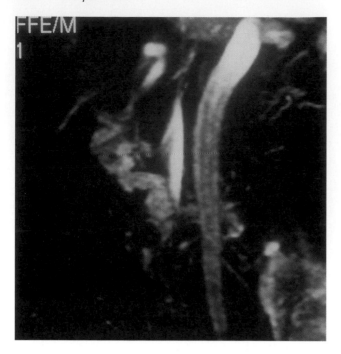

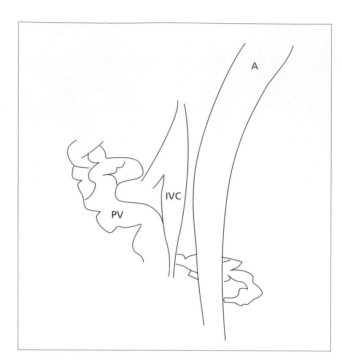

Fig. 10.27. Magnetic resonance angiography in a patient with portal vein thrombosis showing the portal vein replaced by collaterals (PV), the inferior vena cava (IVC) and the aorta (A).

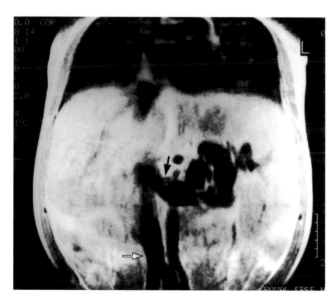

Fig. 10.28. Magnetic resonance angiography showing a spontaneous spleno-renal shunt to the inferior vena cava. Black arrow, renal vein; open arrow, vena cava.

Carbon dioxide wedged venography

Injection of carbon dioxide into a catheter in the wedged hepatic venous position allows an excellent venogram of the hepatic venous and portal venous tree (fig. 10.34) [32].

Portal pressure measurement

A balloon catheter is introduced into the femoral vein and, under fluoroscopic control, into the hepatic vein (fig. 10.35). Measurements are taken in the wedged hepatic venous pressure (WHVP) and free hepatic venous pressure (FHVP) positions by inflating and deflating the balloon in the tip of the catheter [32, 111]. The hepatic venous pressure gradient (HVPG) is the difference between WHVP and FHVP. This is the portal (sinusoidal) venous pressure. The relationship of this to portal venous pressure in a cirrhosis which has a large presinusoidal component, such as primary biliary cirrhosis or autoimmune chronic hepatitis, needs further investigation. The normal HVPG is 5–6 mmHg and values of about 20 mmHg are found in patients with cirrhosis. Measurements can be performed at the same time as transjugular liver biopsy.

HVPG may relate to survival [1] and also to prognosis in patients with bleeding oesophageal varices [110]. Its value in the prediction of variceal bleeding is uncertain. The procedure may be used to monitor therapy, for instance the effect of β-blockers such as propranolol, which should maintain the HVPG at less than 12 mmHg.

Variceal pressure

An *endoscopic pressure guage* may be fixed to the end of the endoscope. The level of venous pressure is a major factor predicting variceal haemorrhage [95].

Pressure may be recorded by *direct puncture* of varices

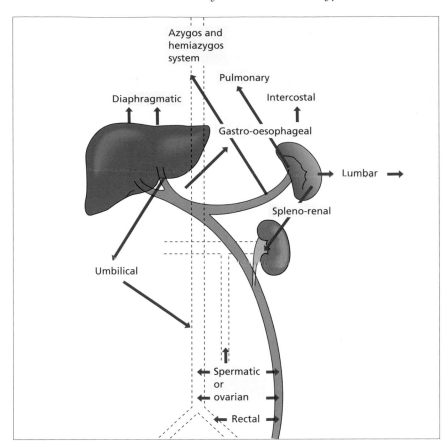

Fig. 10.29. The sites of the collateral circulation in the presence of intra-hepatic portal vein obstruction.

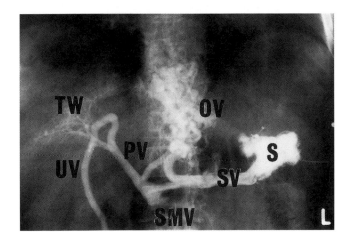

Fig. 10.30. Splenic venogram from a patient with cirrhosis of the liver. The gastro-oesophageal collateral circulation can be seen and the intra-hepatic portal vascular tree is distorted ('tree in winter' appearance). OV, oesophageal veins; PV, portal vein; S, splenic pulp; SMV, superior mesenteric vein; SV, splenic vein; TW, 'tree in winter' appearance; UV, umbilical vein.

at the time of sclerotherapy [61]. It is about 15.5 mmHg in cirrhotic patients, significantly lower than the main portal pressure of about 18.8 mmHg. An *endoscopic balloon* has been developed to measure variceal pressure

and this gives comparable results to direct puncture [49].

Estimation of hepatic blood flow

Constant infusion method

Hepatic blood flow may be measured by a constant infusion of indocyanine green (ICG) and catheterization of the hepatic vein [16, 21]. Flow is calculated by the Fick principle.

Plasma disappearance method

Hepatic blood flow can be measured after an intravenous injection of ICG followed by analysis of the disappearance curve in a peripheral artery and hepatic vein.

If the extraction of a substance is about 100%, for instance, using ^{131}I heat-denatured albumin colloidal complex, hepatic blood flow can be determined by peripheral clearance without hepatic vein catheterization.

In patients with cirrhosis, up to 20% of the blood perfusing the liver may not go through normal channels and hepatic extraction is reduced. In these circumstances, splenomegaly may be a presentation, particularly in children. Peri-umbilical veins are not seen but there may be dilated abdominal wall veins in the left flank.

The liver is normal in size and consistency. Stigmata of hepato-cellular disease, such as jaundice or vascular spiders, are absent. With acute portal venous thrombosis, ascites is early and transient, subsiding as the collateral circulation develops. Ascites is usually related to an additional factor which has depressed hepato-cellular function, such as a haemorrhage or a surgical exploration. It may be seen in the elderly where it is related to the deterioration of liver function with ageing [144].

Hepatic encephalopathy is not uncommon in adults, usually following an additional insult such as haemorrhage, infection or anaesthetic. Chronic encephalopathy may be seen in elderly patients with a particularly large portal-systemic circulation.

Imaging

US shows echogenic thrombus within the portal vein and colour Doppler shows slow flow velocity in the cavernous collaterals and no portal venous signal [70, 108].

CT shows the thrombus as a non-enhancing filling defect within the lumen of the portal vein and dilatation of many small veins at the hilum (fig. 10.38).

MRI shows an area of abnormal signal within the lumen of the portal vein which appears iso-intense on a T_1-weighted image with a more intense signal on a T_2-weighted image (see fig. 5.22).

Angiography in the portal venous phase shows a filling defect or non-opacification of the portal vein. However, the portal vein may not be visualized if blood is diverted away from it into extensive collaterals.

Haematology

Haemoglobin is normal unless there has been blood loss. Leucopenia and thrombocytopenia are related to the enlarged spleen. Circulating platelets and leucocytes, although in short supply, are adequate and function well.

Hypersplenism is not an indication for splenectomy. Blood coagulation is normal.

Serum biochemistry

All the usual tests of 'liver function' are normal. Elevation of serum globulin may be related to intestinal antigens, bypassing the liver through collaterals. Mild pancreatic hypofunction is related to interruption of the venous drainage of the pancreas [153].

Prognosis

This depends on the underlying disease. The outlook is much better than for cirrhosis as liver function is normal. The prognosis is surprisingly good in the child and, with careful management of recurrent bleeding, survival to adult life is expected. The number of bleeds seems to reduce as time passes. Women may bleed in pregnancy but this is unusual; their babies are normal.

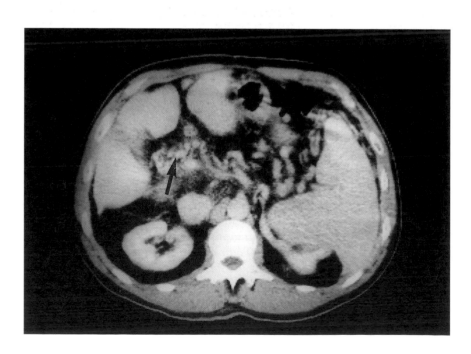

Fig. 10.38. Abdominal CT scan with contrast showing the main portal vein replaced by a leash of small veins (arrow).

Treatment

Any cause must be identified and treated. This may be more important than the portal hypertension. For instance, hepato-cellular carcinoma, invading the portal vein, precludes aggressive therapy for bleeding oeso-phageal varices. If the variceal bleeding is related to polycythaemia rubra vera, reduction of the platelet count must precede any surgical therapy; anticoagulants may be needed.

Prophylactic treatment of varices is not indicated. They may never rupture and as time passes collaterals open up.

With acute portal vein thrombosis, anticoagulant therapy is usually too late as the clot will have under-gone organization. If diagnosed early, anticoagulants may prevent spreading thrombosis.

Children should survive haemorrhage with proper management, including transfusion. Care must be taken to give compatible blood and to preserve peripheral veins. Aspirin ingestion should be avoided. Upper respi-ratory infections should be treated seriously as they seem to precipitate haemorrhage.

Somatostatin infusions may be needed and, occasion-ally, the Sengstaken tube.

Endoscopic sclerotherapy is valuable as an emergency procedure.

Major or recurrent bleeds may be treated by later oblit-erative sclerotherapy. Unfortunately this does not treat the huge gastric fundal varices and the congestive gas-tropathy continues.

Definitive surgery to reduce portal pressure is usually impossible as there are no suitable veins for a shunt. Even apparently normal-looking veins seen on venogra-phy turn out to be in poor condition, presumably related to extension of the original thrombotic process. In chil-dren, veins are very small and difficult to anastomose. Myriads of collateral channels add to the technical difficulties.

Results for all forms of surgery are very unsatisfactory. Splenectomy is the least successful.

A shunt (porta-caval, meso-caval or spleno-caval) is the most satisfactory treatment but usually proves impossible.

When the patient is exsanguinating, despite massive blood transfusion, an oesophageal transection may have to be performed. Here again gastric varices are not treated. Post-operative complications are common.

TIPS is usually impossible.

Splenic vein obstruction

Isolated splenic vein obstruction causes sinistral (left-sided) portal hypertension. It may be due to any of the factors causing portal vein obstruction (fig. 10.39).

Pancreatic disease such as carcinoma (18%), pancreatitis (65%), pseudocyst and pancreatectomy are particularly important [9].

If the obstruction is distal to the entry of the left gastric vein, a collateral circulation bypasses the obstructed splenic vein through short gastric veins into the gastric fundus and lower oesophagus, so reaching the left gastric vein and portal vein. This leads to very promi-nent varices in the fundus of the stomach but few in the lower oesophagus.

The selective venous phase of an angiogram, an enhanced CT scan or MRI are diagnostic. Splenectomy, by blocking arterial inflow, is usually curative but unnec-essary if the patient has not bled from varices [81].

Hepatic arterio-portal venous fistulae

Portal hypertension results from increased portal venous flow. Increase in intra-hepatic resistance due to a rise in portal flow may also be important. Portal zones show thickening of small portal radicles with accompa-nying mild fibrosis and lymphocyte infiltration. The increased intra-hepatic resistance may persist after oblit-eration of the fistula.

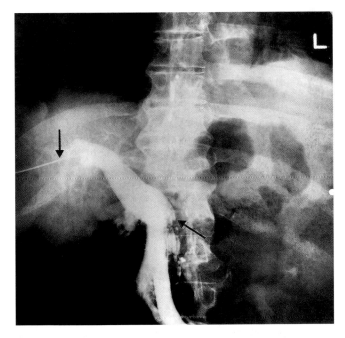

Fig. 10.39. A 64-year-old man with polycythaemia rubra vera. Trans-hepatic portal venogram (transhepatic needle marked by upper arrow) showing a thrombosed splenic vein (marked by the lower arrow) with patent superior mesenteric and portal veins. This patient, after preliminary reduction of red cell and platelet count by radio-active phosphorus, was successfully treated by splenectomy.

in any one varix (fig. 10.51). Complications are more likely with chronic, repeated sclerotherapy than with acute injection to stop bleeding. Factors include the volume of sclerosant used and the Child's grade.

Almost every patient will experience transient fever, dysphagia and chest pain.

Endoscopic variceal ligation (*banding*) is an alternative emergency treatment to endoscopic sclerotherapy. It is superior to sclerotherapy, especially when the varix is spurting rather than oozing [79, 80]. It has fewer complications. These include aspiration pneumonia and large oesophageal ulcers. Vaso-constrictor and blood tranfusion needs are reduced [79, 80]. However, it is more difficult to perform while the patient is bleeding and will probably not replace the more general endoscopic sclerotherapy except in specialized centres.

The technique is based on band ligation of haemorrhoids. The varices are ligated and strangulated by the application of small elastic O rings (fig. 10.52) [75]. A standard end-viewing endoscope loaded with a banding device on its tip is inserted into the lower oesophagus. A varix is identified and aspirated into the device, followed by placement of an elastic band around it by pulling the trip wire. The process is repeated until all the varices are ligated.

Emergency surgery

This has been remarkably reduced with the advent of sclerotherapy, vaso-active drugs, balloon tamponade and, in particular, TIPS. When these fail, or are not available, emergency surgery must be considered. An emergency end-to-side porta-caval shunt is effective in stopping bleeding [102]. Mortality is high in grade C patients, and the post-surgical encephalopathy rate is also high. If bleeding is torrential and recurs after two sclerotherapy sessions, TIPS is the best treatment.

Emergency oesophageal transection may be done by the staple gun technique as an emergency, but not as a prophylatic or elective procedure. Within 2 years, varices recurred, enlarged and frequently re-bled [83].

Prevention of re-bleeding

At 1 year, 25% of Child's grade A, 50% of grade B and 75% of grade C patients with cirrhosis will have re-bled from varices. Prevention is difficult and controversial.

Propranolol reduces re-bleeding in patients with large varices who are in good condition [77]. Patients with decompensated cirrhosis do not respond. Propranolol probably has little effect on survival [104]. It is of value in portal gastropathy.

Chronic variceal sclerotherapy is performed at weekly intervals until all varices are thrombosed. Three to five sessions will probably be needed. After eradication,

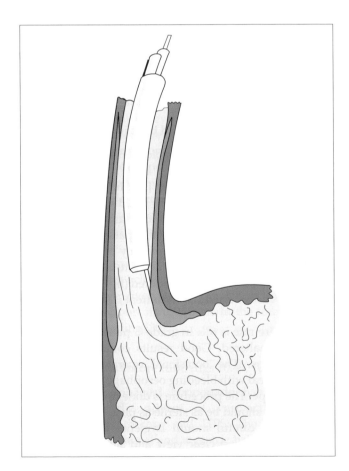

Fig. 10.51. Direct injection of oesophageal varices with an unmodified fibre-optic endoscope.

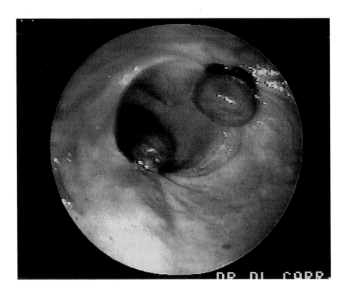

Fig. 10.52. Endoscopic variceal ligation. The varices have been strangulated by an elastic ring introduced via the endoscope.

close endoscopic surveillance and repeated injections to ensure continued eradication are *not* indicated as survival is not increased. Chronic oesophageal sclerotherapy reduces the rate of re-bleeding and the transfusion requirements but has no long-term effect on survival [148]. In good-risk patients, propranolol is as successful as chronic sclerotherapy to obliterate varices [5].

The many complications of chronic sclerotherapy include bleeding from the puncture site, but more usually from remaining varices or deep ulcers that have opened in sub-mucosal channels. Stricture formation is related to chemical oesophagitis, ulceration and acid reflux; impaired swallowing contributes.

Perforation is usually delayed 5–7 days and is probably an extension of the ulcerative process [109].

Pulmonary complications include chest pain, aspiration pneumonia, pleural effusion and mediastinitis [7]. Sclerosant embolizing the lungs may impair respiratory function [123]. Pyrexia and bacteraemia are frequent.

Portal vein thrombosis may affect a subsequent shunt or liver transplantation.

Varices increase at other sites including the stomach, ano-rectal area and percutaneously.

Endoscopic variceal ligation may be the treatment of choice, but variceal recurrence is greater [79, 80].

Chronic sclerotherapy or banding reduces the rate of re-bleeding and transfusion requirements, but has no long-term effect on survival [148]. A shunt, usually porta-caval, or transplant must be considered as rescue when sclerotherapy has failed.

Portal-systemic shunt procedures
(fig. 10.53)

The aim is to reduce portal venous pressure, maintain total hepatic and, particularly, portal blood flow and, above all, not have a high incidence of hepatic encephalopathy. There is no currently available procedure that fulfils all these criteria. Hepatic reserve determines survival. Hepato-cellular function deteriorates after shunting.

Porta-caval

In 1877 Eck [40] first performed a porta-caval shunt in dogs and this remains the most effective way of reducing portal hypertension in man.

The portal vein is joined to the inferior vena cava either end-to-side, with ligation of the portal vein, or side-to-side, maintaining its continuity. The portal blood pressure falls, hepatic venous pressure falls and hepatic arterial flow increases.

Porta-caval shunts are now rare because of the high incidence of post-shunt encephalopathy. Liver function deteriorates due to reduction of portal perfusion. A

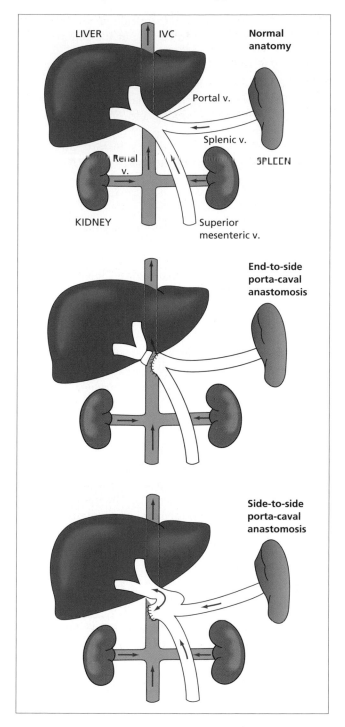

Fig. 10.53. The types of surgical portal-systemic shunt operation performed for the relief of portal hypertension. IVC, inferior vena cava.

subsequent hepatic transplantation can be made more difficult. It is still used, after the bleeding episode has been controlled, in patients with good liver reserves who do not have access to tertiary care or who may have bled from gastric varices. It is useful in some patients with early primary biliary cirrhosis, congenital hepatic fibrosis with good hepato-cellular function and those with portal vein obstruction at the hilum of the liver.

Patients should have had a haemorrhage from proven oesophageal varices. The portal vein must be good and the patient preferably aged less than 50 years. After the age of 40, survival is reduced and encephalopathy is twice as common.

The patient should not have a history of hepatic encephalopathy, and should be Child's grade A or B.

Meso-caval

This is made between the superior mesenteric vein and the inferior vena cava using a Dacron graft (fig. 10.54) [36]. It is technically easy. Shunt occlusion is usual with time and is followed by re-bleeding [36]. It does not interfere with subsequent hepatic transplantation.

Selective 'distal' spleno-renal (fig. 10.55)

Veins feeding the dangerous oesophago-gastric collaterals are divided while allowing drainage of portal blood through short gastric-splenic veins through a spleno-renal shunt to the inferior vena cava. It was hoped that portal perfusion would be maintained but this was not so.

The mortality and encephalopathy results are similar to those reported for non-selective shunts. Better results are reported in non-alcoholic patients and where gastric varices are the main problem [91]. The operation does not interfere with a subsequent liver transplant.

Selective spleno-renal shunt is technically difficult and fewer and fewer surgeons are able or willing to perform it.

General results of portal-systemic shunts

The mortality rate in good-risk patients is about 5%. For poor-risk patients the mortality is 50%.

Bleeding from gastro-oesophageal varices is prevented or at least reduced. Size decreases and oesophageal varices disappear within 6 months to 1 year.

Blood pressure and hepatic blood flow fall so that hepatic function deteriorates. Post-operative jaundice is related to this and to haemolysis. Ankle oedema is due to a fall in portal venous pressure while serum albumin level remains low. Increased cardiac output with failure may contribute. Shunt patency is confirmed by US, CT, MRI, Doppler or angiography.

Hepatic encephalopathy may be transient. Chronic changes develop in 20–40% and personality deterioration in about one-third (Chapter 7). The incidence increases with the size of the shunt. Encephalopathy is more common in older patients

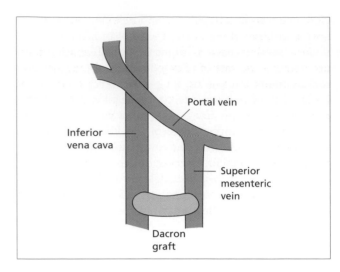

Fig. 10.54. The meso-caval shunt using a Dacron graft.

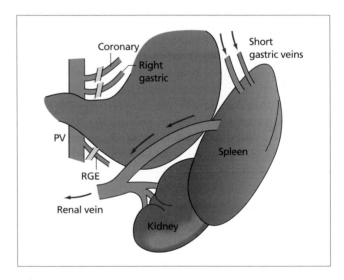

Fig. 10.55. The distal spleno-renal shunt. The veins feeding the varices (coronary, right gastric, right gastro-epiploic — RGE) are ligated. A spleno-renal shunt is made, preserving the spleen; retrograde flow in the short gastric veins is possible. Portal blood flow to the liver is preserved. PV, portal vein.

Myelopathy with paraplegia and parkinsonian cerebellar syndrome are rare (Chapter 7).

TIPS (transjugular intrahepatic portosystemic shunt)

Early attempts to establish intra-hepatic portal-systemic shunts were unsuccessful because the ballooned tract between the hepatic and portal veins did not remain patent. The use of a Palmaz expandable stent allowed maintenance of shunt patency and so the implantation of a metallic stent between an intra-hepatic branch of the portal vein and the hepatic vein radicle (figs 10.56, 10.57) [119, 121, 136].

The usual indication is control of bleeding from oesophageal or gastric varices. Full medical treatment including sclerotherapy and vaso-active drugs are given before TIPS is considered. Results are poor if the patient is actively bleeding. The procedure is performed under sedation and with local anaesthesia. Under US control, the portal bifurcation is located. The middle hepatic vein is catheterized by the transjugular route, and a needle introduced through this catheter into a main portal vein branch. A guide-wire is introduced through the needle and the catheter advanced into the portal vein. The needle is removed and portal venous pressure gradient

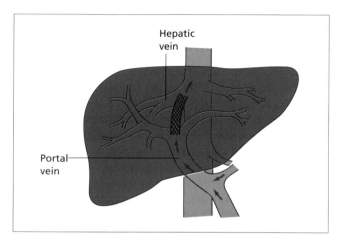

Fig. 10.56. TIPS. An expandable metal stent has been inserted between the portal vein and the hepatic vein producing an intra-hepatic porto-systemic shunt.

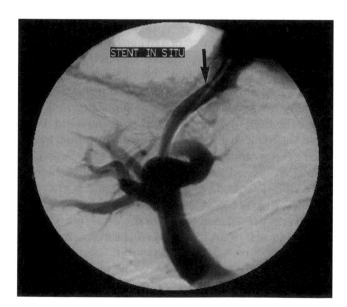

Fig. 10.57. TIPS. A portal venogram showing a porto-hepatic venous shunt; the stent is *in situ* (arrow).

measured. The needle track is balloon-dilated and mesenteric portography performed. A Palmaz metallic balloon expandable stent or a Wallstent self-expanding metal stent is inserted and expanded to 8–12 mm [73]. The diameter is adjusted to achieve a portal pressure gradient of less than 12 mmHg. If portal hypertension persists, a second stent may be placed parallel to the first [58]. US guidance is essential throughout. The time taken is 1–2 h. A subsequent hepatic transplant is not affected by TIPS.

This is a difficult technique and a skilled interventional radiologist must be part of the team. The technical failure rate is about 5–10% (table 10.6). About a third of patients need a second TIPS during the same hospitalization. In 10%, bleeding is uncontrolled by two sessions.

Procedural mortality is less than 1%. Complications include haemorrhage which may be intra-abdominal, biliary or through the liver capsule. The stent may dislocate and have to be retrieved by a looped snare [124].

Infections are prevented by a careful aseptic technique and early removal of central venous lines.

Intravascular haemolysis may be related to damage to erythrocytes by the steel mesh of the stent [128]. Hyperbilirubinaemia developing post-shunt carries a high risk of death or liver transplant [122]. Hypersplenism and, in particular, thrombocytopenia is unaffected [63, 128].

Shunt stenosis and occlusion

The lower pressure gradient between the portal vein and hepatic vein favours occlusion. Early obstruction is due to thrombosis and is related to technical problems [39]. Later stenosis is related to pseudo-intimal hyperplasia and ingrowth of tissue into the shunt lumen [39, 125]. Portal hypertension returns. Cumulative studies show 63% stenosis within the first 6 months and 90% stenosis within 2 years [125]. Prevalence probably depends on the enthusiasm with which shunt patency is investigated.

Follow-up of shunt patency is essential. This may be done by routine portography or Doppler sonography [78]. Duplex sonography may not be sufficiently sensitive to detect patency [103]. Shunt occlusion is treated by

Table 10.6. Reported percentage complications of TIPS

Complication	%
Technical failure	5–10
Portal or splenic vein thrombosis	1–5
Shunt stenosis	33–66
Hepatic encephalopathy	15–30
Worsening liver function	1–5
Chronic haemolysis	1–3

Group. Sclerotherapy for male alcoholic cirrhotic patients who have bled from esophageal varices: results of a randomized multicentre clinical trial. *Hepatology* 1994; **20**: 618.

149 Vianna A, Hayes PC, Moscoso G *et al*. Normal venous circulation of the gastroesophageal junction. A route to understanding varices. *Gastroenterology* 1987; **93**: 876.

150 Viggiano TR, Gostout CJ. Portal hypertensive intestinal vasculopathy: a review of the clinical, endoscopic, and histopathologic features. *Am. J. Gastroenterol.* 1992; **87**: 944.

151 Wanless IR, Peterson P, Das A *et al*. Hepatic vascular disease and portal hypertension in polycythemia vera and agnogenic myeloid metaplasia: a clinicopathological study of 145 patients examined at autopsy. *Hepatology* 1990; **12**: 1166.

152 Webb LJ, Sherlock S. The aetiology, presentation and natural history of extrahepatic portal venous obstruction *Q. J. Med.* 1979; **48**: 627.

153 Webb L, Smith-Laing G, Lake-Bakaar G *et al*. Pancreatic hypofunction in extrahepatic portal venous obstruction. *Gut* 1980; **21**: 227.

154 Weinshel E, Chen W, Falkenstein DB *et al*. Hemorrhoids or rectal varices: defining the cause of massive rectal hemorrhage in patients with portal hypertension. *Gastroenterology* 1986; **90**: 744.

155 Wheatley AM, Zhang X-Y. Intrahepatic modulation of portal pressure and its role in portal hypertension. *Digestion* 1998; **59**: 424.

156 Zacks SL, Sandler RS, Biddle AK *et al*. Decision analysis of transjugular intrahepatic portosystemic shunt vs. distal splenorenal shunt for portal hypertension. *Hepatology* 1999; **29**: 1399.

157 Zoli M, Iervese T, Merkel C *et al*. Prognostic significance of portal haemodynamics in patients with compensated cirrhosis. *J. Hepatol.* 1993; **17**: 56.

Chapter 11
The Hepatic Artery and Hepatic Veins: the Liver in Circulatory Failure

The hepatic artery

The hepatic artery is a branch of the coeliac axis. It runs along the upper border of the pancreas to the first part of the duodenum where it turns upwards between the layers of the lesser omentum, lying in front of the portal vein and medial to the common bile duct. Reaching the porta hepatis it divides into right and left branches. Its branches include the right gastric artery and the gastroduodenal artery. Aberrant branches are common. Surgical anatomy has been defined in donor livers [6]. The common hepatic artery usually rises from the coeliac axis to form the gastroduodenal and proper hepatic artery which divides into right and left branches. A replaced or accessory right hepatic artery may originate from the superior mesenteric artery. A replaced or accessory left hepatic artery may arise from the left gastric artery. Rarely, the entire common hepatic artery arises as a branch of the superior mesenteric or directly from the aorta. Such anomalies are of great importance in liver transplantation.

Anastomoses occur between the right and left branches, with subcapsular vessels of the liver and with the inferior phrenic artery.

Intra-hepatic anatomy

The hepatic artery enters sinusoids adjacent to the portal tracts [17]. Direct arterio-portal venous anastomoses are not seen in man [17].

The hepatic artery forms a capillary plexus around the bile ducts. Interference with this hepatic arterial supply leads to bile duct injury—surgical and laparoscopic (fig. 11.1) [13]. Diseases of the hepatic artery, such as polyarteritis nodosa, may present as biliary strictures [2].

The connective tissue in the portal zones is supplied by the hepatic artery.

Hepatic arterial flow

In man, during surgery, the hepatic artery supplies 35% of the hepatic blood flow and 50% of the liver's oxygen supply [16]. The hepatic arterial flow serves to hold total hepatic blood flow constant. It regulates blood levels of nutrients and hormones by maintaining blood flow, and thereby hepatic clearance, as steady as possible [10].

The proportion of hepatic arterial flow increases greatly in cirrhosis, related to the extent of portal-systemic venous shunting. It is the main blood supply to tumours. A drop in systemic blood pressure from haemorrhage, or any other cause, lowers the oxygen content of the portal vein and the liver becomes more and more dependent on the hepatic artery for oxygen. The hepatic artery and the portal vein adjust the volume of blood and oxygen they supply to the liver according to demand [10].

Hepatic arteriography

Hepatic arteriography is used for the diagnosis of space-occupying lesions including cysts, abscesses and benign and malignant tumours (Chapter 31), as well as vascular lesions such as aneurysms (fig. 11.2) or arteriovenous fistulae. Embolization via the catheter is used for treating tumours and hepatic trauma, and in the management of hepatic arterial aneurysm or arteriovenous fistulae (figs 11.3, 11.4).

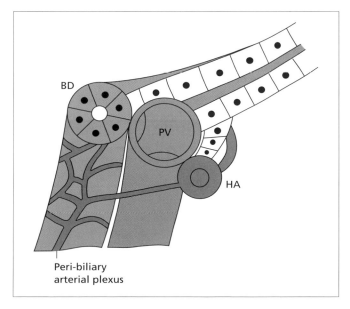

Fig. 11.1. The hepatic artery (HA) forms a peri-biliary plexus supplying the bile duct (BD). PV, portal vein.

In prolonged cholestasis the skin is greenish, possibly due to biliverdin, which does not give the diazo reaction for bilirubin.

Conjugated bilirubin, because of its water solubility and penetration of body fluids, produces more jaundice than unconjugated pigment. This accounts for the more intense colour of hepato-cellular and cholestatic rather than haemolytic jaundice.

Classification of jaundice

Classification is into three types (figs 12.5, 12.6): pre-hepatic, hepatic and cholestatic. There is much overlap, particularly between the hepatic and cholestatic varieties.

Pre-hepatic. There is an increased bilirubin load on the liver cell most usually due to haemolysis. The circulating serum bilirubin is largely unconjugated and the serum transaminase and alkaline phosphatase are normal. Bilirubin cannot be detected in urine. This picture of unconjugated hyperbilirubinaemia is also seen when

there is failure of bilirubin conjugation as in Gilbert's and Crigler–Najjar syndrome.

Hepatic. This is related to failure of the hepatocyte to excrete conjugated bilirubin into bile, presumably as a result of the failure of transport systems across the hepatocyte and the canalicular membrane. Conjugation is intact and therefore there is reflux of conjugated bilirubin into

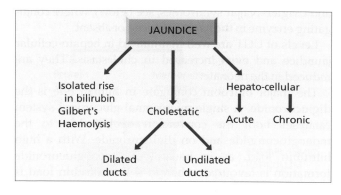

Fig. 12.5. Classification of jaundice.

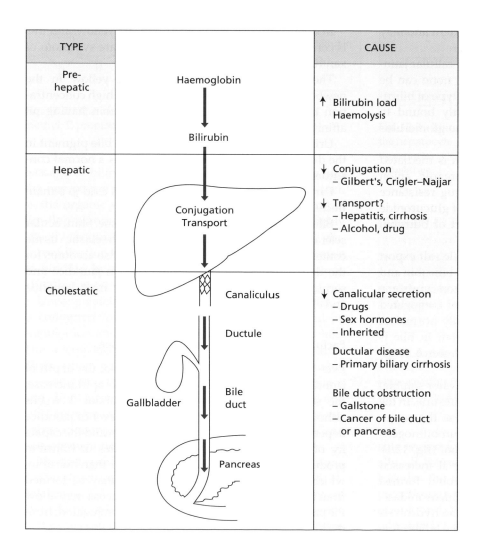

TYPE		CAUSE
Pre-hepatic	Haemoglobin ↓ Bilirubin	↑ Bilirubin load Haemolysis
Hepatic	Conjugation Transport	↓ Conjugation – Gilbert's, Crigler–Najjar ↓ Transport? – Hepatitis, cirrhosis – Alcohol, drug
Cholestatic	Canaliculus Ductule Gallbladder Bile duct Pancreas	↓ Canalicular secretion – Drugs – Sex hormones – Inherited Ductular disease – Primary biliary cirrhosis Bile duct obstruction – Gallstone – Cancer of bile duct or pancreas

Fig. 12.6. Classification and causes of jaundice.

the circulation. Serum biochemistry shows an increase in liver enzymes according to the underlying cause; being predominantly transaminases in viral and drug hepatitis. The jaundice usually comes on rapidly. Fatigue and malaise are conspicuous. If liver damage is severe there may be evidence of liver failure with encephalopathy, fluid retention with oedema and ascites, and bruising both spontaneous and related to venepunctures due to reduced hepatic synthesis of coagulation factors. In the long-standing case, serum albumin levels are reduced.

Cholestatic (Chapter 13). This is due to failure of adequate amounts of bile to reach the duodenum, either through failure of canalicular secretion of bile or physical obstruction to the bile duct at any level. The patient is relatively well, apart from the causative condition, and pruritus is characteristic. The patient becomes increasingly pigmented. The serum shows increases in conjugated bilirubin, biliary alkaline phosphatase, γ-glutamyl transpeptidase (γ-GT), total cholesterol and conjugated bile acids. Steatorrhoea is responsible for weight loss and malabsorption of fat-soluble vitamins A, D, E and K, and calcium.

Diagnosis of jaundice (tables 12.1, 12.2; fig. 12.7)

A careful history and physical examination with routine biochemical and haematological tests are essential. The stool should be inspected and occult blood examination performed. The urine is tested for bilirubin and urobilinogen excess. The place of special tests such as ultrasound, liver biopsy and cholangiography will depend on the category of jaundice.

Clinical history

Occupation should be noted; particularly employment involving alcohol or contact with rats carrying Weil's disease.

Table 12.1. First steps in the diagnosis of the jaundiced patient

Clinical history and examination
Urine, stools
Serum biochemical tests
  bilirubin
  transaminase (AST, ALT)
  alkaline phosphatase, γ-GT
  albumin
  quantitative immunoglobulins
Haematology
  haemoglobin, white cells, platelets
Blood film
Prothrombin time (before and after i.v. vitamin K)
X-ray of chest

ALT, alanine transaminase; AST, aspartate transaminase; γ-GT, γ-glutamyl transpeptidase.

Place of origin (Mediterranean, African or Far East) may suggest carriage of hepatitis B or C.

Family history is important with respect to jaundice, hepatitis and anaemia. Positive histories are helpful in diagnosing haemolytic jaundice, congenital hyperbilirubinaemia and hepatitis.

Contact with jaundiced persons, particularly in nurseries, camps, hospitals and schools, is noted. Close contact with patients on renal units or with drug abusers is recorded, as is any *injection* in the preceding 6 months. 'Injections' include blood tests, drug abuse, tuberculin testing, dental treatment and tattooing as well as blood or plasma transfusions. The patient is asked about previous *drug treatment* with possible hepato-toxic agents. Consumption of *shellfish* and previous *travel* to areas where hepatitis is endemic should be noted.

Previous dyspepsia, fat intolerance and biliary colic suggest choledocholithiasis.

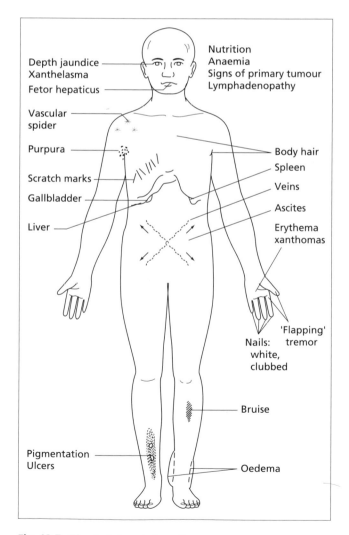

Fig. 12.7. Physical signs in jaundice.

Table 12.2. General features of the common types of acute jaundice

	Gallstones in common bile duct	Carcinoma in peri-ampullary region	Acute viral hepatitis	Cholestatic drug jaundice
Antecedent history	Dyspepsia, previous attack	Nil	Contacts, injections, transfusion or nil	Taking drug
Pain	Constant epigastric, biliary colic or none	Constant epigastric, back or none	Ache over liver or none	None
Pruritus	±	+	Transient	+
Rate of development of jaundice	Slow	Slow	Rapid	Rapid
Type of jaundice	Fluctuates or persistent	Usual but not always	Rapid onset, slow fall with recovery	Variable, usually mild
Weight loss	Slight to moderate	Progressive	Slight	Slight
Examination				
Diathesis	Frequently female, obese	Over 40 years old	Young usually	Often older female, psychotic
Depth of jaundice	Moderate	Deep	Variable	Variable, rash sometimes
Ascites	0	Rarely with metastases	If severe and prolonged	0
Liver	Enlarged, slightly tender	Enlarged, not tender	Enlarged and tender	Slightly enlarged
Palpable gallbladder	0	+ (sometimes)	0	0
Tender gallbladder area	+	0	0	0
Palpable spleen	0	Occasionally	About 20%	0
Temperature	↑	Not usually	↑ onset only	↑ onset
Investigations				
Leucocyte count	↑ or normal	↑ or normal	↓	Normal
Differential leucocytes	Polymorphs ↑	—	Lymphocytes ↑	Eosinophilia at onset
Faeces				
colour	Intermittently pale	Pale	Variable, light to dark	Pale
occult blood	0	±	0	0
Urine: urobilin(ogen)	+	Absent	– Early + Late	– Early
Serum bilirubin (μmol/l)	Usually 50–170	Steady rise to 250–500	Varies with severity	Variable
Serum alkaline phosphatase (times normal)	>3×	>3×	<3×	>3×
Serum aspartate transaminase (times normal)	<5×	<5×	>10×	>5×
Ultrasound and CT	Gallstones ± dilated duct	Dilated ducts ± mass	Splenomegaly	Normal

Jaundice after biliary tract surgery suggests residual calculus, traumatic stricture of the bile duct or hepatitis. Jaundice following the removal of a malignant growth may be due to hepatic metastases. Jaundice due to sepsis and/or shock is common in hospital practice and is often assumed due to viral or drug liver injury [41].

Alcoholics usually have associated features such as anorexia, morning nausea, diarrhoea and mild pyrexia. They may complain of pain over the enlarged liver.

Progressive failure of health and weight loss favour an underlying carcinoma.

The onset is extremely important. Preceding nausea, anorexia and an aversion to smoking (in smokers), followed by jaundice a few days later, suggest viral hepatitis or drug jaundice. Cholestatic jaundice develops more slowly, often with persistent pruritus. Pyrexia with rigors suggests cholangitis associated with gall-stones or biliary stricture.

Dark urine and pale stools precede hepato-cellular or cholestatic jaundice by a few days. In haemolytic jaundice the stools have a normal colour.

In hepato-cellular jaundice the patient feels ill; in cholestatic jaundice he may be inconvenienced only by the itching or jaundice, any other symptoms being due to the cause of the obstruction.

Persistent mild jaundice of varying intensity suggests haemolysis. The jaundice of compensated cirrhosis is usually mild and variable and is associated with normal stools, although patients with superimposed acute 'alcoholic hepatitis' may be deeply jaundiced and pass pale stools.

Biliary colic may be continuous for hours rather than being intermittent. Back or epigastric pain may be associated with pancreatic carcinoma.

Examination (fig. 12.7)

Age and sex. A parous, middle-aged, obese female may have gallstones. The incidence of type A hepatitis decreases as age advances but no age is exempt from type B and C. The probability of malignant biliary obstruction increases with age. Drug jaundice is very rare in childhood.

General examination. Anaemia may indicate haemolysis, cancer or cirrhosis. Gross weight loss suggests cancer. The patient with haemolytic jaundice is a mild yellow colour, with hepato-cellular jaundice is orange, and with prolonged biliary obstruction has a deep greenish hue. A hunched-up position suggests pancreatic carcinoma. In alcoholics, the skin signs of cirrhosis should be noted. Sites to be examined for a primary tumour include breasts, thyroid, stomach, colon, rectum and lung. Lymphadenopathy is noted.

Mental state. Slight intellectual deterioration with minimal personality change suggests hepato-cellular jaundice. Fetor and 'flapping' tremor indicate impending hepatic coma.

Skin changes. Bruising may indicate a clotting defect. Purpuric spots on forearms, axillae or shins may be related to the thrombocytopenia of cirrhosis. Other cutaneous manifestations of cirrhosis include vascular spiders, palmar erythema, white nails and loss of secondary sexual hair.

In chronic cholestasis, scratch marks, melanin pigmentation, finger clubbing, xanthomas on the eyelids (xanthelasmas), extensor surfaces and palmar creases, and hyperkeratosis may be found.

Pigmentation of the shins and ulcers may be seen in some forms of congenital haemolytic anaemia.

Malignant nodules should be sought in the skin. Multiple venous thromboses suggest carcinoma of the body of the pancreas. Ankle oedema may indicate cirrhosis, or obstruction of the inferior vena cava due to hepatic or pancreatic malignancy.

Abdominal examination. Dilated peri-umbilical veins indicate a portal collateral circulation and cirrhosis. Ascites may be due to cirrhosis or to malignant disease. A very large nodular liver suggests cancer. A small liver may indicate severe hepatitis or cirrhosis, and excludes extra-hepatic cholestasis in which the liver is enlarged and smooth. In the alcoholic, fatty change and cirrhosis may produce a uniform enlargement of the liver. The edge is tender in hepatitis, in congestive heart failure, with alcoholism, in bacterial cholangitis and occasionally in malignant disease. An arterial murmur over the liver indicates acute alcoholic hepatitis or primary liver cancer.

In choledocholithiasis the gallbladder may be tender and Murphy's sign positive. A palpable, and sometimes visibly enlarged, gallbladder suggests pancreatic cancer.

The abdomen is carefully examined for any primary tumour. Rectal examination is essential.

Urine and faeces. Bilirubinuria is an early sign of viral hepatitis and drug jaundice. Persistent absence of urobilinogen suggests total obstruction of the common bile duct. Persistent excess of urobilinogen with negative bilirubin supports haemolytic jaundice.

Persistent pale stools suggest biliary obstruction. Positive occult blood favours a diagnosis of ampullary, pancreatic or alimentary carcinoma or of portal hypertension.

Serum biochemical tests

Serum bilirubin confirms jaundice, indicates depth and is used to follow progress. Serum alkaline phosphatase values more than three times normal strongly suggest cholestasis if bone disease is absent and γ-GT is elevated; high values may also be found in patients with non-biliary cirrhosis.

Serum albumin and globulin levels are little changed in jaundice of short duration. In more chronic hepato-cellular jaundice the albumin is depressed and globulin increased. Electrophoretic analysis shows raised α_2- and β-globulins in cholestatic jaundice, in contrast to γ-globulin elevation in hepato-cellular jaundice.

Serum transaminases increase in hepatitis compared with variable but lower levels in cholestatic jaundice. High values may sometimes be found transiently with acute bile duct obstruction due to a stone.

Haematology

A low total leucocyte count with a relative lymphocytosis suggests hepato-cellular jaundice. A polymorph leucocytosis may be found in alcoholic and severe viral hepatitis. Increased leucocyte counts are found with acute cholangitis or underlying malignant disease. If haemolysis is suspected, investigations should include a reticulocyte count, examination of the blood film, erythrocyte fragility, Coombs' test and examination of the bone marrow.

If the prothrombin time is prolonged, vitamin K_1 10mg intravenously for 3 days leads to a return to normal in cholestasis, whereas patients with hepato-cellular jaundice show little change.

Diagnostic routine

Clinical evaluation allows the patient to be categorized into hepato-cellular, infiltrative, possible extra-hepatic biliary obstruction and likely extra-hepatic biliary obstruction [10]. Various algorithms are possible (fig. 12.8). The sequence employed depends on the clinical evaluation, the facilities available and the risk of each investigation. Cost plays a part.

A small proportion of patients with extra-hepatic biliary obstruction are incorrectly diagnosed as having intra-hepatic cholestasis, whereas a larger proportion of patients with intra-hepatic disease are initially thought to have extra-hepatic obstruction.

Computer models are based on clinical history and examination with haematological and biochemical observations made during the first 6h in hospital [29]. These have a performance equalling that of the hepatologist and better than some non-specialist internists. One computer-based system had an overall diagnostic accuracy of 70%, which was the same as experienced hepatologists who, however, reached a correct diagnosis with fewer questions per consultation [7].

Radiology

A chest film is taken to show primary and secondary

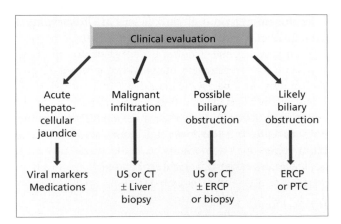

Fig. 12.8. An algorithm for diagnosing jaundice. CT, computed tomography; ERCP, endoscopic retrograde cholangiopancreatography; PTC, percutaneous transhepatic cholangiography; US, ultrasound.

tumours and any irregularity and elevation of the right diaphragm due to an enlarged or nodular liver.

Visualization of the bile ducts

This is indicated if the patient is cholestatic (Chapter 13). The first procedure in distinguishing hepato-cellular from surgical, main duct 'obstructive' jaundice is ultrasound to show whether or not the intra-hepatic bile ducts are dilated (figs 12.8, 13.18). This is usually followed by endoscopic examination (ERCP) although the advances in MRI make non-invasive MRCP an alternative, particularly where there is a relative contraindication to the endoscopic approach (Chapter 32). If direct cholangiography is necessary and ERCP has failed or there has been previous biliary bypass surgery, percutaneous cholangiography is indicated.

Viral markers

These are indicated for hepatitis A and B, cytomegalovirus and Epstein–Barr infections (Chapters 16 and 17). The serum antibody to hepatitis C virus becomes positive only 2–4 months after infection (Chapter 18).

Needle liver biopsy

Acute jaundice rarely merits liver biopsy, which is reserved for the patient who presents diagnostic difficulty and where an intra-hepatic cause is suspected. Deep jaundice is not a contraindication. If dilated bile ducts are shown on imaging, cholangiography is indicated and liver biopsy is inappropriate.

Transjugular or CT- or ultrasound-guided biopsy with plugging of the puncture site in the liver is useful if clotting defects preclude the routine percutaneous technique (Chapter 3).

Acute viral hepatitis is usually diagnosed easily. The greatest difficulty arises in the cholestatic group. However, in most instances an experienced histopathologist can distinguish appearances of intra-hepatic cholestasis, for instance due to drugs or to primary biliary cirrhosis, from the appearances of a block to the main bile ducts.

Laparoscopy

The appearance of a dark green liver with an enormous gallbladder favours extra-hepatic biliary obstruction. Tumour nodules may be seen and needle biopsy may be made under direct vision. A pale yellow–green liver suggests hepatitis and cirrhosis is obvious. The method cannot be relied upon to distinguish extra-hepatic biliary obstruction, especially due to a carcinoma of the main hepatic ducts, from intra-hepatic cholestasis due to drugs.

A photographic record should be taken of the appearances. In the presence of jaundice, peritoneoscopy is safer than needle biopsy but, if necessary, the two procedures may be combined.

Laparotomy

Before the many scanning techniques became available, patients occasionally underwent laparotomy in order to establish the cause of jaundice, with the risk of precipitating acute liver or renal failure. With all the scanning and other diagnostic approaches available laparotomy is inappropriate as a diagnostic approach.

Familial non-haemolytic hyperbilirubinaemias (table 12.3)

Although the upper limit of serum bilirubin is usually taken to be 17 μmol/l (0.8 mg/dl), in some 5% of healthy blood donors higher values (20–50 μmol/l) may be found. When those suffering from haemolysis or from liver disease have been excluded there remain the patients with familial abnormalities of bilirubin metabolism. The commonest is Gilbert's syndrome. Other syndromes can also be identified. The prognosis is excellent. Accurate diagnosis, particularly from chronic liver disease, is important for it enables the patient to be reassured. It is based on family history, duration, absence of stigmata of hepato-cellular disease and of splenomegaly, exclusion of haemolysis, normal serum transaminases and, if necessary, liver biopsy.

Primary hyperbilirubinaemia

This very rare condition is due to increased production of 'early labelled' bilirubin in the bone marrow. The cause is probably the premature destruction of abnormal red cell precursors (ineffective erythrocyte synthesis). The clinical picture is of compensated haemolysis. Peripheral erythrocyte destruction is normal. The condition is probably familial [1].

Gilbert's syndrome

This is named after Augustin Gilbert (1858–1927), a Parisian physician [40]. It is defined as benign, familial, mild, unconjugated hyperbilirubinaemia (serum bilirubin 17–85 μmol/l [1–5 mg/dl]) not due to haemolysis and with normal routine tests of liver function and hepatic histology. It affects some 2–5% of the population.

It may be diagnosed by chance at a routine medical examination or when the blood is being examined for another reason, for instance after viral hepatitis. It has an excellent prognosis. Jaundice is mild and intermittent. Deepening may follow an intercurrent infection or fasting and is associated with malaise, nausea and often discomfort over the liver. These symptoms are probably no greater than in normal controls [21]. There are no other abnormal physical signs; the spleen is not palpable.

Patients with Gilbert's syndrome have a deficiency in hepatic bilirubin glucuronidation—about 30% of normal. The bile contains an excess of bilirubin monoglucuronide over the diglucuronide. The Bolivian squirrel monkey is an animal model for this disorder [26].

The genetic basis for Gilbert's syndrome has been clarified by the finding that the promoter region (A(TA)$_6$TAA) of the gene encoding UGT1*1 (see fig. 12.4) has an additional TA dinucleotide, resulting in a change to (A(TA)$_7$TAA) [3, 19]. It is inherited as autosomal recessive; that is, patients are homozygous for this abnormality.

There is a close relationship between the promoter region genotype and the expression of hepatic bilirubin UGT enzyme activity [27]. Individuals with the 7/7 genotype have the lowest enzyme activity. Heterozygotes (6/7 genotype) have an enzyme activity intermediate between 7/7 and normal wild-type 6/6.

A survey of individuals from eastern Scotland and Canadian Inuit populations have shown homozygosity

Table 12.3. Isolated rise in serum bilirubin

Type	Diagnostic points
Unconjugated	
Haemolysis	Splenomegaly. Blood film. Reticulocytosis. Coombs' test
Gilbert's syndrome	Familial. Serum bilirubin increases with fasting and falls on phenobarbitone administration. Liver biopsy normal but conjugating enzyme reduced. Normal serum transaminases. DNA analysis
Crigler–Najjar syndrome	
type I	No conjugating enzyme in liver. No response to phenobarbitone. Analysis of gene expression. Risk of kernicterus. Liver transplantation effective
type II	Absent or deficient conjugating enzyme in liver. Response to phenobarbitone
Conjugated	
Dubin–Johnson syndrome	Black-liver biopsy. No concentration of cholecystographic media. Secondary rise in BSP test
Rotor type	Normal liver biopsy. Cholecystography normal. BSP test no uptake

BSP, bromsulphalein.

for the genotype A(TA)₇TAA allele in 12–17% of those tested [5]. This genotype may not always correlate with the serum bilirubin because environmental factors, such as alcohol ingestion, influence hepatic bilirubin UGT activity.

Patients with other variations of the A(TA)$_n$TAA allele have also shown elevated serum total bilirubin levels, including the alleles 5/6, 5/7 and 7/8 [5].

In Asians and the Japanese, the frequency of the TATAA box mutations is low, at around 3%. Studies suggest that heterozygosity for mutations in the UGT1*1 gene itself may have a mild hyperbilirubinaemia and appear clinically similar to patients with Gilbert's syndrome [15].

The lengthening of this promoter sequence is thought to interfere with the binding of the transcription factor IID, resulting in reduced UGT1*1 gene expression. However, although a reduced enzyme level is necessary for Gilbert's syndrome, it is not sufficient alone, and other factors such as reduced hepatic intake of bilirubin [24] and occult haemolysis may play a role in the development of hyperbilirubinaemia. Thus there may be a mild impairment of bromsulphalein (BSP) [24] and tolbutamide clearance (a drug that does not need conjugation).

The variant of the TATAA box found in Gilbert's syndrome is a major factor determining the unconjugated hyperbilirubinemia in ABO-incompatible neonates and also neonates with prolonged unconjugated hyperbilirubinaemia [13, 18]. It has also been implicated in persistent unconjugated hyperbilirubinaemia after liver transplantation, due to an abnormal TATAA box in the donor liver [12]. The same variant promoter also appears to influence the level of hyperbilirubinaemia in individuals with inherited haemolytic diseases [30] including β thalassemia where there is also an association with gallstone formation [26].

Specialist diagnostic tests include the increase in serum bilirubin on fasting (fig. 12.9) [22], the fall on taking phenobarbitone which induces the hepatic conjugating enzyme (fig. 12.10), and the increase following intravenous nicotinic acid which raises the osmotic fragility of red blood cells.

Thin layer chromatography shows a significantly higher proportion of unconjugated bilirubin than in normals, chronic haemolysis or chronic hepatitis; this is diagnostic. The fasting serum bile acids are normal or even low. Low values for bilirubin conjugating enzyme are found in liver biopsies. However, Gilbert's syndrome is usually diagnosed with ease without recourse to these specialist methods. The demonstration of a raised bilirubin level that is predominantly unconjugated, with normal liver enzymes and no evidence of haemolysis, is usually sufficient to reassure the patient who is otherwise asymptomatic without abnormal physical signs.

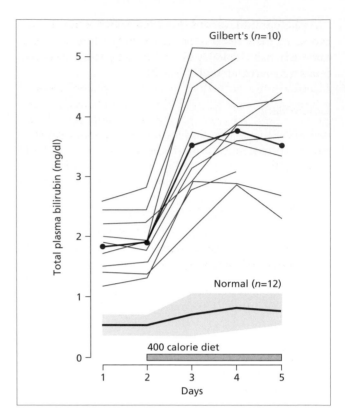

Fig. 12.9. Gilbert's syndrome. The serum unconjugated bilirubin level increases during a 400 calorie diet [22].

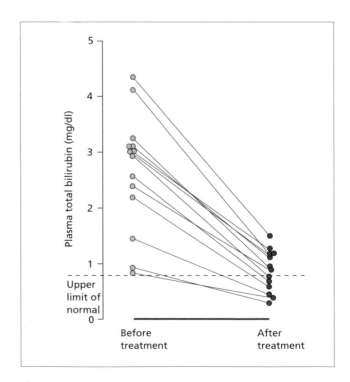

Fig. 12.10. Gilbert's syndrome. The effect of phenobarbitone (60 mg, three times a day) on the serum bilirubin level [2].

Patients with Gilbert's syndrome have a normal life expectancy and reassurance is the only necessary treatment. Hyperbilirubinaemia is life long and not associated with increased morbidity [21].

Serum bilirubin may be reduced by phenobarbitone [2] but, as icterus is rarely obvious, few patients will gain cosmetic benefit from this treatment. 'Sufferers' should be warned that jaundice can follow an intercurrent infection, repeated vomiting or missed meals. The 'sufferer' is a normal risk for life insurance.

Crigler–Najjar syndrome [11, 20]

This extreme form of familial non-haemolytic jaundice is associated with very high serum unconjugated bilirubin values. Inheritance is autosomal recessive. Deficiency of conjugating enzyme can be demonstrated in the liver. Total pigment in the bile is minimal.

Type I

In untreated patients the serum bilirubin is in excess of 350 µmol/l. No bilirubin conjugating enzyme can be detected in the liver. Bile contains only traces of bilirubin conjugates [11]. Since the serum bilirubin levels eventually stabilize, the patient must have some alternative pathway of bilirubin metabolism.

The molecular defect is in one of the five exons (1*1–5) of the bilirubin UGT1*1 gene (see fig. 12.4). Analysis of the Crigler–Najjar type I mutations by expression in COS cells or fibroblasts shows no bilirubin conjugating activity [33].

Around 170 cases of Crigler–Najjar type I have been reported in the world literature [11]. The overall prevalence is unknown. Before phototherapy was used, patients died at between 1 and 2 years of age from kernicterus. In this complication, due to high levels of unconjugated bilirubin, there is staining of basal ganglia and cranial nerve nuclei. Unconjugated bilirubin *in vitro* damages neurons and astrocytes through increased apoptosis [34]. The bilirubin encephalopathy may lead to central deafness, oculomotor palsy, ataxia, choreoathetosis, mental retardation, seizures, spasticity and death. This complication of the Crigler–Najjar syndrome is usually seen in the very young patient but may occur later.

Treatment is by daily phototherapy to keep the serum bilirubin level below 350 µmol/l. Oral calcium phosphate makes phototherapy more effective [38]. There is no response to phenobarbitone. Phlebotomy and plasmapheresis have been used to reduce the serum bilirubin, but with only temporary success. Phototherapy degrades unconjugated bilirubin into products including lumibilirubin, which is water soluble and can be secreted into the bile. Some of the photodegradation products may spontaneously revert to natural isomers of unconjugated bilirubin and the oral administration of calcium salts prevents their reabsorption. An alternative approach to reduce serum bilirubin levels is to inhibit the breakdown of haemoglobin to bilirubin by the enzyme haem oxygenase. Tin protoporphyrin, a haem oxygenase inhibitor, has been demonstrated to give a temporary (5–7 weeks) decrease in plasma unconjugated bilirubin of around 30% [28].

Orthotopic or orthotopic-auxiliary liver transplantation is the only definitive therapy for Crigler–Najjar type I. It has been recommended that this should be performed at a young age, particularly where reliable phototherapy cannot be guaranteed [39]. Phototherapy, although initially successful, becomes less efficient after puberty. There is always a risk of kernicterus because of lack of compliance and/or events that precipitate hyperbilirubinaemia, including infection, drug interactions, trauma and surgical procedures.

In a survey of 57 patients with Crigler–Najjar type I, 37% had received a liver transplant [39]. Twenty-six per cent had suffered brain damage but in half of these damage was mild and liver transplantation was still deemed appropriate.

Experimental treatment using percutaneous, transhepatic intra-portal administration of normal hepatocytes successfully reduced the serum bilirubin and the duration of phototherapy in a case report [9].

In *Gunn rats*, a mutant strain of the Wistar rat, bilirubin UGT is absent and there is unconjugated hyperbilirubinaemia. The genetic defect corresponds to that in Crigler–Najjar type I, with a deletion in the exon common to all UGT enzymes resulting in a premature stop codon which leads to the synthesis of truncated, inactive UGT isoforms. Experimentally, several approaches to gene therapy have been attempted in Gunn rats [37] with varying success. The metabolic defect has been corrected experimentally by site-specific repair using a chimeric oligonucleotide [16].

Type II

Bilirubin conjugating enzyme is reduced to less than 10% of normal in the liver and, although present, is undetectable by the usual methods of analysis. The serum bilirubin usually does not exceed 350 µmol/l. Jaundice is present of about half of patients within the first year of life, but can occur as late as 30 years of age. Acute exacerbations of hyperbilirubinaemia may occur during fasting or intercurrent illnesses and bilirubin encephalopathy can develop [20]. The patients respond dramatically to phenobarbitone and survive into adult life.

DNA analysis of the bilirubin UGT1*1 gene (see fig. 12.4) has shown mutations in exons 1*1–5 [4, 11].

However, expression analysis of these mutants has shown residual enzyme activity—explaining the lower serum bilirubin concentration than found in Crigler–Najjar type I—the presence of glucuronides in bile and the beneficial effect of phenobarbitone.

Some relatives of patients with Crigler–Najjar syndrome have an elevated serum bilirubin concentration, below that of true Crigler–Najjar but higher than that of Gilbert's syndrome [19]. Analysis of the UGT1*1 gene has suggested that these patients are compound heterozygotes, one allele having the Gilbert's TATAA box mutation, and the other having a Crigler–Najjar mutation [3, 36].

Type II is not always benign and phototherapy and phenobarbitone should be given to keep the serum bilirubin level less than 340 µmol/l (26 mg/dl).

The distinction between type I and type II Crigler–Najjar syndrome is made by observing the response to phenobarbitone treatment. There is no response in patients with type I. In patients with type II, the serum bilirubin level falls by more than 25%. There are exceptions to this rule. Some patients with type II do not respond to phenobarbitone. Definitive diagnosis in these patients could be done by *in vitro* expression of mutant DNA from patients in COS cells or fibroblasts, but this is too elaborate and expensive for routine use [33]. An alternative approach is to analyse duodenal bile after phenobarbitone. In type II there is an increase in biliary mono- and diconjugates. In type I only minimal traces of monoconjugate bilirubin are found [35].

Dubin–Johnson syndrome

This is a chronic, benign, intermittent jaundice with conjugated and some unconjugated hyperbilirubinaemia and with bilirubinuria. It is autosomal recessive, and is most frequent in the Middle East among Iranian Jews. The mutation responsible is in the gene encoding cMOAT [23]. The defect in this transporter explains the diagnostic pattern seen in the prolonged BSP test [17]. After intravenous injection of BSP there is an initial fall in serum level which then rises so that the value at 120 min exceeds that seen at 45 min (fig. 12.11) due to regurgitation into the circulation of the glutathione conjugate, which is normally excreted into bile via cMOAT. The defect in this transporter also explains the increased urinary excretion of coproporphyrin I. Studies in the TR⁻ rat, which has a mutation in the homologous canalicular transporter, has allowed characterization of these and other biochemical defects.

The liver, macroscopically, is greenish-black (black-liver jaundice) (fig. 12.12). In sections the liver cells show a brown pigment which is neither iron nor bile (fig. 12.13). There is no correlation between liver pigment and

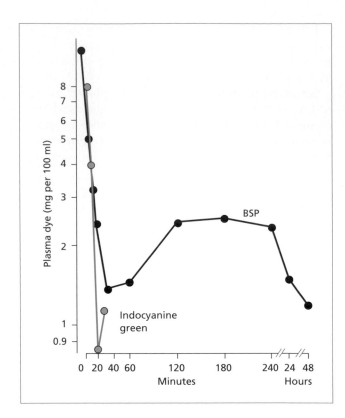

Fig. 12.11. Bromsulphalein (BSP) tolerance test (5 mg/kg i.v.) in a patient with Dubin–Johnson syndrome. At 40 min, the BSP level has almost returned to normal. An increase is then seen at 120, 180 and 240 min. Dye can still be detected in the blood at 48 h. The indocyanine green test is also shown and is normal at 20 min, but also has a tendency to increase at 30 min.

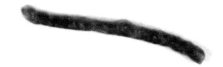

Fig. 12.12. This needle liver biopsy from a patient with Dubin–Johnson syndrome is blackish-brown.

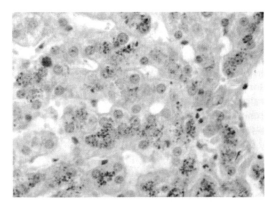

Fig. 12.13. Dubin–Johnson hyperbilirubinaemia. The liver cells and Kupffer cells are packed with a dark pigment which gives the staining reactions of lipofuscin. (H & E, ×275.)

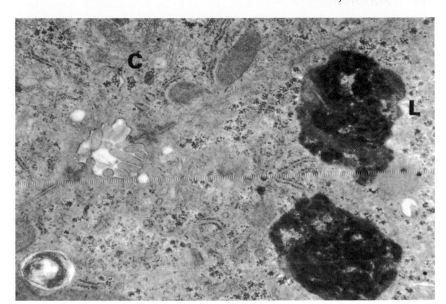

Fig. 12.14. Dubin–Johnson syndrome. Electron microscopy showing normal bile canaliculi with intact microvilli (C). Lysosomes (L) are enlarged, irregularly shaped and contain granular material and often membrane-bound lipid droplets.

serum bilirubin levels. The chemical nature of the pigment is not certain. Previously thought due to melanin, recent data support the proposal that impaired secretion of anionic metabolites of tyrosine, phenylalanine and tryptophan is responsible [14].

Electron microscopy shows the pigment in dense bodies related to lysosomes (fig. 12.14).

Pruritus is absent and the serum alkaline phosphatase and bile acid levels are normal.

The contrast media used in intravenous cholangiography are not transported into bile but ^{99m}Tc-HIDA excretion shows a normal liver, biliary tree and gallbladder.

Rotor type

This is a similar form of chronic familial conjugated hyperbilirubinaemia. It resembles the Dubin–Johnson syndrome, the main difference being the absence of brown pigment in the liver cell [32]. Electron microscopy may show abnormalities of mitochondria and peroxisomes [8].

The condition also differs from the Dubin–Johnson type in that the gallbladder opacifies on cholecystography and there is no secondary rise in the BSP test. The abnormality causing BSP retention appears to be related to a defect in hepatic uptake rather than excretion as originally demonstrated in the Dubin–Johnson syndrome. ^{99m}Tc-HIDA excretion gives no visualization of the liver, gallbladder or biliary tree.

Total urinary coproporphyrins are raised, as in cholestasis.

Family studies make an autosomal inheritance probable. The Rotor type has an excellent prognosis.

The group of familial non-haemolytic hyperbilirubinaemias

There is much overlap between the various syndromes of congenital hyperbilirubinaemia. Patients are found in the same family with conjugated hyperbilirubinaemia, with or without pigment in the liver cells. Pigmented livers have been found in patients with unconjugated hyperbilirubinaemia [6]. In one large family the propositi had the classic Dubin–Johnson picture, but the commonest abnormality in the family was unconjugated hyperbilirubinaemia [6]. In another family, conjugated and unconjugated hyperbilirubinaemia alternated in the same patient [31]. Such observations add to the confusion in separating the groups and in deciding the inheritance.

References

1 Arias IM. Chronic unconjugated hyperbilirubinaemia (CUH) with increased production of bile pigment not derived from the haemoglobin of mature, circulating erythrocytes. *J. Clin. Invest.* 1962; **41**: 1341.

2 Black M, Sherlock S. Treatment of Gilbert's syndrome with phenobarbitone. *Lancet* 1970; **i**: 1359.

3 Bosma PJ, Chowdhury JR, Bakker C *et al.* The genetic basis of the reduced expression of bilirubin UDP-glucuronosyltransferase 1 in Gilbert's syndrome. *N. Engl. J. Med.* 1995; **333**: 1171.

4 Bosma PJ, Goldhoorn B, Elferink RPJO *et al.* A mutation in bilirubin uridine 5′-diphosphate-glucuronosyltransferase isoform 1 causing Crigler–Najjar syndrome Type II. *Gastroenterology* 1993; **105**: 216.

5 Burchell B, Hume R. Molecular genetic basis of Gilbert's syndrome. *J. Gastroenterol. Hepatol.* 1999; **14**: 960.

6 Butt HR, Anderson VE, Foulk WT *et al.* Studies of chronic idiopathic jaundice (Dubin–Johnson syndrome). II. Evalua-

tion of a large family with the trait. *Gastroenterology* 1966; **51**: 619.

7 Camma C, Garofalo G, Almasio P *et al*. A performance evaluation of the expert system 'jaundice' in comparison with that of three hepatologists. *J. Hepatol.* 1991; **13**: 279.

8 Evans J, Lefkowitch J, Lim CK *et al*. Fecal porphyrin abnormalities in a patient with features of Rotor's syndrome. *Gastroenterology* 1981; **81**: 1125.

9 Fox, IJ, Chowdhury JR, Kaufman SS *et al*. Treatment of the Crigler–Najjar syndrome type I with hepatocyte transplantation. *N. Engl. J. Med.* 1998; **338**: 1422.

10 Frank BB. Clinical evaluation of jaundice. A guideline of the patient care committee of the American Gastroenterological Association. *JAMA* 1989; **262**: 3031.

11 Jansen PLM. Diagnosis and management of Crigler–Najjar syndrome. *Eur. J. Paediatr.* 1999; **158** (Suppl. 2): S89.

12 Jansen PLM, Bosma PJ, Bakker C *et al*. Persistent unconjugated hyperbilirubinemia after liver transplantation due to an abnormal bilirubin UDP-glucuronosyltransferase gene promotor sequence in the donor. *J. Hepatol.* 1997; **27**: 1.

13 Kaplan M, Hammerman C, Renbaum P *et al*. Gilbert's syndrome and hyperbilirubinaemia in ABO-incompatible neonates. *Lancet* 2000; **356**: 652.

14 Kitamura T, Alroy J, Gatmaitan Z *et al*. Defective biliary excretion of epinephrine metabolites in mutant (TR⁻) rats: relation to the pathogenesis of black liver in the Dubin–Johnson syndrome and Corriedale sheep with an analogous excretory defect. *Hepatology* 1992; **15**: 1154.

15 Koiwai O, Nishizawa M, Hasada K *et al*. Gilbert's syndrome is caused by heterozygous missense mutation in the gene for bilirubin UDP-glucuronosyltransferase. *Hum. Mol. Gen.* 1995; **4**:1183.

16 Kren BT, Parashar B, Bandyopadhyay P *et al*. Correction of the UDP-glucuronosyltransferase gene defect in the Gunn rat model of Crigler–Najjar syndrome type I with a chimeric oligonucleotide. *Proc. Natl. Acad. Sci. USA* 1999; **96**: 10349.

17 Mandema E, De Fraiture WH, Nieweg HO *et al*. Familial chronic idiopathic jaundice (Dubin–Sprinz disease) with a note on bromsulphalein metabolism in this disease. *Am. J. Med.* 1960; **28**: 42.

18 Monaghan G, McLellan A, McGeehan A *et al*. Gilbert's syndrome is a contributory factor in prolonged unconjugated hyperbilirubinemia of the newborn. *J. Paediatr.* 1999; **134**: 441.

19 Monaghan G, Ryan M, Seddon R *et al*. Genetic variation in bilirubin UDP-glucuronosyltransferase gene promoter and Gilbert's syndrome. *Lancet* 1996; **347**: 578.

20 Nowicki MJ, Poley JR *et al*. The hereditary hyperbilirubinaemias. *Bailliere's Clin. Gastroenterol.* 1998; **12**: 355.

21 Olsson R, Stigendal L. Clinical experience with isolated hyperbilirubinemia. *Scand. J. Gastroenterol.* 1989; **24**: 617.

22 Owens D, Sherlock S. The diagnosis of Gilbert's syndrome: role of the reduced caloric intake test. *Br. Med. J.* 1973; **iii**: 559.

23 Paulusma CC, Kool M, Bosma PJ *et al*. A mutation in the human canalicular multispecific organic anion transporter gene causes the Dublin–Johnson syndrome. *Hepatology* 1997; **25**: 1539.

24 Persico M, Persico, E, Bakker CTM *et al*. Hepatic uptake of

organic anions affects the plasma bilirubin level in subjects with Gilbert's syndrome mutations in UGT1A1. *Hepatology* 2001; **33**: 627.

25 Portman OW, Chowdhury JR, Chowdhury NR *et al*. A non-human primate model of Gilbert's syndrome. *Hepatology* 1984; **4**: 175.

26 Premawardhena A, Fisher CA, Fathiu F *et al*. Genetic determinants of jaundice and gallstones in haemoglobin E β thalassaemia. *Lancet* 2001; **357**: 1945.

27 Raijmakers MTM, Jansen PLM, Steegers EAP *et al*. Association of human liver bilirubin UDP-glucuronyltransferase activity with a polymorphism in the promoter region of the UGT1A1 gene. *J. Hepatol.* 2000; **33**: 348.

28 Rubaltelli FF, Guerrini P, Reddie E *et al*. Tin-protoporphyrin in the management of children with Crigler–Najjar disease. *Paediatrics* 1989; **84**: 728.

29 Saint-Marc Girardin M-F, Le Minor M, Alperovitch A *et al*. Computer-aided selection of diagnostic tests in jaundiced patients. *Gut* 1985; **26**: 961.

30 Sampietro M, Iolascon A. Molecular pathology of Crigler–Najjar type I and II and Gilbert's syndromes. *Haematologica* 1999; **84**: 150.

31 Satler J. Another variant of constitutional familial hepatic dysfunction with permanent jaundice and with alternating serum bilirubin relations. *Acta Hepatosplen.* 1966; **13**: 38.

32 Schiff L, Billing BH, Oikawa Y. Familial nonhemolytic jaundice with conjugated bilirubin in the serum. A case study. *N. Engl. J. Med.* 1959; **260**: 1314.

33 Seppen J, Bosma PJ, Goldhoorn, BG *et al*. Discrimination between Crigler–Najjar type I and II by expression of mutant bilirubin uridine diphosphate glucuronosyl transferase. *J. Clin. Invest.* 1994; **94**: 2385.

34 Silva RFM, Rodrigues CMP, Brites D. Bilirubin-induced apoptosis in cultured rat neural cells is aggravated by chenodeoxycholic acid but prevented by ursodeoxycholic acid. *J. Hepatol.* 2001; **34**: 402.

35 Sinaasappel M, Jansen PLM. The differential diagnosis of Crigler–Najjar disease, types 1 and 2, by bile pigment analysis. *Gastroenterology* 1991; **100**: 783.

36 Strassburg CP, Manns MP. Jaundice, genes and promoters. *J. Hepatol.* 2000; **33**: 476.

37 Tiribelli C, Ostrow JD. New concepts in bilirubin and jaundice: report of the Third International Bilirubin Workshop, April 6–8, 1995, Trieste, Italy. *Hepatology* 1996; **24**: 1296.

38 van der Veere CN, Jansen PLM, Sinaasappel M *et al*. Oral calcium phosphate: a new therapy for Crigler–Najjar disease? *Gastroenterology* 1997; **112**: 455.

39 van der Veere CN, Sinaasappel M, McDonagh AF *et al*. Current therapy of Crigler–Najjar syndrome type I: report of a world registry. *Hepatology* 1996; **24**: 311.

40 Watson KJR, Gollan JL. Gilbert's syndrome. *Clin. Gastroenterol.* 1989; **3**: 337.

41 Whitehead MW, Hainsworth I, Kingham JGC. The causes of obvious jaundice in South West Wales: perceptions versus reality. *Gut* 2001; **48**: 409.

42 Zucker SD, Goessling W, Gollan JL. Kinetics of bilirubin transfer between serum albumin and membrane vesicles. *J. Biol. Chem.* 1995; **270**: 1974.

Chapter 13
Cholestasis

Cholestasis is defined as the failure of normal bile to reach the duodenum. This may be due to pathology anywhere between the hepatocyte and the ampulla of Vater. The term 'obstructive jaundice' is not used, as in many instances no mechanical block can be shown in the biliary tract.

Prolonged cholestasis produces biliary cirrhosis; the time taken for its development varies from months to years. The transition is not reflected in a sudden change in the clinical picture. The term 'biliary cirrhosis' is reserved for a pathological picture. It is diagnosed when there are features of cirrhosis such as nodule formation, encephalopathy or fluid retention.

Anatomy of the biliary system

Bile salts, conjugated bilirubin, cholesterol, phospholipids, proteins, electrolytes and water are secreted by the liver cell into the canaliculus (fig. 13.1). The bile secretory apparatus comprises the *canalicular membrane* with its carrier proteins, the *intra-cellular organelles* and the *cytoskeleton* of the hepatocyte (fig. 13.2). *Tight junctions* between hepatocytes seal the biliary space from the blood compartment.

The canalicular membrane contains carrier proteins which transport bile acids, bilirubin, cations and anions. The microvilli increase the surface area. The organelles include the Golgi apparatus and lysosomes. Vesicles carry proteins such as IgA from the sinusoid to the canaliculus, and newly synthesized cholesterol and phospholipid, and possibly bile acid membrane trans-

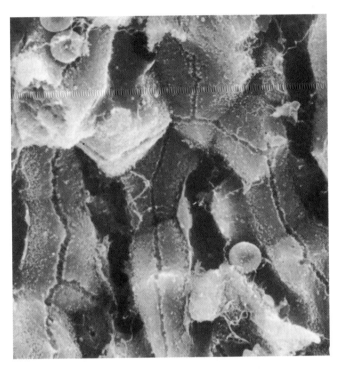

Fig. 13.1. Scanning electron micrograph of the canalicular biliary system.

porters, from the microsomes to the bile canalicular membrane.

The peri-canalicular cytoplasm contains elements of the *cytoskeleton* of the hepatocyte: *microtubules*, *microfilaments* and *intermediate filaments* [84]. Microtubules are

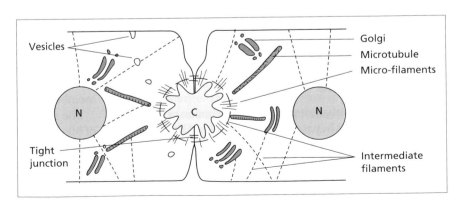

Fig. 13.2. The biliary secretory apparatus. Diagram of the ultrastructure of the bile canaliculus (C), cytoskeleton, and organelles (N, nucleus).

219

biochemistry may not separate them. There is a need for a diagnostic algorithm to differentiate between the two.

Patients with both acute and chronic cholestasis may itch, malabsorb fat and be vitamin K deficient. Chronic cholestatic patients may have in addition hyperlipidaemia and bone disease.

Pathogenesis

Physical obstruction to the bile duct by stone or stricture is straightforward. The pathogenesis of primary biliary cirrhosis and primary sclerosing cholangitis is described elsewhere (Chapters 14 and 15). Drugs, hormones and sepsis affect hepatocyte cytoskeleton and membrane (table 13.1).

Membrane fluidity. Ethinyl oestradiol is known to decrease fluidity of the sinusoidal plasma membrane. This can be prevented experimentally by the methyl donor S-adenosyl-L-methionine (SAME).

Membrane transporters. Endotoxin decreases Na^+/K^+–ATPase activity. Cyclosporin A inhibits ATP-dependent bile acid transport across the canalicular membrane. In an experimental model of the cholestasis associated with colitis, there is decreased expression of the canalicular multi-specific organic anion transporter (cMOAT) possibly due to increased endotoxin levels [50]. Bile acid uptake and secretion by the liver are reduced [87].

Cytoskeleton. Integrity of the canalicular membrane may be altered by disruption of either the *micro-filaments* responsible for canalicular tone and contraction, or the *tight junctions*. Cholestasis due to phalloidin is related to depolymerization of the actin of micro-filaments. Chlorpromazine also affects polymerization of actin. Cytochalasin B and androgens disrupt micro-filaments and canaliculi become less contractile. Oestrogens and phalloidin disrupt tight junctions and this leads to loss of the normal barrier between the intracellular fluid in the space of Disse and canalicular bile, with passage of solutes directly from canaliculus into blood, and vice versa.

Vesicular transport. This depends upon the integrity of microtubules and these can be disrupted by colchicine and chlorpromazine.

Ductular abnormalities. Inflammation and epithelial changes interfere with bile flow but are probably secondary rather than primary.

Table 13.1. Possible cellular mechanisms of cholestasis

Membrane lipid/fluidity	Modified
Na^+/K^+–ATPase/other carriers	Inhibited
Cytoskeleton	Disrupted
Canalicular integrity (membrane, tight junction)	Lost

Effects of retained bile acids

The mechanism of hepato-cellular damage in cholestasis is not fully understood but seems related to the retention of toxic substances, particularly hydrophobic bile acids, which have many effects including the production of oxygen free radicals by mitochondria. Thus although the initial cellular insult may be immunological, toxic or genetic, injury may be exacerbated by bile acids. These not only produce cell necrosis but also trigger apoptosis [74] depending on the concentration of toxic bile acid. Thus, at low concentrations there is apoptosis; at higher concentrations, necrosis. Mitochondrial dysfunction and damage appears involved in both. Ursodeoxycholic acid prevents apoptosis during cholestasis by inhibiting mitochondrial membrane depolarization and channel formation [74]. Aside from cell death, cholestasis impairs enzyme activity. Bile duct ligation decreases mitochondrial respiratory chain enzyme activity and β-oxidation. This does not recover completely after obstruction is relieved [51].

Pathology

Some changes are related to cholestasis itself and depend on its duration. Characteristic changes of specific diseases are not covered here but in the appropriate chapters.

Macroscopically the cholestatic liver is enlarged, green, swollen and with a rounded edge. Nodularity develops late.

Light microscopy. Zone 3 shows marked bilirubin stasis in hepatocytes, Kupffer cells and canaliculi (fig. 13.6). Hepatocytes may show feathery degeneration, possibly due to retention of bile salts, with foamy cells and surrounding mononuclear cells. Cellular necrosis, regeneration and nodular hyperplasia are minimal.

Portal zones (zone 1) show ductular proliferation (fig. 13.7) due to the mitogenic effect of bile salts. Hepatocytes

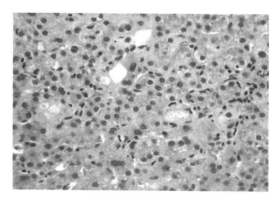

Fig. 13.6. Cholestasis: bile is seen in dilated canaliculi and hepatocytes.

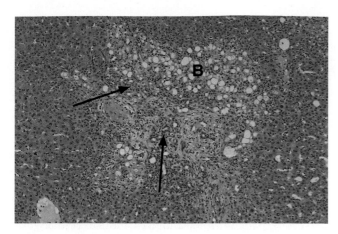

Fig. 13.7. Bile duct obstruction. There is portal tract expansion and ductular proliferation (arrows) with balloon ('feathery') degeneration of surrounding hepatocytes (B). (H & E, ×40.)

transform into bile duct cells and form basement membranes. Reabsorption of bile constituents by ductular cells can result in microlith formation.

Following bile duct obstruction the hepatic changes develop very rapidly. Cholestasis is seen within 36 h. Bile duct proliferation is early; portal fibrosis develops later. After about 2 weeks, duration cannot be related to the extent of hepatic change. *Bile lakes* represent ruptured interlobular ducts.

With ascending cholangitis, histology shows accumulations of polymorphonuclear leucocytes related to bile ducts. The sinusoids also contain numerous polymorphs.

Fibrosis can be seen in zone 1. This is reversible if the cholestasis is relieved. The zone 1 fibrosis extends to meet bands from adjacent zones (fig. 13.8) so that eventually zone 3 is enclosed by a ring of connective tissue (fig. 13.9). In the early stages, the relationship of hepatic vein to portal vein is normal and this distinguishes the picture from biliary cirrhosis. Continuing peri-ductular fibrosis may lead to disappearance of bile ducts and this is irreversible.

Zone 1 oedema and inflammation are related to reflux of bile into lymphatics and to leucotrienes. Mallory bodies can accompany the inflammation and fibrosis in zone 1. Copper-associated protein, demonstrated by orcein staining, is seen in peri-portal hepatocytes.

Class I HLA antigens are normally expressed on hepatocytes. Reports on the pattern of class II expression are conflicting. This HLA antigen seems to be absent on hepatocytes of normal children and present in some patients with autoimmune liver disease and primary sclerosing cholangitis [55].

Biliary cirrhosis follows prolonged cholestasis. Fibrous tissue bands in the portal zones coalesce and the lobules are correspondingly reduced in size. Fibrous bridges join

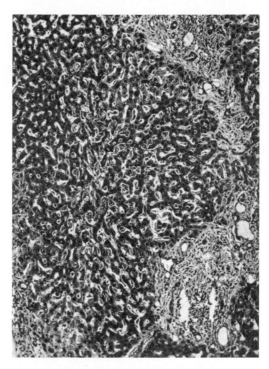

Fig. 13.8. Unrelieved common bile duct obstruction showing bile duct proliferation and fibrosis in the portal tracts, which are becoming joined together. Bile pigment accumulations can be seen in the centrizonal areas. The hepatic lobular architecture is normal. (H & E, ×67.)

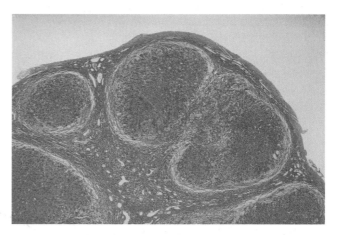

Fig. 13.9. Biliary cirrhosis. Low power view showing marked peri-nodular oedema and partly coalescent nodules—features typical of this condition. (H & E, ×15.)

portal and centrizonal areas (fig. 13.9). Nodular regeneration of liver cells follows, but a true cirrhosis rarely follows biliary obstruction. In total biliary obstruction due to cancer of the head of the pancreas, death ensues before nodular regeneration has had time to develop. Biliary cirrhosis is associated with partial biliary obstruction due, for instance, to benign biliary stricture or primary sclerosing cholangitis.

In biliary cirrhosis the liver is larger and greener than in non-biliary cirrhosis. Margins of nodules are clear-cut rather than moth-eaten. If the cholestasis is relieved the portal zone fibrosis and bile retention disappear slowly.

Electron microscopy. The biliary canaliculi show changes irrespective of the cause. These include dilatation and oedema, blunting, distortion and sparsity of the microvilli. The Golgi apparatus shows vacuolization. Peri-canalicular bile-containing vesicles appear and these represent the 'feathery' hepatocytes seen on light microscopy. Lysosomes proliferate and contain copper bound as a metalloprotein.

The endoplasmic reticulum is hypertrophied; all these changes are non-specific for the aetiology of the cholestasis.

Changes in other organs. The spleen is enlarged and firm due to reticulo-endothelial hyperplasia and increase in mononuclear cells. Later, cirrhosis results in portal hypertension and splenomegaly.

The intestinal contents are bulky and greasy; the more complete the cholestasis, the paler the stools.

The kidneys are swollen and bile stained. Casts containing bilirubin are found in the distal convoluted tubules and collecting tubules. The casts may be heavily infiltrated with cells and the tubular epithelium is disrupted. The surrounding connective tissue may then show oedema and inflammatory infiltration. Scar formation is absent.

Clinical features

Prominent features of cholestasis, both acute and chronic, are itching and malabsorption. Bone disease (hepatic osteodystrophy) and cholesterol deposition (xanthomas, xanthelasmas) are seen with chronic cholestasis, which is also associated with skin pigmentation due to melanin. In contrast to the patient with hepato-cellular disease where there is malaise and physical deterioration, the cholestatic patient feels well. On examination, the *liver* is usually enlarged with a firm smooth non-tender edge. *Splenomegaly* is unusual except in biliary cirrhosis where portal hypertension has developed. Stools are pale.

Pruritus has been attributed to retained bile acids. However, even with the most sophisticated biochemical methods, pruritus did not correlate with the concentration of any naturally occurring bile acid in serum or in skin [29]. Moreover, in terminal liver failure, when pruritus is lost, serum bile acids may still be increased.

The association of pruritus with cholestasis suggests that it is due to some substance normally excreted in the bile. Disappearance of itching when liver cells fail indicates that the agent responsible may be manufactured by the liver. Cholestyramine binds many compounds and thus its success in treating the pruritus of cholestasis does not incriminate one particular agent.

Attention has turned towards agents that may produce itching by a central neurotransmitter mechanism [9, 46].

There is evidence from experimental studies and therapeutic trials that endogenous opioid peptides may be responsible by increasing central opioidergic neurotransmission. Opiate agonists induce opioid receptor mediated scratching activity of central origin. Cholestatic animals in which endogenous opioids accumulate have evidence of increased opioidergic tone, reversible by naloxone. Opiate antagonists reduce scratching in cholestatic patients [6, 89] and may produce opioid withdrawal-like reactions [47].

Opiates are not the only neurotransmitter implicated in itching, however. Ondansetron, a 5-HT$_3$ serotonin receptor antagonist, may also improve itching [60, 75] although not all trials have found significant benefit [61].

Further studies are awaited to unravel the mechanism of this troublesome and occasionally devastating complication of cholestasis, and to find an oral, effective, reliable treatment without side-effects.

Fatigue is a troublesome symptom in 70–80% of patients with chronic cholestatic liver disease, although to what extent this is due to cholestasis as opposed to chronic liver disease *per se* is not clear. It has an impact on quality of life. Experimental data do show behavioural changes in cholestasis and suggest a central mechanism involving serotoninergic neurotransmission and/or neuroendocrine defects in the corticotrophin-releasing hormone axis [9, 80–82]. However, the mechanisms responsible for fatigue in patients with cholestatic liver disease remain speculative [48].

Steatorrhoea is proportional to the degree of jaundice. It is due to the lack of sufficient intestinal bile salts for the absorption of dietary fat and fat-soluble vitamins (A, D, K and E) (figs 13.10, 13.11). Micellar solution of lipid is inadequate. Stools are loose, pale, bulky and offensive. The colour gives a good indication of whether cholestasis is total, intermittent or decreasing.

Fat-soluble vitamins. In short-term cholestasis which requires invasive techniques for investigation and treatment, vitamin K replacement may be necessary to correct the prolonged prothrombin time.

In prolonged cholestasis, plasma vitamin A levels fall. Hepatic storage is normal and the deficiency is due to poor absorption. If cholestasis is sufficiently long standing, hepatic reserves become exhausted and failure of dark adaption follows (night blindness) [86]. Vitamin D deficiency may also occur leading to osteomalacia.

Vitamin E deficiency has been reported in children with cholestasis [77]. The picture is of cerebellar ataxia, posterior column dysfunction, peripheral neuropathy and

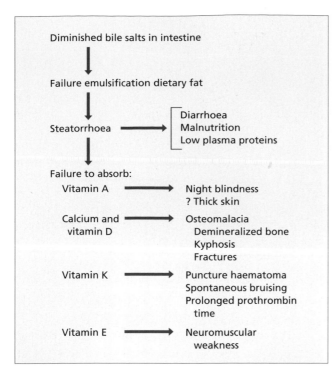

Fig. 13.10. The effects of lack of intestinal bile in chronic cholestatic jaundice.

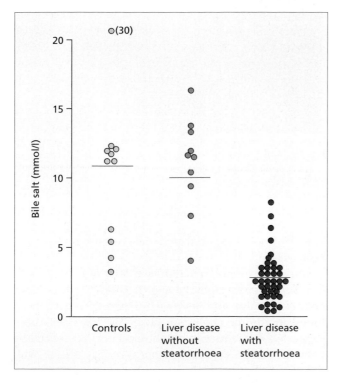

Fig. 13.11. Bile salt concentration of aspirated intestinal contents in patients with non-alcoholic liver disease with and without steatorrhoea [4].

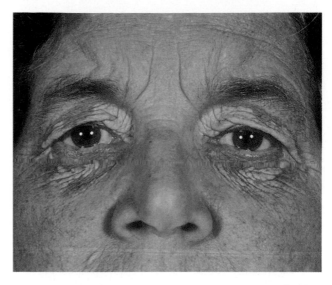

Fig. 13.12. Primary biliary cirrhosis. The patient shows xanthelasma and pigmentation.

retinal degeneration. If the serum bilirubin level exceeds 100 µmol/l (6 mg/dl) almost all adult patients with cholestasis will have subnormal vitamin E levels [45]. However, a specific neurological syndrome does not seem to develop in adults.

Xanthomas. These occur in chronic cholestasis but are seen less frequently than before because of treatment at an earlier stage with liver transplantation. The planous varieties (xanthelasma) are flat or slightly raised, yellow and soft and are usually noted around the eyes (fig. 13.12). They may also be seen in the palmar creases, below the breast and on the neck (fig. 13.13), chest or back. The tuberous lesions, also rarely seen now, appear later and are found on extensor surfaces, on pressure points and in scars. They disappear if serum cholesterol levels fall after cholestasis is relieved or in the late stage of hepatocellular failure.

Hepatic osteodystrophy [36, 90]

Bone disease is a complication of chronic liver disease and in particular chronic cholestasis where it has been studied in most detail. Bone pain and fractures occur. Possible mechanisms are *osteomalacia* and *osteoporosis.* Studies show that osteoporosis is responsible for the bone changes in the majority of patients with primary biliary cirrhosis and primary sclerosing cholangitis, although the potential for osteomalacia exists. A recent study has suggested that risk factors for osteoporosis are low body mass index, steroid treatment, increasing age and female sex rather than cholestasis *per se* [63].

Bone disease manifests as loss of height, back pain (usually mid-thoracic or lumbar), collapsed vertebrae and fractures particularly of ribs with minimal trauma.

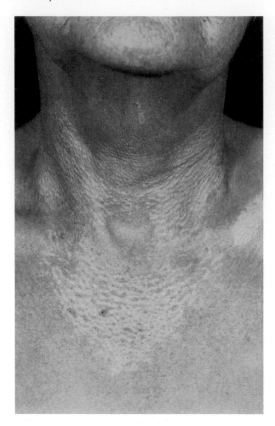

Fig. 13.13. Primary biliary cirrhosis. Xanthomatous skin lesions in the necklace area.

Spinal X-rays may show vertebrae of low density, as well as compression (fig. 13.14).

Bone mineral density may be measured by dual photon absorptiometry. One-third of patients with primary biliary cirrhosis and approximately 10% of those with primary sclerosing cholangitis have a bone density value below the fracture threshold [2, 53]. In patients with primary sclerosing cholangitis, osteoporosis is associated with advanced disease (fig. 13.15) [37].

The pathogenetic mechanism of the bone disease is uncertain, but is likely to be multifactorial. Normal bone homoeostasis depends on the correct balance between bone removal by osteoclasts and bone formation by osteoblasts. Remodelling begins with the retraction of the lining cells (terminally differentiated osteoblasts) from a quiescent area of bone. Osteoclasts attach and resorb bone, forming lacunae. These cells are then replaced by osteoblasts which fill the lacunae with new bone (osteoid), a matrix of collagen and other proteins. The osteoid is then 'mineralized', a process dependent on calcium, and therefore vitamin D. The two main forms of metabolic bone disease are osteoporosis and osteomalacia. In osteoporosis there is loss of bone (both matrix and its mineral). In osteomalacia there is defective mineralization of osteoid. To establish the process leading to bone disease in chronic cholestasis,

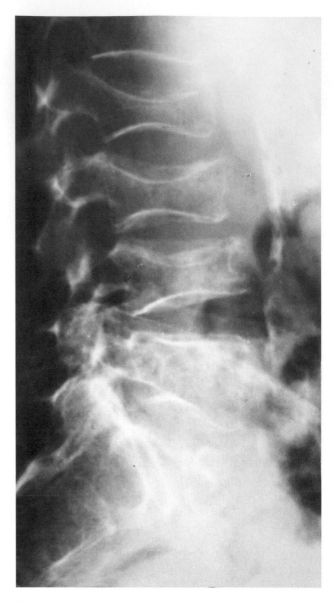

Fig. 13.14. Primary biliary cirrhosis jaundiced for 3 years. Lumbar spine showing very severe biconcave deformities and vertebral compression.

bone biopsy with special analytical techniques has been necessary.

Studies have shown that the majority of patients with hepatic osteodystrophy have *osteoporosis*. Both reduced bone formation and increased resorption have been found in chronic cholestatic liver disease. It has been suggested that reduced formation occurs in pre-cirrhotic patients, with increased resorption in those with advanced disease [36]. In post-menopausal women without liver disease both bone resorption and bone formation are increased, with resorption exceeding formation. This will play a part in patients with primary biliary cirrhosis after the menopause.

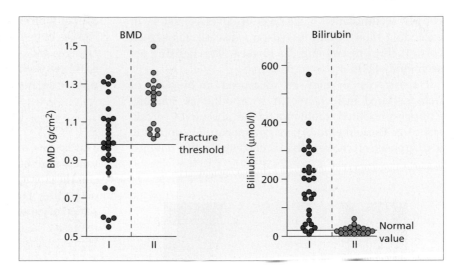

Fig. 13.15. Bone mineral density (BMD) and serum bilirubin concentration in patients with advanced sclerosing cholangitis (group I) and newly diagnosed primary sclerosing cholangitis (group II) [37].

Table 13.2. Factors increasing risk of bone disease in chronic cholestasis

General	Reduced physical activity
	Low body mass index
	Increasing age
	Female sex
	Reduced sunlight exposure
Cholestasis	Vitamin D and K deficiency
	Reduced calcium availability
	Increased serum bilirubin
Genetic	Vitamin D receptor genotype
Hormonal	Menopause/hypogonadism
	Steroid therapy

The cause of osteoporosis in chronic cholestatic liver disease is multifactorial (table 13.2) and not well understood. Factors involved in normal bone metabolism may play a role including vitamin D, calcitonin, parathyroid hormone, growth hormone and sex steroids. External influences in cholestatic patients include immobility, poor nutrition and reduced muscle mass. Vitamin D levels may be reduced due to malabsorption, inadequate diet and reduced exposure to the sun. Treatment with vitamin D, however, does not correct the bone disease. Activation of vitamin D, by 25-hydroxylation in liver and 1-hydroxylation in the kidney, is normal.

In normal individuals and those with primary osteoporosis, allelic polymorphisms of the vitamin D receptor (VDR) gene are related to bone mineral density. VDR genotypes also correlate with the degree of osteoporosis and vertebral fracture in patients with primary biliary cirrhosis [78].

Plasma from patients with jaundice inhibits osteoblast proliferation; unconjugated bilirubin but not bile salts had an inhibitory effect [42].

Treatment with ursodeoxycholic acid does not reduce the rate of bone loss in primary biliary cirrhosis [53]. Liver transplantation results in an improved bone density but this is delayed until 1–5 years after transplant [3]. Before recovery, spontaneous bone fractures are common [23], occurring in 35% of patients with primary biliary cirrhosis in the first year. Corticosteroids used for immunosuppression probably play a part in this increased fracture rate. Vitamin D levels may not return to normal for several months after transplantation and supplementation has been recommended [3].

It is important to measure vitamin D levels in patients with chronic cholestasis since although *osteomalacia* is unusual it may be present and is easily corrected. Isoenzyme analysis of serum alkaline phosphatase will show whether excess bone isoenzyme is present as well as the biliary/liver form. Bone changes cannot be predicted by serum calcium and phosphate values. X-rays may show changes of osteomalacia such as pseudo-fractures and Looser's zones. The hands show rarefaction. Bone biopsy shows wide, uncalcified osteoid seams surrounding the trabeculae. The cause of vitamin D deficiency is probably multiple. Cholestatic patients fail to go out in the sun or take an adequate diet. Absorption is poor due to steatorrhoea. Long-term cholestyramine use may exacerbate the deficiency.

Another manifestation of bone disease is painful *osteoarthropathy* in the wrists and ankles (fig. 13.16) [24]. This is a non-specific complication of chronic liver disease.

Changes in copper metabolism

Approximately 80% of absorbed copper is normally excreted in the bile and lost in the faeces. In all forms of cholestasis, but particularly if it is chronic (as in primary biliary cirrhosis, biliary atresia or sclerosing cholangitis), copper accumulates in the liver to levels equal to or exceeding those found in Wilson's disease. Pigmented corneal rings resembling the Kayser–Fleischer ring are seen rarely [27].

Hepatic copper may be measured in biopsies or demonstrated histochemically by rhodamine staining. Copper-associated protein may be shown by orcein staining. These methods give circumstantial support to a diagnosis of cholestasis. In cholestasis the retained

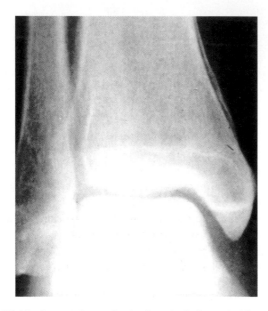

Fig. 13.16. Osteoarthropathy in chronic cholestasis. New subperiosteal bone is seen at the lower end of the tibia.

copper is probably not hepato-toxic. Electron microscopy shows it in electron-dense lysosomes. The organelle changes and oxidative-phosphylation defects associated with cytosolic and mitochondrial copper in Wilson's disease are not observed [31].

Development of hepato-cellular failure

This is slow, and it is remarkable how well the liver cells function in the presence of cholestasis. After 3–5 years of chronic jaundice, liver cell failure is indicated by rapidly deepening jaundice, ascites, oedema and a lowered serum albumin level. Pruritus lessens and the bleeding tendency is not controlled by parenteral vitamin K. Hepatic encephalopathy is terminal.

Extra-hepatic effects (fig. 13.17) [22]

Itching and jaundice are self-evident, but there are numerous other less obvious effects of cholestasis. These have been studied mainly in the context of bile duct obstruction. They may result in serious complications when the patient is stressed by dehydration, blood loss or surgical or non-surgical procedures. Cardio-vascular responses are abnormal and peripheral vaso-constriction in response to hypotension is impaired. The kidneys have an increased susceptibility to hypotension and hypoxic damage [28]. The processes involved in responding to sepsis and in wound healing are impaired. The prolonged prothrombin time is correctable with vitamin K but coagulation may still be abnormal due to platelet dysfunction. The gastric mucosa is more suscep-

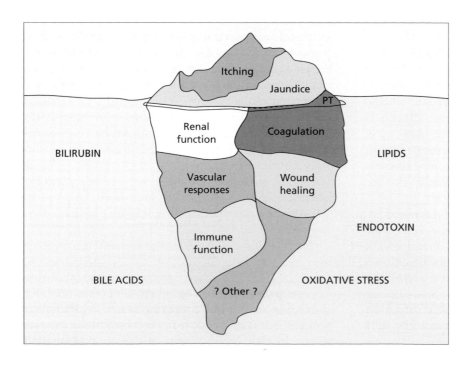

Fig. 13.17. Extra-hepatic effects of cholestasis. Itching and jaundice are obvious (the tip of the iceberg) but there are many other effects for which the clinician should make allowance. Pathogenic factors include bilirubin, bile acids, lipid changes, endotoxaemia and oxidative stress. (PT, prothrombin time.)

tible to ulceration. The cause of these changes is multifactorial. Bile acids and bilirubin have been shown to alter cellular metabolism and function. Changes in serum lipids affect membrane structure and function.

Experimental cholestatic liver disease is associated with increased lipid peroxidation in the kidney, brain and heart [54]. Cholestasis impairs hepatic sinusoidal endothelial cell function [92]. This may be caused by endotoxaemia and release of TNF and IL1 by activated Kupffer cells. Chronic bile duct ligation leads to an increased sensitivity to lipopolysaccharide—a component of the outer membrane of Gram-negative bacteria [35]. N-acetylcysteine may give protection through anti-oxidant pathways [69]. The same agent gives partial protection against renal dysfunction in experimental cholestasis [39].

Thus although deeply jaundiced patients with cholestasis may appear well apart from itching, there are metabolic and functional changes that under the stress of surgical and non-surgical procedures may result in acute renal failure, haemorrhage, wound dehiscence and an increased risk of sepsis.

Haematology

Changes in cholestasis include the appearance of target cells on blood film related to an accumulation of cholesterol in the red cell membrane. This increases red cell surface area and leads to target cell formation.

In extra-hepatic cholestasis, anaemia implies infection, blood loss or malignant disease. A polymorphonuclear leucocytosis suggests cholangitis or underlying neoplastic disease.

Biochemistry

All the constituents of the bile show an increased level in the serum. Conjugation of biliary substances is intact but excretion defective.

The *serum conjugated bilirubin level* is raised. In unrelieved cholestasis the level rises slowly for the first 3 weeks and then fluctuates, always tending to increase. When the cholestasis is relieved, serum bilirubin values fall slowly to normal. This is in part due to the formation of bili-albumin, in which bilirubin and albumin are covalently bound.

The *serum alkaline phosphatase level* is raised, usually to more than three times the upper limit of normal. *Serum γ-glutamyl-transpeptidase levels* are raised. The rises are due to increased synthesis or release of enzymes from liver and biliary plasma membranes.

The total *serum cholesterol* increases but not in all cases. In chronic cholestasis the total serum lipids are greatly increased and this involves particularly phospholipid and total cholesterol. These changes probably reflect increased hepatic synthesis, regurgitation of biliary cholesterol and lecithin into the circulation, and reduced plasma lecithin cholesterol acyl transferase (LCAT) activity. Triglycerides are very slightly increased. In spite of the high lipid content, the serum is characteristically clear and not milky. This may be due to the surface action effect of phospholipid, which keeps the other lipids in solution. Serum cholesterol values fall terminally.

Serum lipoproteins are increased, due to a rise in the low density (α_2, β) fraction. The high density lipoproteins are decreased.

The cholestatic liver secretes a variety of unusual lipoproteins and these can be related to low plasma LCAT levels. The lipoproteins of cholestasis differ from those found in atherosclerosis. Atheroma is not a complication of prolonged cholestasis. The abnormal lipoproteins appear by electron microscopy as disc-shaped particles.

Lipoprotein-X (LP-X) is a spherical particle, 70 nm in diameter, associated with the low density lipoprotein fraction. It is increased in both intra- and extra-hepatic cholestasis but is of no practical diagnostic value.

Bile salts accumulate in the blood in cholestasis.

Serum albumin and globulin concentrations are normal in acute cholestasis. With the development of biliary cirrhosis the serum albumin tends to fall.

The *serum aspartate transaminase* is usually less than 100 iu/l.

Urine. Conjugated bilirubin is present. Urinary urobilinogen is excreted in proportion to the amount of bile reaching the duodenum.

Bacteriology

In the febrile patient with bile duct obstruction or primary sclerosing cholangitis, blood cultures should be performed. Septicaemia, especially due to Gram-negative organisms, complicates patients with duct stones, and those with malignant obstruction or sclerosing cholangitis after invasive procedures. Patients with partial biliary obstruction and cholangitis have a high bacterial population in the bile, rivalling that in the colon. Whether this causes systemic sepsis depends on the biliary pressure and thus the degree of obstruction.

Diagnostic approach

Clinical features from an accurate history and physical examination often suggest the cause of the cholestasis. *Pain* can be related to duct stones, tumour or gallbladder disease. *Fever* and *rigors* may indicate cholangitis due to duct stone or traumatic stricture (*Charcot's intermittent biliary fever*). The patient may have taken *drug treatment* that coincides with the development of cholestasis.

drainage. Itching disappears or is much improved after 24–48 h.

Cholestyramine. This resin will stop itching in 4–5 days in patients with partial biliary obstruction. It is known to bind bile salts in the intestines so eliminating them in the faeces but until the pathogenesis of itching is better understood, its actual mechanism of action will remain speculative. One sachet (4 g) should be given before and one after breakfast so that the arrival of the drug in the duodenum coincides with gallbladder contraction. If necessary, a further dose may be taken before the mid-day and evening meals. The maintenance dose is usually about 12 g/day. The drug causes nausea and there is a reluctance to take it. It is particularly valuable for itching associated with primary biliary cirrhosis, primary sclerosing cholangitis, biliary atresia and biliary stricture. Serum bile acid levels fall. Serum cholesterol drops and skin xanthomas diminish or disappear.

Cholestyramine increases faecal fat even in normal subjects. The dose should be the smallest one that controls pruritus. Hypoprothrombinaemia has developed due to failure to absorb vitamin K.

Cholestyramine may bind calcium, other fat-soluble vitamins and drugs having an entero-hepatic circulation, particularly digoxin. Care must be taken that the cholestyramine and other drugs are given at separate times.

Ursodeoxycholic acid (13–15 mg/kg per day) can reduce itching in patients with primary biliary cirrhosis perhaps by a choleretic effect or by reducing toxic bile salts [71]. Although its use has been associated with biochemical resolution of drug-induced cholestasis [70], it is unproven as an anti-pruritic agent in this and other cholestatic syndromes.

Anti-histamines. These are of value only for their sedative action.

Phenobarbitone may relieve itching in patients resistant to other therapy.

Naloxone, an opiate antagonist given as an intravenous infusion, reduced itching in a randomized controlled trial [6], but is not appropriate for long-term use. An oral opiate antagonist, nalmefene, is also effective [7, 10] and clinical trials of another orally active opiate antagonist, naltrexone, have also shown benefit [89]. Both oral agents are experimental and not yet in clinical use.

Ondansetron reduced itching in small placebo-controlled trials [75] but subsequent studies have questioned its benefit [60, 61].

Propofol, an hypnotic agent given intravenously, has improved itching in 80% of patients [11]. Only short-term benefit has been studied.

S-adenosyl-L-methionine, which among many effects improves membrane fluidity and acts as an antioxidant, has been used to treat cholestatic syndromes [65].

Results are inconsistent and currently this agent remains experimental.

Rifampicin (300–450 mg daily) relieves pruritus within 7 days [19, 30]. This may be by enzyme induction or by inhibition of bile acid uptake. Potential side-effects include increased risk of gallstone formation, reduction in 25-OH-cholecalciferol levels, drug interactions, hepato-toxicity and emergence of resistant organisms, although successful longer term use (mean 18 months) is reported in children without clinical or biochemical toxicity [91]. Patients treated with this agent should be carefully selected and frequently monitored.

Steroids. Glucocorticoids will relieve itching, but at the expense of severe bone thinning particularly in post-menopausal women.

Bright light therapy (10 000 lux) has been studied and found beneficial in a pilot study [8]. Its use is based on the circadian pattern of cholestatic pruritus.

Ileal diversion decreases pruritus and improves quality of life in children with cholestasis and intractable itching [38].

Plasmapheresis. This has been used to treat intractable pruritus associated with hypercholesterolaemia and xanthomatous neuropathy. The procedure is temporarily effective but is costly and labour intensive.

Hepatic transplantation The wide range of partially effective and experimental therapies underlines the difficulty in treating some patients with long-standing cholestasis. Intractable itching may be an indication for liver transplantation.

Nutrition (table 13.5)

The problem is that of intestinal bile salt deficiency. Dietetic advice if available should be taken. Calorie intake should be maintained and protein must be ade-

Table 13.5. Management of chronic cholestasis

Dietary fat (if steatorrhoea)			
reduce neutral fat (40 g daily)			
add medium chain triglycerides (up to 40 g daily)			
Fat-soluble vitamins*	Oral	K	10 mg/day
		A	25 000 U/day
		D	400–4 000 U/day
	i.v.	K	10 mg/month
	i.m.	A	100 000 U/3-monthly
	i.m.	D	100 000 U/month
Calcium			
extra low fat milk			
oral calcium			

*Initial dose and route depend on severity of deficiency and cholestasis, and compliance; maintenance dose depends on response. See text for vitamin E.

quate. In patients with clinically overt steatorrhoea, neutral fat will be poorly tolerated and badly absorbed with reduced calcium absorption. It should be restricted if steatorrhoea is exacerbated and is a clinical problem. Additional fat is supplied by medium chain triglycerides (MCT) as an emulsion, e.g. in a milk shake. In the absence of luminal bile acids, MCT are digested and absorbed quite well into the portal vein as free fatty acids. They can be given as Liquigen (Scientific Hospital Supplies Ltd, UK) or as MCT (coconut) oil for cooking or in salads. Calcium supplements should also be given.

In acute cholestasis, vitamin K deficiency may be shown by prolongation of the prothrombin time. Parenteral vitamin K (10 mg) should be given daily for 2–3 days; the prothrombin time characteristically corrects within a day or two.

In the chronic case, prothrombin time and serum vitamin A and D levels should be monitored, and vitamins A, D and K replaced as necessary. Replacement may be done orally or parenterally depending on the severity of depletion, jaundice and steatorrhoea, and whether the deficiency is corrected. If testing of vitamin levels is not available, empirical replacement is appropriate particularly once the patient becomes jaundiced. Easy bruising suggests prothrombin and thus vitamin K deficiency.

Patients with night blindness may improve with oral rather than intramuscular vitamin A [86]. Vitamin E is not absorbed [1] and dl tocopherol, as the acetate 10 mg daily, is given by injection to children with chronic cholestasis. Others may take 200 mg daily by mouth.

Bone changes [90]

The osteopenia of cholestatic liver disease is predominantly osteoporosis. Malabsorption of vitamin D with subsequent osteomalacia occurs but is less common. Monitoring of serum 25-hydroxyvitamin D levels is necessary; bone densitometry scans will show the degree of osteopenia.

When vitamin D deficiency is detected, treatment is with vitamin D, either 50 000 units orally three times a week [36], or 100 000 units intramuscularly monthly. If serum levels do not become normal on oral therapy, the dose should be increased, or the parenteral route used. Prophylaxis against vitamin D deficiency when vitamin D levels cannot be monitored is empirical but appropriate for the patient with jaundice or long-standing cholestasis without jaundice. Unless serum levels can be monitored, parenteral replacement of vitamin D is more appropriate than the oral route.

In patients with symptomatic osteomalacia, oral or parenteral 1,25-dihydroxyvitamin D_3 appears to be the vitamin D metabolite of choice, but carries a risk of hypercalcaemia. It is biologically very active and has a short half-life. An alternative would be 1α-vitamin D_3 but full metabolic activity only follows hepatic 25-hydroxylation.

Measures should be taken to prevent osteoporosis. These have been little studied in chronic cholestasis. A balanced diet is encouraged with calcium supplements. A daily oral intake of at least 1.5 g elemental calcium should be achieved using effervescent calcium (Sandoz) or calcium gluconate. Patients should be encouraged to take extra skimmed (fat-free) milk and expose themselves to safe levels of sunlight or ultraviolet light. They are also encouraged to be mobile and active, though if osteopenia is severe this may have to be moderated or an exercise programme planned under supervision.

Corticosteroids worsen the process of osteoporosis and should be avoided.

In post-menopausal patients oestrogen replacement therapy is indicated. Such treatment in patients with primary biliary cirrhosis showed no increase in cholestasis while there was a trend towards a reduction in bone loss [17, 62].

Bisphosphonates may be beneficial in cholestatic bone disease. A comparative study between editronate and sodium fluoride (with calcium and vitamin D supplements) favoured editronate, which increased vertebral bone density [33]. Arendronate may be better than editronate in primary biliary cirrhosis patients with osteopenia [68]. Although a limited study of fluoride treatment showed improved bone density in patients with primary biliary cirrhosis [32], larger studies in postmenopausal osteoporosis show no reduction in fractures. Calcitonin has not been shown to be beneficial.

Hepatic bone disease worsens after liver transplantation and calcium and vitamin D supplementation should be continued.

No specific treatment is available for the painful periosteal reactions. Simple analgesics may be of use, and, if arthropathy is present, physiotherapy may be helpful.

References

1 Alvarez F, Landrieu P, Laget P *et al.* Nervous and ocular disorders in children with cholestasis and vitamin A and E deficiencies. *Hepatology* 1983; **3**: 410.

2 Angulo P, Therneau TM, Jorgensen RA *et al.* Bone disease in patients with primary sclerosing cholangitis: prevalence, severity and prediction of progression. *J. Hepatol.* 1998; **29**: 729

3 Argao EA, Balistreri WF, Hollis BW *et al.* Effect of orthotopic liver transplantation on bone mineral content and serum vitamin D metabolites in infants and children with chronic cholestasis. *Hepatology* 1994; **20**: 598.

4 Badley BWD, Murphy GM, Bouchier IAD *et al.* Diminished micellar phase lipid in patients with chronic nonalcoholic liver disease and steatorrhea. *Gastroenterology* 1970; **58**: 781.

5 Baiocchi L, LeSage G, Glaser S et al. Regulation of cholangio-cyte bile secretion. *J. Hepatol.* 1999; **31**: 179.

6 Bergasa NV, Alling DW, Talbot TL et al. Effects of naloxone infusions in patients with pruritus of cholestasis: a double-blind randomized controlled trial. *Ann. Intern. Med.* 1995; **123**: 161.

7 Bergasa NV, Alling DW, Talbot TL et al. Oral nalmefene therapy reduces scratching activity due to the pruritus of cholestasis: a controlled study. *J. Am. Acad. Dermatol.* 1999; **41**: 431.

8 Bergasa NV, Link MJ Keogh M et al. Pilot study of bright-light therapy reflected towards the eyes for pruritus of chronic liver disease. *Am. J. Gastroenterol.* 2001; **96**: 1563.

9 Bergasa NV, Mehlman JK, Jones EA. Pruritus and fatigue in primary biliary cirrhosis. *Bailliere's Clin. Gastroenterol.* 2000; **14**: 643.

10 Bergasa NV, Schmitt JM, Talbot TL et al. Open-label trial of oral nalmefene therapy for the pruritus of cholestasis. *Hepatology* 1998; **27**: 679.

11 Borgeat A, Wilder-Smith OHG, Mentha G. Subhypnotic doses of propofol relieve pruritus associated with liver disease. *Gastroenterology* 1993; **104**: 244.

12 Brenard R, Geubel AP, Benhamou J-P. Benign recurrent intrahepatic cholestasis. *J. Clin. Gastroenterol.* 1989; **11**: 546.

13 Bruguera M, Llach J, Rodes J. Non-syndromic paucity of intrahepatic bile ducts in infancy and idiopathic ductopenia in adulthood: the same syndrome? *Hepatology* 1992; **15**: 830.

14 Bull LN, Juijn JA, Liao M et al. Fine-resolution mapping by haplotype evaluation: the examples of PFIC1 and BRIC. *Human Genet.* 1999; **104**: 241.

15 Bull LN, van-Eijk MJ, Pawlikowska L et al. A gene encoding a P-type ATPase mutated in two forms of hereditary cholestasis. *Nature Genet.* 1998; **18**: 219.

16 Burak KW, Pearson DC, Swain MG et al. Familial idiopathic adulthood ductopenia: a report of five cases in three generations. *J. Hepatol.* 2000; **32**: 159.

17 Crippin JS, Jorgensen RA, Dickson ER et al. Hepatic osteodystrophy in primary biliary cirrhosis: effects of medical treatment. *Am. J. Gastroenterol.* 1994; **89**: 47.

18 Crosbie OM, Crown JP, Nolan NPM et al. Resolution of para-neoplastic bile duct paucity following successful treatment of Hodgkin's disease. *Hepatology* 1997; **26**: 5.

19 Cynamon HA, Andres JM, Iafrate RP. Rifampin relieves pruritus in children with cholestatic liver disease. *Gastroenterology* 1990; **98**: 1013.

20 Degott C, Feldmann G, Larrey D et al. Drug-induced pro-longed cholestasis in adults: a histological semiquantitative study demonstrating progressive ductopenia. *Hepatology* 1992; **15**: 244.

21 Dixon JM, Armstrong CP, Duffey SW et al. Factors affecting morbidity and mortality after surgery for obstructive jaundice: a review of 373 patients. *Gut* 1983; **24**: 845.

22 Dooley JS. Extrahepatic biliary obstruction: systemic effects, diagnosis, management. In Benhamou J-P, Bircher J, McIntre N, Rizzetto M, Rodes J, eds. *Oxford Textbook of Clinical Hepatology*. Oxford University Press, Oxford, 1999, p. 1581.

23 Eastell R, Dickson ER, Hodgson SF et al. Rates of vertebral loss before and after liver transplantation in women with primary biliary cirrhosis. *Hepatology* 1991; **14**: 296.

24 Epstein O, Dick R, Sherlock S. Prospective study of periostitis and finger clubbing in primary biliary cirrhosis and other forms of chronic liver disease. *Gut* 1981; **22**: 203.

25 Faa G, Van Eyken P, Demelia L et al. Idiopathic adulthood ductopenia presenting with chronic recurrent cholestasis. *J. Hepatol.* 1991; **12**: 14.

26 FitzPatrick DR. Zellweger syndrome and associated pheno-types. *J. Med. Genet.* 1996; **33**: 863.

27 Fleming CR, Dickson ER, Hollenhorst RW et al. Pigmented corneal rings in a patient with primary biliary cirrhosis. *Gastroenterology* 1975; **69**: 220.

28 Fogarty BJ, Parks RW, Rowlands BJ et al. Renal dysfunction in obstructive jaundice. *Br. J. Surg.* 1995; **82**: 877.

29 Freedman MR, Holzbach RT, Ferguson DR. Pruritus in cholestasis: no direct causative role for bile acid retention. *Am. J. Med.* 1981; **70**: 1011.

30 Ghent CN, Carruthers SG. Treatment of pruritis in primary biliary cirrhosis with rifampin. Results of a double-blind, crossover, randomized trial. *Gastroenterology* 1988; **94**: 488.

31 Gu M, Cooper JM, Butler P et al. Oxidative-phosphorylation defects in liver of patients with Wilson's disease. *Lancet* 2000; **356**: 469.

32 Guanabens N, Pares A, del Rio L et al. Sodium fluoride prevents bone loss in primary biliary cirrhosis. *J. Hepatol.* 1992; **15**: 345.

33 Guanabens N, Pares A, Monegal A et al. Etidronate vs. fluoride for treatment of osteopenia in primary biliary cirrhosis: preliminary results after 2 years. *Gastroenterology* 1997; **113**: 219.

34 Gubern JM, Sancho JJ, Simo J et al. A randomised trial on the effect of mannitol on postoperative renal function in patients with obstructive jaundice. *Surgery* 1988; **103**: 39.

35 Harry D, Anand R, Holt S et al. Increased sensitivity to endotoxemia in the bile duct-ligated cirrhotic rat. *Hepatology* 1999; **30**: 1198.

36 Hay JE. Bone disease in cholestatic liver disease. *Gastroenterology* 1995; **108**: 276.

37 Hay JE, Lindor KD, Wiesner RH et al. The metabolic bone disease of primary sclerosing cholangitis. *Hepatology* 1991; **14**: 257.

38 Hollands CM, Rivera-Pedrogo FJ, Gonzalez-Vallina R et al. Ileal exclusion for Byler's disease: an alternative surgical approach with promising early results for pruritus. *J. Pediatr. Surg.* 1998; **33**: 220.

39 Holt S, Marley R, Fernando B et al. Acute cholestasis-induced renal failure: effects of antioxidants and ligands for the thromboxane A(2) receptor. *Kidney Int.* 1999; **55**: 271.

40 Jacquemin E, Cresteil D, Manouvrier S et al. Heterozygous nonsense mutation of the MDR3 gene in familial intra-hepatic cholestasis of pregnancy. *Lancet* 1999; **353**: 210.

41 Jacquemin E, De Vree JML, Cresteil D et al. The wide spectrum of multidrug resistance 3 deficiency: from neonatal cholestasis to cirrhosis of adulthood. *Gastroenterology* 2001; **120**: 1448.

42 Janes CH, Dickson ER, Okazaki R et al. Role of hyperbiliru-binaemia in the impairment of osteoblast proliferation asso-ciated with cholestatic jaundice. *J. Clin. Invest.* 1995; **95**: 2581.

43 Jansen PLM, Moller M. Genetic cholestasis: lessons from the molecular physiology of bile formation. *Can. J. Gastroenterol.* 2000; **14**: 233.

44 Jansen PLM, Moller M. The molecular genetics of familial intrahepatic cholestasis. *Gut* 2000; **47**: 1.

45 Jeffrey GP, Muller DPR, Burroughs AK et al. Vitamin E defi-ciency and its clinical significance in adults with primary

biliary cirrhosis and other forms of chronic liver disease. *J. Hepatol.* 1987; **4**: 307.

46 Jones EA, Bergasa NV. The pruritis of cholestasis. *Hepatology* 1999; **29**: 1003.

47 Jones EA, Dekker LR. Florid opioid withdrawal-like reaction precipitated by naltrexone in a patient with chronic cholestasis. *Gastroenterology* 2000; **118**: 431.

48 Jones EA, Yurdaydin C. Is fatigue associated with cholestasis mediated by altered central neurotransmission? *Hepatology* 1997; **25**: 492.

49 Kanno N, LeSage G, Glaser S *et al.* Functional heterogeneity of the intrahepatic biliary epithelium. *Hepatology* 2000; **31**: 555.

50 Kawaguchi T, Sakisaka S, Mitsuyama K *et al.* Cholestasis with altered structure and function of hepatocyte tight junction and decreased expression of canalicular multispecific organic anion transporter in a rat model of colitis. *Hepatology* 2000; **31**: 1285.

51 Krähenbuhl L, Schäfer M, Krähenbuhl S. Reversibility of hepatic mitochondral damage in rats with long-term cholestasis. *J. Hepatol.* 1998; **28**: 1000.

52 Lai ECS, Mok FPT, Fan ST *et al.* Preoperative endoscopic drainage for malignant obstructive jaundice. *Br. J. Surg.* 1994; **81**: 1195.

53 Lindor KD, Janes CH, Crippin JS *et al.* Bone disease in primary biliary cirrhosis: does ursodeoxycholic acid make a difference? *Hepatology* 1995; **21**: 389.

54 Ljubuncic P, Tanne Z, Bomzon A. Evidence of a systemic phenomenon for oxidative stress in cholestatic liver disease. *Gut* 2000; **47**: 710.

55 Lobo-Yeo A, Senaldi G, Portmann B *et al.* Class I and class II major histocompatibility complex antigen expression on hepatocytes: a study in children with liver disease. *Hepatology* 1990; **12**: 224.

56 Marinelli RA, LaRusso NF. Aquaporin water channels in liver: their significance in bile formation. *Hepatology* 1997; **26**: 1081.

57 Marinelli RA, Pham LD, Tietz PS *et al.* Expression of aquaporin-4 water channels in rat cholangiocytes. *Hepatology* 2000; **31**: 1313.

58 Müller M, Jansen PLM. The secretory function of the liver: new aspects of hepatobiliary transport. *J. Hepatol.* 1998; **28**: 344.

59 Morton, DH, Salen G, Batta AK *et al.* Abnormal hepatic sinusoidal bile acid transport in an Amish kindred is not linked to FIC1 and is improved by ursodiol. *Gastroenterology* 2000; **119**: 188.

60 Muller C, Pongratz S, Pidlich J *et al.* Treatment of pruritus of chronic liver disease with the 5-hydroxy-tryptamine receptor type 3 antagonist ondansetron: a randomized, placebo-controlled, double-blind cross-over trial. *Eur. J. Gastroenterol. Hepatol.* 1998; **10**: 865.

61 O'Donohue JW, Haigh C, Williams R. Ondansetron in the treatment of the pruritis of cholestasis: a randomised controlled trial. *Gastroenterology* 1997; **112**: A1349.

62 Olsson R, Mattsson L-A, Obrant K *et al.* Estrogen-progestogen therapy for low bone mineral density in primary biliary cirrhosis. *Liver* 1999; **19**: 188.

63 Ormarsdottir S, Ljunggren O, Mallmin H *et al.* Low body mass and use of corticosteroids, but not cholestasis, are risk factors in patients with chronic liver disease. *J. Hepatol.* 1999; **31**: 84.

64 Oude Elferink RPJ, Groen AK. The role of mdr2 P-glycoprotein in biliary lipid secretion. Cross-talk between cancer research and biliary physiology. *J. Hepatol.* 1995; **23**: 617.

65 Osman E, Owen JS, Burroughs AK. Review article: S-adenosyl-L-methionine—a new therapeutic agent in liver disease? *Aliment. Pharmacol. Ther.* 1993; **7**: 21.

66 Ostrow JD, Mukerjee P, Tiribelli C. Structure and binding of unconjugated bilirubin: relevance for physiological and pathophysiological function. *J. Lipid Res.* 1994; **35**: 1715.

67 Pain JA, Cahill CJ, Gilbert JM *et al.* Prevention of postoperative renal dysfunction in patients with obstructive jaundice: a multicentre study of bile salts and lactulose. *Br. J. Surg.* 1991; **78**: 467.

68 Pares A, Guañabens N, Ros I *et al.* Alendronate is more effective than etidronate for increasing bone mass in osteopenic patients with primary biliary cirrhosis (abstract). *Hepatology* 1999; **30**: 472A.

69 Pastor A, Collado P, Almar M *et al.* Antioxidant enzyme status in biliary obstructed rats: effects of *N*-acetylcysteine. *J. Hepatol.* 1997; **27**: 363.

70 Piotrowicz A, Polkey M, Wilkinson M. Ursodeoxycholic acid for the treatment of flucloxacillin-associated cholestasis. *J. Hepatol.* 1995; **22**: 119.

71 Poupon RE, Poupon R, Balkau B *et al.* Ursodiol for the long-term treatment of primary biliary cirrhosis. *N. Engl. J. Med.* 1994; **330**: 1342.

72 Quigley EMM, Marsh MN, Shaffer JL *et al.* Hepatobiliary complications of total parenteral nutrition. *Gastroenterology* 1993; **104**: 286.

73 Richardet J-P, Mallat A, Zafrani ES *et al.* Prolonged cholestasis with ductopenia after administration of amoxicillin/clavulanic acid. *Dig. Dis. Sci.* 1999; **44**: 1997.

74 Rodrigues CMP, Steer CJ. Mitochondrial membrane perturbations in cholestasis. *J. Hepatol.* 2000; **32**: 135.

75 Schwörer H, Hartmann H, Ramadori G. Relief of cholestatic pruritus by a novel class of drug: 5-hydroxytryptamine type 3 (5-HT3) receptor antagonists; effectiveness of ondansetron. *Pain* 1995; **61**: 33.

76 Setchell KDR, Bragetti P, Zimmer-Nechemias L *et al.* Oral bile acid treatment and the patient with Zellweger syndrome. *Hepatology* 1992; **15**: 198.

77 Sokol RJ, Heubi JE, Iannaccone S *et al.* Mechanism causing vitamin E deficiency during chronic childhood cholestasis. *Gastroenterology* 1983; **83**: 1172.

78 Springer JE, Cole DEC, Rubin LA *et al.* Vitamin D-receptor genotypes as independent genetic predictors of decreased bone mineral density in primary biliary cirrhosis. *Gastroenterology* 2000; **118**: 145.

79 Strazzabosco M. New insights into cholangiocyte physiology. *J. Hepatol.* 1997; **27**: 945.

80 Swain MG, Le T. Chronic cholestasis in rats induces anhedonia and a loss of social interest. *Hepatology* 1998; **28**: 6.

81 Swain MG, Maric M. Defective corticotropin-releasing hormone mediated neuroendocrine and behavioural responses in cholestatic rats: implications for cholestatic liver disease-related sickness behaviours. *Hepatology* 1995; **22**: 1560.

82 Swain MG, Maric M. Improvement in cholestasis-associated fatigue with a serotonin receptor agonist using a novel rat model of fatigue assessment. *Hepatology* 1997; **25**: 291.

83 Trauner M, Meier PJ, Boyer JL. Molecular regulation of hepatocellular transport systems in cholestasis. *J. Hepatol.* 1999; **31**: 165.

84 Tsukada N, Ackerley CA, Phillips MJ. The structure and organization of the bile canalicular cytoskeleton with special reference to actin and actin-binding proteins. *Hepatology* 1995; **21**: 1106.

85 Tygstrup N, Steig BA, Juijn JA *et al.* Recurrent familial intrahepatic cholestasis in the Faeroe Islands. Phenotypic heterogeneity but genetic homogeneity. *Hepatology* 1999; **29**: 506.

86 Walt RP, Kemp CM, Lyness L *et al.* Vitamin A treatment for night blindness in primary biliary cirrhosis. *Br. Med. J.* 1984; **288**: 1030.

87 Weidenbach H, Leiz S, Nussler AK *et al.* Disturbed bile secretion and cytochrome P-450 function during the acute state of experimental colitis in rats. *J. Hepatol.* 2000; **32**: 708.

88 Williams R, Cartter MA, Sherlock S *et al.* Idiopathic recurrent cholestasis: a study of the functional and pathological lesions in four cases. *Q. J. Med.* 1964; **33**: 387.

89 Wolfhagen FJH, Sternieri E, Hop WCJ *et al.* Oral naltrexone treatment for cholestatic pruritus: a double-blind, placebo-controlled study. *Gastroenterology* 1997; **113**: 1264.

90 Wolfhagen FHJ, van Buuren HR, Vleggaar FP *et al.* Management of osteoporosis in primary biliary cirrhosis. *Bailliere's Clin. Gastroenterol.* 2000; **14**: 629.

91 Yerushalmi B, Sokol RJ, Narkewicz MR *et al.* Use of rifampin for severe pruritus in children with chronic cholestasis. *J. Pediatr. Gastroenterol. Nutr.* 1999; **29**: 442.

92 Yoshidome H, Miyazaki M, Shimizu H *et al.* Obstructive jaundice impairs hepatic sinusoidal endothelial cell function and renders liver susceptible to hepatic ischemia/reperfusion. *J. Hepatol.* 2000; **33**: 59.

Chapter 14
Primary Biliary Cirrhosis

Primary biliary cirrhosis (PBC) is a disease of unknown cause in which intra-hepatic bile ducts are progressively destroyed. It was first described in 1851 by Addison and Gull [1] and later by Hanot [37]. The association with high serum cholesterol levels and skin xanthomas led to the term 'xanthomatous biliary cirrhosis'. Ahrens *et al.* [3] termed the condition 'primary biliary cirrhosis'. However, in the early stages nodular regeneration is inconspicuous and cirrhosis is not present.

Aetiology

A profound immunological disturbance has been related to bile duct destruction [31]. Cytotoxic T-cells infiltrate the bile duct epithelium [111] as do class II restricted T4-lymphocytes. The final event is an attack by cytotoxic T-cells on biliary epithelium. Cytokines produced from the activated T-cells contribute to the liver cell damage [61]. Suppressor T-cells are reduced in number and function (fig. 14.1) [7]. Upregulated display of HLA class I antigens and *de novo* expression of HLA class II antigens are compatible with immune-mediated duct destruction [7].

Aberrant expression of HLA class II antigens on bile ducts has been shown, but only in late PBC. This has suggested that the antigen is presented by bile ducts, but this process may take place in the lymph nodes, rather than in the liver. HLA-D8, the autoimmune HLA type, is found in only a minority of patients.

T-helper cells and cytotoxic T-cells are important in pathogenesis. Cytotoxic T-cells may be effective, producing cytokines. However, the Th2 type of CD4 may predominate in the portal zones. This promotes mast cell and eosinophil activation [69]. Analysis of liver-derived T-cell clones shows predominance of Th1 cells, but with considerable heterogeneity [38]. It is possible that in the early stages the Th2 pattern predominates, to be followed by the Th1. The two patterns moreover may convert one to the other.

Epithelioid granulomas suggest a delayed-type hypersensitivity reaction. They are seen in the early, florid stage and may reflect an improved prognosis [55].

Copper is retained in the liver, but in a non-hepato-toxic form.

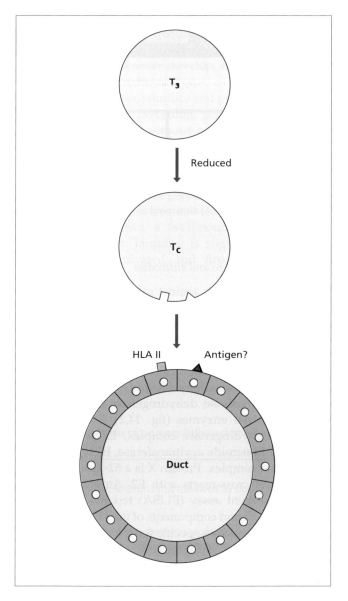

Fig. 14.1. PBC: HLA class II antigens and another unknown antigen are displayed on the bile duct. Suppressor T-cells (T$_s$) are depressed and there is a breach of tolerance to the biliary antigens. Tc, cytotoxic T-cells.

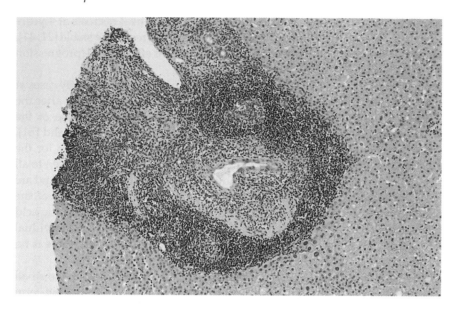

Fig. 14.10. Autoimmune cholangiopathy. Liver biopsy from a young man with mild pruritus, high serum alkaline phosphatase and γ-GT levels. Serum M2 was not detected. Serum ANA was present in high titre. Histology shows damaged zone 1 bile duct with marked inflammation. Appearances resemble PBC. (H & E, ×400.)

10% of patients will need re-transplant, with particularly bad results if this is more than 30 days after the operation [52]. Disease almost certainly recurs in the transplanted liver [5]. Mitochondrial antibody levels increase and the patient may become symptomatic. This is confirmed by finding E2 staining on biliary epithelial cells after the operation [105]. It is, however, difficult to distinguish the features of rejection from recurrent disease which, in any case, is usually non-progressive. Primary malignancies develop later in 10% of patients. In the first 1–3 months, bone density decreases and the results may be catastrophic. The worsening is probably related to bed rest and corticosteroid therapy. After 9–12 months, there is a marked improvement in bone formation and density [25].

Immune cholangiopathy

About 5% of patients presenting with PBC have a negative serum mitochondrial antibody test. Serum antinuclear antibody and anti-actin antibody are usually present in high titre [9, 66]. The patients are usually asymptomatic. Liver histology is identical with that of PBC (fig. 14.10). Prednisolone results in some clinical and biochemical improvement. However, liver histology shows less inflammation, bile duct lesions persist and serum γ-GT levels are very high. These patients provide an overlap between PBC and autoimmune chronic hepatitis.

References

1　Addison T, Gull W. On a certain affection of the skin—vitiligoidea—α plana, β tuberosa. *Guy's Hosp. Rep.* 1851; **7**: 265.

2　Agarwal K, Jones DEJ, Daly AK *et al.* CTL A-4 gene polymorphism confers susceptibility to primary biliary cirrhosis. *J. Hepatol.* 2000: **32**: 538

3　Ahrens EH Jr, Payne MA, Kunkel HG *et al.* Primary biliary cirrhosis. *Medicine (Baltimore)* 1950; **29**: 299.

4　Angulo P, Batts KP, Therneau TM *et al.* Long-term ursodeoxycholic acid delays histological progression in primary biliary cirrhosis. *Hepatology* 1999; **29**: 644.

5　Balan V, Batts KP, Porayko MK *et al.* Histological evidence for recurrence of primary biliary cirrhosis after liver transplantation. *Hepatology* 1993; **18**: 1392.

6　Balasubramaniam K, Grambsch PM, Wiesner RH *et al.* Diminished survival in asymptomatic primary biliary cirrhosis. A prospective study. *Gastroenterology* 1990; **98**: 1567.

7　Ballardini G, Mirakian R, Bianchi FB *et al.* Aberrant expression of HLA-DR antigens on bile duct epithelium in primary biliary cirrhosis: relevance to pathogenesis. *Lancet* 1984; **ii**: 1009.

8　Bassendine MF, Yeaman SJ. Serological markers of primary biliary cirrhosis: diagnosis, prognosis and subsets. *Hepatology* 1992; **15**: 545.

9　Ben-Ari Z, Dhillon AP, Sherlock S. Autoimmune cholangiopathy: part of the spectrum of autoimmune chronic active hepatitis. *Hepatology* 1993; **18**: 10.

10　Bergasa NV, Schmitt JM, Talbot TL *et al.* Open-label trial of oral nalmefene for the pruritus of cholestasis. *Hepatology* 1998; **27**: 679.

11　Bonis PAL, Kaplan M. Methotrexate improves biochemical tests in patients with primary biliary cirrhosis who respond incompletely to ursodiol. *Gastroenterology* 1999; **117**: 397.

12　Brind AM, Bray GP, Portmann BC *et al.* Prevalence and pattern of familial disease in primary biliary cirrhosis. *Gut* 1995; **36**: 615.

13　Bruguera M, Llach J, Rodés J. Nonsyndromic paucity of intrahepatic bile ducts in infancy and idiopathic ductopenia in adulthood: the same syndrome? *Hepatology* 1992; **15**: 830.

14　Burroughs AK, Rosenstein IJ, Epstein O *et al.* Bacteriuria and primary biliary cirrhosis. *Gut* 1984; **25**: 133.

15　Buscher H-P, Zietzschnmann Y, Gerok W. Positive responses to methotrexate and ursodeoxycholic acid in patients with primary biliary cirrhosis responding insufficiently to ursodeoxycholic acid alone. *J. Hepatol.* 1993; **18**: 9.

16 Bush A, Mitchison H, Walt R *et al.* Primary biliary cirrhosis and ulcerative colitis. *Gastroenterology* 1987; **92**: 2009.

17 Butler P, Valle F, Hamilton-Miller JMT *et al.* M2 mitochondria antibodies and urinary rough mutant bacteria in patients with primary biliary cirrhosis and in patients with recurrent bacteriuria. *J. Hepatol.* 1993; **17**: 408.

18 Cauch-Dudek K, Abbey S, Stewart DE *et al.* Fatigue in primary biliary cirrhosis. *Gut* 1998; **43**: 705.

19 Chen C-Y, Lu C-L, Chiu C-F *et al.* Primary biliary cirrhosis associated with mixed type autoimmune haemolytic anaemia and sicca syndrome: a case report and review of the literature. *Am. J. Gastroenterol.* 1997; **92**: 1547.

20 Christensen E, Grunson B, Neuberger J. Optimal timing of liver transplantation for patients with primary biliary cirrhosis: use of prognostic modelling. *J. Hepatol.* 1999; **30**: 285.

21 Degott C, Zafrani ES, Callard P. Histopathological study of primary biliary cirrhosis and the effects of ursodeoxycholic acid treatment on histology progression. *Hepatology* 1999; **29**: 1007.

22 Dickson ER, Grambsch PM, Fleming TR et al. Prognosis in primary biliary cirrhosis: model for decision making. *Hepatology* 1989; **10**: 1.

23 Donaldson PT. TNF gene polymorphisms in primary biliary cirrhosis: a critical appraisal. *J. Hepatol.* 1999; **31**: 366.

24 Dörner T, Held C, Trebeljahr G *et al.* Serologic characteristics in primary biliary cirrhosis associated with sicca syndrome. *Scand. J. Gastroenterol.* 1994; **29**: 655.

25 Eastell R, Dickson ER, Hodgson SF *et al.* Rates of vertebral bone loss before and after liver transplantation in women with primary biliary cirrhosis. *Hepatology* 1991; **14**: 296.

26 Epstein O, Dick R, Sherlock S. Prospective study of periostitis and finger clubbing in primary biliary cirrhosis and other forms of chronic liver disease. *Gut* 1981; **22**: 203.

27 Epstein O, Fraga E, Sherlock S. Importance of clinical staging for prognosis in primary biliary cirrhosis. *Gut* 1985; **26**: A1126.

28 Feizi T, Naccarato R, Sherlock S *et al.* Mitochondrial and other tissue antibodies in relatives of patients with biliary cirrhosis. *Clin. Exp. Immunol.* 1972; **10**: 609.

29 Flannery GR, Burroughs AK, Butler P. Antimitochondrial antibodies in primary biliary cirrhosis recognize both specific peptides and shared epitopes of the M2 family of antigens. *Hepatology* 1989; **10**: 370.

30 Fox RA, Scheuer PJ, James DG *et al.* Impaired delayed hypersensitivity in primary biliary cirrhosis. *Lancet* 1969; **i**: 959.

31 Gershwin ME, Mackay IR. Primary biliary cirrhosis: paradigm or paradox for autoimmunity. *Gastroenterology* 1991; **100**: 822.

32 Gores GJ, Wiesner RH, Dickson ER *et al.* Prospective evaluation of esophageal varices in primary biliary cirrhosis: development, natural history and influence on survival. *Gastroenterology* 1989; **96**: 1552.

33 Goudie BM, Burt AD, Macfarlane GJ *et al.* Risk factors and prognosis in primary biliary cirrhosis. *Am. J. Gastroenterol.* 1989; **84**: 713.

34 Goulis J, Leandro G, Burroughs AK. Randomized controlled trials of ursodeoxycholic acid therapy for primary biliary cirrhosis: a meta-analysis. *Lancet* 1999; **354**: 1653.

35 Guanaben SN, Pare SA, Monegal A *et al.* Etidronate vs. fluoride for treatment of osteopenia in primary biliary cirrhosis: preliminary results after 2 years. *Gastroenterology* 1997; **113**: 219.

36 Hall S, Axelsen PH, Larson DE *et al.* Systemic lupus erythematosus developing in patients with primary biliary cirrhosis. *Ann. Intern. Med.* 1984; **100**: 388.

37 Hanot V. *Etude sur une Forme de Cirrhose Hypertrophique de Foie (Cirrhose Hypertrophique avec Ictère Chronique).* Baillière, Paris, 1876.

38 Harada K, Van de Water J, Leung PSC *et al. In situ* nucleic acid hybridization of cytokines in primary biliary cirrhosis: predominance of the Th1 subset. *Hepatology* 1997; **25**: 791.

39 Haydon GH, Neuberger J. PBC: an infectious disease? *Gut* 2000; **47**: 586.

40 Heathcote EJ. Management of primary biliary cirrhosis. *Hepatology* 2000; **31**: 1005.

41 Heathcote EJ. Cutch-Dudek K, Walker V *et al.* The Canadian multicenter double-blind randomized controlled trial of ursodeoxycholic acid in primary biliary cirrhosis. *Hepatology* 1994; **19**: 1149.

42 Hendrikse M, Rigney F, Giaffer MH *et al.* Low-dose methotrexate in primary biliary cirrhosis. Long-term results of a placebo-controlled trial. *Hepatology* 1997; **26**: 248A.

43 Hopf U, Möller B, Stemerowicz R *et al.* Relation between *Escherichia coli* R (rough) forms in gut, lipid A in a liver, and primary biliary cirrhosis. *Lancet* 1989; **ii**: 1419.

44 Howard MJ, Fuller C, Broadhurst RW *et al.* Three-dimensional structure of the major autoantigen in primary biliary cirrhosis. *Gastroenterology* 1998; **115**: 139.

45 Howel D, Metcalf JV, Gray J *et al.* Cancer risk in primary biliary cirrhosis: a study in northern England. *Gut* 1999; **45**: 756.

46 Jones DEJ, Metcalf JV, Collier JD *et al.* Hepatocellular carcinoma in primary biliary cirrhosis and its impact on outcomes. *Hepatology* 1997; **26**: 1138.

47 Jones DEJ, Palmer JM, James OFW et al. T-cell responses to components of pyruvate dehydrogenase complex in primary biliary cirrhosis. *Hepatology* 1995; **21**: 995.

48 Jones DEJ, Watt FE, Metcalf JV *et al.* Familial primary biliary cirrhosis revisited: a geographically based population study. *J. Hepatol.* 1999; **30**: 402.

49 Joplin RE, Johnson GD, Matthews JB *et al.* Distribution of pyruvate dehydrogenase dihydrolipoamide acetyltransferase (PDC-E2) and another mitochondrial marker in salivary gland and biliary epithelium from patients with primary biliary cirrhosis. *Hepatology* 1994; **19**: 1375.

50 Kew MC, Varma RR, Dos Santos HA *et al.* Portal hypertension in primary biliary cirrhosis. *Gut* 1971; **12**: 830.

51 Kilmurry MR, Heathcote EJ, Cauch-Dudek K *et al.* Is the Mayo model for predicting survival useful after the introduction of ursodeoxycholic acid treatment for primary biliary cirrhosis? *Hepatology* 1996; **23**: 1148.

52 Kim WR, Wiesner RH, Therneau TM *et al.* Optimal timing of liver transplantation for primary biliary cirrhosis. *Hepatology* 1998; **28**: 33.

53 Kingham JGC, Parker DR. The association between primary biliary cirrhosis and coeliac disease: a study of relevant prevalence. *Gut* 1998; **42**: 120.

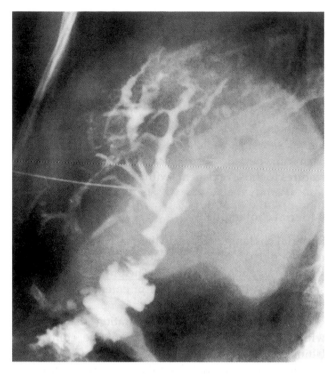

Fig. 15.10. Percutaneous cholangiography following choledocho-jejunostomy. There is no obstruction to flow of contrast into the jejunum but an intra-hepatic sclerosing cholangitis, marked by strictures and beading, has developed.

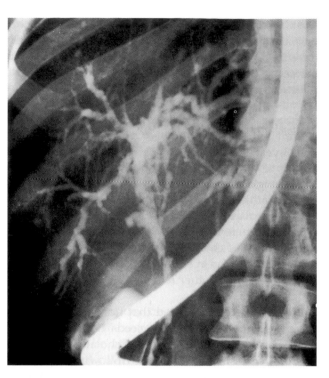

Fig. 15.11. ERCP showing distortion of the intra-hepatic biliary tree with irregularities in a patient with severe skin sepsis following burning. The picture resembles PSC.

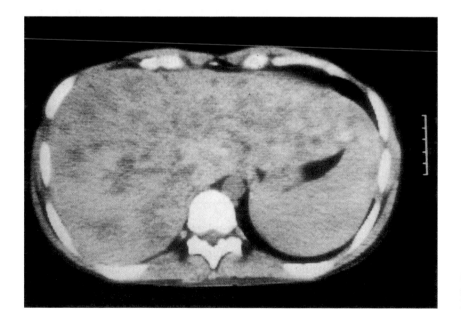

Fig. 15.12. CT from the same patient as in fig. 15.11 showing multiple space-occupying lesions due to metastatic bacterial abscesses.

malities [16, 24]. The usual causative organism is cytomegalovirus or cryptosporidia alone or in combination. *Cryptococcus, Candida albicans* and *Klebsiella pneumoniae* may be associated [15].

Abnormalities of the biliary system are associated with AIDS. In one series, 20 of 26 patients with AIDS and biliary problems had markedly abnormal cholangiograms. In 14 of these, the pattern was of sclerosing cholangitis with or without papillary stenosis.

PSC and AIDS cholangiopathy differ in the inflammatory infiltration surrounding the diseased bile ducts. In PSC, it is rich in T_4-lymphocytes, the subpopulation specifically depleted in patients with AIDS [60].

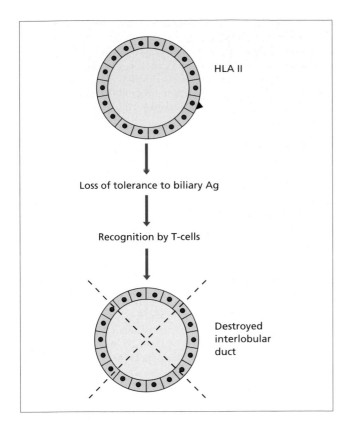

Fig. 15.13. Hepatic rejection (graft-versus-host disease). HLA class antigens are displayed on the bile duct. There is loss of tolerance to biliary antigens (Ag) which are recognized by cytotoxic T-cells and the interlobular ducts are destroyed.

Graft-versus-host disease

Aberrant expression of HLA class II antigen on bile ducts is seen in the transplanted human liver undergoing rejection and in patients with graft-versus-host disease following allogenic bone marrow transplantation (fig. 15.13). Rejection is marked by progressive non-suppurative cholangitis culminating in disappearance of interlobular bile ducts. The bile duct epithelium is penetrated by mononuclear cells with focal necrosis and rupture of the epithelium. Similar lesions are found in graft-versus-host disease following allogenic bone marrow transplantation. In one such patient, marked cholestatic jaundice lasted 10 years, and serial liver biopsies confirmed progressive biliary-type fibrosis and cirrhosis [35]. She ultimately died in liver failure.

Vascular cholangitis

The bile ducts are richly supplied by the hepatic artery which forms a peri-biliary vascular plexus. Interference leads to ischaemic necrosis of the bile ducts, both extra- and intra-hepatic, and to their ultimate disappearance. Injury to hepatic arterial branches, for instance during cholecystectomy, leads to ischaemia of the duct wall, damage to the ductal mucosa and entry of bile into the duct wall so causing fibrosis and stricture [66]. A similar sequence can complicate hepatic transplantation [74], especially if the segment of the recipient duct is too short and thus deprived of its arterial supply.

Biliary ischaemia secondary to intimal thickening of hepatic arterioles is a rare feature of chronic allograft rejection in man.

Diffuse small vessel arteritis, part of a systemic vasculitis, can be followed by bile duct loss.

Floxuridine (5-FUDR) can be infused by pump into the hepatic artery for the treatment of colo-rectal hepatic metastases. Biliary strictures can follow [33, 45]. The picture resembles PSC. The loss of bile ducts may be so severe that hepatic transplantation becomes necessary.

Drug-related cholangitis

Caustic cholangitis can be related to the injection of a scolicidal solution into a hydatid cyst. Only a part of the biliary tree is usually affected [5]. Within months the strictures result in jaundice, biliary cirrhosis and portal hypertension.

Histiocytosis X

A cholangiographic picture identical with that of PSC may complicate histiocytosis X [68]. The biliary lesions progress from a hyperplastic to a granulomatous, xanthomatous and, finally, a fibrotic stage. Clinically, the picture resembles PSC.

References

1 Aadlund E, Schrumpf E, Fausa O *et al.* Primary sclerosing cholangitis: a long-term follow up study. *Scand. J. Gastroenterol.* 1987; **22**: 655.
2 Abu-Elmagd KM, Malinchoc M, Dickson ER *et al.* Efficacy of hepatic transplantation in patients with primary sclerosing cholangitis. *Surg. Gynecol. Obstet.* 1993; **177**: 335.
3 Angulo P, Lindor KD. Primary sclerosing cholangitis. *Hepatology* 1999; **30**: 325.
4 Bass NM, Chapman RW, O'Reilly A *et al.* Primary sclerosing cholangitis associated with angioimmunoblastic lymphadenopathy. *Gastroenterology* 1983; **85**: 420.
5 Belghiti J, Benhamou J-P, Heuly S *et al.* Caustic sclerosing cholangitis. A complication of the surgical treatment of hydatid disease of the liver. *Arch. Surg.* 1986; **121**: 1162.
6 Berquist A, Glaumann H, Persson B *et al.* Risk factors and clinical presentation of hepatobiliary carcinoma in patients with primary sclerosing cholangitis: a case–control study. *Hepatology* 1998; **27**: 311.
7 Boberg KM, Schrumpf E, Fausa O *et al.* Hepatobiliary disease in ulcerative colitis. An analysis of 18 patients with hepatobiliary lesions classified as small-duct primary sclerosing cholangitis. *Scand. J. Gastroenterol.* 1994; **29**: 744.
8 Bodenheimer HC, LaRusso NF, Thayer WR *et al.* Elevated

circulating immune complexes in primary sclerosing cholangitis. *Hepatology* 1983; **3**: 150.

9　Broome U, Lofberg R, Veress B *et al.* Primary sclerosing cholangitis and ulcerative colitis: evidence for increased neoplastic potential. *Hepatology* 1995; **22**: 1404.

10　Broome U, Olsson R, Loof L *et al.* Natural history and prognostic factors in 305 Swedish patients with primary sclerosing cholangitis. *Gut* 1996; **38**: 610.

11　Campbell WL, Ferris JV, Holbart BL *et al.* Biliary tract carcinoma complicating primary sclerosing cholangitis: evaluation with CT, cholangiography, US and MR imaging. *Radiology* 1998; **207**: 41.

12　Cangemi JR, Wiesner RH, Beaver SJ *et al.* Effect of proctocolectomy for chronic ulcerative colitis on the natural history of primary sclerosing cholangitis. *Gastroenterology* 1989; **96**: 790.

13　Chapman RWG, Arborgh BAM, Rhodes JM *et al.* Primary sclerosing cholangitis—a review of its clinical features, cholangiography and hepatic histology. *Gut* 1980; **21**: 870.

14　Chapman RWG, Varghese Z, Gaul R *et al.* Association of primary sclerosing cholangitis with HLA-B8. *Gut* 1983; **24**: 38.

15　Cockerill FR, Hurley DV, Malagelada JR *et al.* Polymicrobial cholangitis and Kaposi's sarcoma in blood product transfusion-related acquired immune deficiency syndrome. *Am. J. Med.* 1986; **80**: 1237.

16　Davis JJ, Heyman MB, Ferrell L *et al.* Sclerosing cholangitis associated with chronic cryptosporidiosis in a child with a congenital immunodeficiency disorder. *Am. J. Gastroenterol.* 1987; **82**: 1196.

17　Di Palma JA, Strobel CT, Farrow JG. Primary sclerosing cholangitis associated with hyperimmunoglobulin M immuno-deficiency (dysgammaglobulinemia). *Gastroenterology* 1986; **91**: 464.

18　Dickson ER, Murtaugh PA, Wiesner RH *et al.* Primary sclerosing cholangitis: refinement and validation of survival models. *Gastroenterology* 1992; **103**: 1893.

19　Donaldson PT, Farrant JM, Wilkinson ML *et al.* Dual association of HLA DR2 and DR3 with primary sclerosing cholangitis. *Hepatology* 1991; **13**: 129.

20　El-Shabrawi M, Wilkinson ML, Portmann B *et al.* Primary sclerosing cholangitis in childhood. *Gastroenterology* 1987; **92**: 1226.

21　Ernst O, Asselah T, Sergent G *et al.* MR cholangiography in primary sclerosing cholangitis. *Am. J. Roentgenol.* 1998; **171**: 1027.

22　Farges O, Malassagne B, Sebagh M *et al.* Primary sclerosing cholangitis: liver transplantation or biliary surgery. *Surgery* 1995; **117**: 146.

23　Farrant JM, Hayllar KM, Wilkinson ML *et al.* Natural history and prognostic variables in primary sclerosing cholangitis. *Gastroenterology* 1991; **100**: 1710.

24　Gremse DA, Bucuvalas JC, Bongiovanni GL. Papillary stenosis and sclerosing cholangitis in an immunodeficient child. *Gastroenterology* 1989; **96**: 1600.

25　Haagsma EB, Mulder AHL, Bouw ASH *et al.* Neutrophil cytoplasmic autoantibodies after liver transplantation in patients with primary sclerosing cholangitis. *J. Hepatol.* 1993; **19**: 8.

26　Harrison RF, Davies MH, Neuberger JM *et al.* Fibrous and obliterative cholangitis in liver allografts: evidence of recurrent primary sclerosing cholangitis. *Hepatology* 1994; **20**: 356.

27　Hobson CH, Butt TJ, Ferry DM *et al.* Enterohepatic cir-

culation of bacterial chemotactic peptide in rats with experimental colitis. *Gastroenterology* 1988; **94**: 1006.

28　Howell DA, Beveridge RP, Bosco J *et al.* Endoscopic needle aspiration biopsy at ERCP in the diagnosis of biliary strictures. *Gastrointest. Endosc.* 1992; **38**: 531.

29　Ito K, Mitchell DG, Outwater EK *et al.* Primary sclerosing cholangitis. MR imaging features. *Am. J. Roentgenol.* 1999; **172**: 1527.

30　Kaplan MM. Toward better treatment of primary sclerosing cholangitis. *N. Engl. J. Med.* 1997; **336**: 719.

31　Keeffe EB. Diagnosis of primary sclerosing cholangitis in a blood donor with elevated serum alanine aminotransferase. *Gastroenterology* 1989; **96**: 1358.

32　Keiding S, Hansen SB, Rasmussen HH *et al.* Detection of cholangiocarcinoma in primary sclerosing cholangitis by positron emission tomography. *Hepatology* 1998; **28**: 700.

33　Kemeny MM, Battifora H, Blayney DW *et al.* Sclerosing cholangitis after continuous hepatic artery infusion of FUDR. *Ann. Surg.* 1985; **202**: 176.

34　Kim WR, Poterucha JJ, Wiesner RH *et al.* The relative role of the Child–Pugh classification and the Mayo natural history in the assessment of survival in patients with primary sclerosing cholangitis. *Hepatology* 1999; **29**: 1643.

35　Knapp AB, Crawford JM, Rappeport JM *et al.* Cirrhosis as a consequence of graft-versus-host disease. *Gastroenterology* 1987; **92**: 513.

36　Kono K, Ohnishi K, Omata M *et al.* Experimental portal fibrosis produced by intraportal injection of killed nonpathogenic *Escherichia coli* in rabbits. *Gastroenterology* 1998; **94**: 787.

37　Kurzawinski TR, Deery A, Dooley JS *et al.* A prospective study of biliary cytology in 100 patients with bile duct strictures. *Hepatology* 1993; **18**: 1399.

38　Lee JG, Schutz SM, England RE *et al.* Endoscopic therapy of sclerosing cholangitis. *Hepatology* 1995; **21**: 661.

39　Lee Y-M, Kaplan MM. Primary sclerosing cholangitis. *N. Engl. J. Med.* 1995; **332**: 924.

40　Lefkowitch JH. Primary sclerosing cholangitis. *Arch. Intern. Med.* 1982; **142**: 1157.

41　Lichtman SN, Sartor RB, Keku J *et al.* Hepatic inflammation in rats with experimental small intestinal bacterial overgrowth. *Gastroenterology* 1990; **98**: 414.

42　Lindor KD for the Mayo Primary Sclerosing Cholangitis-Ursodeoxycholic Acid Study Group. Ursodiol for primary sclerosing cholangitis. *N. Engl. J. Med.* 1997; **336**: 691.

43　Loftus EV Jr, Aguilar HI, Sandborn WJ *et al.* Risk of colorectal neoplasia in patients with primary sclerosing cholangitis and ulceraive colitis following orthotropic liver transplantation. *Hepatology* 1998; **27**: 685.

44　Loftus EV Jr, Sandborn WJ, Tremaine WJ *et al.* Risk of colorectal neoplasia in patients with primary sclerosing cholangitis. *Gastroenterology* 1996; **110**: 432.

45　Ludwig J, Kim CH, Wiesner RH *et al.* Floxuridine-induced sclerosing cholangitis: an ischemic cholangiopathy? *Hepatology* 1989; **9**: 215.

46　Ludwig J, MacCarty RL, LaRusso NF. Intrahepatic cholangiectases and large duct obliteration in primary sclerosing cholangitis. *Hepatology* 1986; **6**: 560.

47　MacCarty RL, LaRusso NF, Wiesner RH *et al.* Primary sclerosing cholangitis: findings on cholangiography and pancreatography. *Radiology* 1983; **149**: 39.

48　Mandal A, Dasgupta A, Jeffers L *et al.* Autoantibodies in sclerosing cholangitis against a shared peptide in biliary and colon epithelium. *Gastroenterology* 1994; **106**: 185.

49 Martin FM, Rossi RL, Nugent FW *et al*. Surgical aspects of sclerosing cholangitis: results in 178 patients. *Ann. Surg.* 1990; **212**: 551.

50 Mehal WZ, Dennis Lo Y-M, Wordsworth BP *et al*. HLA DR4 is a marker for rapid disease progression in primary sclerosing cholangitis. *Gastroenterology* 1994; **106**: 160.

51 Minuk GY, Hershfield NB, Lee WY *et al*. Reticulo-endothelial system Fc receptor-mediated clearance of IgG-tagged erythrocytes from the circulation of patients with idiopathic ulcerative colitis and chronic liver disease. *Hepatology* 1986; **6**: 1.

52 Nashan B, Schlitt HJ, Tusch G *et al*. Biliary malignancies in primary sclerosing cholangitis: timing for liver transplantation. *Hepatology* 1996; **23**: 1105.

53 Naveh Y, Mendelsohn H, Spira G *et al*. Primary sclerosing cholangitis associated with immunodeficiency. *Am. J. Dis. Child.* 1983; **137**: 114.

54 Neuberger J, Gunson B, Komolmit P *et al*. Pretransplant prediction of prognosis after liver transplantation in primary sclerosing cholangitis using a Cox regression model. *Hepatology* 1999; **29**: 1375.

55 Nichols JC, Gores GJ, LaRusso NF *et al*. Diagnostic role of serum CA 19-9 for cholangiocarcinoma in patients with primary sclerosing cholangitis. *Mayo Clin. Proc.* 1993; **68**: 874.

56 Olsson R, Danielsson Å, Järnerot G *et al*. Prevalence of primary sclerosing cholangitis in patients with ulcerative colitis. *Gastroenterology* 1991; **100**: 1319.

57 Porayko MK, Wiesner RH, LaRusso NF *et al*. Patients with asymptomatic primary sclerosing cholangitis frequently have progressive disease. *Gastroenterology* 1990; **98**: 1594.

58 Rahn RH III, Koehler RE, Weyman PJ *et al*. CT appearance of sclerosing cholangitis. *Am. J. Roentgenol.* 1983; **141**: 549.

59 Rasmussen HH, Fallingborg JF, Mortensen PB *et al*. Hepatobiliary dysfunction and primary sclerosing cholangitis in patients with Crohn's disease. *Scand. J. Gastroenterol.* 1997; **32**: 604.

60 Roulot D, Valla D, Brun-Vezinet F *et al*. Cholangitis in the acquired immuno-deficiency syndrome: report of two cases and review of the literature. *Gut* 1987; **28**: 1653.

61 Schrumpf E, Abdelnoor M, Fausa O *et al*. Risk factors in primary sclerosing cholangitis. *J. Hepatol.* 1994; **21**: 1061.

62 Seibold F, Weber P, Klein P *et al*. Clinical significance of antibodies against neutrophils in patients with inflammatory bowel disease and primary sclerosing cholangitis. *Gut* 1992; **33**: 657.

63 Shetty K, Rybicki L, Carey WD. The Child–Pugh classification as a prognostic indicator for survival in primary sclerosing cholangitis. *Hepatology* 1997; **25**: 1049.

64 Steckman M, Drossman DA, Lesesne HR. Hepatobiliary disease that precedes ulcerative colitis. *J. Clin. Gastroenterol.* 1990; **6**: 425.

65 Steinhart AH, Simons M, Stone R *et al*. Multiple hepatic abscesses: cholangiographic changes simulating sclerosing cholangitis and resolution after percutaneous drainage. *Am. J. Gastroenterol.* 1990; **85**: 306.

66 Terblanche J, Allison HE, Northover JMA. An ischemic basis for biliary strictures. *Surgery* 1983; **94**: 52.

67 Terjung B, Herzog V, Worman HJ *et al*. Atypical antineutrophil cytoplasmic antibodies with perinuclear fluorescence in chronic inflammatory bowel diseases and hepatobiliary disorders colocalize with nuclear lamina proteins. *Hepatology* 1998; **28**: 332.

68 Thompson HH, Pitt HA, Lewin KJ *et al*. Sclerosing cholangitis and histocytosis X. *Gut* 1984; **25**: 526.

69 Van Hoogstraten HJF, Wolfhagen FJH, van de Meebert PC *et al*. Ursodeoxycholic acid therapy for primary sclerosing cholangitis: results of a 2-year randomized controlled trial to evaluate single versus multiple daily doses. *J. Hepatol.* 1998; **29**: 417.

70 Wee A, Ludwig J. Pericholangitis in chronic ulcerative colitis: primary sclerosing cholangitis of the small bile ducts? *Ann. Intern. Med.* 1985; **102**: 581.

71 Wiesner RH, Grambsch PM, Dickson ER *et al*. Primary sclerosing cholangitis: natural history, prognostic factors and survival analysis. *Hepatology* 1989; **10**: 430.

72 Wiesner RH, LaRusso NF, Dozois RR *et al*. Peristomal varices after proctocolectomy in patients with primary sclerosing cholangitis. *Gastroenterology* 1986; **90**: 316.

73 Wilschanski M, Chait P, Wade JA *et al*. Primary sclerosing cholangitis in 32 children: clinical, laboratory, and radiographic features. *Hepatology* 1995; **22**: 1415.

74 Zajko AB, Campbell WL, Logsdon GA *et al*. Cholangiographic findings in hepatic artery occlusion after liver transplantation. *Am. J. Roentgenol.* 1987; **149**: 485.

Chapter 16
Viral Hepatitis: General Features, Hepatitis A, Hepatitis E and Other Viruses

The first reference to epidemic jaundice has been ascribed to Hippocrates. The earliest record in Western Europe is in a letter written in 751 AD by Pope Zacharias to St Boniface, Archbishop of Mainz. Since then there have been numerous accounts of epidemics, particularly during wars. Hepatitis was a problem in the Franco-Prussian War, the American Civil War and World War I. In World War II huge epidemics occurred, particularly in the Middle East and Italy [11].

There are many varieties of hepatitis (table 16.1). Hepatitis A is a self-limited, faecally spread disease. Hepatitis B is a parenterally transmitted disease that often becomes chronic. Hepatitis D is parenterally spread and affects only those with a hepatitis B infection. Hepatitis C is a parenterally spread disease with a high chronicity rate. Hepatitis E is enterically spread, usually via water, and causes a self-limited hepatitis in developing countries. There is increasing evidence for other viral causes of hepatitis.

Pathology

All forms of viral hepatitis have a basic pathology. The essential lesion is an acute inflammation of the entire liver [2]. Hepatic cell necrosis is associated with leucocytic and histiocytic reaction and infiltration. Zone 3 shows the necrosis most markedly and the portal tracts the greatest cellularity (figs 16.1, 16.2, 16.3). The sinusoids show mononuclear cellular infiltration, polymorphs and eosinophils. Surviving liver cells retain their glycogen. Fatty change is rare. Zone 3 liver cells may show eosinophilic change (*acidophil bodies*), ballooning pleomorphism and giant multi-nucleated cells may be present. Mitoses are sometimes prominent. Zone 3 cholestasis may be found. Focal 'spotty' necrosis may be seen. Bile duct proliferation is usual and damage is an occasional feature [7].

The reticulin framework is usually well preserved even in the midst of extreme disorganization. It provides a scaffolding when the liver cells regenerate. Inflammatory cells disappear gradually, and some new zone 1

Table 16.1. Viral hepatitis A, B, C, D and E contrasted

	HAV	HBV	HCV	HDV	HEV
Genome	RNA	DNA	RNA	RNA	RNA
Family	Picorna	Hepadna	Flavi : Pesti	Viroid	Calici
Incubation (days)	15–45	30–180	15–150	30–180	15–60
Transmission	Faecal	Blood	Blood	Blood	Faecal
	Oral	Saliva	Saliva	—	Oral
Acute attack	Depends on age	Mild or severe	Usually mild	Mild or severe	Usually mild
Rash	Yes	Yes	Yes	Yes	Yes
Serum diagnosis	IgM anti-HAV	IgM anti-HBc	Anti-HCV	IgM anti-HDV	IgM anti-HEV
		HBsAg	HCV RNA		
		HBV DNA			
Peak ALT	800–1000	1000–1500	300–800	1000–1500	800–1000
Up and down	No	No	Yes	No	No
Prevention	Vaccine	Vaccine	—	—	—
Chronicity	No	Yes	Yes	Yes	No
Treatment	Symptomatic	Symptomatic	Symptomatic	Symptomatic	Symptomatic
		?Antivirals	?Antivirals	?Antivirals	

ALT, alanine aminotransferase

Table 17.3. Groups in which acute and chronic type B hepatitis should be suspected

---

Immigrants from Mediterranean countries, Africa or the Far East
Drug abusers
Homosexual men
Neonates of HBsAg-positive mothers
Hospital staff
Patients with
    renal failure
    reticuloses
    cancer
    organ transplants
Staff and patients of hospitals for the mentally retarded
Post-transfusion

---

itive patients receiving hepatic transplants and accounts for re-infection of the graft.

Epidemiology (table 17.3)

The disease is transmitted parenterally or by intimate, often sexual, contact. The carrier rate of HBsAg varies worldwide from 0.1 to 0.2% in Britain, the USA and Scandinavia, to more than 3% in Greece and southern Italy and even up to 10–15% in Africa and the Far East. If anti-HBs is measured, the rate of exposure to hepatitis B in any community is much higher. Carriage of HBsAg is even higher in some isolated communities: 45% in Alaskan Eskimos [47] and 85% in Australian Aborigines.

In high carriage rate areas, infection is acquired by passage from the mother to the neonate. The infection is usually not via the umbilical vein, but from the mother at the time of birth and during close contact afterwards. The chance of transmission increases as term approaches and is greater from HBeAg-positive than HBeAg-negative mothers. Antigenaemia develops in the baby within 2 months of birth and tends to persist [9].

In high endemic areas, such as Africa, Greece and the Far East, the transmission is in childhood and probably horizontal through kissing, shared utensils such as toothbrushes and razors, and injections [49]. Contact in pre-school day-care centres is possible. Sexual contacts in the family are at risk.

Infection among homosexual men is related to duration of homosexual activity, number of sexual contacts and anal contact.

Blood-sucking arthropods such as mosquitoes or bed bugs may be important vectors, particularly in the tropics, although insecticide spraying of dwellings has had no effect on HBV infection [50].

The MHC class II allele DRB1*1302 is associated with protection against persistent HBV in children and adults in the Gambia [63].

Blood transfusion continues to cause hepatitis B in countries where donor blood is not screened. Transmission is more likely with blood from paid donors than from volunteers.

Opportunities for parenteral infection exist in the use of instruments for dental treatment, ear piercing and manicures, neurological examination, prophylactic inoculations, subcutaneous injections, acupuncture, tattooing and autohaemotherapy [69].

Parenteral drug abusers develop hepatitis from using shared, unsterile equipment. The mortality may be very high in this group. Multiple attacks are seen and chronicity is frequent. Liver biopsy may show, in addition to acute or chronic hepatitis, foreign material, such as chalk, injected with illicit drugs.

Hospital staff in contact with patients, and especially patients' blood, usually have a higher carrier rate than the general community. This applies particularly to staff on renal dialysis or oncology units. Patients are immunosuppressed and, on contracting the disease, become chronic carriers. The patient's attendant is infected from contact with blood parenterally, such as from pricking or through skin abrasions. Surgeons and dentists are particularly at risk in operating on HBsAg-positive patients with a positive HBeAg. Holes in gloves and cuts on hands are common. Wire sutures may be a particular hazard in penetrating the skin.

Spread from a health-care worker is usually through a surgeon performing complex invasive procedures [70]. In the UK, proof of immunity (through vaccination or past infection) is required of all surgeons and other medical staff performing invasive procedures. Students have to show certificates of immunization and immunity on registration for a medical or dental course.

Use of standard cleansing procedures means that HBV infection is not spread by endoscopes.

Institutionalized mentally retarded children (especially with Down's syndrome) and their attendants have a high carrier rate [35].

Clinical course (fig. 17.11)

The course may be anicteric. Sub-clinical episodes are extremely frequent. The non-icteric case is more liable to become chronic than the icteric one.

The usual acute clinical attack, diagnosed in the adult, tends to be more severe than for HAV or HCV infections. The overall picture is, however, similar. The self-limited, benign, icteric disease usually lasts less than 4 months. Jaundice rarely exceeds 4 weeks. Occasionally, a prolonged benign course is marked by increased serum transaminase values for more than 100 days. Relapses are rare. Cholestatic hepatitis with prolonged deep jaundice is unusual.

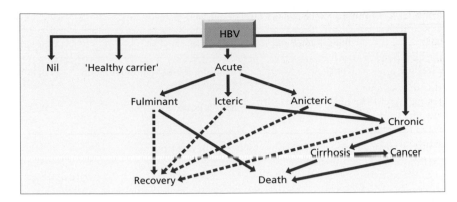

Fig. 17.11. The effect of exposure to HBV.

There may be features suggesting immune complex disease. This is shown in the prodromal period by a serum sickness-like syndrome. This develops about a week before jaundice. It can be associated with an icteric or an anicteric attack. The syndrome has also been described with chronic hepatitis B. Fever is usual. The skin lesion is urticarial, and rarely, in children, a papular acrodermatitis develops. The arthralgia is symmetrical, non-migratory and affects small joints. Serum rheumatoid factor is negative. It is usually transitory but can persist.

A fulminant course of hepatitis B in the first 4 weeks is related to an enhanced immune response with more rapid clearing of the virus. Antibodies to surface and 'e' antigen increase, and multiplication of the virus ceases. In fulminant hepatitis B, the surface antigen may be in low titre or undetectable. The diagnosis may be made only by finding serum IgM anti-HBc.

Another viral hepatitis, superimposed on the symptomless HBV carrier, may precipitate a fulminant course. The new agent may be HAV, HDV or HCV.

Sub-acute hepatic necrosis is marked by increasingly severe disease evolving over 1–3 months.

Extra-hepatic associations

These are often associated with circulating immune complexes containing HBsAg. The accompanying liver disease is usually mild. Acute and chronic type B hepatitis can develop in patients with agammaglobulinaemia.

Polyarteritis. This involves largely medium and small arteries and appears early in the course of the disease. Immune complexes containing HBsAg are found in the vascular lesions and their blood levels correlate with disease activity. Polyarteritis is a rare complication of hepatitis B [46]. Plasmapheresis and adenine arabinoside have been used for treatment [65].

Glomerulonephritis. This has been associated with HBV infection, largely in children [43]. Liver disease is minimal. The patients are usually HBsAg positive. Immune complexes of HBsAg and HBsAb, HBcAg and anti-HBc or HBeAg and anti-HBe are found in glomerular basement membranes [66]. In children, interferon treatment may lead to a remission. Remission may precede HBeAg seroconversion to anti-HBe. In children, the glomerulonephritis usually resolves spontaneously in 6 months to 2 years. In adults the disease is slowly but relentlessly progressive in one-third and the response to interferon is disappointing [37].

Essential mixed cryoglobulinaemia is a rare association of HBV infection although very frequent in HCV (Chapter 18).

The *Guillain–Barré syndrome* has been reported with HBsAg-containing immune complexes in serum and cerebrospinal fluid [55].

HBV carriers

Approximately 10% of patients contracting hepatitis B as adults and 98% of those infected as neonates will not clear HBsAg from the serum within 6 months (see fig. 17.8). Such patients become carriers and this is likely to persist. Reversion to a negative HBsAg is rare, but may develop in old age. Males are six times more likely to become carriers than females.

The dilemma of a person, such as a hospital worker, carrying the antigen and coming from an area where it is prevalent is a very difficult one. Hospital staff who develop HBsAg-positive hepatitis and clear the antigen from the blood are immune to type B hepatitis. If they become carriers, the position is difficult.

'Healthy' carriers may show changes on liver biopsy ranging from non-specific minimal abnormalities through to chronic hepatitis and cirrhosis. The extent of the changes is not reflected by serum biochemical tests and may only be revealed by liver biopsy. The carrier presenting by chance is likely to have minor hepatic changes compared to the patient presenting to a gastroenterology department where more serious liver disease is probable. In a survey of patients found to be HBsAg positive at blood donation, 95% had near normal

Table 17.4. Immunoprophylaxis of viral hepatitis B

Type	Immunoglobulin	Indication	Regime
B (adults)	HBIG	Exposure to HBsAg-positive blood Sexual consorts	0.06 ml/kg, as soon as possible, combined with first dose of vaccine*
B (neonates)	HBIG	HBsAg-positive mother	0.5 ml, as soon as possible, combined with first dose of vaccine†

*Full course of vaccine given if subject is anti-HBc negative.
†Full course of vaccine given.

liver biopsies and only 1.6% proceeded to chronic hepatitis or cirrhosis [22].

Chronic organic sequelae

Exposure to HBV can have difficult results (fig. 17.11). Some patients are immune and have no clinical attack; they presumably have anti-HBs. In others, an acute attack develops, varying from anicteric to fulminant. Previously normal people usually clear the antigen from the serum within about 4–6 weeks from the onset of symptoms. Chronic liver disease is associated with persistent antigenaemia. In general, the more florid and acute the original attack, the less likely the chronic sequelae.

If the patient survives a fulminant attack of viral hepatitis, ultimate recovery is complete without the development of chronic disease. Chronicity is more likely in those with immunological incompetence such as neonates, homosexual men, patients with AIDS, leukaemia and cancer, renal failure or those receiving immunosuppressive treatment.

Prevention

Hepatitis B immunoglobulin (HBIG)

HBIG is a hyperimmune serum globulin with a high antibody titre. It is effective for passive immunization if given prophylactically or within hours of infection (table 17.4) [60]. Hepatitis vaccine should always be given with HBIG, particularly if the subject is at risk of re-infection. It is indicated for sexual contacts of acute sufferers, babies born to HBsAg-positive mothers and victims of parenteral exposure (needle stick) to HBsAg-positive blood (tables 17.5, 17.6).

Repeated HBIG injections are being used to prevent re-infection of a donor liver inserted into an HBV DNA positive patient (Chapter 38).

HBV vaccines

Available vaccines are prepared from the non-infectious outer surface of the virus HBsAg. The plasma derived and the recombinant are equally effective and safe.

Table 17.5. Indication for hepatitis vaccination

Surgical and dental staff including medical students
Hospital and laboratory staff in contact with blood
Patients and staff in departments of oncology and haematology, kidney, mental subnormality and liver disease
Mental subnormality
Accidental exposure to HBsAg-positive blood
Close family and sexual contacts of HBsAg-positive carriers
Babies born to HBsAg-positive mothers
Children as part of 'Expanded Program on Immunization' (EPI)
Drug abusers
Homosexually active men
Travellers to high-risk areas

Table 17.6. Prophylaxis of persons accidentally exposed to possibly infectious blood

• **Check** donor blood for HBsAg; victim's blood for HBsAg and HBcAb
• **Give at once** 0.06 ml/kg HBIG plus first dose of hepatitis B vaccine

	HBsAg	HBcAb	Further action to victim
Victim	−ve	+ve	None: immune
Donor	+ve		Continue vaccine course
	−ve		None or continue vaccine course if victim is at risk of further hepatitis B exposure

Hepatitis B vaccines are effective in preventing hepatitis B in promiscuous homosexual men (fig. 17.12) [62], haemodialysis patients, Down's syndrome and other mentally retarded patients, health-care workers, babies born to HBsAg-positive mothers' and those not already immune in Alaska [47]. In Gambia, vaccination of infants was 84% effective against HBV infection and 94% effective against chronic carriage [71]. A 12-year follow-up of infants vaccinated in Senegal showed that 81% who received a booster at school age had anti-HBs. The protective efficacy of the vaccine was 88% [18].

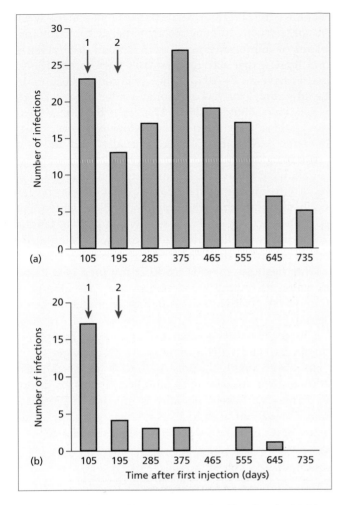

Fig. 17.12. Efficacy of hepatitis B vaccine. Results of a double-blind trial of the efficacy of hepatitis B vaccine in 1083 homosexual men. Distribution of infections in recipients of (a) placebo and (b) vaccine over 735 days. Arrows show time of first and second injections. (Modified from [62].)

In healthy individuals the recombinant vaccine is given in a dose of 10 µg (1 ml) intramuscularly, repeated at 1 month with a booster at 6 months. This induces sufficient antibody response in at least 94% of individuals. It is given intramuscularly into the arm.

Pre-testing. Vaccination is unnecessary if the person has a positive HBsAb or HBcAb.

The cost-effectiveness of pre-testing to save vaccine depends on the prevalence of serum B markers in a community.

The finding of an isolated serum anti-HBs does not necessarily mean immunity to hepatitis B. A positive serum anti-HBc is preferable as this detects infected as well as immune persons.

Duration of protection. Protection probably persists after the anti-HBs response has declined to undetectable levels. Immunological memory provides continued protection [64]. However, a booster should be considered at

Table 17.7. Failure of antibody response to hepatitis B vaccine

Age > 50 years
Underlying disease
HIV positive
Genetics (HLA-B8)
Buttock injection
Frozen vaccine
Unknown

5–7 years after the initial course if the subject is still being exposed to hepatitis B [24]. Antibody levels at the time of the booster dose may give a good indication of a duration of adequate antibody titres.

Antibody response

The long-term protection depends on the antibody response, which is 85–100% in healthy young subjects. Anti-HBs should be measured 1–3 months after completion of the basic course of vaccine.

Non-responders have peak anti-HBs levels of <10 iu/l and lack protection.

Low responders have peak anti-HBs levels of 10–100 iu/l and generally lack detectable anti-HBs levels within about 5–7 years. They may respond to a further booster of double the dose of vaccine.

Good responders have peak anti-HBs >100 iu/l and usually have long-term immunity.

Failure to develop adequate antibodies may be related to freezing the vaccine or giving it into the buttock, rather than the deltoid region. A poor antibody response is seen in the aged and in the immunocompromised, including HIV-positive persons (table 17.7). They should be given doses of 20 µg.

Approximately 5–10% of normal persons have an absent or poor antibody responses. Some may respond to a booster.

Indications for vaccination (see table 17.5)

The need for vaccination depends on the chance of being exposed to hepatitis B [52]. Vaccination is mandatory for health-care staff in close contact with hepatitis B patients, particularly those working on renal dialysis units, liver units, haemophilia and oncology units, genitourinary departments treating homosexual men or those working in homes for the mentally retarded. Surgeons and dentists and their assistants, medical students and laboratory workers regularly exposed to blood are candidates. The vaccine should be given to medical personnel going overseas to areas where the prevalence of hepatitis B is high.

Acute sufferers from hepatitis B are highly infectious and their sexual contacts should be vaccinated and given HBIG. Sexual and family contacts of HBV carriers should be vaccinated after their antibody status has been determined.

Promiscuous homosexual men, if they are not immune, should be vaccinated. The same rule applies to drug abusers.

Babies born to HBsAg-positive and, particularly, HBeAg-positive mothers should be vaccinated and given immune globulin at birth. Even in countries with a lower carrier rate, it is essential to screen all pregnant women for HBsAg and not only those with a high risk of being carriers. If possible, the pregnant woman should be tested at 14 weeks of gestation and supplemented at delivery by rapid screening of those who escaped routine prenatal care [28].

The introduction of HBV vaccine has had a disappointing effect on the overall prevalence of HBV in the USA. Transmission amongst homosexual men has fallen, but intravenous drug abuse has increased with spread to non-abuser social and sexual contacts. Healthcare workers show a reduction of HBV.

The addition to infant vaccination of targeting adolescents will give preventative protection before the subject is exposed to risk factors such as sexual lifestyle, abuse of drugs or joining the healthcare profession.

Unfortunately, integration of HBV vaccination into all extended immunization programmes is not being implemented, whether because of cost or apathy. Some of the richest countries in the world are the most to blame, although the programme is cost-effective, even in low-risk countries.

Other vaccines

The most simple vaccine is derived from heat-inactivated plasma containing HBsAg, and is based on the original observation of Krugman [35] who boiled infectious HBV-positive serum and showed that it protected against hepatitis B. This vaccine is relatively crude, highly immunogenic and inexpensive.

The pre-S region. A mutation in the surface (S) has been associated with infants born to carrier mothers becoming HBV positive, despite successful vaccination. The mutation is in the 'a' determinant of S to which the vaccine promotes antibodies (see figs 17.5, 17.6). New vaccines will contain pre-S1 and pre-S2 domains and may be effective in those failing to respond to conventional vaccination. They may also be useful in those who fail to show an adequate antibody response to standard vaccination [75].

Chronic hepatitis B

Chronic hepatitis B is found predominantly in males. Features associated with an increased risk of HBV include ethnic origin, sexual contacts of sufferers, work in contact with human blood, patients having transplants or immunosuppressive treatment, drug abusers and homosexual activity. Neonates born to an HBeAg carrier have an 80–90% chance of chronic infection. In healthy adults, the risk of chronicity after an acute attack is very low (about 5.5%) [32]. There may be none of these associations. The condition may follow unresolved acute hepatitis B. The acute attack is usually mild and of a 'grumbling' type.

Following the attack, serum transaminase levels fluctuate with intermittent jaundice. The patient may be virtually symptom-free with only biochemical evidence of continued activity, and may simply complain of fatigue and being generally unwell—the diagnosis being made after a routine medical check.

The diagnosis may be made at the time of a blood donation or routine blood screen when the HBsAg is found to be positive and serum transaminases modestly raised.

Chronic hepatitis is often a silent disease. Symptoms do not correlate with the severity of liver damage.

In about one-half, presentation is as established chronic liver disease with jaundice, ascites or portal hypertension. Encephalopathy is unusual at presentation. The patient usually gives no history of a previous acute attack of hepatitis. Some present as hepato-cellular carcinoma.

Clinical relapse and reactivation

An apparently stable patient may have a clinical relapse. This is marked by increasing fatigue and, usually, rises in serum transaminase values. Relapse may be related to seroconversion from an HBeAg-positive state to an HBeAg-negative one (fig. 17.13). Liver biopsy shows an acute interface hepatitis which ultimately subsides and the serum transaminase values fall.

Seroconversion may be spontaneous in 10–15% of patients per annum or it may follow antiviral therapy. HBV DNA can remain positive even when anti-HBe has

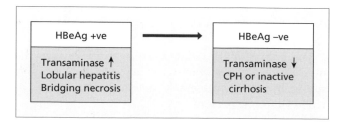

Fig. 17.13. Changes in a patient with chronic hepatitis B on conversion from HBeAg positive to HBeAg negative. CPH, chronic persistent hepatitis.

developed. In some HBeAg-positive patients, flare-ups of viral replication and transaminase elevation are found without eventual clearing of HBeAg.

Spontaneous reactivation from HBeAg negative to HBeAg and HBV DNA positive has also been described. The clinical picture ranges from absence of manifestations to fulminant liver failure. Reactivation is particularly severe in HIV-positive patients.

Reactivation may be marked serologically simply by finding a positive IgM anti-HBc.

Reactivation can follow cancer chemotherapy, low-dose methotrexate to treat rheumatoid arthritis [25], organ transplantation or administration of corticosteroids to HBeAg-positive patients.

Severe exacerbations have been associated with pre-core mutants [54] where HBV DNA is present, but 'e' antigen is absent.

The patient may be superinfected with HDV. This leads to a marked acceleration in the progress of chronic hepatitis.

Superinfection with HAV or HCV must also be considered.

Finally, any deterioration in a HBV carrier should raise the possibility of hepato-cellular carcinoma.

Laboratory tests

Serum bilirubin, aspartate transaminase and gamma-globulin are only moderately increased. Serum albumin is usually normal. At time of presentation, features of hepato-cellular disease are usually mild. Smooth muscle antibody, if present, is in low titre. Serum mitochondrial antibody is negative.

Serum HBsAg is present. In the later stages, HBsAg may be detected with difficulty in the blood yet IgM anti-HBc is usually present. HBe antigen or antibody and HBV DNA are variably detected.

HBV DNA can be detected by the PCR technique even in the plasma of people negative for HBsAg [69].

Needle liver biopsy

Hepatic histology varies widely and includes chronic hepatitis, active cirrhosis and hepato-cellular carcinoma. There are no constant diagnostic features, unless HBsAg is demonstrated as 'ground glass' cells by the orcein method or HBcAg by immunoperoxidase. The amount of replicating virus in the serum does not correlate with the degree of histological activity [51].

Course and prognosis

The clinical course varies considerably (fig. 17.14). Many patients remain in a stable, compensated state. This is particularly so in the asymptomatic and where hepatic histology shows only a mild, chronic hepatitis.

Clinical deterioration in a previously stable HBV carrier can have varying explanations. The patient may be converting from a replicative to an integrated state. This is usually followed by a remission which may be permanent, serum enzyme levels falling into the normal

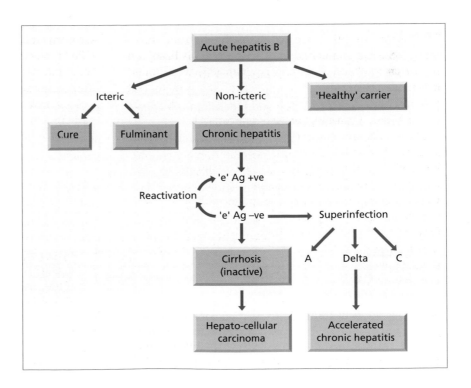

Fig. 17.14. The natural history of HBV infection.

range and liver histology improving; 10–20% per year may follow this course.

Prognosis is proportional to the severity of the underlying liver disease. Women have less severe liver disease. Age over 40 years and ascites are bad signs. There seem to be geographical and age-related differences in the natural history. HBV DNA positive Italian children have a 70% chance, before they are adults, of becoming HBeAb positive and HBV DNA negative with normalization of the transaminases irrespective of previous antiviral therapy; 25% will clear HBsAg [9, 10]. In contrast, only 2% of healthy Chinese carriers or chronic hepatitis patients cleared HBsAg in a mean of 4.0±2.3 years [41].

Patients aged over 40 years, HBeAg negative and with established cirrhosis are more likely to clear HBsAg.

In general, the prognosis for the healthy HBV carrier is good. A 16-year follow-up of asymptomatic HBV carriers from Montreal, showed that they remained asymptomatic and the risk of death from HBV-related cirrhosis and/or hepato-cellular carcinoma was low. The annual clearance rate for HBsAg was 0.7% [68]. Similarly, HBsAg carriers with normal transaminase levels in Italy have an excellent prognosis. A mortality follow-up of sufferers in the 1942 epidemic of HBV in the American army, showed a slight excess for hepato-cellular cancer. However, the mortality from non-alcoholic chronic liver disease was less [19]. Very few immunocompetent adult males became carriers.

Recurrence of HBV in the graft is usual after liver transplantation in patients with HBV infection, especially if HBV DNA and HBeAg positive (Chapter 38).

Treatment

The patient must be counselled concerning personal infectivity. This is particularly important if he or she is HBeAg positive. Close family and sexual contacts should be checked for HBsAg and HBcAb and, if negative, hepatitis B vaccination should be offered.

Bed rest is not helpful. Physical fitness is encouraged by graduated exercises. Diet is normal. Alcohol should be avoided as this enhances the effects of HBsAg carriage. However, one or two glasses of wine or beer a day are allowed if this is part of the patient's lifestyle.

The majority of patients with chronic hepatitis B lead normal lives. Strong reassurance will prevent introspection by the patient.

Antiviral therapy

The aim is to control infectivity, eradicate the virus and prevent the development of cirrhosis. However, permanent loss of HBeAg and HBV DNA are unusual and HBsAg usually persists. Treatment does result in a reduction of infectivity and of necrotic inflammation in

Table 17.8. Factors determining the response of patients with chronic hepatitis B to antiviral therapy

---

Good
Female
Heterosexual
Compliant
Recent infection
High serum transaminases
'Active' liver biopsy
High HBV DNA

Bad
Homosexual
HIV positive
Disease acquired early
Oriental

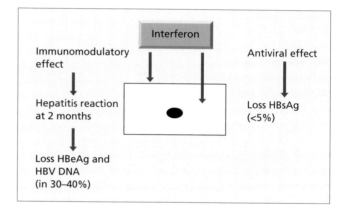

Fig. 17.15. Interferon, used to treat chronic hepatitis B, acts as an immunomodulatory agent resulting in loss of circulating HBeAg and HBV DNA in 30–40% of cases, and to a lesser extent as an antiviral agent resulting in loss of HBsAg in less than 5% of cases.

the liver. Thus cirrhosis may be prevented and with it the risk of hepatocellular carcinoma.

Those most likely to respond have a history of acute hepatitis, high serum ALT and low serum HBV levels (table 17.8).

Interferon-α (IFN-α). This is licensed to treat chronic HBV infection. It acts immunologically by enhancing the display of HLA class I antigens and increasing mechanisms to destroy diseased hepatocytes (fig. 17.15). It also has antiviral effects.

The usual regime in the USA is 5 million units daily or 10 million units three times a week by injection for 16 weeks. Extending the duration or using higher doses does not seem to increase the response rate.

Early symptomatic side-effects, usually temporary, occur 4–8h after the injection during the first week and are relieved by analgesics (table 17.9). Later, psychiatric complications, especially in those with pre-existing

Table 17.9. Interferon side-effects

Early
Flu-like
Myalgia, usually temporary
Headaches
Nausea

Late
Fatigue
Muscle aches
Irritability
Anxiety and depression
Weight loss
Diarrhoea
Alopecia
Bone-marrow suppression
Bacterial infections
Autoimmune autoantibodies
Optic tract neuropathy
Lichen planus worsens

Table 17.10. The effect of interferon for HBeAg-positive patients: meta-analysis (15 studies) [72]

	Loss (%)	
	HBsAg	HBeAg
Interferon	7.8	33
Spontaneous	1.8	12

nervous diseases, indicate cessation of therapy. Autoimmune changes develop 4–6 months after starting and include positive serum ANA, AMA and anti-thyroid antibodies. Pre-existing antibodies against thyroid microsomes are a contraindication to starting interferon. Bacterial infections develop, especially in cirrhotics.

A positive response is shown by loss of HBeAg and HBV DNA with a transient rise in transaminases at about 8 weeks as infected cells are lysed (fig. 17.15). Interferon results in a sustained loss of HBeAg and HBV DNA in only 30–40% of Caucasian patients, but progression of the disease seems to be prevented (table 17.10) [53, 72]. These results apply to white adults, in good health and with compensated liver disease. Only 17% of Chinese patients lose HBeAg and become HBV DNA negative [44].

Patients with decompensated cirrhosis suffer severe side-effects, particularly infections. Some patients may respond to low doses (e.g. 1 million units, three times a week).

Interferon-α has resulted in long-term remission of patients with chronic HBV with glomerulonephritis [15].

About 25% of patients with the pre-core HBV mutant (HBeAg negative, HBV DNA positive) respond to treatment.

After relapse, re-treatment with interferon is sometimes successful [13].

Lamivudine. This nucleoside analogue inhibits reverse transcriptase and HBV DNA polymerase enzymes necessary for HBV replication.

Nucleoside analogues interfere with mitochondrial function and can cause severe side-effects. These led to the withdrawal of one, fialuridine, which caused fatalities [45]. Fortunately, lamivudine is only a weak inhibitor of the cellular enzymes required for mitochondrial DNA replication and serious side-effects have not been reported.

Lamivudine is given orally in a dose of 100–300 mg daily. It is cleared by the kidney and adjustments may be necessary in those with impaired kidney function.

Controlled trials have shown that after 1 year of treatment (100–300 mg daily), 70–100% of patients will become HBV DNA negative as shown by PCR. Seventeen per cent of Caucasian or Chinese patients show HBeAg seroconversion and this increases to 24% after 2 years of treatment [36]. Histology improves and, in the majority, serum ALT falls.

Results are better in those with higher ALT levels [14]. Those with initially normal ALT levels should probably not be treated.

After 1 year, 45% of initially positive patients have lost HBV DNA with normal ALT, but only 15% remain HBV DNA negative 16 weeks after stopping therapy [59]. Exacerbations after stopping therapy are due to viral resistance (mutants) and to recrudescence of viraemia [31]. This can lead to hepatic decompensation [6, 40]. It is difficult to decide when to stop therapy. This could probably be done following HBeAg seroconversion and 18 months of therapy [20, 21].

Cirrhotic patients, especially if decompensated, must be treated cautiously, although in some patients biochemical tests and Child's grade may so improve that liver transplant becomes possible [67].

Lamivudine (300 mg daily) inhibits HBV replication in HIV-infected patients. However, lamivudine-resistant HBV may occur in 20% of patients per year [5].

Combination therapy. The combination of lamivudine with interferon increases the HBeAg seroconversion rate [58]. Ribavirin may be added [16]. In Chinese patients, the combination of lamivudine with famciclovir was superior to monotherapy [39].

In preliminary studies, priming with prednisolone enhanced the efficacy of subsequent lamivudine therapy [42].

Lamivudine resistance. Unfortunately, lamivudine therapy is followed by viral resistance in a high proportion of cases. This develops, with return of viral replication in 27% of patients at 1 year, and 58% after 2 years of treatment.

The resistance is marked by amino acid mutations in the highly conserved YMDD motifs of the active site of the polymerase [2, 40]. These mutants impair HBV replication, but the virus is still pathogenic.

Use in liver transplantation. Pre-transplant prophylaxis and treatment of post-transplant recurrence may improve the outlook for liver transplanation [26, 56]. Lamivudine should be continued in liver transplant patients who develop resistance.

Other therapies

Adenofivir (dipivoxil) inhibits HBV polymerase and is under trial but renal toxicity is a problem.

Lobucavir gave initially encouraging results, but animal carcinogenicity is urging caution.

Experimental agents including *EMS 200 475*, a novel guanosine analogue, have not reached clinical trials [33].

Immunotherapy

Patients with chronic HBV lack a long-term polyclonal non-specific T-cell response. This can be stimulated by repeated doses of standard recombinant HBV vaccines [17].

DNA-based vaccines are being tested to provide a specific T-cell response and induce cell-mediated immunity [30].

Molecular therapy

These therapies attempt to interfere directly with viral replication. Antisense oligonucleotides and antisense RNA bind to specific RNA targets causing arrest of translation and degradation.

Ribosomes are RNA enzymes that catalyse RNA cleavage and splicing reactions.

Permanent negative mutants and intracellular antibodies interfere with nucleocapsid assembly. All these molecular therapies are in the pre-clinical phase of development.

Outstanding problems

There are many uncertainties in the management of chronic HBV. How should patients be selected to receive interferon as opposed to lamivudine? Lamivudine should be given for at least 2 years, but for how long? When should the drug be withdrawn because of success or failure? Lamivudine resistance inhibits its use, but the clinical significance of the mutants that develop remains uncertain.

Screening for hepato-cellular carcinoma

Patients who are HBsAg positive with chronic hepatitis or cirrhosis, especially if male and more than 45 years old, should be screened regularly so that hepato-cellular carcinoma may be diagnosed early when surgical resection may prove possible (see Chapter 31). Serum α-fetoprotein should be measured and ultrasound examination performed at 6-monthly intervals.

References

1 Akahane Y, Yamanaka T, Suzuki H *et al.* Chronic active hepatitis with hepatitis B virus DNA and antibody against e antigen in the serum. Disturbed synthesis and secretion of e antigen from hepatocytes due to a point mutation in the precore region. *Gastroenterology* 1990; **99**: 1113.

2 Atkins M, Gray DF. Lamivudine resistance in chronic hepatitis. *J. Hepatol.* 1998; **28**: 169.

3 Baker BL, Di Bisceglie AM, Kaneko S *et al.* Determination of hepatitis B virus DNA in serum using the polymerase chain reaction: clinical significance and correlation with serological and biochemical markers. *Hepatology* 1991; **13**: 632.

4 Bartolome J, Moraleda G, Molina J *et al.* Hepatitis B virus DNA in liver and peripheral blood mononuclear cells during reduction in virus replication. *Gastroenterology* 1990; **99**: 1745.

5 Benhamou Y, Mochet M, Thibault V *et al.* Long-term incidence of hepatitis B virus resistance to lamivudine in human immunodeficiency virus-infected patients. *Hepatology* 1999; **30**: 1302.

6 Bessesen M, Ives D, Condrea YL *et al.* Chronic active hepatitis B exacerbations in human immunodeficiency virus-infected patients following development of resistance to withdrawal of lamivudine. *Clin. Infect. Dis.* 1999; **28**: 1302.

7 Bloom HE. Variants of hepatitis B, C and D viruses: molecular biology and clinical significance. *Digestion* 1995; **56**: 85.

8 Blumberg BS, Alter HJ, Visnich S. A 'new' antigen in leukaemia sera. *JAMA* 1965; **191**: 541.

9 Bortolotti F, Cardrobbi P, Crivellaro C *et al.* Long-term outcome of chronic type B hepatitis in patients who acquire hepatitis B virus infection in childhood. *Gastroenterology* 1990; **99**: 805.

10 Bortolotti F, Jara P, Barbera C *et al.* Long-term effect of alpha interferon in children with chronic hepatitis B. *Gut* 2000; **46**: 715.

11 Brunetto MR, Stemler M, Schodel F *et al.* Identification of HBV variants which cannot produce precore derived HBeAg and may be responsible for severe hepatitis. *Ital. J. Gastroenterol.* 1989; **21**: 151.

12 Carman WF, Hadziyannis S, McGarvey MJ *et al.* Mutation preventing formation of hepatitis B e antigen in patients with chronic hepatitis B infection. *Lancet* 1989; **ii**: 588.

13 Carreno V, Marcellin P, Hadziyannis S *et al.* Retreatment of chronic hepatitis B e antigen-positive patients with recombinant interferon alfa-2a. *Hepatology* 1999; **29**: 277.

14 Chien RN, Liaw Y-F, Atkins M. Pre-therapy alanine transferase level as a determinant for hepatitis B e antigen seroconversion during lamivudine therapy in patients with chronic hepatitis B. *Hepatology* 1999; **30**: 770.

15 Conjeevaram HS, Hoofnagle JH, Austin HA *et al.* Long-term outcome of hepatitis B virus-related glomerulonephritis after therapy with interferon alfa. *Gastroenterology* 1995; **109**: 540.

16 Cotonat T, Quiroga JA, Lopez-Alcorocho JM *et al.* Pilot study of combination therapy with ribavirin and interferon alfa for the retreatment of chronic hepatitis B e antibody-positive patients. *Hepatology* 2000; **31**: 502.

17 Couillin I, Pol S, Mancini M *et al.* Specific vaccine therapy in chronic hepatitis B: induction of specific T-cell proliferative responses for envelope antigens. *J. Infect. Dis.* 1999; **180**: 15.

18 Coursaget P, Leboulleux D, Soumare M *et al.* Twelve-year follow-up study of hepatitis B immunization of Senegalese infants. *J. Hepatol.* 1994; **21**: 250.

19 Di Bisceglie AM, Goodman ZD, Ishak KG *et al.* Long-term clinical and histopathological follow-up of clinical post-transfusion hepatitis. *Hepatology* 1991; **14**: 969.

20 Dienstag JL, Schiff ER, Mitchell M *et al.* Extended lamivudine retreatment for chronic hepatitis B: maintenance of viral suppression after discontinuation of therapy. *Hepatology* 1999; **30**: 1082.

21 Dienstag JL, Schiff ER, Wright TL *et al.* Lamivudine as initial treatment for chronic hepatitis B in the United States. *N. Engl. J. Med.* 1999; **341**: 1256.

22 Dragosics B, Ferenci P, Hitchman E *et al.* Long-term follow-up study of asymptomatic HBsAg-positive voluntary blood donors in Austria: a clinical and histological evaluation of 242 cases. *Hepatology* 1987; **7**: 302.

23 Dudley FJ, Fox RA, Sherlock S. Cellular immunity and hepatitis associated (Australia) antigen liver disease. *Lancet* 1972; **i**: 743.

24 European Consensus Group of Hepatitis B Immunity. Are booster immunizations needed for lifelong hepatitis B immunity? *Lancet* 2000; **255**: 561.

25 Flowers MA, Heathcote J, Wanless IR *et al.* Fulminant hepatitis as a consequence of reactivation of hepatitis B virus infection after discontinuation of low-dose methotrexate therapy. *Ann. Intern. Med.* 1990; **112**: 381.

26 Grellier L, Mutimer D, Ahmed M *et al.* Lamivudine prophylaxis against reinfection in liver transplantation for hepatitis B cirrhosis. *Lancet* 1996; **348**: 1212.

27 Grob P. Introduction to epidemiology and risk of hepatitis B. *Vaccine* 1995; **13**: 514.

28 Grosheide PM, Wladimiroff JW, Heijtink RA *et al.* Proposal for routine antenatal screening at 14 weeks for hepatitis B surface antigen. *Br. Med. J.* 1995; **311**: 1197.

29 Haruna Y, Hayashi N, Katayama K *et al.* Expression of X protein and hepatitis B virus replication in chronic hepatitis. *Hepatology* 1991; **13**: 418.

30 Heathcote J, McHutchinson J, Lee S *et al.* A pilot study of the CY-1899 T-cell vaccine in subjects chronically infected with the hepatitis B virus. *Hepatology* 1999; **30**: 531.

31 Honkoop P, de Man RA, Niesters HGM *et al.* Acute exacerbation of chronic hepatitis B virus infection after withdrawal of lamivudine therapy. *Hepatology* 2000; **32**: 635.

32 Hyams KC. Risks of chronicity following acute hepatitis B virus infection: a review. *Clin. Infect. Dis.* 1995; **20**: 992.

33 Innaimo SF, Seifer M, Bissacchi GS *et al.* Identification of EMS-200475 as a potent and selective inhibitor of hepatitis B virus. *Antimicrob. Agents Chemother.* 1997; **41**: 1444.

34 Joller-Jemelka HI, Wicki AN, Grob PJ. Detection of HBs antigen in 'anti-HBe alone' positive sera. *J. Hepatol.* 1994; **21**: 269.

35 Krugman S, Overby LR, Mushahwar IK *et al.* Viral hepatitis type B: studies on natural history and prevention re-examined. *N. Engl. J. Med.* 1979; **300**: 101.

36 Lai CL, Chien RN, Leung NW *et al.* A one-year trial of lamivudine for chronic hepatitis B. *N. Engl. J. Med.* 1998; **339**: 61.

37 Lai KN, Li PKT, Lui SF *et al.* Membranous nephropathy related to hepatitis B virus in adults. *N. Engl. J. Med.* 1991; **324**: 1457.

38 Lau JYN, Wright TL. Molecular virology and pathogensis of hepatitis B. *Lancet* 1992; **342**: 1335.

39 Law GKK, Tsang M, Hou J *et al.* Combination therapy with lamivudine and famciclovir for chronic hepatitis B-infected Chinese patients: a viral dynamics study. *Hepatology* 2000; **32**: 394.

40 Liaw Y-F, Chien RN, Leung N *et al.* Acute exacerbations and hepatitis B virus clearance after emergence of YMDD motif mutation during lamivudine therapy. *Hepatology* 1998; **30**: 567.

41 Liaw Y-F, Sheen I-S, Chen T-J *et al.* Incidence, determinants and significance of delayed clearance of serum HbsAg in chronic hepatitis B virus infection: a prospective study. *Hepatology* 1991; **13**: 627.

42 Liaw Y-F, Tsai S-L, Chien R-N *et al.* Prednisolone priming enhances Th1 response and efficacy of subsequent lamivudine therapy in patients with chronic hepatitis B. *Hepatology* 2000; **32**: 604.

43 Lin C-Y. Hepatitis B virus-associated membranous nephropathy: clinical featuers, immunological profiles and outcome. *Nephron* 1990; **55**: 37.

44 Lok ASF, Ma OCK, Lau JYN. Interferon alpha therapy in patients with chronic hepatitis B patients treated with interferon alfa. *Gastroenterology* 1993; **105**: 1883.

45 McKenzie R, Fruied MW, Sallie R *et al.* Hepatic failure and lactic acidosis due to fialuridine (FIAU), an investigational nucleoside analogue for chronic hepatitis B. *N. Engl. J. Med.* 1995; **333**: 1099.

46 McMahon BJ, Heyward WL, Templin DW *et al.* Hepatitis B-associated polyarteritis nodosa in Alaskan Eskimos: clinical and epidemiologic features and long-term follow-up. *Hepatology* 1989; **9**: 97.

47 McMahon BJ, Rhoades ER, Hayward WL *et al.* A comprehensive programme to reduce the incidence of hepatitis B virus infection and its sequelae in Alaskan natives. *Lancet* 1987; **ii**: 1134.

48 Marcellin P, Martinot-Peignoux M, Loriot M-A *et al.* Persistence of hepatitis B virus DNA demonstrated by polymerase chain reaction in serum and liver after loss of HBsAg induced by antiviral therapy. *Ann. Intern. Med.* 1990; **112**: 227.

49 Mayans MV, Hall AJ, Inskip HM *et al.* Risk factors for transmission of hepatitis B virus to Gambian children. *Lancet* 1990; **336**: 1107.

50 Mayans MV, Hall AJ, Inskip HM *et al.* Do bedbugs transmit hepatitis B? *Lancet* 1994; **343**: 761.

51 Mills CT, Lee E, Perillo R. Relationship between histology, aminotransferase levels, and viral replication in chronic hepatitis B. *Gastroenterology* 1990; **99**: 519.

52 MMWR. Protection against viral hepatitis. Recommendations of the Immunization Practices Advisory Committee (ACIP). *MMWR* 1990; **39**: 1.

53 Niederau C, Heintges T, Lange S *et al.* Long-term follow-up of HBeAg-positive patients treated with interferon alfa for chronic hepatitis B. *N. Engl. J. Med.* 1996; **334**: 1422.

54 Omata M, Ehata T, Yokosuka O *et al.* Mutations in the precore region of hepatitis B virus DNA in patients with fulminant and severe hepatitis. *N. Engl. J. Med.* 1991; **324**: 1699.

55 Penner E, Maida E, Mamoli B *et al*. Serum and cerebrospinal fluid immune complexes containing hepatitis B surface antigen in Guillain–Barré syndrome. *Gastroenterology* 1982; **82**: 576.

56 Perrilllo R, Rakela J, Dienstag J *et al*. Multicentre study of lamivudine therapy for hepatitis B after liver transplantation. *Hepatology* 1999; **29**: 1581.

57 Sanchez-Quijano A, Jauregui JI, Leal M *et al*. Hepatitis B virus occult infection in subjects with persistent isolated anti-HBc reactivity. *J. Hepatol.* 1993; **17**: 288.

58 Schalm SW, Heathcote J, Cianciar AJ *et al*. Lamivudine and interferon combination treatment of patients with chronic hepatitis B infection: a randomized trial. *Gut* 2000; **46**: 562.

59 Schiff E, Karavalcin S, Grimm I *et al*. A placebo-controlled study of lamivudine and interferon alpha-2b in patients with chronic hepatitis B who previously failed interferon therapy. *Hepatology* 1998; **28**: 388A.

60 Seeff LB, Koff RS. Passive and active immunoprophylaxis of hepatitis B. *Gastroenterology* 1984; **86**: 958.

61 Shindo M, Okuno T, Arai K *et al*. Detection of hepatitis B virus DNA in paraffin-embedded liver tissues in chronic hepatitis B or non-A, non-B hepatitis using the polymerase chain reaction. *Hepatology* 1991; **13**: 167.

62 Szmunes SW, Stevens CE, Harley EJ *et al*. Hepatitis B vaccine: demonstration of efficacy in a controlled trial in a high-risk population in the United States. *N. Engl. J. Med.* 1980; **303**: 833.

63 Thursz MR, Kwiatkowski D, Allsopp CEM *et al*. Association between an MHC class II allele and clearance of hepatitis B virus in The Gambia. *N. Engl. J. Med.* 1995; **332**: 1065.

64 Tilzey AJ. Hepatitis B vaccine boosting: the debate continues. *Lancet* 1995; **345**: 1000.

65 Trepo CG, Ouzan D. Successful therapy of polyarteritis due to hepatitis B virus by combination of plasma exchanges and adenine arabinoside therapy. *Hepatology* 1985; **5**: 1022 (abstract).

66 Venkatasehan VS, Lieberman K, Kim DU *et al*. Hepatitis B-associated glomerulonephritis: pathology, pathogenesis and clinical course. *Medicine (Baltimore)* 1990; **69**: 200.

67 Villeneuve J-P, Condreay LD, Bernard W *et al*. Lamivudine treatment for decompensated cirrhosis resulting from chronic hepatitis B. *Hepatology* 2000; **31**: 207.

68 Villeneuve J-P, Desrochers M, Infante-Rivard C *et al*. Long-term, follow-up study of asymptomatic hepatitis B surface antigen-positive carriers in Montreal. *Gastroenterology* 1994; **106**: 1000.

69 Webster GJM, Hallett R, Whalley SA *et al*. Molecular epidemiology of a large outbreak of hepatitis B linked to auto-haemotherapy. *Lancet* 2000; **356**: 379.

70 Welch J, Webster M, Tilzey AJ *et al*. Hepatitis B infections after gynaecological surgery. *Lancet* 1989; **i**: 205.

71 Whittle HC, Maine N, Pilkington J *et al*. Long-term efficacy of continuing hepatitis B vaccination in two Gambian villages. *Lancet* 1995; **345**: 1089.

72 Wong DKH, Chung AM, O'Rourke K *et al*. Effects of alpha-interferon in patients with hepatitis B antigen-positive chronic hepatitis B. A meta analysis. *Ann. Intern. Med.* 1993; **119**: 312.

73 Yamada G, Takaguchi K, Matsueda K *et al*. Immunoelectron microscopic observation of intrahepatic HBeAg in patients with chronic hepatitis B. *Hepatology* 1990; **12**: 133.

74 Yoffe B, Burns DK, Bhatt HS *et al*. Extra-hepatic hepatitis B virus DNA sequences in patients with acute hepatitis B infection. *Hepatology* 1990; **12**: 187.

75 Zuckerman JN, Sabin C, Craig FM *et al*. Immune response to a new hepatitis B vaccine in healthcare workers who had not responded to standard vaccine: randomised double blind dose–response study. *Br. Med. J.* 1997; **314**: 329.

Hepatitis delta virus (HDV)

The delta agent is a very small (36 nm) RNA particle coated with HBsAg (fig. 17.16) [19]. It is not able to replicate on its own, but is capable of infection when activated by the presence of HBV. It resembles satellite viruses of plants which cannot replicate without another specific virus. The interaction between the two viruses is very complex. Synthesis of HDV may depress the appearance of hepatitis B viral markers in infected cells and even lead to the elimination of active hepatitis B viral replication.

The delta virus is a single-stranded, circular, antisense RNA. It is highly infectious and can induce hepatitis in an HBsAg-positive host.

There are at least three genotypes having variable geographical distribution and clinical associations [6, 28].

HBV and HDV infection may be simultaneous (*co-infection*) or HDV may infect a chronic HBsAg carrier (*superinfection*) (figs 17.17, 17.18).

Epidemiology

HDV infection is not a new disease. Analysis of stored blood shows it to have been present in the American army in 1947, in Los Angeles since 1967 [7] and in liver specimens from Brazil in the 1930s.

HDV infection is strongly associated with intravenous

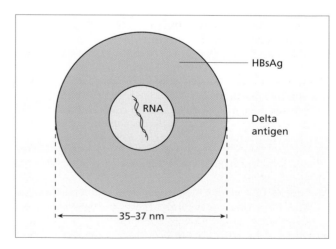

Fig. 17.16. Delta antigen is a small RNA particle coated by HBsAg.

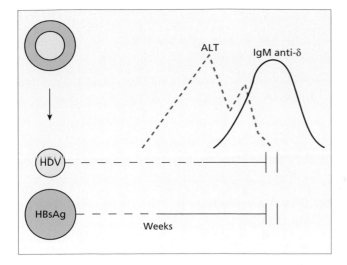

Fig. 17.17. Simultaneous infection with HBV and HDV results in acute hepatitis B with a rise in alanine transaminase (ALT). HDV infection follows with a second peak of ALT and the appearance of IgM anti-delta in the blood. Clearing of HBsAg is associated with clearing of delta [19].

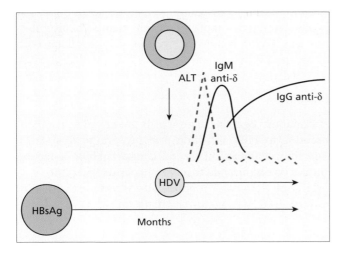

Fig. 17.18. HDV infection in an HBsAg carrier results in an attack of acute hepatitis with the appearance of IgM anti-delta followed by IgG anti-delta in the blood [19].

drug abuse [15], but can affect all risk groups for HBV infection. It is infrequent in homosexual men [26] but can affect health-care workers, transfusion recipients, haemophiliacs, immigrants and the developmentally disabled [12]. HDV can spread heterosexually [15]. Intra-family spread has been noted in southern Italy [3]. Children can be affected. HDV infection may be reactivated by HIV infection.

HDV infection is worldwide, but is particularly found in southern Europe, the Balkans, the Middle East, South India, Taiwan and parts of Africa. An endemic area has been identified in Okinawa, Japan [22].

Epidemics of HDV infection have been reported from the Amazon Basin, Brazil (Labrea fever) [2], Colombia

Table 17.11. The diagnosis of delta virus infection

| | Acute co-infection | | |
	Early	Convalescence	Chronic
Serum			
IgG anti-delta	+	+ (low titre)	+ (high titre)
IgM anti-delta	+ (late)	–	+
HDAg	+	–	+
HDV RNA	+	–	+
Liver			
HDAg	+	–	–
HDV RNA	+	–	+

(Santa Marta hepatitis) [4], Venezuela [11] and Equatorial Africa. In these areas children of the indigent population are affected and mortality is high.

Along with HBV, HDV infection is declining rapidly. This is particularly true in Italy [20, 25]. Universal HBV vaccination is particularly important in reducing the prevalence.

Diagnosis (table 17.11)

Acute delta hepatitis is diagnosed by rising titres of serum IgG anti-HDV (anti-delta).

Co-infection is diagnosed by finding serum IgM anti-HDV in the presence of high-titre IgM anti-HBc. These markers appear at 1 week, and IgM anti-HDV is gone by 5–6 weeks but may last for up to 12 weeks [1]. When serum IgM anti-HDV disappears, serum IgG anti-HDV is found. There may be a window period between the disappearance of one and the detection of the other. Loss of IgM anti-HDV confirms the resolution of HDV infection, whereas persistence predicts chronicity [9].

HBsAg is positive, but often in low titre and may be undetectable. Serum IgM anti-HBc is also suppressed. Unless delta markers are sought, the patient may be misdiagnosed as having acute hepatitis C.

Superinfection with HDV is marked by the early presence of serum IgM anti-HDV, usually at the same time as early IgG anti-HDV and both antibodies persist [5]. These patients are usually IgM anti-HBc negative, but may have low titres of this antibody. Sufferers of chronic delta infection with chronic hepatitis and active cirrhosis usually have a positive serum IgM anti-HDV.

Serum and liver HDV RNA, by staining or PCR, are found in delta antibody-positive patients with acute and chronic HDV infection [16, 27].

Clinical features (figs 17.17, 17.18)

With *co-infection*, the acute delta hepatitis is usually self-limited as HDV cannot outlive the transient HBs antigenaemia. The long-term outlook is therefore good. The

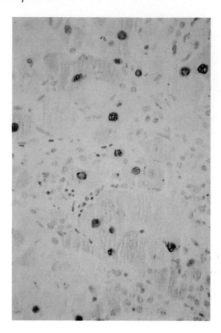

Fig. 17.19. Fulminant acute delta virus hepatitis (Labrea hepatitis) in a 3-year-old girl from northern Brazil who died with fulminant hepatitis after 3 days' symptoms. An autopsy liver sample shows microvesicular fatty change in large hepatocytes with central nucleus (Morular, vegetable-type cells). (Immunoperoxidase, × 500.)

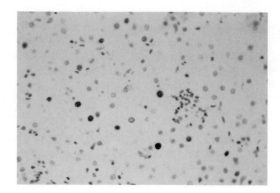

Fig. 17.20. Delta virus hepatitis: immunoperoxidase staining showing delta in the hepatocyte nuclei (× 100).

clinical picture is usually indistinguishable from hepatitis B alone. However, a biphasic rise in aspartate transaminase may be noted, the second rise being due to the acute effects of delta [8].

With *superinfection*, the acute attack may be severe and even fulminant, or may be marked only by a rise in serum transaminase levels. HDV infection should always be considered in any HBV carrier, usually clinically stable, who has a relapse.

HDV infection reduces active hepatitis B viral synthesis and patients are usually HBeAg and HBV DNA negative. Between 2 and 10% lose HBsAg. However, chronic delta hepatitis is usual and this results in acceleration towards cirrhosis.

Episodes of reactivation with delta viraemia can develop [10]. If hepatitis B viraemia persists, the outcome is worse [24]. Hepato-cellular cancer seems less common in HBsAg carriers with HDV. This may be due to inhibition of hepatitis B or rapid progression so that the patient dies before the cancer develops. However, when delta is found with late-stage chronic liver disease it does not seem to influence survival and hepato-cellular cancer may be a complication in these patients.

Hepatic histology

Inflammation and focal confluent and bridging necrosis are marked. Acidophil bodies are seen.

The South American and Equatorial African epidemics are marked by microvesicular fat in hepatocytes, intense eosinophilic necrosis and large amounts of delta antigen within the liver (fig. 17.19) [4]. These changes have also been noted in a New York drug abuser with HDV infection [14]. Morular (plant-like) cells may be seen.

Using immunoperoxidase, delta antigen is shown in hepatocyte nuclei, more in chronic than in acute infection (fig. 17.20). It falls with cirrhosis. It correlates with viraemia [27].

Prevention

Vaccination against hepatitis B makes the recipient immune to HBV infection and protects against HDV infection. Patients likely to contract HDV infection should be encouraged to have a hepatitis B vaccine.

HBV carriers must be educated concerning the risks of acquiring HDV by continued drug abuse.

Treatment

Treatment is unsatisfactory. High doses of interferon given for long periods result in reductions of AST but recurrence is usual [18, 21].

Lamivudine does not improve disease activity or lower HDV RNA levels in patients with chronic delta hepatitis [13].

Patients receiving a liver transplant for HDV and HBV end-stage liver disease show reduced HBV recurrence [17]. The hepatocytes contain large amounts of HDV but hepatitis develops only if there is persistent infection with HBV (Chapter 38). The HDV virion in the post-transplantation setting is typical HDV and requires the helper function of HBV infection [23].

References

1 Aragona M, Macagno S, Caredda F *et al.* Serological

response to the hepatitis delta virus in hepatitis D. *Lancet* 1987; **i**: 478.

2 Bensabath G, Hadler SC, Soares MCP *et al.* Hepatitis delta virus infection and Labrea hepatitis. Prevalence and role in fulminant hepatitis in the Amazon Basin. *JAMA* 1987; **258**: 479.

3 Bonino F, Caporaso N, Dentico P *et al.* Familiar clustering and spreading of hepatitis delta virus infection. *J. Hepatol.* 1985; **1**: 221.

4 Buitrago B, Popper H, Hadler SC *et al.* Specific histological features of Santa Marta hepatitis: a severe form of hepatitis delta-virus infection in northern South America. *Hepatology* 1986; **6**: 1285.

5 Buti M, Amengual J, Esteban R *et al.* Serological profile of tissue autoantibodies during acute and chronic delta hepatitis. *J. Hepatol.* 1989; **9**: 345.

6 Cortrina M, Buti M, Jardi R *et al.* Hepatitis delta genotypes in chronic delta infection in the north-east of Spain (Catalonia). *J. Hepatol.* 1998; **28**: 971.

7 De Cock KM, Govindarajan S, Chin KP *et al.* Delta hepatitis in the Los Angeles area: a report of 126 cases. *Am. Intern. Med.* 1986; **105**: 108.

8 Govindarajan S, De Cock KM, Redeker AG. Natural course of delta superinfection in chronic hepatitis B virus-infected patients: histopathologic study with multiple liver biopsies. *Hepatology* 1986; **6**: 640.

9 Govindarajan S, Gupta S, Valinluck B *et al.* Correlation of IgM antihepatitis D virus (HDV) to HDV RNA in sera of chronic HDV. *Hepatology* 1989; **10**: 34.

10 Govindarajan S, Smedile, A, De Cock KM *et al.* Study of reactivation of chronic hepatitis delta infection. *J. Hepatol.* 1989; **9**: 204.

11 Hadler SC, De Monzon M, Ponzetto A *et al.* Delta virus infection and severe hepatitis: an epidemic in the Yupca Indians of Venezuela. *Ann. Intern. Med.* 1984; **100**: 339.

12 Hershow RC, Chomel BB, Graham DR *et al.* Hepatitis D virus infection in Illinois state facilities for the developmentally disabled. *Ann. Intern. Med.* 1989; **110**: 779.

13 Lau DT-Y, Doo E, Park Y *et al.* Lamivudine for chronic delta hepatitis. *Hepatology* 1999; **30**: 546.

14 Lefkowitch JH, Goldstein H, Yatto R *et al.* Cytopathic liver injury in acute delta virus hepatitis. *Gastroenterology* 1987; **92**: 1262.

15 Lettau LA, McCarthy JG, Smith MH *et al.* Outbreak of severe hepatitis due to delta and hepatitis B viruses in parenteral drug abusers and their contacts. *N. Engl. J. Med.* 1987; **317**: 1256.

16 Madejón A, Castillo I, Bartolomé J *et al.* Detection of HDV-RNA by PCR in serum of patients with chronic HDV infection. *J. Hepatol.* 1990; **11**: 381.

17 Ottobrelli A, Marzano A, Smedile A *et al.* Patterns of hepatitis delta virus reinfection and disease in liver transplantation. *Gastroenterology* 1991; **101**: 1649.

18 Porres JC, Carreño V, Bartolomé J *et al.* Treatment of chronic delta infection with recombinant human interferon alpha 2c at high doses. *J. Hepatol.* 1989; **9**: 338.

19 Rizzetto M. The delta agent. *Hepatology* 1983; **3**: 729.

20 Rosina F, Conoscitore P, Cuppone R *et al.* Changing pattern of chronic hepatitis D in Southern Europe. *Gastroenterology* 1999; **117**: 163.

21 Rosina F, Pintus C, Meschievitz C *et al.* A randomized controlled trial of a 12-month course of recombinant human interferon-alpha in chronic delta (type D) hepatitis: a multicentre Italian study. *Hepatology* 1991; **13**: 1052.

22 Sakugawa H, Nakasone H, Shokita H *et al.* Seroepidemiological study of hepatitis delta virus infection in Okinawa, Japan. *J. Med. Virol.* 1995; **45**: 312.

23 Smedile A, Casey JL, Cote PJ *et al.* Heptatitis D viremia following orthotopic liver transplantation involves a typical HDV virion with a hepatitis B surface antigen envelope. *Hepatology* 1998; **27**: 1723.

24 Smedile A, Rosina F, Saracco G *et al.* Hepatitis B virus replication modulates pathogenesis of hepatitis D virus in chronic hepatitis D. *Hepatology* 1991; **13**: 413.

25 Stroffolini T, Ferrigno L, Cialdea L *et al.* Incidence and risk factors of acute delta hepatitis in Italy: results from a national surveillance system. *J. Hepatol.* 1994; **21**: 1123.

26 Weisfuse IB, Hadler SC, Fields HA *et al.* Delta hepatitis in homosexual men in the United States. *Hepatology* 1989; **9**: 872.

27 Wu J-C, Chen T-A, Huang Y-S *et al.* Natural history of hepatitis D viral superinfection: significance of viremia detected by polymerase chain reaction. *Gastroenterology* 1995; **108**: 796.

28 Wu J-C, Choo K-B, Chen C-M *et al.* Genotyping of hepatitis D virus by restriction-fragment length polymerase and relation to outcome of hepatitis D. *Lancet* 1995; **346**: 939.

Chapter 18
Hepatitis C Virus

The ability to diagnose hepatitis virus A and B infection did not resolve the problem of acute and chronic hepatitis. A third major category had always been suspected but, in the absence of a diagnostic test, had been designated non-A, non-B virus hepatitis. A third type has now been identified and called hepatitis C virus (HCV) [119]. This followed identification of a viral clone of the HCV virus from chimpanzee liver which had been infected with non-A, non-B virus [119]. An antibody test followed. Hepatitis C is a major health problem [20]. Global prevalence of chronic hepatitis C is estimated to average 3% (ranging from 0.1 to 5% in different countries). There are some 175 million chronic HCV carriers throughout the world, of which an estimated 2 million are in the USA and 5 million in Western Europe. HCV accounts for 20% of cases of acute hepatitis, 70% of cases of chronic hepatitis, 40% of cases of end-stage cirrhosis, 60% of cases of hepato-cellular carcinoma and 30% of liver transplants. It is the most frequent indication for hepatic transplantation. The incidence of new symptomatic infections has been estimated to be 1–3 per 100 000 persons annually. The actual incidence is obviously much higher as the majority of cases are asymptomatic. The incidence is declining as transmission by blood products has now been reduced to near zero.

Universal precautions have markedly reduced transmission in medical settings. Intravenous drug use remains the main mode of transmission; but this route of transmission is diminishing due to a heightened awareness of the risk of needle sharing and, in some countries, the availability of needle-exchange programmes. However, a huge backlog of infected patients continue to progress towards cirrhosis and hepato-cellular carcinoma. The cost of investigating and treating these patients remains and continues to be enormous.

Molecular virology

The structure and replicating cycle are still incompletely understood due to the lack of an efficient cell culture system.

HCV has been classified as a member of the *flaviviridae* family. The other members include classical flaviviruses such as yellow fever, dengue and bovine diarrhoea virus. All members of this family are small-sized enveloped viruses containing antisense single-stranded RNA encoding viral polyprotein (fig. 18.1) [26]. The viral genome is composed of a 5′ non-coding region, a long open reading frame encoding a polyprotein precursor of about 3000 amino acids, and a 3′ non-coding region. The 5′ non-coding region is highly conserved. Because of this and the crucial role played in the translation of the viral polyprotein, the 5′ non-coding region has become a target for the development of nucleic acid-based antiviral agents such as antisense oligonucleotides and ribosomes. The structural proteins include the core protein and two envelope glycoproteins, E1 and E2.

HCV quasi-species

HCV exists within an individual as a mixture of closely related, yet heterogeneous viral sequences known as *quasi-species*. Although mutations occur throughout the entire genome, studies have focused on the hypervariable region, HV01, located at the end terminus of the E2NS1 region. The degree of diversity is related to the progression of liver disease [50]. Mutations follow therapy allowing HCV to escape antiviral effects [45]. Lower heterogeneity increases the response to antiviral therapy for there are fewer variants to evade immune surveillance and so resist treatment [60].

Genotypes

HCV shows considerable heterogeneity, particularly in the viral envelope. Using sequence comparisons, known variants of HCV collected from different parts of the world can be divided into six main genotypes. There are at least 50 more closely related variants [106]. There is considerable geographical variation in the prevalence of the various genotypes (table 18.1).

The major clinical difference between genotypes is the response to antiviral therapy. Sustained response to interferon-α alone or in combination with ribavirin is markedly less for genotype 1 than for genotypes 2 and 3 [15]. Suggestions that genotype 1b results in more serious hepatic disease have not been confirmed [93].

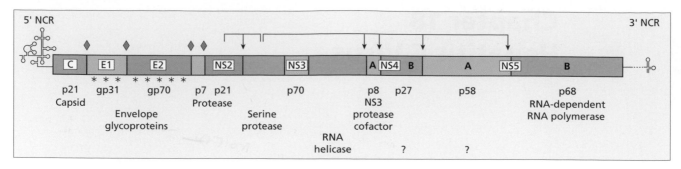

Fig. 18.1. The hepatitis C viral genome. Asterisks in the E1 and E2 region indicate glycosylation of the envelope proteins. Diamonds denote cleavages of the HCV polyprotein precursor by the endoplasmic reticulum signal peptidase. Arrows indicate cleavages by HCV NS2–3 and NS3 proteases. NCR, non-coding region. (From [83].)

Table 18.1. Geographical distribution of HCV genotypes

Area	Type
Europe	1, 2, 3
Australia	1, 2, 3
USA	1, 2, 3
Far East	1, 2
Middle East	4
North Africa	4
South Africa	5
Southeast Asia	6

Type 4, largely found in the Middle East, is also associated with a poor response to interferon.

Other types are not routinely investigated. The method depends on sequence analysis of different regions of the genome [106]. It identifies infection with the genotypes likely to be encountered in Europe, other Western countries and Japan. The investigation is costly. It is used as a preliminary to starting antiviral therapy. Genotype 1 implies worse results and indicates therapy for 1 year, rather than 6 months (see tables 18.5 and 6) [20].

Serological tests

Serological tests for HCV detect antibodies to viral antigens. ELISA is satisfactory for routine screening, particularly of blood donors; it is less sensitive in haemodialysis and immunocompromised patients.

cDNA PCR has been used to detect hepatitis C viral sequences (HCV RNA) in liver and serum [34]. PCR is a supersensitive technique which is complicated, time-consuming and costly. It is also subject to interlaboratory error [125]. It will not achieve routine general use.

The quantitative method is branched DNA (bDNA) signal amplification [63]. It is costly, generally available and easy to perform although less sensitive than PCR. The bDNA signal amplification method is based on hybridization with specific probes in the 5′ non-coding region which are used to capture the HCV bDNA on the

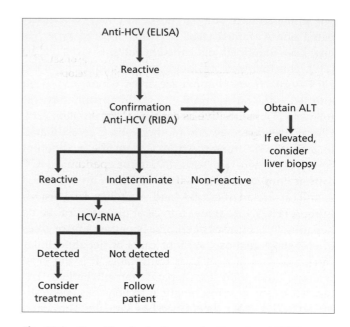

Fig. 18.2. Algorithm for further evaluation of anti-HCV ELISA-positive specimens [27].

surface of the tube. The lower limit of detection is 2×10^5 HCV genome equivalents/ml. The bDNA method is less sensitive than the Amplicor method and may not be sensitive enough to detect virus in all pre-treatment samples.

The Amplicor HCV kit amplifies HCV RNA in a single reaction using the fairly stable enzyme rTth DNA polymerase [67]. The detection limit is 1000 genome equivalents/ml. Either this or the bDNA technique can be used to follow therapy [77, 78].

In low-risk settings such as blood banks and other general screening situations, approximately 25% of ELISA-positive tests may be false. A supplemental specificity test such as a strip immunoblot assay (RIBA) is recommended (fig. 18.2). Then, quantitative HCV RNA should be performed if anti-HCV positivity is confirmed.

In high-risk populations, and in clinical settings where HCV is suspected, a positive ELISA should be confirmed by a quantitative HCV RNA.

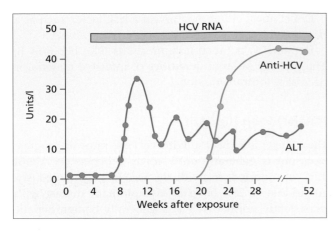

Fig. 18.3. The serology of hepatitis C infection with a chronic course. Note that HCV RNA appears early, before the rise in alanine transferase (ALT) and persists. Anti-HCV positivity is delayed, appearing between 11 and 20 weeks of the onset. ALT shows characteristic fluctuations as chronicity develops.

The ELISA is positive as early as 11 weeks after infection and always within 20 weeks of the onset (fig. 18.3). In patients with acute hepatitis of unknown cause, an ELISA should be performed first. If hepatitis A and B tests are negative, quantitative HCV RNA must be performed. In ELISA-negative patients with chronic hepatitis of unknown cause, particularly in haemodialysis and immunocompromised patients, a quantitative HCV RNA test is essential.

Immune response

The virus-specific CD4+ and Th1+ T-cell response, that eliminates the virus during the acute stage, has to be maintained permanently to achieve long-term control of the virus [39, 86].

There is no association between the course of the disease and the HLA class I alleles (HLA A, B, C) which present viral antigens to CD8+ cytotoxic T-cells. However, there is a significant association between HLA class II alleles (DR, DQ and DP) and protection from HCV chronicity. HLA class II alleles DRB1*1101 and DQB1*0301 are associated with viral clearance [110].

Serological tests for autoantibodies (antinuclear, smooth muscle and rheumatoid factor) may be weakly positive, but have not been shown to have a causative role [66].

Epidemiology

Blood transfusion

Hepatitis C is carried by about 0.01–2% of blood donors worldwide [4, 103, 105]. The risk factors associated with acute hepatitis C in the USA are present or past injecting

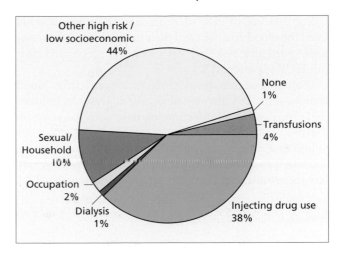

Fig. 18.4. Risk factors associated with acute hepatitis C in the USA (1990–1993). These include sexual or household contacts, health-care employment, multiple exposures to blood and injecting drug abuse. Other high-risk patients include low socioeconomic status and multiple sexual partners. (From the Sentinel Counties, Centers for Disease Control and Prevention [4].)

of drugs, previous transfusions, health-care employment, sexual/household contact and a low socioeconomic status (fig. 18.4) [4]. Egypt seems to have the highest prevalence in blood donors [1]. Anti-HCV was found in 12% of rural primary children, 22.1% of army recruits and 16.4% in children with hepato-splenomegaly [1].

The introduction of second-generation screening for anti-HCV has greatly reduced the incidence of post-transfusion hepatitis [31, 41, 54].

Other blood products

Thalassaemics, because of repeated blood transfusions, have an anti-HCV prevalence of between 10 and 50%.

Until about 1964, therapeutic coagulation factors contained HCV. This has resulted in a prevalence of nearly 100% HCV in haemophiliac patients receiving unsterilized large-pool coagulation factors [70, 117]. Introduction of vapour-heated and recombinant clotting factors has controlled this method of spread.

Patients with primary hypogammaglobulinaemia have developed hepatitis C after treatment with contaminated immunoglobulin [13, 122].

Contaminated anti-rhesus D immunoglobulin has caused large outbreaks of HCV in Ireland [92] and Germany [30].

Parenteral exposure

The chances of HCV after a needle-stick exposure to a patient with a positive HCV, RNA is 3–10% [82, 107].

Dentists are at risk of acquiring HCV, presumably from the blood and saliva of their patients. Oral surgeons are at particular risk [59]. An infected surgeon can transmit HCV to patients [32].

Dialysis patients develop HCV, not only from blood transfusions, but also by negligent dialysis techniques [89]. The chances of infection increase with the years on dialysis.

Injecting drug users using shared needles and syringes account for most HCV in the USA [85]. The injection may have occurred many years ago, forgotten by the patient [21].

Sexual and intra-familial spread

This is believed to be very low. In most population studies, anti-HCV does not appear until the age of 16 years. This would suggest that sexual transmission is important [108]. There are geographical differences in reported prevalence of sexual transmission. However, consorts of anti-HCV positive haemophiliac patients have tested positive and HCV has been linked with multiple sexual partners [5]. But in a Spanish study, only 6% of heterosexual contacts of injecting drug users were positive [31].

Serum samples of 94 husbands of women with HCV following infection with contaminated immunoglobulin showed no HCV RNA [79]. Only three of their 231 children showed serological evidence of HCV.

Where one member is HCV positive, those with a steady partner should not change their sexual practices. Those with multiple partners should use safe sex methods. Prevalence in homosexuals is 3%, in prostitutes 6% and in heterosexuals attending a sexually transmitted disease clinic 4%.

Intra-familial spread is rare but has been reported with the same strain of HCV [50, 58].

Vertical transmission is infrequent. It is greater if the mother is serum HCV RNA positive [88]. Transmission may be increased by concomitant maternal HIV infection [126]. Infection is more likely if the mother suffers an acute attack in the last trimester. Breast milk does not transmit HCV [72]. Babies born to anti-HCV positive mothers usually have circulating antibody for 6 months, presumably due to passive transfer, but HCV RNA is absent.

In those with no obvious risk factors

Where did the disease come from in the millions of carriers without risk factors? Family spread is possible but rare. Infection may be through sharing razors, toothbrushes or unsterile syringes and needles with infected people. Other possibilities include past abuse of intravenous drugs and folk remedies such as acupuncture and cutting skin using non-sterilized knives [58].

Direct questioning may reveal a risk factor such as a past blood transfusion or intravenous drug abuse.

Hepatitis C is much less infectious than hepatitis B. The passage of large quantities of infective material is necessary for transmission.

Natural history (fig. 18.5)

Hepatitis C is a disease with varying rates of progression, but is generally only slowly progressive. About 15% of infected individuals recover spontaneously. An additional 25% have an asymptomatic disease with persistently normal ALT and generally benign hepatic histology [20]. Hence, 40% of patients recover or have a benign outcome. The majority of those with raised ALT and evidence of chronic hepatitis, have only mild histological changes and the long-term outcome is unknown, but probably most of them will not succumb to the liver disease [3]. About 20% of patients develop cirrhosis in 10–20 years. The incidence of hepato-cellular carcinoma is 1–4% per year in patients with cirrhosis.

Other co-factors such as hepatitis B and D are associated with more serious disease [64]. Alcohol is also an important risk factor and intake should be recorded [91].

Clinical course [73]

Acute hepatitis C

Descriptions are largely based on findings in transfused patients where the time of infection is certain. Clinical presentation of disease after other modes of transmission, such as intravenous drug addiction, is not well documented.

The incubation period is about 7–8 weeks (range 2–26 weeks). Prodromal symptoms are rare. Only 20% of patients become icteric. The symptoms resemble those of

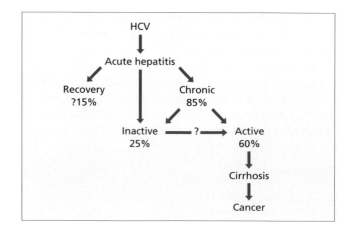

Fig. 18.5. The natural history of HCV infection.

other forms of viral hepatitis. Serum HCV RNA becomes positive 1–2 weeks after infection. At 7–8 weeks, serum ALT is moderately increased to about 15 times the upper limit of normal. Clinical diagnosis is rarely made and this depends on viral markers. Icteric hepatitis is rare and fulminant hepatic failure is controversial [51]. The anti-HIV positive patient may have a rapidly progressive course [76].

Those with self-limited disease develop a normal serum ALT and HCV RNA becomes negative. Anti-HCV persists for many years. Aplastic anaemic [9], agranulocytosis and peripheral neuropathy may be complications.

Chronic hepatitis C

About 85% of those infected with HCV will not clear the virus and will develop chronic hepatitis of varying severity (fig. 18.5) [73]. Viral load fluctuates and in many patients declines with time [33]. The disease is an indolent one extending over many years.

Chronic hepatitis with normal ALT

This is seen in approximately one-third of patients despite detectable HCV RNA in serum. The patients are often diagnosed by chance at the time of blood donation, routine medical check or during investigation for another condition. In most instances, hepatic histology shows only mild disease. HCV RNA is lower than in those with a raised ALT; hepatic fibrosis progression and activity are also lower [53].

Chronic hepatitis with elevated ALT

The severity of the liver disease varies considerably.

Mild chronic hepatitis affects 50% [73]. The main symptom is fatigue associated with musculo-skeletal pain [10]. When HCV is diagnosed the quality of life falls [96]. Part of this may be the result of labelling. There is no correlation between symptoms, ALT levels and the hepatic histological score.

The course is a slow one, marked by fluctuating transaminases over many years. Each elevation probably represents an episode of HCV viraemia, perhaps due to quasi-species.

Moderate or severe chronic hepatitis is seen in about 50% of newly diagnosed patients with a raised ALT. There are no abnormal physical signs and the ALT is usually 2–10 times the upper limit of normal, but this is a poor marker of disease activity [46]. Serum bilirubin, albumin and prothrombin time are usually normal. Serum HCV RNA values exceeding 10^5 genome equivalents per ml correlate with active disease.

If possible, viral genotype should be checked. Type 1b may be related to increased severity, worse response to antivirals, recurrence after liver transplantation and the possible development of cancer. Type 4 is related to antiviral failure.

Serum autoantibodies should be sought for diagnosis from autoimmune chronic hepatitis and especially if interferon therapy is being considered.

Liver biopsy remains the most accurate way of distinguishing mild from moderate or severe chronic hepatitis.

Cirrhosis

Within two or three decades, cirrhosis develops in 20–30% of HCV-infected patients. It is usually clinically silent and features of end-stage liver disease are late. It may be discovered by liver biopsy in the asymptomatic patient or present as variceal haemorrhage or jaundice. Evidence of portal hypertension is rare; splenomegaly is present in only one-half the patients at presentation. Bleeding from oesophageal varices is unusual until late on. Thrombocytopenia develops as the spleen size increases and this is a good indication that cirrhosis has developed.

Hepato-cellular carcinoma (Chapter 31)

This is generally associated with cirrhosis. It can be found in the compensated case and can be clinically silent for long periods. Screening for hepato-cellular carcinoma is done by 6-monthly serum α-fetoprotein levels and ultrasound of the liver. These should be performed in all cirrhotic patients, particularly if male and more than 40 years old.

Hepatic histology

This is not diagnostic but often makes a characteristic pattern [99]. The most striking feature is the presence of lymphoid aggregates or follicles in the portal tracts, either alone or as part of a general inflammatory infiltration of the tracts (figs 18.6, 18.7) [99]. The aggregates comprise a core of B-cells mixed with many T-helper/inducer lymphocytes. The outer ring is predominantly T-suppressor/cytotoxic lymphocytes [37]. Their presence does not correlate with features of autoimmunity. The prevalence of bile duct damage varies amongst different series [8]. Interface hepatitis is mild but lobular cellular activity is usual. Fatty change is found in 75% of cases, though the mechanism is unclear. The characteristic picture is of mild chronic hepatitis. Chronic hepatitis can exist with cirrhosis or the picture may simply be that of inactive cirrhosis. Appearances bear no relationship to duration or to the transaminase levels at presentation.

Genotypes 1b and 4 have been associated with more liver complications [81]. However, this might not be an independent factor, but rather an indicator of longer duration and hence worse hepatic function and more fibrosis.

Viral load does not seem to influence the prognosis. Markers of hepatitis B infection and of HIV worsen the prognosis [12].

Increased alcohol intake is associated with decreased survival. However, this is difficult to assess as patients may reduce their consumption when told of the diagnosis of HCV infection.

Serum albumin is an important indicator of complications such as liver failure and hepato-cellular cancer, and the need for liver transplantation. Patients with a serum albumin level of less than 3 g/dl have a 75% chance of liver transplant or liver-related death after 5 years [56]. Serum bilirubin is also associated with liver-related death and transplant, but to a lesser extent than albumin. Correlation with ALT is poor, but very high values are serious. Liver failure and hepato-cellular cancer are rarely seen less than 20 years after infection. Many patients avoid these complications. Identification of those with severe progressive disease is essential so that cirrhosis and hepato-cellular cancer can be prevented.

Prevention: vaccines

The problem is the lack of an animal model for testing, other than the chimpanzee. A reproducible culture system to propagate the virus is lacking.

Efforts have been made to generate recombinant vaccines by expressing part of the individual structural proteins in soluble form. Unfortunately, the antibody response to these recombinant envelope proteins is late and weak and they do not confer immunity to heterologous or homologous HCV infection [17].

DNA-based immunization is promising in the animal model, but further work is needed against HCV structural proteins in man [61].

HCV-like particles have been synthesized in insects and are capable of inducing a humoral response targeted against various regions of HCV structural proteins [11]. They may be vaccine candidates. Exogenous stimulation of T-cell responses may be a strategy. T-cell epitopes within the core and NS3 and NS4 domains are immunodominant and conserved. They may be ideal components of preventative or therapeutic T-cell vaccines [62].

Treatment (fig. 18.9)

Selection of patients [20] (table 18.4)

Liver biopsy should be performed. Patients with moderate or severe necro-inflammation and/or fibrosis should

Table 18.4. Possible factors predicting a favourable response to antiviral therapy in chronic HCV infection

Host
Age less than 45 years
Female
Non-obese
Duration of infection less than 5 years
No co-infection with HBV
Not immunosuppressed
No alcoholism
ALT modestly increased
Normal γ-glutamyl transpeptidase
Liver biopsy: low activity score
No cirrhosis
Liver iron low

Virus
Low serum HCV RNA
Genotype 2 or 3

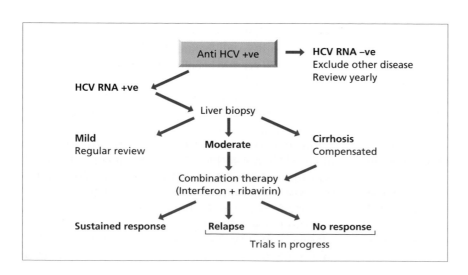

Fig. 18.9. Algorithm for management of the HCV-positive patient.

be considered [87]. It is difficult to decide on treatment in patients with mild hepatic histological changes. These patients should be monitored regularly and, if possible, regression assessed by a further liver biopsy performed about 3 years later [73].

Age. The physiological age is more important than the chronological. General health and cardiovascular status must be considered.

Clinical status. There is a poor correlation between liver histology and clinical status. Symptoms do lessen in patients who achieve a sustained loss of HCV RNA after treatment.

Viraemia. Those with levels exceeding 2 million genome equivalents/ml are less likely to respond, but should not be denied treatment.

Genotype. If possible, this should be recorded. Those with genotype 1 respond less well than genotype 2 or 3 but should not be denied therapy. The lower response in genotype 1 has been attributed to amino acid variations in the NS5A protein of the HCV [84].

HIV co-infection. Therapy can be given in stabilized patients (CD4+ count exceeding 200). Drug interactions should be considered.

Cirrhosis. Compensated patients can be treated. In general, those who are decompensated are excluded.

Persistently normal ALT. Underlying liver disease is usually mild and treatment is withheld. Follow-up of ALT is necessary every 4–6 months.

Acute HCV infection. The decision to treat is not yet certain, but with only a small chance of spontaneous recovery (about 15%), the patient and physician may decide on therapy.

Children [97]. They respond to interferon in a similar fashion to adults and should be accepted using the same guidelines. The effects on growth are not clear. Data for combination are awaited.

Contraindications. These include active, heavy alcohol intake. Active intravenous drug abusers are excluded because of re-infection risk and poor compliance. Those with histologically mild disease may be excluded, particularly if older and with co-morbid conditions.

Monitoring therapy

If possible, liver biopsy is performed. Genotype is recorded. Quantitative tests for HCV RNA are done before treatment and, if possible, after 3 months treatment, at the end of treatment and 6 months later [20].

All patients should be tested for thyroid function before treatment and at regular intervals.

Because of the risk of teratogenicity with ribavirin, women of reproductive potential should have a negative pregnancy test. Men and women should practice safe sex during therapy and for 6 months afterwards.

A full blood count is performed before treatment and at weekly intervals for 4 weeks, then every 3 months during therapy and 6 months later. Baseline ultrasound of the liver should be performed to assess liver size and shape, splenomegaly, portal vein diameter and any space-occupying lesions.

Evaluation of response

In the assessment of efficacy an end of treatment response (ETR) must be distinguished from a sustained response (SR) when HCV-RNA is negative and ALT normal 6 months after stopping treatment. Thus after an ETR, a proportion of patients relapse. Once SR is achieved, relapse is unusual and the long-term outcome is good [74].

Selection of therapy

Previously untreated patients

The combination of interferon-α with ribavirin is the current standard of care for chronic hepatitis C where there is no contraindication [20, 23]. A higher SR using pegylated interferon-α with ribavirin has recently been reported for genotype 1 [71]. Pegylated interferon is more convenient for patients. This combination is becoming accepted as the current choice for untreated patients.

Interferon-ribavirin combination. Ribavirin is an oral guanosine analogue with a broad spectrum of activity against RNA and DNA viruses, including the flavivirus family. It also has immunomodulatory effects. Used alone in patients with chronic HCV, it decreases transaminase levels and hepatic histology may improve, but HCV RNA levels do not fall. Relapse occurrs after withdrawal of therapy. When combined with interferon-α, the antiviral effect is enhanced.

Two large randomized trials in previously untreated (naïve) patients compared combination therapy (interferon-α_{2b} and ribavirin) against monotherapy with interferon-α_{2b} for 48 weeks [69, 94]. Both studies showed more than a two-fold greater SR with combination therapy than with monotherapy (38 v 13%, and 43 v 19%). One of the trials compared 24 weeks of treatment [69]. The SR with combined therapy was 31%, and with interferon monotherapy, 6%. Histological improvement was greater in those receiving combination therapy.

An analysis of six other randomized controlled trials in previously untreated patients showed that combined interferon-ribavirin resulted in an approximately three-fold increase in SR over interferon alone (table 18.5) [98]. Although patients with genotype 1 still had a lower SR than genotype 2 and 3, results were a considerable improvement compared with interferon therapy alone.

The recommended dose of ribavirin is 1000–1200 mg (depending on body weight <75 kg or >75 kg) daily by mouth in two doses. Interferon-α is given in a dose of 3 million units three times a week by injection (table 18.6). After 24 weeks of treatment, if HCV RNA by PCR is still positive, treatment is stopped since there is little likelihood of response after this time. If HCV RNA is negative, patients with genotype 1 receive a further 24 weeks of treatment, since SR is higher after 48 than 24 weeks (e.g. 28% versus 16%) [69]. In HCV-RNA negative patients with genotype 2 or 3, treatment is stopped since for these genotypes SR after 24 weeks is similar to that after 48 weeks of therapy (64 v 66%) [69].

Data have shown that SR differs according to the viral load, defined in studies as less than or greater than 2×10^6 genome equivalents/ml. This measure is not, however, currently used to direct the duration of therapy, because of naturally occurring fluctuations in viral load over time, and the variability of quantitative HCV RNA assays.

Combination therapy adds considerably to the cost. It is cost effective, however, if genotype is assessed and therapy continued to 1 year only in those who are genotype 1 and have achieved negative HCV RNA at 24 weeks [124].

Absolute contraindications to combination therapy. Interferon-α should not be used if there is psychiatric disease (psychosis, severe depression, risk of suicide), neutropenia or thrombocytopenia, coronary artery disease or cardiac arrhythmias, decompensated cirrhosis, or renal transplantation. These also rule out interferon monotherapy. Ribavirin should not be used in the absence of a reliable form of contraception or during pregnancy, if there is anaemia or renal insufficiency, or if there is severe heart disease. A minimum baseline of haemoglobin >12 g/dl, neutrophils $>1.5 \times 10^9$/l and platelets $>75 \times 10^9$/l is required.

Adverse effects to combination therapy. These are frequent and often lead to dose reduction. In one study, of those randomized to combination therapy for 48 weeks, 21% discontinued treatment because of side effects [69]. Ribavirin causes dose-dependent haemolysis due to membrane oxidative damage [25], and haemoglobin and serum bilirubin must be monitored during therapy. Haemoglobin can drop by 3–4 g/dl and precipitate symptoms of ischaemic heart disease in those susceptible. Ribavirin is also hyperuricaemic.

The side effects of interferon are described in Chapter 17 (see table 17.8). HCV patients with anti-LKM antibodies may have an increased risk of an adverse hepatic reaction with interferon. Patients must be monitored closely for possible liver dysfunction [111]. Positive pretherapy serum thyroid autoantibodies are a risk factor for subsequent thyroid dysfunction [75, 116].

Pegylated interferon-ribavirin combination. Pegylated interferon is interferon-α covalently bound to a large 40-kDa or 12-kDa branched polyethylene glycol moiety. After one dose, interferon is still present in serum 1 week later [40]. This eliminates the large fluctuations in serum concentration seen with non-pegylated interferons, which have a short half-life, disappearing from blood between daily administration. Treatment based on low doses of standard interferon-α, administered three times a week, is associated with troughs between the doses allowing viral replication to rebound post-injection (day 2) [109]. Thus the estimated half-life of free HCV virions is 2.7 hours. 12×10^6 virions are produced each day. Troughs of interferon concentration facilitate the emergence of resistant forms. Various strategies have been

Table 18.5. Percentage sustained response in six trials of interferon (IFN)–ribavirin (RV) therapy in cirrhotic and non-cirrhotic patients with chronic HCV infection [98]

Patients	Treatment	Genotype 1	Genotype 2 and 3
No cirrhosis	IFN	8	24
	IFN + RV	23	65
Cirrhosis	IFN	1	5
	IFN + RV	7	24

Table 18.6. Chronic hepatitis C: interferon and ribavirin therapy

Pre-treatment
Serum HCV RNA by PCR
Liver biopsy
Genotype
Routine biochemistry
Routine haematology
Prothrombin time
Abdominal ultrasound
Thyroid antibodies/function

Regimen for 6 months
Interferon-α 3 million units, three times a week*
Ribavirin 1000–1200 mg daily

End of 6 months' treatment

HCV RNA positive	Stop therapy	
HCV RNA negative	Genotype 1	Genotype 2, 3
	Continue 6 more months	Stop therapy

6 months' post-treatment
Serum HCV RNA
Serum ALT

*Pegylated interferon-α if available (see text)

tried to avoid these troughs, including daily large doses [118]. However, compliance and cost were disadvantages.

Pegylated interferon-α has a more sustained antiviral effect. Weekly dosage has the advantage of improved patient convenience and compliance.

The combination of pegylated interferon-α_{2b} (1.5 μg/kg/week) with ribavirin (800 mg/day) for 48 weeks had a significantly higher SR compared with standard interferon-α_{2b} and ribavirin (54% versus 47%) [71]. This benefit was seen particularly in patients with genotype 1 (42% versus 33%), and those without bridging fibrosis/cirrhosis (57% versus 49%). Dose reduction because of adverse effects was necessary in 42% and 34% of patients respectively. Optimization of the dose of the two drugs will require further study [65, 71]. The recommendations for duration of treatment are being assessed in current series.

Patients with contraindications to or side effects from ribavirin

Interferon-α monotherapy is appropriate for these patients. Studies using pegylated interferon-α show it to be more effective than standard interferon. A course of 180 μg weekly pegylated interferon-α_{2a} for 48 weeks gave a 39% SR compared with 19% for standard interferon [127]. In another study pegylated interferon-α_{2b} (1.0 μg/kg/week) for 48 weeks gave an SR of 25% compared with 12% for standard interferon [65]. There was a slightly higher rate of dose reduction and drug discontinuation in those given pegylated interferon in some but not all studies [48, 65, 127].

If standard interferon-α is used the dose is 3 million units by injection three times a week for 12 months. Treatment should be stopped in those not recording a negative HCV RNA after 3 months. Re-treatment of relapsers may be considered if the HCV RNA was undetectable at the end of the first course. Prolonged therapy to 60 weeks may increase the percentage with SR. Long-term therapy may be especially useful in those with high pre-treatment viral load.

Table 18.7. Compensated HCV cirrhosis: once weekly (180 μg) pegylated interferon-α_{2a} compared with thrice weekly non-pegylated interferon [48]

	% ETR	% SR
Pegylated	44	30
Non-pegylated	14	8

ETR, end of treatment response; SR, sustained response.

Patients with compensated HCV cirrhosis

Combination therapy with ribavirin and interferon-α is more effective than interferon-α alone (table 18.5) [69, 94, 98]. The overall results with pegylated interferon/ribavirin are similar to non-pegylated interferon/ribavirin [71]. If ribavirin cannot be used, monotherapy with pegylated interferon-α_{2a} (180 μg/kg/week) has a higher SR than standard interferon after 48 weeks treatment (30% versus 8%) (table 18.7) [48].

Treatment of patients who have relapsed after interferon monotherapy

These patients benefit from combination therapy. In a randomized trial, the SR after combination therapy with ribavirin (49%) was superior to retreatment with interferon-α_{2b} (5%) [24]. In patients with a contraindication to ribavirin, longer courses of higher dose interferon or pegylated interferon-α alone are options [20].

There are currently no guide-lines for the treatment of patients who relapse after combination therapy, or who do not respond to combination or interferon monotherapy [23].

Consensus interferon is genetically engineered to contain the commonest amino acids in natural interferons and may be useful in relapsers or non-responders to previous interferon-α therapy [47]. Further trials are needed to find optimal approach for these patients.

Other treatments

Ursodeoxycholic acid does not affect HCV RNA clearance or liver histology [7]. *Amantadine* has been used in combination with interferon-α. There is conflicting evidence of efficacy and at present there is no clear role for this combination [128].

New antiviral agents. Knowledge of the molecular biology of HCV has led to the identification of specific functions associated with particular regions of the virus. Treatments may be targeted to inhibit specifically encoded functions. These include antisense oligonucleotides targeted against the ribosomal binding site of the 5′ non-translated region of the HCV genome [68]. Protease and helicase inhibitors are under development. Unfortunately, they have not reached the stage of clinical trials. Inosine monophosphate dehydrogenase (IMPDH) inhibitors are being tested.

Conclusion

Combination therapy with interferon-α and ribavirin is the current standard of care for chronic hepatitis C. This offers a 30–65% chance of sustained virological

It is characterized by female predominance, hyperglobulinaemia, positive circulating autoantibodies, and association with HLA-DR3 and HLA-DR4 [30]. Those with known aetiological factors, such as virus, drugs and alcohol, are excluded. The condition usually responds to immunosuppressive treatment. Classification into various types is made on the basis of circulating autoantibody patterns (table 19.9) [21].

In general, those with no known aetiology are more florid clinically and have higher serum transaminase and γ-globulin levels with more active liver histology than those with a known aetiology; the response to corticosteroid therapy is better.

Type 1 (formerly called lupoid)

This type covers the vast majority of patients with autoimmune chronic hepatitis. It is associated with high circulating titres of anti-DNA and anti-actin (smooth muscle). This type will be described in detail later as a prototype.

Type 2

This is associated with autoantibodies against liver–kidney microsomes (LKM) type 1. It is subdivided into types 2a and 2b.

Type 2a [20]. Cytochrome mono-oxygenase P450 2D6 is the target antigen. Antibodies react specifically with an amino acid sequence. This is absent in patients with non-specific reactivity such as HCV. It is associated with a severe chronic hepatitis. Other autoantibodies are usually absent. The disease largely affects girls, mainly in Europe and not the USA. There is a good response to corticosteroid treatment. Extra-hepatic immunological diseases such as diabetes can be found. The disease may be fulminant in children.

Table 19.9. Chronic liver disease with circulating autoantibodies

Type	Antibody				
	ANA	SMA	LKM	AMA	SLA
1 ('lupoid')	+++	+++	–	–	++
2a	–	–	+++	–	
2b (HCV)	–	–	+	–	
3	+	+	–	–	++
Autoimmune cholangiopathy	+++	+	–	–	
Primary biliary cirrhosis	–	±	–	+++	

ANA, antinuclear antibody; SMA, smooth muscle (actin) antibody; LKM, liver-kidney microsomal antibody; AMA, anti-mitochondrial antibody; SLA, soluble liver antigen.

Type 2b. Antibodies to LKM-1 are found in up to 7% of patients with chronic hepatitis C infection in Europe, but not in the USA or the UK. The antibody reacts with cytochrome P450 2D6 related to shared antigenic sites (molecular mimicry). However, more detailed analysis of the microsomes shows that anti-LKM-1 antibody from patients with HCV is directed against different antigenic sites on the P450 2D6 proteins than those with autoimmune LKM positivity [40]. Patients with type 2b tend to be male and older. There is no clear association with other autoimmune diseases and they respond better to antiviral than immunosuppressive therapy.

Type 3. This is characterized by antibodies to soluble liver antigen (SLA) and to liver and pancreas antigen (LPA) [28]. Patients lack anti-LKM but may have ANA. Anti-SLA could be a marker for type 1 autoimmune chronic hepatitis [9]. The target antigen for SLA/LPA autoantibodies has been cloned [39].

Chronic hepatitis D

Some patients with chronic delta virus infection have a circulating autoantibody against LKM-3. The microsomal target is uridine diphosphate glucuronyl transferase [31]. The relationship of this autoantibody to disease progression is uncertain.

Primary biliary cirrhosis and immune cholangitis

These cholestatic syndromes are marked by serum mitochondrial antibodies in the case of primary biliary cirrhosis (Chapter 14) and to DNA and actin in the case of immune cholangitis (Chapter 14) [2].

Chronic autoimmune hepatitis (type 1)

In 1950, Waldenström [38] described a chronic hepatitis occurring predominantly in young people, especially women. The syndrome has since been given various titles [1]. It is now termed 'chronic autoimmune hepatitis'. The condition seems to be decreasing, but this may simply be due to more accurate diagnosis of other causes of chronic hepatitis, for instance drug-related or hepatitis B or C.

Aetiology

The aetiology is unknown. Immunological changes are conspicuous. Serum γ-globulin levels are grossly elevated. The finding of a positive LE cell test in about 15% led to the term 'lupoid hepatitis'. Tissue antibodies are found in a high proportion of patients.

Chronic (lupoid) hepatitis is not the same as classical systemic lupus erythematosus [16] for the liver rarely shows any lesions in classical lupus. Moreover, the smooth muscle antibody and the mitochondrial antibody are not present in the blood of patients with systemic lupus erythematosus.

Immunological mechanisms and autoantibodies [28]

Autoimmune chronic hepatitis is a disease of disordered immunoregulation marked by a defect in suppressor (regulatory) T-cells. This results in the production of autoantibodies against hepatocyte surface antigens. It is uncertain whether the defect in the immune regulatory apparatus is primary or secondary to an acquired change in the antigenicity of the tissues.

The mononuclear infiltrate in the portal zones consists of B-lymphocytes and helper T-cells with relatively fewer cytotoxic/suppressor cells. This is consistent with the view that antibody-dependent cytotoxicity is the main effector mechanism (fig. 19.9).

Patients have persistently high titres of circulating measles antibodies. This is likely to be due to hyperfunction of the immune system and not to reactivation of persistent virus [24].

The nature of the target antigens on the hepatocyte membrane is unknown. Cell-mediated immunity to membrane proteins has been shown. Liver membrane-specific activated T-cells in peripheral blood may be important in the autoimmune attack of chronic hepatitis.

Patients show many serum autoantibodies. Their role in pathogenesis is not known but they are of great diagnostic value. There is no evidence that antibodies against cellular antigens can themselves mediate the autoimmune attack.

Antinuclear antibody is present in the serum of about 80% of patients. The homogeneous (diffuse) and speckled patterns of immunofluorescence are equal. The speckled form is more frequent in younger patients with higher serum transaminase values [10].

Smooth muscle (actin) antibody is present in about 70% of patients, and in about 50% of patients with primary biliary cirrhosis. It is also present in low titre in patients with acute type A or B viral hepatitis or with infectious mononucleosis. Titres exceeding 1:40 are rare except in autoimmune chronic hepatitis type 1. The antigen is related to the S-actin of smooth and skeletal muscle. It is also present in cell membranes and in the cytoskeleton of the liver cell. SMA can therefore be regarded as a result of liver cell injury.

Human asialo-glycoprotein receptor autoantibodies. The antigen is a component of liver-specific protein (LSP). The presence is closely linked to inflammation and activity [37].

Mitochondrial antibody. This is usually absent or in only low titre.

Genetics [11, 15]

The female sex predominance (8:1) is similar to other autoimmune diseases. The disease can be familial [19].

Effector T-lymphocytes recognize antigen only if presented on the surface of the damaged hepatocyte by autologous HLA molecules (fig. 19.10) [15]. The interac-

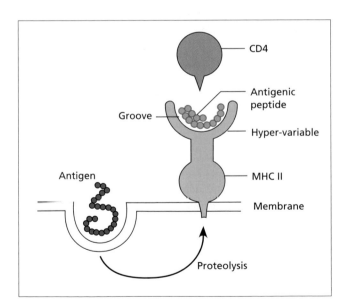

Fig. 19.10. Immunogenetics of autoimmune liver disease: the postulated antigen enters the liver cell by endocytosis. The HLA class II molecule fuses with the antigen-containing endosome. The antigen is broken down to peptides by proteolysis. The HLA class II peptide–complex is transported to the plasma membrane expressed in a groove and presented to the CD4 lymphocyte. The hyper-variability of HLA class II in the groove may predispose to autoimmune chronic hepatitis.

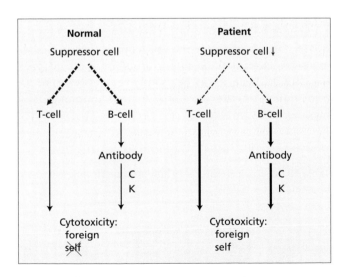

Fig. 19.9. The mechanism of immunological hepatocyte injury in autoimmune chronic hepatitis. In the patient, related to a defect in T-suppressor (regulatory) cells, cytotoxicity is directed not only against foreign antigens but also against self. C, cytotoxic T-cell; K, killer T-cell.

tion between the HLA molecule, the antigenic peptide presented in its groove and the T-cell receptor are crucial. Certain alleles at the HLA loci predispose individuals to related disease. Only the predisposition is inherited not the disease itself which must be triggered by an antigen.

The major histocompatibility complex (MHC) is located on the short arm of chromosome 6. MHC class I and II genes are highly polymorphic. In autoimmune hepatitis type 1, there is a dual association for white people with either HLA-A1-B8-DR3 or HLA-DR4. In Japanese patients the association is predominantly with HLA-DR4. Only limited data are available for autoimmune hepatitis type 2. Analysis of the hyper-variable region of HLA class II indicates that lysine at position 71 is crucial for autoimmune hepatitis type 1 in white people, whereas position 13 is important for Japanese.

The complement genes are also polymorphic and are known as HLA class III genes. The MHC class III allele, C4A-QO, is significantly increased in autoimmune hepatitis type 1 and 2. In the future, HLA typing may be used to identify susceptibility to autoimmune chronic hepatitis. However, recognition of the nature of the antigenic peptide in the HLA groove which is presented to the lymphocyte is essential for further progress.

Hepatic pathology

The lesion is a severe chronic hepatitis. Activity is variable and some areas may be near normal.

Cellular infiltrates, largely lymphocytes and plasma cells, are seen in zone 1 and infiltrating between the liver cells. Aggressive septum formation isolates groups of liver cells as rosettes. Fatty change is inconspicuous. Areas of collapse may be seen. The connective tissue encroaches on the parenchyma. Cirrhosis develops rapidly and is usually of the large nodular type. The chronic hepatitis and the cirrhosis seem to develop almost simultaneously.

As time passes the activity subsides, the cellularity decreases, the necrosis lessens and the fibrosis becomes denser. At necropsy in the long-standing case, the lesion is an inactive cirrhosis. In most cases, however, careful search will reveal areas of interface necrosis and rosette formation.

During remissions, the disease remains inactive, regeneration appears inadequate as the architecture is not restored to normal and the pattern of injury remains detectable.

Cirrhosis is present early in only one-third of patients but is usually present 2 years after the onset [33]. Repeated episodes of necrosis with further stromal collapse and fibrosis lead to a more severe cirrhosis. Eventually the liver becomes small and grossly cirrhotic.

Clinical features (table 19.10)

The condition is predominantly, but not exclusively, one of young people with a peri-pubertal peak and a further increase between the fourth and sixth decades. Three-quarters are female.

The onset is usually insidious, the patient feels generally unwell and is noticed to be jaundiced. In about a quarter of cases the disease seems to present as a typical attack of acute viral hepatitis. It is only when the jaundice persists that the physician is alerted to the possibility of a more chronic liver disorder. It is unclear whether the disease can be initiated by acute viral hepatitis, or whether this is simply an intercurrent infection in a patient with long-standing chronic hepatitis.

In most instances, the hepatic lesion on presentation does not agree with the stated duration of symptoms. Chronic hepatitis must remain asymptomatic for some months or possibly years before jaundice becomes overt and the diagnosis is made. Patients may be recognized sooner if a routine examination reveals stigmata of liver disease or if biochemical tests of liver function are found to be abnormal.

Although the serum bilirubin level is usually increased, some are anicteric. Frank jaundice is often episodic. Rarely, deep cholestatic jaundice is seen.

Amenorrhoea is usual and regular menses is a good sign. However, if a period does occur it may be associated with an increase of symptoms and deepening of jaundice. Epistaxis, bleeding gums and bruising with minimal trauma are other complaints.

Examination shows a tall girl, often above normal stature, and generally looking healthy (fig. 19.11). Spider naevi are virtually constant. They tend to be small and to come and go with changes in the activity of the disease. Livid cutaneous striae may sometimes be found on the thighs, lateral aspect of the abdominal wall, and also, in severe cases, on the upper arms, breasts and back (fig. 19.12). The face may be rounded even before the administration of corticosteroids. Acne is prominent and hirsutism may be seen.

Table 19.10. Typical features of autommune chronic active hepatitis

Usually female
Age 15–25 years or menopause
Serum
transaminases × 10
γ-globulin × 2
Liver biopsy: active, non-diagnostic
ANA > 1 : 40 diffuse
Anti-actin > 1 : 40
Dramatic response to corticosteroids

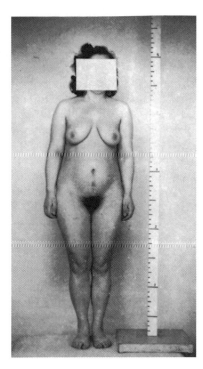

Fig. 19.11. Active juvenile cirrhosis. Well-developed girl with good nutrition.

Abdominal examination in the early stages shows a firm liver edge some 4 cm below the right costal margin. The left lobe may be disproportionately enlarged. In the later stages the liver becomes impalpable. The spleen is usually enlarged. Ascites, oedema and hepatic encephalopathy are late features.

Recurrent episodes of active liver disease punctuate the course.

Associated conditions

Chronic autoimmune active hepatitis is not a condition confined to the liver (table 19.11).

In those who are particularly ill, there may be sustained pyrexia [33]. Such patients may also have an acute, recurrent, non-deforming, migrating polyarthritis of the large joints. In most cases, pain and stiffness are present without marked swelling. The changes usually resolve completely.

Associated skin conditions include allergic capillaritis, acne, erythema, LE-type changes and purpura.

Splenomegaly may be present, often with generalized lymphadenopathy, presumably related to lymphoid hyperplasia.

Renal biopsy often shows mild glomerulitis. Immune complexes in the glomeruli are restricted to those with kidney disease. Glomerular antibodies in about half the patients are unrelated to the extent of renal damage.

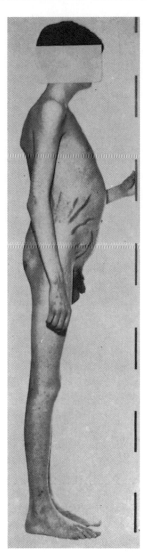

Fig. 19.12. Active chronic 'lupoid' hepatitis. Note the appearance of a tall boy with ascites and striae on the abdominal wall and upper arms.

Table 19.11. Associated lesions in 81 cases of autoimmune chronic hepatitis [33]

Purpura	2
Erythemas	4
Arthralgia	9
Lymphadenopathy	2
Pulmonary infiltrates	7
Pleurisy	2
Rheumatic heart disease	4
Ulcerative colitis	5
Diabetes	3
Hashimoto's thyroiditis	2
Renal tubular defects	3
Lupus kidney	3
Haemolytic anaemia	1

Pulmonary changes include pleurisy, transitory pulmonary infiltrations and collapse. A mottled chest radiograph may be related to dilated precapillary blood vessels. Multiple pulmonary arteriovenous anastomoses are also found (Chapter 6). Fibrosing alveolitis is another possibility.

Primary pulmonary hypertension has been described in one patient with multi-system involvement [5].

Endocrine changes include a cushingoid appearance, acne, hirsutism and cutaneous striae. Boys may develop gynaecomastia. Hashimoto's thyroiditis may be seen and other thyroid abnormalities include myxoedema and thyrotoxicosis. Patients develop diabetes mellitus, before and after diagnosis of the chronic hepatitis.

Mild anaemia, leucopenia and thrombocytopenia are associated with the enlarged spleen. A positive Coombs' test with haemolytic anaemia is another rare complication. Rarely, a hypereosinophilic syndrome is associated [7].

Ulcerative colitis presents either with the chronic active hepatitis or after it.

Hepato-cellular cancer is reported but is very rare [4].

Biochemistry

This picture is of very active disease (see table 19.10). Apart from the hyperbilirubinaemia of about 2–10 mg/dl (35–170 μmol/l), the serum γ-globulin levels are more than twice the upper limit of normal (fig. 19.13). Electrophoresis shows a polyclonal gammopathy, rarely monoclonal. Serum transaminases are usually more than 10 times increased. Serum albumin is maintained until the later stages of liver failure. During the course transaminases and γ-globulin levels fall spontaneously.

Serum α-fetoprotein levels may be increased to greater than twice the upper limit of normal. Levels fall with corticosteroid therapy.

Haematology

Thrombocytopenia and leucopenia are frequent even before the late stage of portal hypertension and very large spleen. A mild anaemia is also usual. Prothrombin time is often prolonged even in the early stages when hepato-cellular function seems preserved.

Needle biopsy of the liver

This is very valuable, but may prove difficult to perform because of the coagulation defect. Transjugular liver biopsy may be needed. If biopsy is possible, classic severe chronic hepatitis is seen.

Differential diagnosis (fig. 19.14)

Needle liver biopsy may be required to determine whether *cirrhosis* is present.

The distinction from *hepatitis B positive chronic hepatitis* is made by testing for hepatitis B markers.

Patients with *hepatitis C* may have circulating autoantibodies. Using first-generation HCV-antibody testing, some are false positive related to high serum globulin values, but even second-generation tests sometimes read positive. Patients with HCV may have circulating autoantibodies to LKM-1 (see table 19.9).

The distinction from *Wilson's disease* is vital. A family history of liver disease is important. Presentation is often with haemolysis and ascites. Slit lamp examination of the cornea should be performed to look for Kayser–Fleischer rings. Confirmation of the diagnosis is made by finding a reduced serum copper and caeruloplasmin and increased urinary copper values. Liver copper is increased.

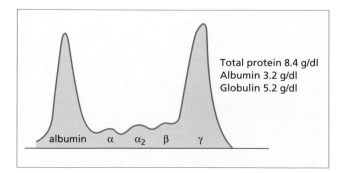

Total protein 8.4 g/dl
Albumin 3.2 g/dl
Globulin 5.2 g/dl

albumin   α   α₂   β   γ

Fig. 19.13. Electrophoresis of the serum proteins. Note the very high γ-globulin.

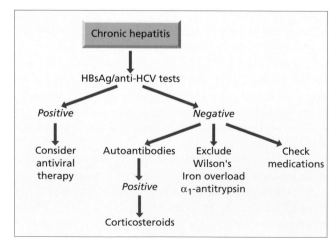

Fig. 19.14. The differential diagnosis and management of chronic hepatitis.

Ingestion of *drugs*, such as nitrofurantoin, methyl dopa or isoniazid, must be excluded.

Chronic hepatitis may coexist with *ulcerative colitis*. A distinction must be made between this combination and *sclerosing cholangitis* where serum alkaline phosphatase values are usually increased and serum smooth muscle antibodies are absent. ERCP is diagnostic.

Alcoholic liver disease. The history, stigmata of chronic alcoholism and large tender liver are helpful diagnostic points. Liver histology shows fat (a rare association of autoimmune hepatitis), alcoholic hyaline, focal polymorphs infiltration and maximal liver damage in zone 3.

Haemochromatosis should be excluded by serum transferrin saturation and ferritin determination.

Treatment

Clinical trials have shown that corticosteroid treatment prolongs life in severe chronic autoimmune type 1 hepatitis [6, 29, 36].

Benefit is greatest in the first 2 years (figs 19.15, 19.16) [25]. Fatigue lessens, appetite improves, fever and arthralgias are controlled. The menses return. Serum bilirubin, transaminase and γ-globulin levels usually fall. The changes are so dramatic as to be virtually diagnostic of autoimmune chronic hepatitis. Hepatic histology shows decreased inflammatory activity but the progression from chronic hepatitis to cirrhosis is not prevented.

Liver biopsy must precede therapy. If coagulation defects prohibit this procedure the biopsy must be done as soon as possible after a remission has been induced by corticosteroids.

The usual dose is 30 mg/day prednisolone (or 40 mg prednisone) for 1 week reducing to a maintenance dose of 10–15 mg daily (table 19.12).

Biochemical and histological remission can usually be achieved within 6 months. Prednisolone therapy usually extends over 2–3 years or longer, usually for life (table 19.13). Premature withdrawal leads to relapse [18]. Although control is usually re-established within 1 or 2 months, there are occasional fatalities.

Prednisone may be used but in a slightly higher dose. Alternate day prednisolone is not recommended as the incidence of serious complications is higher and histological remission less frequent.

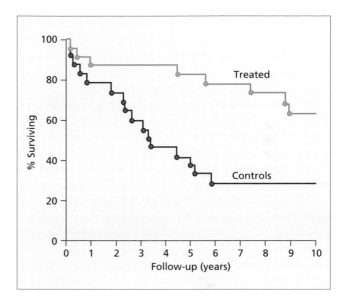

Fig. 19.16. Later results of the Royal Free Hospital trial of prednisolone in chronic autoimmune hepatitis. Note the improved survival in the treated group [25].

Table 19.12. Prednisolone in autoimmune chronic hepatitis

First week
10 mg prednisolone three times a day (30 mg/day)

Second and third weeks
Reduce prednisolone to maintenance dose (10–15 mg/day)

Every month
Clinical check—liver tests

At 6 months
Full check—clinical and biochemical

No remission
Continue maintenance dose for 6 more months, consider adding azathioprine (50–100 mg/day)
Maximum dose—20 mg prednisolone with 100 mg azathioprine

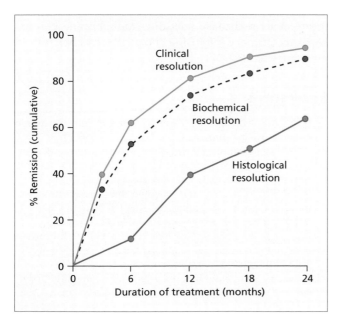

Fig. 19.15. The effect of prednisolone treatment in severe chronic autoimmune hepatitis.

Table 19.13. Autoimmune chronic hepatitis: duration of prednisolone treatment

At least 2 years until
Serum
ANA is negative
bilirubin
γ-globulin normal
transaminase
Liver biopsy inactive (usually more than 2 years)

Patients with milder forms, usually middle-aged or elderly men and women, may be maintained with lower doses of prednisolone as steroid side-effects are particularly undesirable in these patients.

Complications of treatment include facial mooning, acne, obesity, hirsutism and striae. These are particularly unwanted by female patients. More serious complications include growth retardation in those younger than 10 years, with diabetes and serious infections.

Bone loss is found even with only 10 mg prednisolone daily and is related to duration of therapy. Calcium supplementation may be indicated and physical activity encouraged. Bone density scans are done every 1–2 years. Post-menapausal women are given hormone replacement therapy.

Side-effects are rare if the dose of prednisolone is not more than 15 mg daily. If this is exceeded or serious complications have arisen, alternative measures must be considered.

If 20 mg prednisolone daily has not produced a remission, azathioprine 50–100 mg daily may be added. It is not given as routine. Continual use of such a drug over many months or even years has obvious disadvantages. Other indications for azathioprine include gross cushingoid features, associated diseases such as diabetes and other side-effects at doses required to induce remission.

Azathioprine in a higher dose (2 mg/kg body weight) has been given alone to those who have been in complete remission for at least 1 year on the combination [23]. Side-effects include arthralgias, myelosuppression and an increased risk of cancer.

Cyclosporine has been used in a patient resistant to corticosteroid therapy [17]. This toxic drug should not be given except as a last resort when conventional therapy has failed.

Hepatic transplantation is considered when corticosteroids have failed to induce a remission or in the late stages where the complications of cirrhosis have developed. The survival rate is comparable to that of patients who enter a remission after corticosteroids [34]. Autoimmune chronic hepatitis may recur after the transplant [14].

Course and prognosis

This is extremely variable. The course is a fluctuant one marked by episodes of deterioration when jaundice and malaise are increased. The ultimate effect is inevitably cirrhosis with very few exceptions.

The 10-year survival is 63% [25]. After an initial remission following 2 years of corticosteroid therapy, one-third achieve a 5-year remission while two-thirds relapse and have to be re-treated. Further corticosteroids have more side-effects. The mean survival is 12.2 years. Mortality is greatest during the first 2 years when the disease is most active. Sustained remission is more likely if the patient is diagnosed early and if immunosuppression is adequate. Corticosteroid therapy prolongs life, but most patients eventually reach the end-stage of cirrhosis.

Post-menopausal women respond to initial corticosteroid therapy but have more long-term complications.

Patients who are DR3 allotypes present earlier than DR4, they enter remission less frequently and tend to relapse. They need more transplants [11].

Oesophageal varices are an uncommon initial finding. Nevertheless, bleeding from oesophageal varices and hepato-cellular failure are the usual causes of death.

Pregnancy in patients with chronic active hepatitis is discussed later (Chapter 27).

Syncytial giant-cell hepatitis

This chronic hepatitis was once considered to be related to paramyxoma infection [32]. However, this could not be confirmed. The condition is probably related to many forms of liver disease including autoimmune chronic hepatitis, primary sclerosing cholangitis and hepatitis C virus infection [13, 27].

References

1 Bearn AG, Kunkel HG, Slater RJ. The problem of chronic liver disease in young women. *Am. J. Med.* 1956; **21**: 3.
2 Ben-Ari Z, Dhillon AP, Sherlock S. Autoimmune cholangiopathy: part of the spectrum of autoimmune chronic active hepatitis. *Hepatology* 1993; **18**: 10.
3 Brunt EM. Grading and staging: the histopathological lesions of chronic hepatitis: the Knodell histology activity index and beyond. *Hepatology* 2000; **31**: 241.
4 Burroughs AK, Bassendine MF, Thomas HC et al. Primary liver cell cancer in autoimmune chronic liver disease. *Br. Med. J.* 1981; **282**: 273.
5 Cohen N, Mendelow H. Concurrent 'active juvenile cirrhosis' and 'primary pulmonary hypertension'. *Am. J. Med.* 1965; **39**: 127.
6 Cook GC, Mulligan R, Sherlock S. Controlled prospective trial of corticosteroid therapy in active chronic hepatitis. *Q. J. Med.* 1971; **40**: 159.
7 Croffy B, Kopelman R, Kaplan M. Hypereosinophilic

syndrome. Association with chronic active hepatitis. *Dig. Dis. Sci.* 1988; **33**: 233.

8 Czaja AJ. Chronic active hepatitis: the challenge for a new nomenclature. *Ann. Intern. Med.* 1993; **119**: 510.

9 Czaja AJ, Manns MP, McFarlane IG *et al.* Autoimmune hepatitis: the investigational and clinical challenges. *Hepatology* 2000; **31**: 1194.

10 Czaja AJ, Nishioka M, Morshed SA *et al.* Patterns of nuclear immunofluorescence and reactivities to recombinant nuclear antigens in autoimmune hepatitis. *Gastroenterology* 1994; **107**: 200.

11 Czaja AJ, Strettel MDJ, Thomson LJ et al. Associations between alleles of the major histocompatibility complex and type 1 autoimmune hepatitis. *Hepatology* 1997; **25**: 317.

12 Desmet VJ, Gerber M, Hoofnagle JH *et al.* Classification of chronic hepatitis: diagnosis, grading and staging. *Hepatology* 1994; **19**: 1513.

13 Devaney K, Goodman ZD, Ishak KG. Post infantile giant-cell transformation in hepatitis. *Hepatology* 1992; **16**: 327.

14 Devlin J, Donaldson P, Portmann B *et al.* Recurrence of autoimmune hepatitis following liver transplantation. *Liver Transplant Surg.* 1995; **1**: 162.

15 Donaldson P, Doherty D, Underhill J *et al.* The molecular genetics of autoimmune liver disease. *Hepatology* 1994; **20**: 225.

16 Gurian LE, Rogoff TM, Ware AJ *et al.* The immunological diagnosis of chronic active 'auto-immune' hepatitis: distinction from systemic lupus erythematosus. *Hepatology* 1985; **5**: 397.

17 Hayams JS, Ballows M, Leichtner AM. Cyclosporin treatment of autoimmune chronic active hepatitis. *Gastroenterology* 1987; **93**: 890.

18 Hegarty JE, Nouri Aria KT, Portmann B *et al.* Relapse following treatment withdrawal in patients with autoimmune chronic active hepatitis. *Hepatology* 1983; **3**: 685.

19 Hodges S, Loboyeo A, Donaldson P *et al.* Autoimmune chronic active hepatitis in a family. *Gut* 1991; **32**: 299.

20 Homberg JC, Abuaf N, Bernard O *et al.* Chronic active hepatitis associated with antiliver/kidney microsome antibody type 1: a second type of 'autoimmune' hepatitis. *Hepatology* 1987; **7**: 1333.

21 International Autoimmune Hepatitis Group. Report: review of criteria for diagnosis of autoimmune hepatitis. *J. Hepatol.* 1999; **31**: 929.

22 Ishak KG. Pathologic features of chronic hepatitis: a review and update. *Am. J. Clin. Pathol.* 2000; **113**: 40.

23 Johnson PJ, McFarlane IG, Williams R. Azathioprine for long-term maintenance of remission in autoimmune hepatitis. *N. Engl. J. Med.* 1995; **333**: 958.

24 Kalland K-H, Endresen C, Haukenes G *et al.* Measles-specific nucleotide sequences and autoimmune chronic active hepatitis. *Lancet* 1989; **1**: 1390 (letter).

25 Kirk AP, Jain S, Pocock S *et al.* Late results of Royal Free Hospital controlled trial of prednisolone therapy in hepatitis B surface antigen-negative chronic active hepatitis. *Gut* 1980; **21**: 78.

26 Knodell RG, Ishak KG, Black WC *et al.* Formulation and application of a numerical scoring system for assessing histological activity in asymptomatic chronic active hepatitis. *Hepatology* 1981; **4**: 431.

27 Lau JYN, Konkoulis G, Mieli-Vergano G *et al.* Syncytial giant-cell hepatitis: a specific disease entity? *J. Hepatol.* 1992; **15**: 216.

28 Manns MP, Strassburg CP. Autoimmune hepatitis: clinical challenges. *Gastroenterology* 2001; **120**: 1502.

29 Murray-Lyon IM, Stern RB, Williams R. Controlled trial of prednisone and azathioprine in active chronic hepatitis. *Lancet* 1973; **i**: 735.

30 Obermayer-Straub P, Strassburg CP, Manns MP. Autoimmune hepatitis. *J. Hepatol.* 2000; **32** (suppl. 1); 181.

31 Philipp T, Durazzo M, Trautwein C *et al.* Recognition of uridine diphosphate glucuronyl transferases by LKM-3 antibodies in chronic hepatitis D. *Lancet* 1994; **344**: 578.

32 Phillips MJ, Blendis LM, Paucell S *et al.* Syncytial giant-cell hepatitis. Sporadic hepatitis with distinctive pathologic features, a severe clinical course and paramyxoviral features. *N. Engl. J. Med.* 1991; **324**: 455.

33 Read AE, Harrison CV, Sherlock S. 'Juvenile cirrhosis'; part of a system disease. The effect of corticosteroid therapy. *Gut* 1963; **4**: 378.

34 Sanchez-Urdazpal L, Czaja AJ, Van Hock B *et al.* Prognostic features and role of liver transplantation in severe corticosteroid-treated autoimmune chronic active hepatitis. *Hepatology* 1991; **15**: 215.

35 Sherlock S. Chronic hepatitis and cirrhosis. *Hepatology* 1984; **4**: 25S.

36 Soloway RD, Summerskill WH, Baggenstoss AH *et al.* Clinical, biochemical, and histological remission of severe chronic active liver disease: a controlled study of treatments and early prognosis. *Gastroenterology* 1972; **63**: 820.

37 Treichel U, Poralla T, Hess G *et al.* Autoantibodies to human asialoglycoprotein receptor in autoimmune-type chronic hepatitis. *Hepatology* 1990; **11**: 606.

38 Waldenström J. *Leber, Blutproteine und Nahrungsweiss Stoffwechs Krh*, Sonderband: XV, p. 8. Tagung, Bad Kissingen, 1950.

39 Wies I, Brunner S, Henninger J *et al.* Identification of target antigen for SLA/LP autoantibodies in autoimmune hepatitis. *Lancet* 2000; **355**: 1510.

40 Yamamoto AM, Cresteil D, Homberg JC *et al.* Characterization of antiliver–kidney microsome antibody (anti-LKM I) from hepatitis C virus-positive and virus-negative sera. *Gastroenterology* 1993; **104**: 1762.

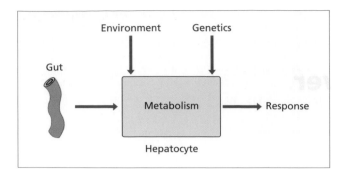

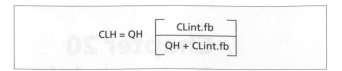

Fig. 20.3. Formula for calculating clearance (CLH) of a drug by the liver. CLint, intrinsic clearance; fb, plasma protein binding; QH, liver blood flow [10].

Fig. 20.2. The response of the liver to drugs depends on an interplay between absorption, environmental factors and genetics.

Table 20.1. Classification of hepatic drug reactions

Type	Features	Examples
Zone 3 necrosis	Dose dependent, multi-organ failure	Carbon tetrachloride Paracetamol Halothane
Mitochondrial cytopathies	Affects children Reye's-like syndrome Cirrhosis	Valproate
Steato-hepatitis	Long half-life Cirrhosis	Perhexiline Amiodarone
Acute hepatitis	Bridging necrosis Short term, acute Long term, chronic	Methyl dopa Isoniazid Halothane Ketoconazole
General hypersensitivity	Often with granulomas	Sulphonamides Quinidine Allopurinol
Fibrosis	Portal hypertension Cirrhosis	Methotrexate Vinyl chloride Vitamin A
Cholestasis		
canalicular	Dose dependent, reversible	Sex hormones
hepato-canalicular	Reversible 'obstructive' jaundice	Chlorpromazine Erythromycin Nitrofurantoin Azathioprine
ductular	Age-related. Renal failure	Benoxyprofen
Vascular		
Veno-occlusive disease	Dose dependent	Irradiation Cytotoxics
Sinusoidal dilatation and peliosis		Azathioprine Sex hormones
Hepatic vein obstruction	Thrombotic effect	Sex hormones
Portal vein obstruction	Thrombotic effect	Sex hormones
Biliary		
Sclerosing cholangitis	Cholestasis	Hepatic arterial FUDR
Gallbladder sludge	Biliary colic	Ceftriaxone
Neoplastic		
Focal nodular hyperplasia	Benign. Presents space-occupying lesion	Sex hormones
Adenoma	May rupture. Usually regress	Sex hormones
Hepato-cellular carcinoma	Very rare Relatively benign	Danazol Sex and anabolic hormones

FUDR, 5-fluoro-2′-deoxyuridine.

Table 20.2. Classification of drugs based on pharmacokinetic parameters obtained in normal subjects [70]

	Hepatic extraction	Protein binding	Effect of shunting on systemic availability	Examples
Enzyme limited, binding insensitive	Low	Low (<90%)	0	Antipyrine Amobarbital Caffeine Theophylline Aminopyrine
Enzyme limited, binding sensitive	Low	High (>90%)	0	Chlordiazepoxide Diazepam Diphenylhydantoin Indomethacin Phenylbutazone Rifampicin Tolbutamide Warfarin
Flow and enzyme sensitive	Medium	No effect	+	Acetaminophen Chlorpromazine Isoniazid Merperidine Metoprolol Nortriptyline Quinidine
Flow limited	High	No effect	+++	Galactose Indocyanine green Labetalol Lidocaine Morphine Pentazocine Propoxyphene Propranolol Verapamil

green is one such drug. These drugs are usually highly lipid soluble. If liver blood flow falls, for instance due to cirrhosis or heart failure, the systemic effect of the high first-pass rate drug will be enhanced. Administration of drugs such as propranolol or cimetidine which lower hepatic blood flow will have a similar effect.

Because of its high first-pass uptake, a drug such as glyceryl trinitrate has to be given sublingually to avoid entry into the portal vein. Similarly, lignocaine has to be given intravenously.

Drugs with a low intrinsic clearance, such as theophylline, depend on enzyme function. Changes in hepatic blood flow have little effect.

Plasma protein binding limits the presentation of the drug to hepatic enzymes. This will be affected by changes in the synthesis and degradation of plasma proteins.

Hepatic drug metabolism

Phase 1. The main drug-metabolizing system resides in the microsomal fraction of the liver cell (smooth endoplasmic reticulum). The enzymes concerned are mixed function mono-cytochrome C reductase and cytochrome P450. Reduced NADPH in the cytosol is a co-factor. The drug is rendered more polar by hydroxylation or oxidation. Alternative phase 1 drug-metabolizing reactions include the conversion of alcohol to acetaldehyde by alcohol dihydrogenases found mainly in the cytosolic fraction.

Enzyme inducers include barbiturates, alcohol, anaesthetics, hypoglycaemic and anti-convulsant agents, griseofulvin, rifampicin, phenylbutazone and meprobamate. Enlargement of the liver following the introduction of drug therapy can be related to enzyme induction.

Phase 2. These biotransformations involve conjugation of the drug or drug metabolite with a small endogenous molecule. The enzymes concerned are usually

of FIAU into the mitochondrial genome in place of thymidine [107].

Fulminant hepatitis with severe lactate acidosis has been reported in HIV-infected patients on *didanosine* (ddI) [10]. Some of the side-effects of *azidothymidine* (AZT) and *23-dideoxycitidine* (ddC) are probably due to inhibition of mitochondrial DNA synthesis.

Lamivudine has not resulted in serious liver damage. It does not inhibit mitochondrial DNA replication in intact cells [148].

Bacillus cereus

Emetic toxin in contaminated food can cause fulminant liver failure due to mitochondrial toxicity [87].

Steato-hepatitis

The reaction termed *non-alcoholic steato-hepatitis* (NASH) histologically resembles acute alcoholic hepatitis with sometimes, in addition, electron microscopic evidence of lysosomal phospholipidosis. Mallory's hyaline is found in zone 3 in distinction to true alcoholic hepatitis.

Perhexiline maleate

Perhexiline maleate, an anti-anginal drug now withdrawn, has been associated with hepatic histology resembling acute alcoholic hepatitis. Patients with this reaction lack a gene concerned with the oxidation of debrisoquine. The defect leads to a deficiency of a monoxygenase reaction in liver microsomes.

Amiodarone

This anticardiac–dysrhythmia drug has caused toxic damage to lung, cornea, thyroid, peripheral nerves and liver [155]. Abnormal biochemical tests of liver function are found in 15–50% of patients receiving it [121].

Hepato-toxicity usually develops more than 1 year after starting therapy but can occur within 1 month. The spectrum is wide, from isolated asymptomatic transaminase elevations to a fulminant fatal disorder. Hepatotoxicity is usually marked by an increase in serum transaminases and rarely by jaundice. Symptoms may be absent and toxicity detected only by routine monitoring; hepatomegaly is not constant. Severe cholestasis may be a feature. Fatal cirrhosis can develop. Children can be affected.

Amiodarone has a very large volume of distribution and a very long half-life, so that blood levels may remain raised for many months after withdrawal of therapy (fig. 20.14). Amiodarone and its major metabolite, *N*-desethyl-amiodarone, are present in the liver for several months after stopping the drug [138]. The incidence and severity

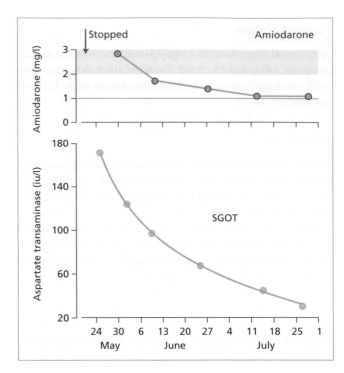

Fig. 20.14. Aspartate transaminase (SGOT) and blood amiodarone levels in a 63-year-old physician. Note the persistence of blood amiodarone levels 2 months after stopping therapy.

of side-effects correlates with the serum concentration, and the dose must be kept between 210 and 600 mg daily.

Amiodarone is iodinated and this results in an increased density on a CT scan. This does not correlate with hepatic injury.

Hepatic histology shows an acute alcoholic hepatitis-like picture with fibrosis and, sometimes, pronounced bile ductular proliferation. Electron microscopy shows phospholipid-laden lysosomal lamellar bodies containing myelin figures (fig. 20.15) [78]. These are constantly found in amiodarone-treated patients and signify drug exposure, not drug toxicity. Swollen granular zone 3 macrophages, presumably iodine-laden lysosomal bodies, may be an early marker of amiodarone hepatotoxicity. Either the drug itself or its main metabolite probably inhibit lysosomal phospholipases responsible for catabolizing phospholipids.

A similar phospholipidosis can be found with *parenteral nutrition* and complicating *trimethoprim–cotrimoxazole* therapy (Septrin, Bactrim) [93].

Synthetic oestrogens

A picture of 'alcoholic hepatitis' has been associated with massive doses of synthetic oestrogen used to treat prostatic cancer [132].

Calcium channel blockers

Nifedipine has been associated with steato-hepatitis but more evidence is required. Diltiazem has been associated with fevers, headache and abnormal transaminases within 18 days of starting treatment. Liver biopsy shows many well-defined granulomas [125].

Fibrosis

Fibrosis forms part of most drug reactions, but in some it may be the predominant feature. The fibrous tissue is deposited in the Disse space, where it obstructs sinusoidal blood flow, causing non-cirrhotic portal hypertension and hepato-cellular dysfunction. The lesion is related to toxic drug metabolites and is usually in zone 3, an exception being methotrexate where the damage is in zone 1.

Methotrexate

Hepato-toxicity results from a toxic metabolite of microsomal origin which induces fibrosis and ultimately cirrhosis (fig. 20.16). Primary liver cancer can develop. Hepato-toxicity is likely to follow long-term therapy, usually for psoriasis, rheumatoid arthritis or leukaemia. The risk seems to be lower in rheumatoid patients than in those with psoriasis [161]. Symptomatic liver disease is rare. Serial liver biopsies usually show benign appearances but three of 45 patients with rheumatoid arthritis developed serious liver disease [109]. Fibrosis may be graded from mild, which is probably insignificant, to significant and even to cirrhosis when the drug should be stopped.

Fibrosis is dose and duration dependent. When given in three 5-mg doses at 12-h intervals each week (i.e. 15 mg/week), it seems safe. Baseline liver biopsies are only indicated in those at particular risk, having significant alcohol intake or a history of liver disease. Serum transaminases are a poor reflection of underlying liver disease but should be monitored monthly; increases indicate that a liver biopsy should be done. In all cases a routine liver biopsy should be performed at 2 years or when the cumulative dose of methotrexate exceeds 1.5 g.

Ultrasound may be useful in detecting fibrosis and indicating stopping therapy. Hepatic transplantation has been performed for severe methotrexate hepato-toxicity [44].

Other cytotoxic drugs

These have a wide range of hepato-toxicity. The liver, however, is surprisingly resistant to injury by cytotoxic drugs, perhaps due to its low proliferative rate and extensive detoxifying capabilities.

Cytotoxic drugs cause rises in serum transaminases if large amounts are given. Drugs such as methotrexate, azathioprine and cyclophosphamide cause zone 3 necrosis, fibrosis and cirrhosis. Mild sclerosis of some portal zones results in the picture of idiopathic portal hypertension after cytotoxic therapy for leukaemia [134].

Veno-occlusive disease (VOD) is associated with cyclophosphamide, busulphan and irradiation. *Cholestasis* may be dose-related due to such drugs as cytosine arabinoside, or *hepato-canalicular* due to azathioprine. *Sinusoidal dilatation, peliosis* and *tumours* are associated with sex and anabolic hormone therapy. One drug

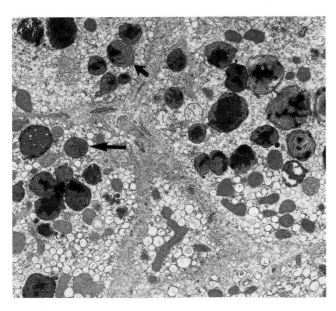

Fig. 20.15. Amiodarone hepato-toxicity: electron microscopy of the liver showing lysosomal lamellar bodies containing myelin figures (arrows).

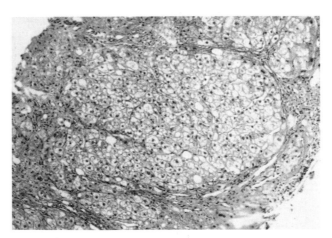

Fig. 20.16. Methotrexate liver injury. The zonal architecture is maintained. The portal zones are expanded with fibrous tissue and mononuclear cells. The hepatocytes show fatty change. (H & E, ×65.)

may enhance the toxicity of another, for instance 6-mercaptopurine effects are worsened by doxorubicin.

Long-term use of cytotoxic agents in recipients of renal transplants or in children with acute lymphatic leukaemia leads to chronic hepatitis, fibrosis and portal hypertension.

Arsenic

The organic, trivalent compounds are particularly poisonous. Arsenic trioxide 1% (Fowler's solution) given for long periods for the treatment of psoriasis has resulted in non-cirrhotic portal hypertension [100]. Acute, probably homicidal, arsenic poisoning can cause perisinusoidal fibrosis and VOD [66].

Arsenic in drinking water and native drugs in India may be related to 'idiopathic' portal hypertension. The liver

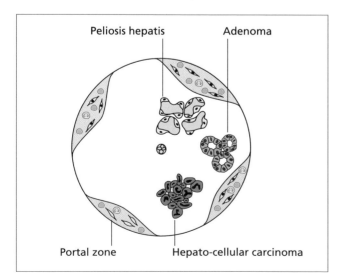

Fig. 20.17. Arsenic hepato-toxicity following treatment of psoriasis. Zone 1 is expanded by fibrosis and sclerosis of portal vein radicles. (Mallory's trichrome stain.)

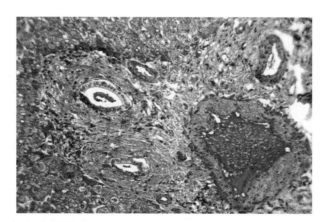

Fig. 20.18. Toxic effects of vinyl chloride, arsenic and thorotrast on the liver.

shows portal tract fibrosis and sclerosis of the portal vein branches (fig. 20.17). Angiosarcoma is a complication.

Vinyl chloride

Workers exposed to vinyl chloride monomer over many years develop hepato-toxicity (fig. 20.18). The earliest change is a sclerosis of portal venules in zone 1 of the liver with the clinical changes of splenomegaly and portal hypertension. Later associations include angiosarcoma of the liver and peliosis hepatis. Early histological alterations indicative of vinyl monomer exposure are focal hepato-cellular and focal mixed hepatocyte and sinusoidal cell hyperplasia. These are followed by sub-capsular portal and perisinusoidal fibrosis.

Vitamin A

Vitamin A is being increasingly used in dermatology, by food faddists, in cancer prevention and for hypogonadism. Toxicity develops with as little as 25 000 iu daily over 6 years or 50 000 iu daily for 2 years [42]. It is potentiated by alcohol abuse.

The patient presents with nausea, vomiting, hepatomegaly, abnormal biochemical tests and portal hypertension. Ascites, either exudate or transudate, may develop. Histology shows hyperplasia of fat-storing (Ito) cells with vacuoles which fluoresce under ultraviolet light. Fibrosis and cirrhosis may develop [42].

Vitamin A is slowly metabolized from the hepatic stores and may be identified in the liver months after stopping treatment.

Retinoids

These vitamin A derivatives are used largely in dermatology. Etretinate, which is structurally similar to retinol, has caused severe hepatic reactions. Hepato-toxicity has also been reported with its metabolite, acitretin [151], and with isotretinoin.

Vascular changes

Sinusoidal dilatation

Focal dilatation of zone 1 sinusoids may complicate contraceptive or anabolic steroid therapy. This can cause hepatomegaly and abdominal pain with rises in serum enzymes. Hepatic arteriography shows stretched, attenuated branches of the hepatic artery with a patchy parenchymal pattern where areas of contrast alternate with areas which are not well filled.

The condition regresses on stopping the hormone.

A similar change may complicate azathioprine given after renal transplantation and this may be followed 1–3 years later by fibrosis and cirrhosis.

Peliosis hepatis

The large blood-filled cavities may or may not be lined with sinusoidal cells (fig. 20.19). They are distributed randomly, the diameter varying from 1 mm to several centimetres [168]. Electron microscopy shows the passage of red blood cells through the endothelial barrier and perisinusoidal fibrosis may develop. These alterations might constitute the primary event [167].

Peliosis has been described in patients taking oral contraceptives, in men having androgenic and anabolic steroids, and following tamoxifen. Peliosis has been reported in recipients of renal transplants. It has also complicated danazol therapy.

Veno-occlusive disease (VOD)

Small, zone 3 hepatic veins are particularly sensitive to toxic damage, reacting by sub-endothelial oedema and subsequent collagenization. The disease was originally described from Jamaica due to toxic injury to the minute hepatic veins by pyrrolizidine alkaloids taken as *Senecio* in medicinal bush teas. It has since been described from India [146], Israel, Egypt and even Arizona. It has been related to contamination of wheat [146].

The disease is marked by an acute stage with painful hepatomegaly, ascites and inconspicuous jaundice. The patient may recover, die or pass into a sub-acute stage of hepatomegaly and recurrent ascites. The chronic type resembles any other cirrhosis. Diagnosis is made by liver biopsy.

Azathioprine induces endotheliitis. Its long-term use in kidney and liver transplant recipients is associated with sinusoidal dilatation, peliosis, VOD and nodular regenerative hyperplasia [141].

Cytotoxic therapy especially with cyclophosphamide BNCU, azathioprine, busulphan, VP-16 and total body irradiation exceeding 12 Gy are associated with VOD. VOD follows high-dose cytoreductive therapy in bone marrow recipients [136]. There is widespread damage to zone 3 structures including hepatocytes, sinusoids and particularly small hepatic venules. It is marked by jaundice, painful hepatomegaly and weight gain (ascites). In 25% of patients it is severe with death occurring within 100 days.

Hepatic irradiation. The liver has a low tolerance to radiotherapy. Radiation hepatitis increases when doses reach or exceed 35 Gy to the whole organ delivered as 10 Gy/week. VOD appears 1–3 months after completion of therapy. It may be transient or death may ensue from liver failure. Histologically, zone 3 haemorrhage is seen with hepatic venules showing fibrosis and obliteration.

Hepatic vein occlusion (Budd–Chiari syndrome) has been reported following oral contraceptives, and after azathioprine in a renal transplant patient (Chapter 11) [150].

Acute hepatitis

The reaction is immuno-allergic. A drug metabolite binds covalently to a particular membrane P450. This metabolite–P450 acts as neoantigen and stimulates the immune system to form autoantibodies (fig. 20.20) [122]. In metabolically and immunologically susceptible subjects, the immune reaction is severe enough to destroy the hepatocyte.

Only a very small proportion of patients taking the drug will have this reaction. There is usually no method of predicting who will be susceptible. The reaction is unrelated to dose, but is commoner after multiple exposures. The onset is delayed until about 1 week after exposure, and it usually appears within 12 weeks of starting therapy.

The reaction is usually hepatic, the clinical picture resembling acute viral hepatitis. Biochemical tests indicate hepato-cellular damage. Serum γ-globulins are increased.

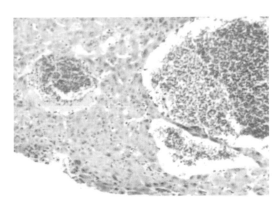

Fig. 20.19. Peliosis hepatis. A dilated blood space is seen with no clear-cut wall.

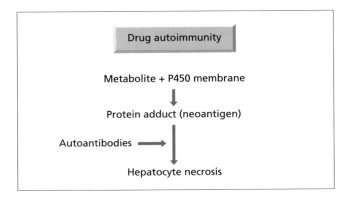

Fig. 20.20. Possible mechanism of drug-related autoimmune hepatocyte necrosis.

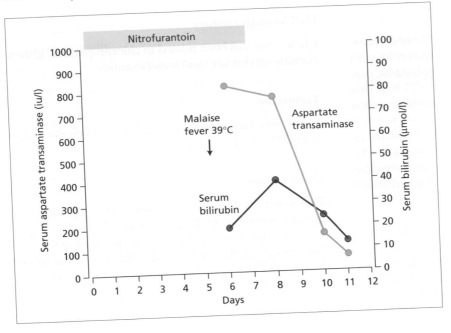

Fig. 20.28. Nitrofurantoin therapy for a urinary tract infection was followed 5 days later by a systemic reaction with jaundice. On stopping the drug the patient recovered rapidly.

Bile duct stricture can follow 10 years after upper abdominal *radiotherapy* [20].

Hepatic nodules and tumours

These are discussed more fully in Chapter 30.

Hepatic adenomas can be associated with sex hormones, particularly oral birth control pills [7]. The incidence is falling as the present pill contains reduced amounts of hormone. If possible, treatment should be conservative as the tumour may show spontaneous regression when hormones are stopped. Pregnancy is avoided.

Women taking hormones, particularly for many years, should be warned of the possibility of adenoma development. If adenoma is diagnosed, the woman must be warned of the possibility of rupture and the significance of any unexplained right upper quadrant pain or swelling in the abdomen. Surgery may be needed for complications, particularly intra-peritoneal or intra-tumour bleeding, severe abdominal pain and anaemia.

Hepato-cellular carcinoma

There is a low, but probably increased, risk of hepato-cellular carcinoma in women receiving oral contraceptives for 8 years or more. The tumour develops in a non-cirrhotic liver, metastases rarely and does not infiltrate [51]. Young women with oral contraceptive exposure tend to survive longer, have fewer symptoms and lower serum α-fetoprotein levels than those developing hepato-cellular carcinoma without exposure to hormones. Tumours are more vascular and haemoperitoneum is commoner.

Adenomas and carcinoma have been associated with *danazol* [39].

Vascular lesions may accompany adenoma or focal nodular hyperplasia. Large arteries and veins are present in excess, sinusoids may be focally dilated and *peliosis* may be present.

Focal nodular hyperplasia does not have such a strong association with hormones as adenoma. It affects both sexes, including children, but especially women in their reproductive years, some of whom may never have taken sex hormones. Asymptomatic patients should be observed regularly. In the symptomatic, stopping the hormones may lead to the lesion regressing. In others, and in particular those with complications, surgical resection is indicated.

Androgenic and *anabolic steroids* can be associated with adenoma, peliosis, nodular regenerative hyperplasia and particularly hepato-cellular carcinoma. Angiosarcoma may be associated. The drugs may be given for aplastic anaemia, hypopituitarism, eunuchoidism, impotency, in female transexuals [160] and in athletes to increase muscle mass [26]. Hepato-cellular cancer is much more frequent with male than female hormone therapy, perhaps due to the much larger doses given. The incidence of hepatic abnormality may be very high, in one series 19 of 60 patients given methyltestosterone showed abnormal liver function tests [160].

Angiosarcoma may follow androgenic anabolic steroids, vinyl chloride, thorotrast and inorganic arsenic.

Epithelioid haemangio-endothelioma is a rare malignant vascular tumour that has been related to oral contraceptive use [29] and to vinyl chloride [41].

Conclusions

Before marketing a new drug, testing must be done on both an acute and chronic basis and on more than one species or strain. Both the drug and its known metabolites must be used. The albumin-binding properties of the drug must be noted. The role of the drug as a hepatic enzyme-inducer must be studied. Clinical trials must include regular pre- and post-treatment estimations of serum bilirubin and transaminase levels. A needle liver biopsy, after informed consent, is particularly helpful in establishing the relation between a drug and liver injury and in determining the type of injury.

The serum transaminases may rise during the first 4 weeks of therapy only to subside despite the drug being continued. When a hepatic reaction is possible, as with isoniazid, it is wise to check serum transaminases 3 and 4 weeks after commencing treatment. If more than three times increased, the drug should be stopped. If less, a further value is taken 1 week later when an increase is an indication for stopping the drug. Continuance of therapy once a hepatic reaction has commenced is the commonest cause of a fatal outcome.

The safety of a drug which causes transient rises in transaminases and apparently no other hepatic effects remains obscure. Many valuable drugs in widespread use fall into this category. In many instances, challenge is the only method of linking a drug with a hepatic reaction, but if its consequence is likely to be serious, this is ethically impossible. However, reporting agencies and drug manufacturers should pay particular attention to the results of inadvertent challenge and to the effects of withdrawing the drug (de-challenge).

Intake of a drug, such as paracetamol, within the therapeutic range, may cause liver injury if the patient is ingesting another drug, such as alcohol, which by enzyme induction increases the production of hepatotoxic metabolites.

An iatrogenic cause must be considered in any patient presenting with any clinical pattern of hepato-biliary disease. This is particularly so with a picture suggesting viral hepatitis in a middle-aged or elderly patient, especially a woman. In the absence of evidence supporting genuine viral hepatitis, the cause is very frequently drug-related.

Widespread recognition of the relation between a drug and a hepatic reaction would follow increased reporting to agencies such as the Committee for Safety of Medicines in the UK, or Medwatch in the USA.

Some catastrophies would be avoided if clinical trials included subjects of all ages, from children to old people, and those with liver disease.

References

1 Altraif I, Lilly L, Wanless IR *et al.* Cholestatic liver disease with ductopenia (vanishing bile duct syndrome) after administration of clindamycin and trimethoprim-sulfamethoxazole. *Am. J. Gastroenterol.* 1994; **89**: 1230.
2 Amitrano L, Gigliotti T, Guardascione MA *et al.* Enoxacin acute liver injury. *J. Hepatol.* 1992; **15**: 270.
3 Andreu V, Mas A, Bruguara M *et al.* Ecstasy: a common cause of severe acute hepatotoxicity. *J. Hepatol.* 1998; **29**: 394.
4 Assal F, Spahr L, Hadangue A *et al.* Tolcapone and fulminant hepatitis. *Lancet* 1998; **352**: 958 (letter).
5 Ault A. Troglitazone may cause irreversible liver damage. *Lancet* 1997; **350**: 1451.
6 Banks AT, Zimmerman HJ, Ishak KG *et al.* Diclofenac-associated hepatotoxicity: analysis of 180 cases reported to the Food and Drug Administration as adverse reactions. *Hepatology* 1995; **22**: 821.
7 Baum JK, Bookstein JJ, Holtz F *et al.* Possible association between benign hepatomas and oral contraceptives. *Lancet* 1973; **ii**: 926.
8 Bernal W, Wendon J, Rela M *et al.* Use and outcome of liver transplantation in acetaminophen-induced acute liver failure. *Hepatology* 1998; **27**: 1050.
9 Berson A, Renault S, Letteron P *et al.* Uncoupling of rat and human mitochondria: a possible explanation for tacrine-induced liver dysfunction. *Gastroenterology* 1996; **110**: 1878.
10 Bissuel F, Bruneel F, Harbersetzer F *et al.* Fulminant hepatitis with severe lactate acidosis in HIV-infected patients on didanosine therapy. *J. Intern. Med.* 1994; **235**: 367.
11 Black M, Mitchell JR, Zimmerman HJ *et al.* Isoniazid-associated hepatitis in 114 patients. *Gastroenterology* 1975; **69**: 289.
12 Black M, Rabin L, Schatz N. Nitrofurantoin-induced chronic active hepatitis. *Ann. Intern. Med.* 1980; **92**: 62.
13 Blake JC, Sawyer AM, Dooley JS *et al.* Severe hepatitis caused by cyproterone acetate. *Gut* 1990; **31**: 556.
14 Bonkovsky HL, Kane RE, Jones DP *et al.* Acute hepatitis and renal toxicity from low doses of acetaminophen in the absence of alcohol abuse or malnutrition: evidence for increased susceptibility to drug toxicity due to cardiopulmonary and renal insufficiency. *Hepatology* 1994; **19**: 1141.
15 Bossard R, Stieger B, O'Neill B *et al.* Ethinylestradiol treatment induces multiple canalicular membrane alterations in rat liver. *J. Clin. Invest.* 1993; **91**: 2714.
16 Bridger S, Henderson K, Glucksman F *et al.* Deaths from low dose paracetamol poisoning. *Br. Med. J.* 1998; **316**: 1724.
17 Callaghan R, Desmond PV, Paull P *et al.* Hepatic enzyme activity is the major factor determining elimination rate of high-clearance drugs in cirrhosis. *Hepatology* 1993; **18**: 54.
18 Cameron RG, Feuer G, de la Iglesia FA, eds. *Drug-induced Hepatotoxicity.* Springer, Berlin, 1996.
19 Castiella A, Lopez Dominguez L, Txoperena G *et al.* Indication for liver transplantation in *Amanita phalloides* poisoning. *Presse Med.* 1993; **22**: 117 (letter).
20 Cherqui D, Palazzo L, Piedbois P *et al.* Common bile duct

stricture as a late complication of upper abdominal radiotherapy. *J. Hepatol.* 1994; **21**: 693.

21 Chien R-N, Yang L-J, Lin P-Y *et al.* Hepatic injury during ketoconazole therapy in patients with onychomycosis: a controlled cohort study. *Hepatology* 1997; **25**: 103.

22 Ching CK, Smith PG, Long RG. Tamoxifen associated hepatocellular damage and agranulocytosis. *Lancet* 1992; **339**: 940 (letter).

23 Cicogani C, Malavolti M, Morselli-Labate AM *et al.* Flutamide-induced toxic hepatitis. Potential utility of ursodeoxycholic acid administration in toxic hepatitis. *Dig. Dis. Sci.* 1996; **41**: 2219.

24 Clark JA, Zimmerman HJ, Tanner LA. Labetalol hepatotoxicity. *Ann. Intern. Med.* 1990; **113**: 210.

25 Corbella X, Vadillo M, Cabellos C *et al.* Hypersensitivity hepatitis due to pyrazinamide. *Scand. J. Infect. Dis.* 1995; **27**: 93.

26 Creagh TM, Rubin A, Evans DJ. Hepatic tumours induced by anabolic steroids in an athlete. *J. Clin. Pathol.* 1988; **41**: 441.

27 Dalton TA, Perry RS. Hepatotoxicity associated with sustained-release niacin. *Am. J. Med.* 1992; **93**: 102.

28 De Graaf EM, Oosterveld M, Tjabbes T *et al.* A case of tizanidine-induced hepatic injury. *J. Hepatol.* 1996; **25**: 772.

29 Dean PJ, Haggitt RC, O'Hara CJ. Malignant epithelioid haemangioendothelioma of the liver in young women: relationship to oral contraceptive use. *Am. J. Surg. Pathol.* 1985; **9**: 695.

30 Degott C, Feldmann G, Larrey D *et al.* Drug-induced prolonged cholestasis in adults: a histological semiquantitative study demonstrating progressive ductopenia. *Hepatology* 1992; **15**: 244.

31 Diaz D, Febre I, Daujat M *et al.* Omeprazole is an aryl hydrocarbon-like inducer of human hepatic cytochrome P-450. *Gastroenterology* 1990; **99**: 737.

32 Dincsoy HP, Saelinger DA. Haloperidol-induced chronic cholestatic liver disease. *Gastroenterology* 1982; **83**: 694.

33 Durand F, Bernuau J, Pessayre D *et al.* Deleterious influence of pyrazinamide on the outcome of patients with fulminant or subfulminant liver failure during antituberculous treatment, including isoniazid. *Hepatology* 1995; **21**: 929.

34 Dykhuizen RS, Brunt PW, Atkinson P *et al.* Ecstasy induced hepatitis mimicking viral hepatitis. *Gut* 1995; **36**: 939.

35 Eliasson E, Stal P, Oksanon A *et al.* Expression of autoantibodies to specific cytochromes P450 in a case of disulfiram hepatitis. *J. Hepatol.* 1998; **29**: 819.

36 Ellis AJ, Wendon JA, Portmann B *et al.* Acute liver damage and ecstasy ingestion. *Gut* 1996; **38**: 454.

37 Fairley CK, McNeil JJ, Desmond P *et al.* Risk factors for development of flucloxacillin associated jaundice. *Br. Med. J.* 1993; **306**: 233.

38 Farrell GC. *Drug-induced Liver Disease.* Churchill Livingstone, Edinburgh, 1994.

39 Fermand JP, Levy Y, Bouscary D *et al.* Danazol-induced hepatocellular adenoma. *Am. J. Med.* 1990; **88**: 529.

40 Fidler H, Dhillon A, Gertner D *et al.* Chronic ecstasy (3, 4-methylenedioxymeta-amphetamine) abuse: a recurrent and unpredictable cause of severe acute hepatitis. *J. Hepatol.* 1996; **25**: 563.

41 Gelin M, Van de Stadt J, Rickaert F *et al.* Epithelioid haemangioendothelioma of the liver following contact with vinyl chloride. *J. Hepatol.* 1989; **8**: 99.

42 Geubel AP, De Galocsy C, Alves N *et al.* Liver damage caused by therapeutic vitamin A administration: estimate of dose-related toxicity in 41 cases. *Gastroenterology* 1991; **100**: 1701.

43 Gil ML, Ramirez MC, Terencio MC *et al.* Immunochemical detection of protein adducts in cultured human hepatocytes exposed to diclofenac. *Biochem. Biophys. Acta* 1995; **1272**: 140.

44 Gilbert SC, Klintmalm G, Menter A *et al.* Methotrexate-induced cirrhosis requiring liver transplantation in three patients with psoriasis. A word of caution in the light of the expanding use of this 'steroid-sparing' agent. *Arch. Intern. Med.* 1990; **150**: 889.

45 Goldstein PE, Deviere J, Cremer M. Acute hepatitis and drug-induced lupus induced by minocycline treatment. *Am. J. Gastroenterol.* 1997; **92**: 143.

46 Gonzalez FJ, Skoda RC, Kimura S *et al.* Characterization of the common genetic defect in humans deficient in debrisoquine metabolism. *Nature* 1988; **331**: 442.

47 Gough A, Chapman S, Wagstaff K *et al.* Minocycline induced autoimmune hepatitis and systemic lupus erythematosus-like syndrome. *Br. Med. J.* 1996; **312**: 169.

48 Harrison PM, Keays R, Bray GP *et al.* Improved outcome of paracetamol-induced fulminant hepatic failure by late administration of acetylcysteine. *Lancet* 1990; **335**: 1572.

49 Hassanein T, Razack A, Gavaler JS *et al.* Heatstroke: its clinical and pathological presentation, with particular attention to the liver. *Am. J. Gastroenterol.* 1992; **87**: 1382.

50 Hautekeete ML, Kockx MM, Naegels S *et al.* Cholestatic hepatitis related to quinolones: a report of two cases. *J. Hepatol.* 1995; **23**: 759 (letter).

51 Henderson BE, Preston-Martin S, Edmondson HA *et al.* Hepatocellular carcinoma and oral contraceptives. *Br. J. Cancer* 1983; **48**: 437.

52 Hjelm M, de Silva LVK, Seakins JWT *et al.* Evidence of inherited urea cycle defect in a case of fatal valproate toxicity. *Br. Med. J.* 1986; **292**: 23.

53 Hoet P, Graf MLM, Bourdi M *et al.* Epidemic of liver disease caused by hydrochlorofluorocarbons used as ozone-sparing substitutes of chlorofluorocarbons. *Lancet* 1997; **350**: 556.

54 Hoyumpa AM, Schenker S. Is glucuronidation truly preserved in patients with liver disease? *Hepatology* 1991; **13**: 786.

55 International Group. Guidelines for diagnosis of therapeutic drug-induced liver injury in liver biopsies. *Lancet* 1974; **i**: 854.

56 Kadmon M, Klünemann C, Böhme M *et al.* Inhibition by cyclosporin A of adenosine triphosphate-dependent transport from the hepatocyte into bile. *Gastroenterology* 1993; **104**: 1507.

57 Kawahara H, Marceau N, French SW. Effects of chlorpromazine and low calcium on the cytoskeleton and the secretory function of hepatocytes *in vitro*. *J. Hepatol.* 1990; **10**: 8.

58 Keeffe EB, Reis TC, Berland JE. Hepatotoxicity to both erythromycin estolate and erythromycin ethylsuccinate. *Dig. Dis. Sci.* 1982; **27**: 701.

59 Keeffe EB, Sunderland M, Gabourel JD. Serum gamma-glutamyl transpeptidase activity in patients receiving chronic phenytoin therapy. *Dig. Dis. Sci.* 1986; **31**: 1056.

60 Keiding S. Drug administration to liver patients: aspects of liver pathophysiology. *Semin. Liver Dis.* 1995; **15**: 268.

61 Kelly BD, Heneghan MA, Bennani F *et al.* Nitrofurantoin-

induced hepatotoxicity mediated by CD8+ T-cells. *Am. J. Gastroenterol.* 1998; **93**: 819.

62 Kharasch ED, Hankins D, Mautz D *et al.* Identification of the enzyme responsible for oxidative halothane metabolism: implications for prevention of halothane hepatitis. *Lancet* 1996; **347**: 1367.

63 Kohlroser J, Mathai J, Reichheld J *et al.* Hepatotoxicity due to troglitazone: a report of two cases and review of adverse events reported to the United States Food and Drug Administration. *Am. J. Gastroenterol.* 2000; **95**: 272.

64 Kowdley KV, Keeffe EB, Fawaz KA. Prolonged cholestasis due to trimethoprim sulfamethoxazole. *Gastroenterology* 1992; **102**: 2148.

65 Kretz-Rommel A, Boelsterli UA. Cytotoxic activity of T-cells and non-T-cells from diclofenac-immunized mice against cultured syngeneic hepatocytes exposed to diclofenac. *Hepatology* 1995; **22**: 213.

66 Labadie H, Stoessel P, Callard P *et al.* Hepatic veno-occlusive disease and perisinusoidal fibrosis secondary to arsenic poisoning. *Gastroenterology* 1990; **99**: 1140.

67 Labowitz JK, Silverman WB. Cholestatic jaundice induced by ciprofloxacin. *Dig. Dis. Sci.* 1997; **42**: 192.

68 Lake-Bakkaar G, Scheuer PJ, Sherlock S. Hepatic reactions associated with ketoconazole in the United Kingdom. *Br. Med. J.* 1987; **294**: 419.

69 Larrey D. Hepatotoxicity of herbal remedies. *J. Hepatol.* 1997; **26** (Suppl. 1): 47.

70 Larrey D, Branch RA. Clearance by the liver: current concepts in understanding the hepatic disposition of drugs. *Semin. Liver Dis.* 1983; **3**: 285.

71 Larrey D, Geneve J, Pessayre D *et al.* Prolonged cholestasis after cyproheptadine-induced acute hepatitis. *J. Clin. Gastroenterol.* 1987; **9**: 102.

72 Larrey D, Hadengue A, Pessayre D *et al.* Carbamazepine-induced acute cholangitis. *Dig. Dis. Sci.* 1987; **32**: 554.

73 Larrey D, Vial T, Micaleff A *et al.* Hepatitis associated with amoxycillin-clavulanic acid combination report of 15 cases. *Gut* 1992; **33**: 368.

74 Larrey D, Vial T, Pauwels A *et al.* Hepatitis after germander (*Teucrium chamaedrys*) administration: another instance of herbal medicine hepatotoxicity. *Ann. Intern. Med.* 1992; **117**: 129.

75 Lavrijsen AP, Balmus KJ, Nugteren-Huying WM *et al.* Hepatic injury associated with itraconazole. *Lancet* 1992; **340**: 251 (letter).

76 Lazaros GA, Papatheodonridis GV, Delladatsima JK *et al.* Terbinafine-induced cholestatic liver disease. *J. Hepatol.* 1996; **24**: 753.

77 Lee WM. Drug-induced hepatotoxicity. *N. Engl. J. Med.* 1995; **333**: 1121.

78 Lewis JH, Ranard RC, Caruso A *et al.* Amiodarone hepatotoxicity: prevalence and clinicopathologic correlations among 104 patients. *Hepatology* 1989; **9**: 679.

79 Lewis JH, Zimmerman HJ, Ishak KG *et al.* Enflurane hepatotoxicity: a clinicopathologic study of 24 cases. *Ann. Intern. Med.* 1983; **98**: 984.

80 Liaw Y-F, Huang M-J, Fan K-D *et al.* Hepatic injury during propylthiouracil therapy in patients with hyperthyroidism. A cohort study. *Ann. Intern. Med.* 1993; **118**: 424.

81 Loeper J, Descatoire V, Letteron P *et al.* Hepatotoxicity of germander in mice. *Gastroenterology* 1994; **106**: 464.

82 Loeper J, Descatoire V, Maurice M *et al.* Presence of functional cytochrome P-450 on isolated rat hepatocyte plasma membrane. *Hepatology* 1990; **11**: 850.

83 Luis A, Rodriguez G, Bruno H *et al.* Risk of acute liver injury associated with the combination of amoxycillin and clavulanic acid. *Arch. Intern. Med.* 1996; **156**: 1327.

84 MacFarlane B, Davies S, Mannan K *et al.* Fatal acute fulminant liver failure due to clozapine: a case report and review of clozapine-induced hepatotoxicity. *Gastroenterology* 1997; **112**: 1707.

85 Macilwain C. NIH, FDA seek lessons from hepatitis B drug trial deaths. *Nature* 1993; **364**: 275.

86 Maganto P, Traber PG, Rusnell C *et al.* Long-term maintenance of the adult pattern of liver-specific expression for P-450b, P450e, albumin and α-fetoprotein genes in intrasplenically transplanted hepatocytes. *Hepatology* 1990; **11**: 585.

87 Mahler H, Pasi A, Kramer JM *et al.* Fulminant liver failure in association with the emetic toxin of *Bacillus cereus*. *N. Engl J Med.* 1997; **336**: 1142.

88 Makin AJ, Wendon J, Williams R. A 7 year experience of severe acetaminophen-induced hepatotoxicity (1987–93). *Gastroenterology* 1995; **109**: 1907.

89 Malka D, Pham B-N, Courvalin J-C *et al.* Acute hepatitis caused by alverine associated with antilamin A and C autoantibodies. *J. Hepatol.* 1997; **27**: 399.

90 Martin JL, Plevak DJ, Flannery KD *et al.* Hepatotoxicity after desflurane anaesthesia. *Anaesthesiology* 1995; **83**: 1125.

91 Mitchell JR, Zimmerman HJ, Ishak KG *et al.* Isoniazid liver injury: clinical spectrum, pathology and probable pathogenesis. *Ann. Intern. Med.* 1976; **84**: 181.

92 Mondardini A, Pasquino P, Bernardi P *et al.* Propafenone-induced liver injury: report of a case and review of the literature. *Gastroenterology* 1993; **104**: 1524.

93 Muñoz SJ, Martinez-Hernandez A, Maddrey WC. Intrahepatic cholestasis and phospholipidosis associated with the use of trimethoprim-sulfamethoxazole. *Hepatology* 1990; **12**: 342.

94 Murphy R, Swartz R, Watkins PB. Severe acetaminophen toxicity in a patient receiving isoniazid. *Ann. Intern. Med.* 1990; **113**: 799.

95 Mutimer DJ, Ayres RCS, Neuberger JM *et al.* Serious paracetamol poisoning and the results of liver transplantation. *Gut* 1994; **35**: 809.

96 Myers JL, Augur NA Jr. Hydralazine-induced cholangitis. *Gastroenterology* 1984; **87**: 1185.

97 Nadir A, Agrawal S, King PD *et al.* Acute hepatitis associated with the use of a Chinese herbal product, Ma-huang. *Am. J. Gastroenterol.* 1996; **91**: 1436.

98 Nehra A, Mullick F, Ishak KG *et al.* Pemoline-associated hepatic injury. *Gastroenterology* 1990; **99**: 1517.

99 Neuschwander-Tetri BA, Isley WL, Oki JC *et al.* Troglitazone-induced hepatic failure leading to liver transplantation. *Ann. Intern. Med.* 1998; **129**: 38.

100 Nevens F, Fevery J, Van Steenbergen W *et al.* Arsenic and noncirrhotic portal hypertension. A report of eight cases. *J. Hepatol.* 1990; **11**: 80.

101 Njoku D, Laster MJ, Gong DH *et al.* Biotransformation of halothane, enflurane, isoflurane and desflurane to trifluoroacetylated liver proteins: association between protein acylation and hepatic injury. *Anaesth. Analg.* 1997; **84**: 173.

102 Noseda A, Borsch G, Muller K-M *et al.* Methimazole-associated cholestatic liver injury: case report and brief literative review. *Hepatogastroenterology* 1986; **33**: 244.

103 O'Grady JG. Paracetamol-induced acute liver failure: prevention and management. *J. Hepatol.* 1997; **26** (Suppl. 1): 41.

104 Ozenne G, Manchon ND, Doucet J *et al.* Carbimazole-induced acute cholestatic hepatitis. *J. Clin. Gastroenterol.* 1989; **11**: 95.

105 Pande JN, Singh SPN, Khilnani GC *et al.* Risk factors for hepatotoxicity from antituberculosis drugs: a case–control study. *Thorax* 1996; **51**: 132.

106 Park HZ, Lee SP, Schy AL. Ceftriaxone-associated gallbladder sludge. Indentification of calcium-ceftriaxone salt as a major component of gallbladder precipitate. *Gastroenterology* 1991; **100**: 1665.

107 Parker WB, Cheng YC. Mitochondrial toxicity of antiviral nucleoside analogs. *J. NIH Res.* 1994; **6**: 57.

108 Paterson D, Kerlin P, Walker N *et al.* Piroxicam-induced submassive necrosis of the liver. *Gut* 1992; **33**: 1436.

109 Phillips CA, Cera PJ, Mangan TF *et al.* Clinical liver disease in patients with rheumatoid arthritis taking methotrexate. *J. Rheumatol.* 1992; **19**: 229.

110 Phillips MJ, Oda M, Mak E *et al.* Microfilament dysfunction as a possible cause of intrahepatic cholestasis. *Gastroenterology* 1975; **69**: 48.

111 Picciotto A, Campo N, Brizzolara R *et al.* Chronic hepatitis induced by Jin Bu Huan. *J. Hepatol.* 1998; **28**: 165.

112 Pinto HC, Baptista A, Camilo ME *et al.* Tamoxifen-associated steatohepatitis—report of three cases. *J. Hepatol.* 1995; **23**: 95.

113 Powell-Jackson PR, Tredger JM, Williams R. Progress report, hepatotoxicity to valproate: a review. *Gut* 1984; **25**: 673.

114 Rabinovitz M, Van Thiel DH. Hepatotoxicity of non-steroidal anti-inflammatory drugs. *Am. J. Gastroenterol.* 1992; **87**: 1696.

115 Rabkin MJ, Corless CL, Orloff SL *et al.* Liver transplantation for disulfiran-induced hepatic failure. *Am. J. Gastroenterol.* 1998; **93**: 830.

116 Rahmat J, Gelfand RL, Gelfand MC *et al.* Captopril-associated cholestatic jaundice. *Ann. Intern. Med.* 1985; **102**: 56.

117 Ratanasavanh D, Beaune P, Morel F *et al.* Intralobular distribution and quantification of cytochrome P-450 enzymes in human liver as a function of age. *Hepatology* 1991; **13**: 1142.

118 Read AE, Harrison CV, Sherlock S. Chronic chlorpromazine jaundice: with particular reference to its relationship to primary biliary cirrhosis. *Am. J. Med.* 1961; **31**: 249.

119 Redlich CA, West AB, Fleming L *et al.* Clinical and pathological characteristics of hepatotoxicity associated with occupational exposure to dimethylformamide. *Gastroenterology* 1990; **99**: 748.

120 Reynolds TB, Lapin AC, Peters RL *et al.* Puzzling jaundice. Probable relationship to laxative ingestion. *JAMA* 1970; **211**: 86.

121 Rinder HM, Love JC, Wexler R. Amiodarone hepatotoxicity. *N. Engl. J. Med.* 1986; **314**: 321.

122 Robin MA, Le Roy M, Descatoire V *et al.* Plasma membrane cytochromes P450 as neoantigens and autoimmune targets in drug-induced hepatitis. *J. Hepatol.* 1997; **26** (Suppl. 1): 23.

123 Rosellini SR, Costa PL, Gaudio M *et al.* Hepatic injury related to enalapril. *Gastroenterology* 1989; **97**: 810.

124 Rosenberg WMC, Ryley NG, Trowell JM *et al.* Dextropropoxyphene-induced hepatotoxicity: a report of nine cases. *J. Hepatol.* 1993; **19**: 470.

125 Sarachek NS, London RL, Matulewicz TJ. Diltiazem and granulomatous hepatitis. *Gastroenterology* 1985; **88**: 1260.

126 Scheider DM, Klygis LM, Tsang T-K *et al.* Hepatic dysfunction after repeated isoflurane administration. *J. Clin. Gastroenterol.* 1993; **17**: 168.

127 Schenker S, Bay M. Drug disposition and hepatotoxicity in the elderly. *J. Clin. Gastroenterol.* 1994; **18**: 232.

128 Schenker S, Martin RR, Hoyumpa AM. Antecedent liver disease and drug toxicity. *J. Hepatol.* 1999; **31**: 1098.

129 Schidt FV, Rochling FA, Casey DL *et al.* Acetaminophen toxicity in an urban country hospital. *N. Engl. J. Med.* 1997; **337**: 1112.

130 Schultz JC, Adamson JS Jr, Workman WW *et al.* Fatal liver disease after intravenous administration of tetracycline in high dosage. *N. Engl. J. Med.* 1963; **269**: 999.

131 Seeff LB, Cuccherini BA, Zimmerman HJ *et al.* Acetaminophen hepatotoxicity in alcoholics: a therapeutic misadventure. *Ann. Intern. Med.* 1986; **104**: 399.

132 Seki K, Minami Y, Nishikawa M *et al.* 'Non-alcoholic steatohepatitis' induced by massive doses of synthetic oestrogen. *Gastroenterol. Jpn* 1983; **18**: 197.

133 Sheikh NM, Philen RM, Love LA. Chaparral-associated hepatotoxicity. *Arch. Intern. Med.* 1997; **157**: 913.

134 Shepherd P, Harrison DJ. Idiopathic portal hypertension associated with cytotoxic drugs. *J. Clin. Pathol.* 1990; **43**: 216.

135 Shiffman ML, Keith FB, Moore EW. Pathogenesis of ceftriaxone-associated biliary sludge. *In vitro* studies of calcium-ceftriaxone binding and solubility. *Gastroenterology* 1990; **99**: 1772.

136 Shulman HM, Fisher LB, Schoch G *et al.* Venoocclusive disease of the liver after marrow transplantation: histological correlates of clinical signs and symptoms. *Hepatology* 1994; **19**: 1171.

137 Silva MO, Roth D, Reddy KR et al. Hepatic dysfunction accompanying acute cocaine intoxication. *J. Hepatol.* 1991; **12**: 312.

138 Simon JB, Manley PN, Brien JF *et al.* Amiodarone hepatotoxicity simulating alcoholic liver disease. *N. Engl. J. Med.* 1984; **311**: 167.

139 Steele MA, Burk RF, DesPrez RM. Toxic hepatitis with isoniazid and rifampicin. A meta-analysis. *Chest* 1991; **99**: 465.

140 Sterling MJ, Kane M, Grace ND. Pemoline-induced autoimmune hepatitis. *Am. J. Gastroenterol.* 1996; **91**: 2233.

141 Sterneck M, Wiesner R, Ascher N *et al.* Azathioprine hepatotoxicity after liver transplantation. *Hepatology* 1991; **14**: 806.

142 Stricker BHCh, Blok APR, Babany G *et al.* Fibrin ring granulomas and allopurinol. *Gastroenterology* 1989; **96**: 1199.

143 Stricker BHC, Blok APR, Bronkhorst FB *et al.* Ketoconazole-associated hepatic injury: a clinicopathological study of 55 cases. *J. Hepatol.* 1986; **3**: 399.

144 Stricker BHC, Spoelstra P. *Drug-induced Hepatic Injury.* Elsevier, Amsterdam, 1985.

145 Taggart HMcA, Alderdice JM. Fatal cholestatic jaundice in elderly persons taking benoxaprofen. *Br. Med. J.* 1982; **284**: 1372.

146 Tameda Y, Hamada M, Takase K *et al.* Fulminant hepatic failure caused by ecarazine hydrochloride (a hydralazine) derivative. *Hepatology* 1996; **23**: 465.

147 Tarazi EM, Harter JG, Zimmerman HJ *et al.* Sulindac-associated hepatic injury: analysis of 91 cases reported to the Food and Drug Administration. *Gastroenterology* 1993; **104**: 569.

148 Tyrrell DLJ, Mitchell MC, De Man RA *et al.* Phase II trial of

lamivudine for chronic hepatitis B. *Hepatology* 1993; **18**: 112 A.

149 Ussery XT, Henar EL, Black DD *et al*. Acute liver injury after protracted seizures in children. *J. Paediatr. Gastroenterol. Nutr.* 1989; **9**: 421.

150 Valla D, Le MG, Poynard T *et al*. Risk of hepatic vein thrombosis in relation to recent use of oral contraceptives: a case–control study. *Gastroenterology* 1986; **90**: 807

151 Van Ditzhuijsen TJM, van Haelst UJGM, van Dooren-Greebe RJ. Severe hepatotoxic reaction with progression to cirrhosis after use of a novel retinoid (acitretin). *J. Hepatol.* 1990; **11**: 185.

152 Van Steenbergen W, Peeters P, De Bondt J *et al*. Nimesulide-induced acute hepatitis: evidence from six cases. *J. Hepatol.* 1998; **29**: 135.

153 Van Steenbergen W, Vanstapel MJ, Desmet V *et al*. Cimetidine-induced liver injury. Report of three cases. *J. Hepatol.* 1985; **1**: 359.

154 Van't Wout JW, Herrmann WA, de Vries RA *et al*. Terbinafine-associated hepatic injury. *J. Hepatol.* 1994; **21**: 115.

155 Vorperian VR, Havighurst TC, Miller S *et al*. Adverse effects of low dose amiodarone: a meta-analysis. *J. Am. Coll. Cardiol.* 1997; **30**: 791.

156 Wanless IR, Dore S, Gopinath N *et al*. Histopathology of cocaine hepatotoxicity. Report of four patients. *Gastroenterology* 1990; **98**: 497.

157 Watkins PB. The role of cytochromes P-450 in cyclosporin metabolism. *J. Am. Acad. Dermatol.* 1990; **23**: 1301.

158 Watkins PB. Role of cytochromes P-450 in drug metabolism and hepatotoxicity. *Semin. Liver Dis.* 1990; **10**: 235.

159 Watkins PB, Zimmerman HJ, Knapp MJ *et al*. Hepatotoxic effects of tacrine administration in patients with Alzheimer's disease. *JAMA* 1994; **271**: 992.

160 Westaby D, Ogle SJ, Paradinas FJ *et al*. Liver damage from long-term methyltestosterone. *Lancet* 1977; **ii**: 261.

161 Whiting-O'Keefe QE, Fye KH, Sack KD. Methotrexate and histological hepatic abnormalities: a meta-analysis. *Am. J. Med.* 1991; **90**: 711.

162 Woolf GM, Petrovic LM, Rojter SE *et al*. Acute hepatitis associated with the Chinese herbal product Jin Bu Huan. *Ann. Intern. Med.* 1994; **121**: 729.

163 Wysowski DK, Freiman JP, Tourtelot JB *et al*. Fatal and non-fatal hepatotoxicity associated with flutamide. *Ann. Intern. Med.* 1993; **118**: 860.

164 Yamamoto M, Ogawa K, Morita M *et al*. The herbal medicine Inchin-ko-to inhibits liver cell apoptosis induced by transforming growth factor B1. *Hepatology* 1996; **23**: 552.

165 Yamamoto T, Suou T, Hirayama C. Elevated serum aminotransferase induced by isoniazid in relation to isoniazid acetylator phenotype. *Hepatology* 1986; **6**: 295.

166 Yao F, Behling CA, Saab S *et al*. Trimethoprim-sulfamethoxazole-induced vanishing bile duct syndrome. *Am. J. Gastroenterol.* 1997; **92**: 167.

167 Zafrani ES, Cazier A, Baudelot A-M *et al*. Ultra-structural lesions of the liver in human peliosis: a report of 12 cases. *Am. J. Pathol.* 1984; **114**: 349.

168 Zafrani ES, Pinaudeau Y, Dhumeaux D. Drug-induced vascular lesions of the liver. *Arch. Intern. Med.* 1983; **143**: 495.

169 Zimmerman HJ. *The Adverse Effects of Drugs and Other Chemicals on the Liver*, 2nd edn. Raven Press, New York, 1999.

170 Zimmerman HJ, Maddrey WC. Acetaminophen (paracetamol) hepatotoxicity with regular intake of alcohol: analysis of instances of therapeutic misadventure. *Hepatology* 1995; **22**: 767.

regulate the intermediate metabolism of amino acids, proteins, carbohydrates, lipids and minerals. They interact with classical hormones such as glucocorticoids. Since many cytokines exert growth factor like activity, in addition to their specific pro-inflammatory effects, the distinction between cytokines and growth factors is somewhat artificial. No growth factor or cytokine acts independently.

The liver, predominantly the Kupffer cells, produces pro-inflammatory cytokines such as TNF-α, IL1 and IL6 (fig. 6.9). The liver also clears circulating cytokines, so limiting their systemic action. Failure of clearance may account for some of the immunological changes in cirrhosis. Cytokines may also inhibit hepatic regeneration.

Cytokine production is mediated through activation of monocytes and macrophages by endotoxin of gut origin. In cirrhosis, endotoxaemia is enhanced by increased gut permeability and depressed Kupffer cells which normally prevent uptake of endotoxin by the hepatocyte for detoxification and elimination. Cytokine overproduction mediates some of the systemic changes of cirrhosis, such as fever and anorexia. Fatty acid synthesis is increased by TNF-α, IL1, and interferon-α (IFN-α) with resultant fatty liver.

IL6, IL1 and TNF-α induce hepatic acute-phase protein synthesis with production, amongst others, of C-reactive protein, amyloid A, haptoglobin, complement B and α1-antitrypsin.

The remarkable hepatocyte regenerative capacity after such insults as viral hepatitis or hepatic resection is probably initiated by growth factors interacting with specific receptors on cell surfaces.

Hepatocyte growth factor (HGF) is the most potent stimulator of DNA synthesis in mature hepatocytes, and triggers liver regeneration after injury. It is produced not only by liver cells (including stellate cells) but also in other tissues and by tumours [13]. Production is regulated by several factors including IL1α and IL1β, as well as TGF-β1 and glucocorticoids. It stimulates the growth of other cell types including melanocytes and haemopoietic cells.

Epidermal growth factor (EGF) is formed in regenerating hepatocytes. EGF receptors have a high density on hepatocyte membranes and are also found in the nucleus. EGF uptake is greatest in zone 1 (peri-portal) where regeneration is most active.

TGF-α has a 30–40% sequence homology with EGF and can bind to EGF receptors so initiating hepatocyte replication.

TGF-β1 is probably the major inhibitor of hepatocyte proliferation and is strongly expressed in non-parenchymal cells during liver regeneration. Experimentally TGF-β1 exerts both positive and negative effects, depending on the cell type and culture conditions.

TGF-β inhibits and EGF stimulates amino acid uptake by cultured hepatocytes.

Monitoring fibrogenesis

The proteins and metabolites of connective tissue metabolism spill over into the plasma where they can be measured. Unfortunately, results reflect fibrosis generally and may not give information specifically about hepatic fibrosis.

Aminoterminal *procollagen type III peptide* (PIII-P) is cleaved off the procollagen molecule in the synthesis of a collagen type III fibril. In studies of patients with chronic liver disease there is a relationship between the serum concentration and the degree of hepatic fibrosis [2, 35]. However, because of overlap the value of a single measurement in an individual patient is not of practical diagnostic value. Serum levels may be useful in monitoring hepatic fibrosis particularly in the alcoholic [59]. However increased levels may reflect inflammation and necrosis rather than fibrosis alone.

Many other assays have been studied—the number reflecting the absence of a reliable marker of fibrosis—including hyaluronan, TIMP-1 [42], integrin-β1, YKL-40 [35] and MMP-2 [55]. Urinary desmosine and hydroxylysylpyridinoline, markers of elastin and collagen breakdown, also correlate with hepatic fibrosis [2]. In general, however, these serum and urinary estimations are largely of experimental interest and are infrequently used clinically. Liver biopsy cannot currently be replaced by these markers to assess the degree of fibrosis in the individual patient.

Classification of cirrhosis

Morphological classification

Three anatomical types of cirrhosis are recognized: micronodular, macronodular and mixed.

Micronodular cirrhosis is characterized by thick, regular septa, by regenerating small nodules varying little in size, and by involvement of every lobule (figs 21.5, 21.6). The micronodular liver may represent impaired capacity for regrowth as in alcoholism, malnutrition, old age or anaemia.

Macronodular cirrhosis is characterized by septa and nodules of variable sizes and by normal lobules in larger nodules (figs 21.7, 21.8). Previous collapse is shown by juxtaposition in the fibrous scars of three or more portal tracts. Regeneration is reflected by large cells with large nuclei and by cell plates of varying thickness.

Regeneration in a micronodular cirrhosis results in a macronodular or *mixed* appearance. With time, micronodular cirrhosis often converts to macronodular.

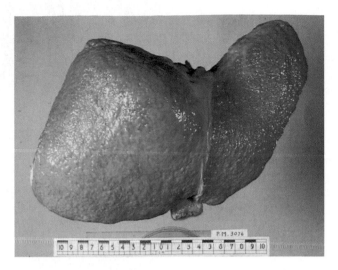

Fig. 21.5. The small finely nodular liver of micronodular cirrhosis.

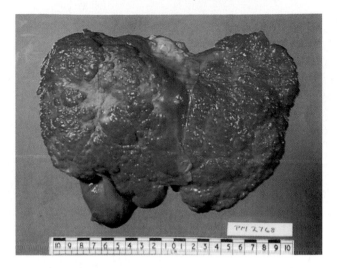

Fig. 21.7. The grossly distorted coarsely nodular liver of macronodular cirrhosis.

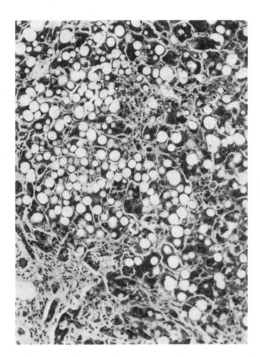

Fig. 21.6. Micronodular cirrhosis. Gross fatty change. The liver cells are often necrotic. Fibrous septa dissect the liver. (H & E, ×135.)

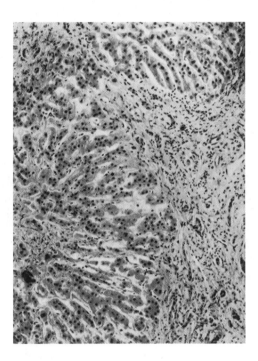

Fig. 21.8. Macronodular cirrhosis. Nodules of regenerating liver cells of different sizes are intersected by fibrous bands of various widths containing proliferating bile ducts. Fatty change is not seen. (H & E, ×135.)

Aetiology (table 21.1)

1 Viral hepatitis types B ± delta; C.
2 Alcohol.
3 Metabolic, e.g. haemochromatosis, Wilson's disease, α_1-antitrypsin deficiency, type IV glycogenosis, galactosaemia, congenital tyrosinosis, non-alcoholic steatohepatitis, intestinal bypass.
4 Prolonged cholestasis, intra- and extra-hepatic.
5 Hepatic venous outflow obstruction, e.g. veno-occlusive disease, Budd–Chiari syndrome, constrictive pericarditis.
6 Disturbed immunity (autoimmune hepatitis).
7 Toxins and therapeutic agents, e.g. methotrexate, amiodarone.
8 Indian childhood cirrhosis.

Other possible factors to be considered include the following.

Table 21.1. Aetiology and definitive treatment of cirrhosis

Aetiology	Treatment
Viral hepatitis (B, C and D)	?Antivirals
Alcohol	Abstention
Metabolic	
iron overload	Venesection. Desferrioxamine
copper overload (Wilson's disease)	Copper chelator
α_1-antitrypsin deficiency	?Transplant
type IV glycogenesis	?Transplant
galactosaemia	Withdraw milk and milk products
tyrosinaemia	Withdraw dietary tyrosine. ?Transplant
Cholestatic (biliary)	Relieve biliary obstruction. ?Transplant
Hepatic venous outflow block	
Budd–Chiari syndrome	Relieve main vein block. ?Transplant
heart failure	Treat cardiac cause
Autoimmune hepatitis	Prednisolone
Toxins and drugs, e.g. methotrexate, amiodarone	Identify and stop
Indian childhood cirrhosis	?Penicillamine
Cryptogenic	—

Malnutrition (Chapter 25).

Infections. Malarial parasites do not cause cirrhosis. The coexistence of malaria and cirrhosis probably reflects malnutrition and viral hepatitis in the community.

Syphilis causes cirrhosis in neonates but not in adults.

In schistosomiasis, the ova excite a fibrous tissue reaction in the portal zones. The association with cirrhosis in certain countries is probably related to other aetiological factors, for example hepatitis C.

Granulomatous lesions. Focal granuloma in such conditions as brucellosis, tuberculosis and sarcoidosis heal with fibrosis, but the liver does not show nodular regrowth.

Cryptogenic cirrhosis. The aetiology is unknown and this is clearly a heterogeneous group. Frequency varies in different parts of the world; in the UK it is about 5–10%, whereas in other areas such as France or in urban parts of the USA where alcoholism is prevalent the proportion is lower. As specific diagnostic criteria appear, so the percentage falls. The advent of testing for hepatitis B and C transferred many previously designated cryptogenic cirrhotics to the post-hepatitic group. Estimations of serum smooth muscle and mitochondrial antibodies and better interpretation of liver histology separate others into the autoimmune chronic hepatitis–primary biliary cirrhosis category. Some of the remainder may be alcoholics who deny alcoholism or have forgotten that they ever consumed alcohol. There remains a hard core of patients in whom the cirrhosis remains cryptogenic. Some of these have features suggesting that non-alcoholic steatohepatitis is responsible [15, 67].

Mechanisms are discussed in individual chapters. The clinical and pathological picture may be that of a 'chronic hepatitis' which has proceeded to cirrhosis.

Anatomical diagnosis

The diagnosis of cirrhosis depends on demonstrating widespread nodules in the liver combined with fibrosis. This may be done by *direct visualization*, for instance at laparotomy or laparoscopy. However, laparotomy should never be used to diagnose cirrhosis because it may precipitate liver failure even in those with very well-compensated disease.

Laparoscopy visualizes the nodular liver and allows directed liver biopsy (fig. 21.9).

Radio-isotope scanning may show decreased hepatic uptake, an irregular pattern and uptake by spleen and bone marrow. Nodules are not identified.

Using *ultrasound*, cirrhosis is suggested by liver surface nodularity (fig. 5.5) and portal vein mean flow velocity [27]. The caudate lobe is enlarged relative to the right lobe. However, ultrasound is not reliable for the diagnosis of cirrhosis. Regenerating nodules may be shown as focal lesions [39]. These should be considered malignant unless proved otherwise by serial imaging and α-fetoprotein levels.

CT scan is cost-effective for the diagnosis of cirrhosis and its complications (fig. 21.10). Liver size can be assessed and the irregular nodular surface seen. Benign regenerative nodules are not visualized by CT. Fatty change, increased density due to iron and a space-occupying lesion can be recognized. After intravenous contrast, the portal vein and hepatic veins can be identified in the liver, and a collateral circulation with splenomegaly may give confirmation to the diagnosis of

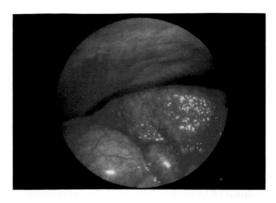

Fig. 21.9. Laparoscopy showing the nodular liver of cirrhosis. Note gallbladder to the left.

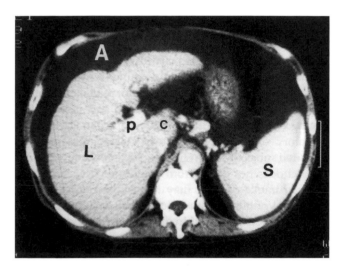

Fig. 21.10. CT scan, after intravenous contrast, in cirrhosis shows ascites (A), small liver with irregular surface (L), enlarged caudate lobe (c), patent portal vein (p) and splenomegaly (S).

Table 21.2. Staining of connective tissue collagen in biopsies

Type	Site	Stained by
I	Portal zones, central zones, broad scars	Van Giesen
II	Sinusoids (elastic tissue)	Elastin
III	Reticulin fibres (sinusoids, portal zones)	Silver
IV	Basement membranes	PAS

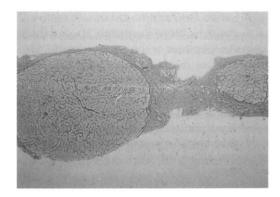

Fig. 21.11. Liver biopsy in cirrhosis: the specimen is small but nodules are shown outlined by reticulin. (Reticulin stain, ×40.)

portal hypertension. Large collateral vessels, usually peri-splenic or para-oesophageal, may add confirmation to a clinical diagnosis of chronic porto-systemic encephalopathy. Ascites can be seen. The CT scan provides an objective record useful for following the course. Directed biopsy of a selected area can be performed safely.

Biopsy diagnosis of cirrhosis may be difficult. Reticulin and collagen stains are essential for the demonstration of a rim of fibrosis around the nodule (fig. 21.11, table 21.2).

Helpful diagnostic points include absence of portal tracts, abnormal vascular arrangements, hepatic arterioles not accompanied by portal veins, the presence of nodules with fibrous septa, variability in liver cell size and appearance in different areas, and thickened liver cell plates [72].

Since neither liver biopsy nor scanning have a diag-nostic sensitivity greater than 90% (ultrasound, 87%; liver biopsy, 62%) [27], it has been proposed that ultrasound be done before liver biopsy is performed [71]. If cirrhosis is suspected on ultrasound (or clinical findings) at least two separate liver biopsy specimens should be taken for histology. If histology does not show cirrhosis but the specimen shows fragmentation, fibrosis or architectural disruption, this together with the ultrasound result should allow a diagnosis of cirrhosis to be made [71].

Functional assessment

Liver failure is assessed by such features as jaundice, ascites (Chapter 9), encephalopathy (Chapter 7), low serum albumin, and a prothrombin deficiency not corrected by vitamin K.

Portal hypertension (Chapter 10) is shown by splenomegaly, oesophageal varices and by the newer methods of measuring portal pressure.

Evolution is monitored by serial clinical, biochemical and histological observations, and classified as progressing, regressing or stationary.

Clinical cirrhosis (table 21.3)

Cirrhosis, apart from other features peculiar to the cause, results in two major events: hepato-cellular failure (Chapters 6, 7 and 9) and portal hypertension (Chapter

walls (*cirrhotic glomerular sclerosis*). Deposits of IgA are most frequent (fig. 21.12) [58, 60]. These are particularly found with alcoholic liver disease. The changes are usually latent, but occasionally are associated with proliferative changes and the clinical manifestations of glomerular involvement. Chronic hepatitis C infection is associated with cryoglobulinaemia and membranoproliferative glomerulonephritis [34].

16 *Infections.* Bacterial infections are frequent due to reduced immune defence mechanisms and impaired reticulo-endothelial cell phagocytic activity. Bacteraemia, pneumonia and urinary tract infections are common. Patients with ascites are prone to spontaneous bacterial peritonitis (SBP) (Chapter 9) present in 10–20% of patients with ascites admitted to hospital [57]. Spontaneous bacterial empyaema in a pre-existing hydrothorax may occur in the absence of SBP [82]. In the cirrhotic with febrile coma, bacterial meningitis should be considered [64]. Nasal carriage of *Staphylococcus aureus* is increased in cirrhotic patients [16].

Sepsis should always be suspected in cirrhotic patients with unexplained pyrexia or deterioration. Empirical treatment with a broad-spectrum antibiotic is often necessary after appropriate specimens have been taken for microbiological culture. After gastrointestinal haemorrhage the risk of sepsis is greater in Child C rather than Child A/B grade cirrhotics (53 vs. 18%). Prophylactic antibiotics (ciprofloxacin and augmentin) reduced the incidence of sepsis in Child C cirrhotics to 13% [63].

There has been a resurgence of tuberculosis, and tuberculous peritonitis is therefore still encountered but often not suspected.

17 *Drug metabolism.* In cirrhotics the effect of drugs is generally increased due to reduced elimination [29]. There are two particular causes: reduced hepatocyte mass rather than enzyme activity [50], and the shunting

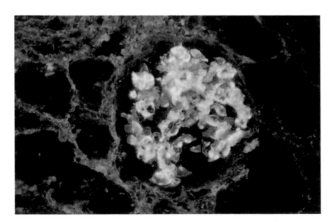

Fig. 21.12. IgA nephropathy: renal biopsy showing IgA deposition in glomerulus of cirrhotic patient (alcohol-related) with creatinine clearance of 20 ml/min and proteinuria (immunostaining with FITC rabbit antihuman IgA).

of blood past the liver. For drugs with a high hepatic extraction ratio (high first-pass effect) predicting the therapeutic effect after oral administration is difficult, due to the variation in the degree of shunting (both porto-systemic and intra-hepatic) between patients. The clinical effect of low extraction drugs in cirrhotics is more dependent on hepato-cellular function and therefore more predictable. Overall drug dosage should be reduced according to the severity of liver disease.

Other components of the metabolic pathway may alter drug handling in cirrhosis including absorption, tissue distribution, protein binding, biliary secretion, enterohepatic circulation and target-organ responsiveness.

18 *Diabetes mellitus.* While up to 80% of cirrhotics are glucose intolerant, only 10–20% are truly diabetic. The prevalence of diabetes is greater among those with hepatitis C or alcohol-related cirrhosis compared with those with cholestatic cirrhosis [84].

19 *Sleep disturbance.* Patients with cirrhosis have abnormalities of sleep pattern, unrelated to hepatic encephalopathy. This may be related to a tendency for being active in the evening, and having a delayed bedtime and wake-up time [19]. This seems part of a broader abnormality of circadian rhythm [12].

Hyperglobulinaemia

Elevation of the total serum globulin, and particularly gamma level, is a well-known accompaniment of chronic liver disease. Electrophoresis shows a polyclonal gamma response, but rarely a monoclonal picture may be seen. The increased γ-globulin values may be related in part to increased tissue autoantibodies, such as smooth muscle antibody. However, the major factor seems to be failure of the damaged liver to clear intestinal antigens (fig. 21.13). Patients with cirrhosis show increased serum antibodies to gastrointestinal tract antigens, particularly *Escherichia coli*. Such antigens bypass the liver through portal-systemic channels or through the internal shunts developing around the cirrhotic nodules. Once in the systemic circulation they provoke an increased antibody response from such organs as the spleen. Systemic endotoxaemia may arise similarly. Polymeric IgA and IgA–antigen complexes of gut origin can also reach the systemic circulation. Suppressor T-lymphocyte function is depressed in chronic liver disease and this would reduce the suppression of B-lymphocytes and so favour antibody production.

Compensated cirrhosis

The disease may be discovered at a routine examination or biochemical screen, or at operation undertaken for some other condition (fig. 21.14). Cirrhosis may be suspected if the patient has mild pyrexia, vascular

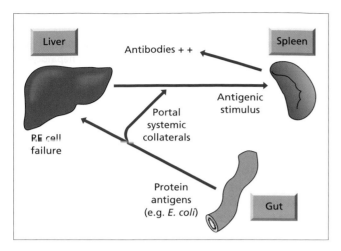

Fig. 21.13. A possible mechanism for the increased serum antibody (and globulin) levels in cirrhosis. Protein antigens from the gut bypass reticulo-endothelial (RE) Kupffer cells in the liver and present an antigenic stimulus to other organs, particularly the spleen, so increasing serum antibodies.

spiders, palmar erythema, or unexplained epistaxis or oedema of the ankles. Firm enlargement of the liver and splenomegaly are helpful diagnostic signs. Vague morning indigestion and flatulent dyspepsia may be early features in the alcoholic cirrhotic. Confirmation should be sought by biochemical tests, scanning and, if necessary, by liver biopsy.

Biochemical tests may be quite normal in this group. The most frequent changes are a slight increase in the serum transaminase or γ-GT level.

Diagnosis is confirmed by *needle liver biopsy*.

These patients may remain compensated until they die from another cause. Some proceed, in a period from months to years, to the stage of hepato-cellular failure. In others the problem is of portal hypertension with oesophageal bleeding. Portal hypertension may be present even with normal liver function tests. The course in the individual patient is very difficult to predict.

Decompensated cirrhosis

The patient usually seeks medical advice because of ascites and/or jaundice. General health fails with weakness, muscle wasting and weight loss. Continuous mild fever (37.5–38°C) is often due to Gram-negative bacteraemia, to continuing hepatic cell necrosis or to a complicating liver cell carcinoma. A liver flap may be present. Cirrhosis is the commonest cause of hepatic encephalopathy.

Jaundice implies that liver cell destruction exceeds the capacity for regeneration and is always serious. The deeper the jaundice the greater the inadequacy of liver cell function.

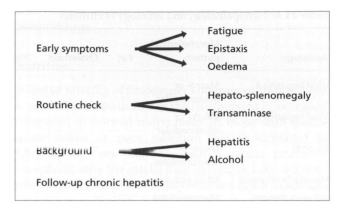

Fig. 21.14. Presentation of 'compensated' hepatic cirrhosis.

The skin may be pigmented. Clubbing of the fingers is occasionally seen. Purpura over the arms, shoulders and shins may be associated with a low platelet count. Spontaneous bruising and epistaxes reflect a prothrombin deficiency. The circulation is over-active. The blood pressure is low. Sparse body hair, vascular spiders, palmar erythema, white nails and gonadal atrophy are common.

Ascites is usually preceded by abdominal distension. Oedema of the legs is frequently associated.

The liver may be enlarged, with a firm regular edge, or contracted and impalpable. The spleen may be palpable.

The differential diagnosis of hepatic encephalopathy, ascites and jaundice are described in Chapters 7, 9 and 12.

Laboratory findings

Haematology. There is usually a mild normocytic, normochromic anaemia; it is occasionally macrocytic. Gastrointestinal bleeding leads to hypochromic anaemia. The leucocyte and platelet counts are reduced ('hypersplenism'). The prothrombin time is prolonged and does not return to normal with vitamin K therapy. The bone marrow is macronormoblastic. Plasma cells are increased in proportion to the hyperglobulinaemia.

Serum biochemical changes. In addition to the raised serum bilirubin level, albumin is depressed and γ-globulin raised. The serum alkaline phosphatase is usually raised to about twice normal; very high readings are occasionally found, particularly with alcoholic cirrhosis. Serum transaminase values may be increased.

Urine. Urobilinogen is present in excess; bilirubin is also present if the patient is jaundiced. The urinary sodium excretion is diminished in the presence of ascites, and in a severe case less than 5 mmol/l is passed daily.

microtubules, a process that can be inhibited by microtubule disruptive drugs such as *colchicine*. Trials have suggested benefit [36] but evidence is not sufficiently strong to recommend the use of long-term colchicine for patients with cirrhosis.

Surgical procedures [25]

All operations in cirrhotic patients carry a high risk and a high mortality. Surgery in non-bleeding cirrhotic patients has an operative mortality of 30% and an additional morbidity rate of 30%. These are related to Child's grade—mortality being 10% in grade A, 31% in grade B, and 76% in grade C patients. Operations on the biliary tract, for peptic ulcer disease or for colon resection have a particularly bad prognosis. Predictive features of a poor outcome include a low serum albumin, the presence of infection and a prolonged prothrombin time. The surgical risk in patients with chronic liver disease emphasizes the need for a careful pre-operative evaluation.

Upper abdominal surgery increases the difficulty, and should be avoided in potential candidates for liver transplantation (Chapter 38).

References

1 Adler M, Verset D, Bouhdid H *et al.* Prognostic evaluation of patients with parenchymal cirrhosis. *J. Hepatol.* 1997; **26**: 642.

2 Afdhal NH, Keaveny AP, Cohen SB *et al.* Urinary assays for desmosine and hydroxylysylpyridinoline in the detection of cirrhosis. *J. Hepatol.* 1997; **27**: 993.

3 Altman C, Grange J-D, Amiot X *et al.* Survival after a first episode of spontaneous bacterial peritonitis. Prognosis of potential candidates for orthotopic liver transplantation. *J. Gastroenterol. Hepatol.* 1995; **10**: 47.

4 Alvaro D, Angelico M, Gandin C *et al.* Physico-chemical factors predisposing to pigment gallstone formation in liver cirrhosis. *J. Hepatol.* 1990; **10**: 228.

5 Andersen H, Borre M, Jakobsen J *et al.* Decreased muscle strength in patients with alcoholic liver cirrhosis in relation to nutritional status, alcohol abstinence, liver function, and neuropathy. *Hepatology* 1998; **27**: 1200.

6 Angeli P, Albino G, Carraro P *et al.* Cirrhosis and muscle cramps: evidence of a causal relationship. *Hepatology* 1996; **23**: 264.

7 Armonis A, Patch D, Burroughs A. Hepatic venous pressure measurement: an old test as a new prognostic marker in cirrhosis? *Hepatology* 1997; **25**: 245.

8 Bauer TM, Schwacha H, Steinbrückner B *et al.* Diagnosis of small intestinal bacterial overgrowth in patients with cirrhosis of the liver: poor performance of the glucose breath hydrogen test. *J. Hepatol.* 2000; **33**: 382.

9 Benyon RC, Arthur MJP. Extracellular matrix degradation and the role of hepatic stellate cells. *Semin. Liver Dis.* 2000; (in press).

10 Benyon RC, Iredale JP. Is liver fibrosis reversible? *Gut* 2000; **46**: 443.

11 Bernardi M, Calandra S, Colantoni A *et al.* Q-T interval prolongation in cirrhosis: prevalence, relationship with sever-

12 Blei AT, Zee P. Abnormalities of circadian rhythmicity in liver disease. *J. Hepatol.* 1998; **29**: 832–835.

13 Boros P, Miller CM. Hepatocyte growth factor: a multifunctional cytokine. *Lancet* 1995; **345**: 293.

14 Bustamante J, Rimola A, Ventura P-J *et al.* Prognostic significance of hepatic encephalopathy in patients with cirrhosis. *J. Hepatol.* 1999; **30**: 890.

15 Caldwell SH, Oelsner DH, Iezzoni JC *et al.* Cryptogenic cirrhosis: clinical characterization and risk factors for underlying disease. *Hepatology* 1999; **29**: 664.

16 Chapoutot C, Pageaux G-P, Perrigault P-F *et al. Staphylococcus aureus* nasal carriage in 104 cirrhotic and control patients: a prospective study. *J. Hepatol.* 1999; **20**: 249.

17 Christensen E. Prognostic models in chronic liver disease: validity, usefulness and future role. *J. Hepatol.* 1997; **26**: 1414.

18 Christensen E, Schlichting P, Anderson PK *et al.* Updating prognosis and therapeutic evaluation in cirrhosis with Cox's multiple regression model for time-dependent variables. *Scand. J. Gastroenterol.* 1986; **21**: 163.

19 Córdoba J, Cabrera J, Lataif L *et al.* High prevalence of sleep disturbance in cirrhosis. *Hepatology* 1998; **27**: 339.

20 Dickinson CJ. The aetiology of clubbing and hypertrophic osteoarthropathy. *Eur. J. Clin. Invest.* 1993; **23**: 330.

21 Dillon JF, Nolan J, Thomas H *et al.* The correction of autonomic dysfunction in cirrhosis by captopril. *J. Hepatol.* 1997; **26**: 331.

22 Fernández-Rodriguez CM, Prada IR, Prieto J *et al.* Circulating adrenomedullin in cirrhosis: relationship to hyperdynamic circulation. *J. Hepatol.* 1998; **29**: 250.

23 Finucci G, Tirelli M, Bellon S *et al.* Clinical significance of cholelithiasis in patients with decompensated cirrhosis. *J. Clin. Gastroenterol.* 1990; **12**: 538.

24 Fleckenstein JF, Frank SM, Thuluvath PJ. Presence of autonomic neuropathy is a poor prognostic indicator in patients with advanced liver disease. *Hepatology* 1996; **23**: 471.

25 Friedman LS. The risk of surgery in patients with liver disease. *Hepatology* 1999; **29**: 1617.

26 Friedman SL, Maher JJ, Bissell DM. Mechanisms and therapy of hepatic fibrosis: report of the AASLD single topic basic research conference. *Hepatology* 2000; **32**: 1401.

27 Gaiani S, Gramantieri L, Venturoli N *et al.* What is the criterion for differentiating chronic hepatitis from compensated cirrhosis? A prospective study comparing ultrasonography and percutaneous liver biopsy. *J. Hepatol.* 1997; **6**: 979.

28 Henriksen JH, Møller S, Schifter S *et al.* Increased arterial compliance in decompensated cirrhosis. *J. Hepatol.* 1999; **31**: 712.

29 Huet P-M, Villeneuve J-P, Fenyves D. Drug elimination in chronic liver diseases. *J. Hepatol.* 1997; **26** (Suppl. 2): 63.

30 Infante-Rivard C, Esnaola S, Villeneuve J-P *et al.* Clinical and statistical validity of conventional prognostic factors in predicting short-term survival among cirrhotics. *Hepatology* 1987; **7**: 660.

31 Iredale JP, Benyon RC, Pickering J *et al.* Mechanisms of spontaneous resolution of rat liver fibrosis: hepatic stellate cell apoptosis and reduced hepatic expression of metalloproteinase inhibitors. *J. Clin. Invest.* 1998; **102**: 538.

32 Italian Multicentre Cooperative Project. Nutritional status in cirrhosis. *J. Hepatol.* 1994; **21**: 317.

33 Iwao T, Oho K, Sakai T *et al.* Splanchnic and extrasplanchnic

ity, and aetiology of the disease and possible pathogenic factors. *Hepatology* 1998; **27**: 28.

arterial haemodynamics in patients with cirrhosis. *J. Hepatol.* 1997; **27**: 817.

34 Jefferson JA, Johnson RJ. Treatment of hepatitis C-associated glomerular disease. *Semin. Nephrol.* 2000; **20**: 286.

35 Johansen JS, Christoffersen P, Møller S *et al.* Serum YKL-40 is increased in patients with hepatic fibrosis. *J. Hepatol.* 2000; **32**: 911.

36 Kershenobich D, Vargas F, Garcia-Tsao G *et al.* Colchicine in the treatment of cirrhosis of the liver. *N. Engl. J. Med.* 1988; **318**: 1709.

37 Kitada T, Seki S, Ikeda K *et al.* Clinicopathological characterization of prion: a novel marker of activated human hepatic stellate cells. *J. Hepatol.* 2000; **33**: 751.

38 Kojima H, Tsujimoto T, Uemura M *et al.* Significance of increased plasma adrenomedullin concentration in patients with cirrhosis. *J. Hepatol.* 1998; **28**: 840.

39 Kondo F, Ebara M, Sugiura N *et al.* Histological features and clinical course of large regenerative nodules: evaluation of their precancerous potential. *Hepatology* 1990; **12**: 592.

40 Krowka MJ. Hepatopulmonary syndromes. *Gut* 2000; **46**: 1.

41 Li D, Friedman SL. Liver fibrogenesis and the role of hepatic stellate cells: new insights and prospects for therapy. *J. Gastroenterol. Hepatol.* 1999; **14**: 618.

42 Li J, Rosman AS, Leo MA *et al.* Tissue inhibitor of metalloproteinase is increased in the serum of precirrhotic and cirrhotic alcoholic patients and can serve as a marker of fibrosis. *Hepatology* 1994; **19**: 1418.

43 Liu H, Lee SS. Cardiopulmonary dysfunction in cirrhosis. *J. Gastroenterol. Hepatol.* 1999; **14**: 600.

44 Lochs H, Plauth M. Liver cirrhosis: rationale and modalities for nutritional support—the European Society of Parenteral and Enteral Nutrition consensus and beyond. *Curr. Opin. Clin. Nutr. Metabol. Care* 1999; **2**: 345.

45 Ma Z, Lee SS. Cirrhotic cardiomyopathy: getting to the heart of the matter. *Hepatology* 1996; **24**: 451.

46 Ma Z, Zhang Y, Huet P-M *et al.* Differential effects of jaundice and cirrhosis on α-adrenoceptor signalling in three rat models of cirrhotic cardiomyopathy. *J. Hepatol.* 1999; **30**: 485.

47 McIntyre N. The Child–Turcotte and Child–Pugh classification. In: Reichen J, Poupon RE, eds. *Surrogate Markers to Assess Efficacy of Treatment in Chronic Liver Disease.* Kluwer Academic Publishers, London, 1996, p. 69.

48 Madden AM, Bradbury W, Morgan MY. Taste perception in cirrhosis: its relationship to circulating micronutrients and food preferences. *Hepatology* 1997; **26**: 40.

49 Madden AM, Morgan MY. Resting energy expenditure should be measured in patients with cirrhosis, not predicted. *Hepatology* 1999; **30**: 655.

50 Meyer B, Luo H, Bargetzi M *et al.* Quantification of intrinsic drug-metabolizing capacity in human liver biopsy specimens: support for the intact-hepatocyte theory. *Hepatology* 1991; **13**: 475.

51 Moreau R, Lebrec D. Endogenous factors involved in the control of arterial tone in cirrhosis. *J. Hepatol.* 1995; **22**: 370.

52 Morencos FC, De Las Heras Castano G, Ramos LM *et al.* Small bowel bacterial overgrowth in patients with alcoholic cirrhosis. *Dig. Dis. Sci.* 1996; **41**: 552.

53 Morrison WL, Bouchier IAD, Gibson JNA *et al.* Skeletal muscle and whole-body protein turnover in cirrhosis. *Clin. Sci.* 1990; **78**: 613.

54 Muller MJ, Boker KHW, Selberg O. Are patients with liver cirrhosis hypermetabolic? *Clin. Nutr.* 1994; **13**: 131.

55 Murawaki Y, Yamada S, Ikuta Y *et al.* Clinical usefulness of serum matrix metalloproteinase-2 concentration in patients with chronic viral liver disease. *J. Hepatol.* 1999; **30**: 1090.

56 Naschitz JE, Slobodin G, Lewis RJ *et al.* Heart diseases affecting the liver and liver diseases affecting the heart. *Am. Heart J.* 2000; **140**: 111.

57 Navasa M, Rimola A, Rods J. Bacterial infections in liver disease. *Semin. Liver Dis.* 1997; **17**: 323.

58 Newell GC. Cirrhotic glomerulonephritis: incidence, morphology, clinical features, and pathogenesis. *Am. J. Kidney Dis.* 1987; **9**: 183.

59 Niemela O, Risteli L, Sotaniemi EA *et al.* Aminoterminal propeptide of type III procollagen in serum in alcoholic liver disease. *Gastroenterology* 1983; **85**: 254.

60 Noble-Jamieson G, Thiru S, Johnston P *et al.* Glomerulonephritis with end-stage liver disease in childhood. *Lancet* 1992; **339**: 706.

61 Pardo A, Bartoli R, Lorenzo-Zúniga V *et al.* Effect of cisapride on intestinal bacterial overgrowth and bacterial translocation in cirrhosis. *Hepatology* 2000; **31**: 858.

62 Pateron D, Beyne P, Laperche T *et al.* Elevated circulating cardiac troponin I in patients with cirrhosis. *Hepatology* 1999; **29**: 640.

63 Pauwels A, Mostefa-Kara N, Debenes B *et al.* Systemic antibiotic prophylaxis after gastrointestinal haemorrhage in cirrhotic patients with a high risk of infection. *Hepatology* 1996; **24**: 802.

64 Pauwels A, Pines E, Abboura M *et al.* Bacterial meningitis in cirrhosis: review of 16 cases. *J. Hepatol.* 1997; **27**: 830.

65 Piche T, Schneider SM, Tran A *et al.* Resting energy expenditure in chronic hepatitis C. *J. Hepatol.* 2000; **33**: 623.

66 Plauth M, Merli M, Kondrup J *et al.* ESPEN guidelines for nutrition in liver disease and transplantation. *Clin. Nutr.* 1997; **16**: 43.

67 Poonawala A, Nair S, Thuluvath PJ. Prevalence of obesity and diabetes in patients with cryptogenic cirrhosis: a case-control study. *Hepatology* 2000; **32**: 689.

68 Pozzi M, Carugo S, Boari G *et al.* Evidence of functional and structural cardiac abnormalities in cirrhotic patients with and without ascites. *Hepatology* 1997; **26**: 1131.

69 Richardson RA, Davidson HI, Hinds A *et al.* Influence of the metabolic sequelae of liver cirrhosis on nutritional intake. *Am. J. Clin. Nutr.* 1999; **69**: 331.

70 Rudolph KL, Chang S, Millard M *et al.* Inhibition of experimental liver cirrhosis in mice by telomerase gene delivery. *Science* 2000; **287**: 1253.

71 Schalm SW. The diagnosis of cirrhosis: clinical relevance and methodology. *J. Hepatol.* 1997; **27**: 1118.

72 Scheuer PJ, Lefkowitch JH. *Liver Biopsy Interpretation*, 2th edn. London: WB Saunders, 2000, p. 173.

73 Sheen I-S, Liaw Y-F. The prevalence and incidence of cholecystolithiasis in patients with chronic liver diseases: a prospective study. *Hepatology* 1989; **9**: 538.

74 Simpson KJ, Lukacs NW, Colletti L *et al.* Cytokines and the liver. *J. Hepatol.* 1997; **27**: 1120.

75 Siringo S, Burroughs AK, Bolondi L *et al.* Peptic ulcer and its course in cirrhosis: an endoscopic and clinical prospective study. *J. Hepatol.* 1995; **22**: 633.

76 Siringo S, Vaira D, Menegatti M *et al.* High prevalence of *Helicobacter pylori* in liver cirrhosis. Relationship with clinical and endoscopic features and the risk of peptic ulcer. *Dig. Dis. Sci.* 1997; **42**: 2024.

dation motivate stellate cells to produce collagen. Cytokines are also important [2].

Cytokines

A complex relationship exists between endotoxins, stellate cell activation and release of cytokines and chemokines. Endotoxins are increased in the blood of alcoholics [33]. This is related to increased intestinal bacterial flora, increased gut permeability and reduced endotoxin scavenging by the reticulo-endothelial system (fig. 22.7). The endotoxin releases a battery of cytokines [33]. Cytokines IL1, IL2 and TNF-α are released from non-parenchymal cells. In alcoholic hepatitis, TNF-α produced by monocytes is increased. IL8, the neutrophilic chemotactic factor, might be related to the neutrophilia and hepatic polymorph infiltration. It is also possible that the stimulus for cytokine production comes from alcohol-induced or alcohol-injured hepatocytes.

The biological effects of certain cytokines resemble the clinical manifestations of acute alcoholic liver disease (table 22.5). Cytokines stimulate fibroblast production. TGF-β activates collagen production from stellate cells [52]. TNF-α can depress P450 drug metabolism, induce cell surface expression of HLA antigens and cause hepato-toxicity.

Morphological changes

The changes are usually classified into fatty liver, alcoholic hepatitis and cirrhosis.

Fatty liver (steatosis) (figs 22.8, 22.9)

The fat accumulates in zones 3 and 2. In the more severely affected, the fatty change is diffuse. The fat may be in macrovesicular (large droplet) form. Less often it is in microvesicular (small droplet) form.

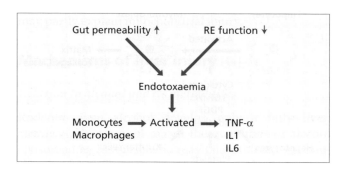

Fig. 22.7. The relation of gut permeability and reticulo-endothelial (RE) function to endotoxaemia and cytokine production.

Table 22.5. The biological effects of cytokine-inducers of the acute phase response compared with the changes seen in acute alcoholic liver disease (ALD)

Change	ALD	Cytokines
Fever	+	+
Anorexia	+	+
Muscle wasting	+	+
Hypermetabolism	+	+
Neutrophilia	+	+
Decreased albumin	+	+
Collagen disposition	+	+
Increased triglycerides	+	+
Decreased bile flow	+	+
Shock	+	+

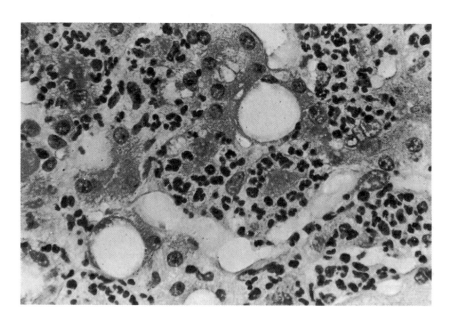

Fig. 22.8. Acute alcoholic hepatitis. Liver cells undergoing necrosis and containing clumps of Mallory's hyaline are surrounded by cuffs of polymorphonuclear cells. There is fatty change. (H & E, ×120.)

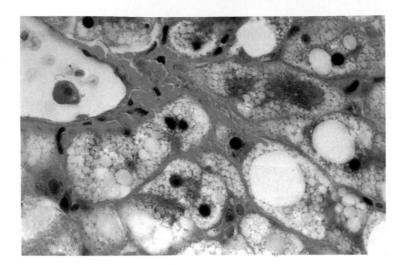

Fig. 22.9. Acute alcoholic hepatitis. Hepatocytes are ballooned and contain micro- and macrovesicular fat and clumps of purplish-red Mallory's alcoholic hyaline. (Chromophobe aniline blue, ×100.)

Large fat droplets appear in hepatocytes within 3–7 days of excess alcohol ingestion. Microvesicular fat represents mitochondrial damage and more active lipid synthesis by the hepatocyte. Hepatic mitochondrial DNA deletion is associated [27].

The fatty change can be quantified as follows:

+   less than 25% of liver cells contain fat
++   25–50% of liver cells contain fat
+++   50–75% of liver cells contain fat
++++ more than 75% of liver cells contain fat.

Alcoholic hepatitis

The full picture of a florid, acute alcoholic hepatitis is relatively rare. There are all gradations of severity. The hepatitis may be separate or combined with an established cirrhosis.

Balloon degeneration. Hepatocytes are swollen with granular cytoplasm often dispersed into fine strands. The nucleus is small and hyperchromatic. Steatosis, is usually macrovesicular, but with some microvesicular change. The ballooning is due to retention of water and to failure of the microtubular excretion of protein from the hepatocyte.

Acidophilic bodies represent apoptosis.

Mallory bodies are seen by haematoxylin and eosin as purplish-red intra-cytoplasmic inclusions [37, 38]. They may be more obvious with Masson's trichrome or chromophobe aniline blue stains (fig. 22.9). They consist of clumped organelles—largely intermediate filaments. They target the hepatocyte for destruction. The Mallory-containing cell is surrounded by a satellite of polymorphs (fig. 22.8).

Giant mitochondria form globular intra-cytoplasmic inclusions seen by light microscopy using a Masson trichrome stain.

Sclerosing hyaline necrosis. Collagen deposition is maximal in zone 3. The fibres are peri-sinusoidal and enclose normal or ballooned hepatocytes. The pericellular fibrosis is like lattice or chicken wire and has been termed 'creeping collagenosis' (fig. 22.10) [23].

Collagenization of the space of Disse is shown by electron microscopy (fig. 22.11). The number and porosity of the sinusoidal lining is reduced [35]. These changes interfere with the exchange of substances between plasma and the hepatocyte cell membrane and contribute to portal hypertension [29]. Lesions in terminal and sublobular veins include lymphocytic phlebitis, gradual obliteration and veno-occlusion [30].

Portal zone changes are inconspicuous and mild chronic inflammation is seen only in the advanced case. Marked zone 1 fibrosis suggests a complicating chronic pancreatitis (fig. 22.12) [58].

Cholestasis in bile canaliculi is a feature of all types of alcoholic liver disease. It is strongly associated with decreased survival [60].

The *histological patterns* form a spectrum from minimal alcoholic hepatitis to an advanced, probably irreversible, picture, where necrosis is more extensive and scars form. Alcoholic hepatitis is a precursor of cirrhosis.

Hyperplastic nodules develop in those who reduce their alcohol consumption [28].

Cirrhosis

Classically, cirrhosis of the alcoholic is micronodular (fig. 22.13). No normal zonal architecture can be identified, and zone 3 venules are difficult to find. The formation of nodules is often slow because of a presumed inhibitory effect of alcohol on hepatic regeneration. The amount of fat is variable and acute alcoholic hepatitis may or may not coexist. With continuing necrosis and replacement

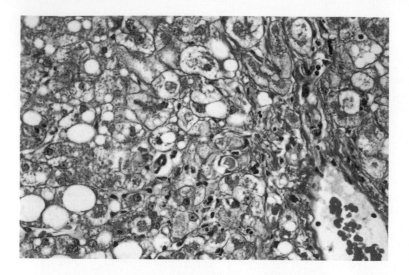

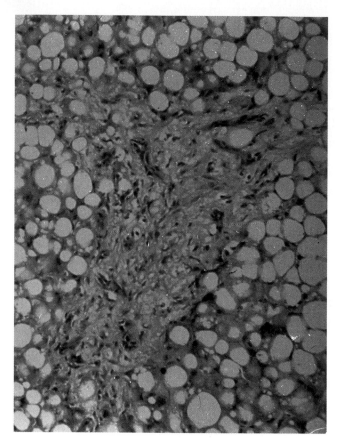

Fig. 22.10. Advanced zone 3 collagenosis with fatty change. A thickened hepatic vein can be seen bottom right. (Chromophobe aniline blue,×100.)

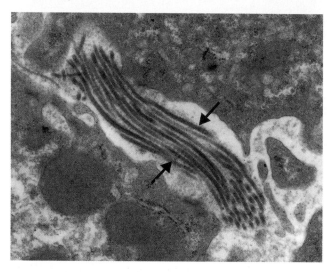

Fig. 22.11. Electron micrograph of liver in a patient with alcoholic liver disease. Note the deposition of collagen fibrils in Disse's space (arrowed). This could interfere with oxygen and metabolite exchange between blood and hepatocytes.

Fig. 22.12. Portal zone (zone 1) with marked fibrosis and fatty change in the hepatocytes. This patient suffered from chronic alcoholic pancreatitis with partial biliary obstruction. (H & E, ×120.)

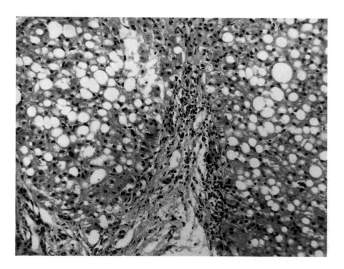

Fig. 22.13. Cirrhosis of the alcoholic. Fibrous bands divide the liver into small regular nodules. Fatty change is conspicuous. (H & E,×120.)

Table 22.6. Alcoholism—the CAGE questionaire

C	Have you felt the need to cut down?
A	Annoyed at the suggestion of a drinking problem
G	Guilty of excess drinking
E	Drink (eye opener) in the morning

fibrosis, the cirrhosis may progress from a micro- to a macronodular pattern, but this is usually accompanied by a reduction in steatosis. When this end-stage picture is reached, an alcoholic aetiology is difficult to confirm on histological grounds.

Cirrhosis may follow peri-cellular fibrosis without apparent hepatic necrosis and inflammation. Zone 3 myofibroblastic proliferation and collagen deposition may be the first lesions in the sequence of events leading to alcoholic cirrhosis.

Increased hepatic iron is found in approximately one-third of alcohol subjects [24]. This is partly due to increased intestinal absorption and to the iron content of beverages, especially wine. Free radical mediated toxicity contributes.

Early recognition

This depends on a high index of suspicion. If alcoholism is suspected, the CAGE questionnaire should be used (table 22.6). One point is scored for each positive response. Scores of 2 or more suggest alcohol-related problems. A patient may present with non-specific digestive symptoms such as anorexia, morning nausea with dry retching, diarrhoea, vague right upper abdominal pain and tenderness or pyrexia.

The patient may seek medical advice because of the effects of alcoholism such as social disruption, poor work performance, accidents, violent behaviour, fits, tremulousness or depression.

The diagnosis may be made when hepatomegaly, a raised serum transaminase or γ-glutamyl transpeptidase (γ-GT) level or macrocytosis are discovered at a routine examination, for instance at a life insurance check-up or during investigation of another condition.

Physical signs may be non-contributory, although tender hepatomegaly, prominent vascular spiders and associated features of alcoholism may be helpful. The clinical features do not reflect the hepatic histology and biochemical tests of liver function may be normal.

Investigation

Biochemical tests [54]

Serum transaminase levels rarely exceed 300 iu/l. AST (SGOT), which is derived from alcoholic damage to mitochondria or smooth muscle, is more increased than the ALT (SGPT) which is confined to the liver. In alcoholic liver disease, the AST:ALT ratio usually exceeds 2. This is partially explained by the depletion in alcoholics of pyridoxal 5-phosphate, the biologically active form of vitamin B_6 which is necessary for the activity of both enzymes and is depleted in alcoholics.

The serum γ-GT is a widely used screening test for alcohol abuse. The rise results mainly from enzyme induction, although hepato-cellular damage and cholestasis may contribute. There are many false positives due to other factors, such as drugs, other diseases and the patient having a value at the upper limit of the normal range.

Serum alkaline phosphatase may be markedly increased (greater than four times normal) especially in those with severe cholestasis and alcoholic hepatitis. Serum IgA values may be very high.

Blood and urinary alcohol levels can be used in the clinic to refute the individual who has a high blood alcohol level but denies imbibing.

Non-specific serum changes in acute and chronic alcoholism include elevations in uric acid, lactate and triglyceride, and reductions in glucose and magnesium. Hypophosphataemia is related to a renal tubular defect, independent of liver function impairment [3]. Low serum tri-iodothyronine (T_3) levels presumably reflect decreased hepatic conversion of thyroxine to T_3. Levels correlate inversely with the severity of alcoholic liver disease.

Type III collagen can be estimated by the serum procollagen type III peptides. Serum type IV collagen and laminin estimate components of basement membranes. Results of these three tests correlate with disease severity, degree of alcoholic hepatitis and alcohol intake [59].

Other serum tests are markers of alcohol abuse rather than alcoholic liver damage. They include serum glutamate dehydrogenase, the mitochondrial isoenzyme of aspartate transaminase. Serum carbohydrate-deficient (de-sialylated) transferrin levels may be a useful marker of excessive alcohol intake irrespective of liver disease but this test is not generally available [6].

Even sensitive biochemical methods may fail to reveal alcoholic liver damage and liver biopsy is necessary in cases of doubt.

Haematological changes

Macrocytosis (MCV) greater than 95 fl is presumably due to a direct effect of alcohol on bone marrow. Deficiencies of folate and vitamin B_{12} contribute in the malnourished. The combination of a raised MCV and serum γ-GT will identify 90% of alcohol-dependent patients.

Liver biopsy

This confirms liver disease and identifies alcohol abuse as the likely cause (table 22.7). The dangers of the liver damage can be emphasized more forcibly to the patient.

Table 22.7. Liver biopsy in alcoholic patients

Diagnosis: exclude
    chronic viral hepatitis (hepatitis C virus)
    genetic haemochromatosis
Prognosis
    fatty change
    alcoholic hepatitis
    cirrhosis
Enforce abstinence

Liver biopsy is important prognostically. Fatty change alone is not nearly so serious as peri-venular sclerosis, which is a precursor of cirrhosis [80]. An established cirrhosis can be confirmed.

Non-alcoholic steato-hepatitis (*NASH*) may be due to various causes. In contrast to the alcoholic, the lesion is largely peri-portal (Chapter 25).

Portal hypertension

Splenomegaly is not prominent. Portal hypertension and gastrointestinal bleeding, however, are frequent at all stages. Bleeding is not only from oesophageal varices but from duodenal ulcers, gastritis and Mallory–Weiss lower oesophageal tears following repeated vomiting.

The portal hypertension may be related to cirrhosis. Fatty change and zone 3 collagenosis (peri-venular sclerosis) lead to a pre-sinusoidal portal hypertension [30]. Collagenization of the space of Disse raises portal pressure. Enlargement of hepatocytes probably plays little part.

Scanning

With severe alcoholic hepatitis or cirrhosis, isotopes are hardly taken up by the liver because the blood shunts past the reticulo-endothelial cells.

Ultrasound will not detect minimal change, fat or fibrosis. However, in more advanced disease, the liver is diffusely abnormal and the changes correlate with those seen on liver biopsy.

CT and MRI scanning are very useful in demonstrating fatty liver (see fig. 22.16), irregular liver surface, splenomegaly, portal collateral circulation, ascites and pancreatitis. It may show alcoholic pseudo-tumour (fig. 22.14).

Clinical syndromes

Fatty liver

The patients are usually asymptomatic, the diagnosis being made when an enlarged, smooth, firm liver is dis-

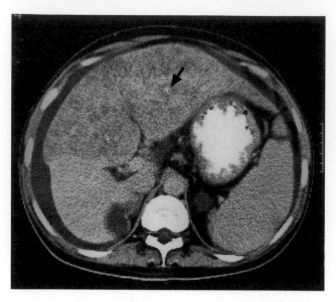

Fig. 22.14. Alcoholic pseudo-tumour. A mass was felt in the upper abdomen and a liver tumour was suspected. This CT scan (enhanced oral contrast) shows features suggestive of hepato-cellular carcinoma (arrowed). Directed needle biopsy showed only acute alcoholic hepatitis. This is a rare type of alcoholic hepatitis, affecting particularly one part of the liver.

covered. Liver function tests may be normal or the transaminases and alkaline phosphatase slightly increased. If the alcoholic fatty liver is sufficiently severe to merit admission to hospital the patient has usually been drinking heavily for some time and is anorexic. There may be nausea and vomiting with peri-umbilical, epigastric or right upper quadrant pain. Clinically, the fatty liver patient cannot be separated from one with mild alcoholic hepatitis. Needle liver biopsy is essential to diagnose alcoholic hepatitis.

Acute alcoholic hepatitis

In the very mildest case, the diagnosis may be made only by a liver biopsy in an asymptomatic patient who is misusing alcohol and has shown abnormal serum enzyme tests and macrocytosis.

Patients in the next category complain only of fatigue, anorexia and weight loss. There is tender hepatomegaly and usually pyrexia. The patient may be obese, but some features of malnutrition are present in 90% of patients.

In the more severe case, the patient has usually been drinking particularly heavily and not eating. The severe hepatic decompensation may be precipitated by vomiting, diarrhoea, an intercurrent infection or prolonged anorexia.

Intake of quite modest doses of paracetamol may precipitate the alcoholic into severe hepatitis (fig. 22.15). Transaminase levels are enormous [89].

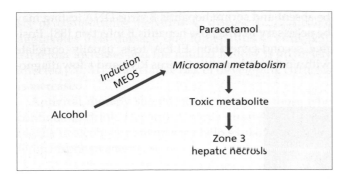

Fig. 22.15. Alcohol, by inducing microsomal metabolism, enhances the effects of toxic metabolites of drugs such as paracetamol (acetaminophen) on the liver.

Severe alcoholic hepatitis is marked by pyrexia, anorexia, jaundice and repeated vomiting. The patient may experience pain over a very enlarged tender liver. In about half, an arterial murmur may be heard over the liver. Florid vascular spiders are usual. There may be signs of liver failure such as ascites, encephalopathy and a bleeding diathesis. The blood pressure is usually low with a hyperdynamic circulation. Signs of vitamin deficiencies, such as beri beri or scurvy, are usual in the malnourished.

Diarrhoea with steatorrhoea can be related to decreased biliary excretion of bile salts, to pancreatic insufficiency and to a direct, toxic effect of alcohol on the intestinal mucosa.

Patients with acute fatty liver may die suddenly in shock, attributable to pulmonary fat emboli. Sudden deaths have also been reported in hypoglycaemia.

Gastrointestinal haemorrhage is frequently from a local gastric or duodenal lesion, rather than related to portal hypertension.

Acute alcoholic hepatitis may be confused with acute viral hepatitis. Helpful diagnostic points are the history, the florid vascular spiders, the very large liver and the leucocytosis.

Laboratory tests

Serum transaminases are increased, but rarely to greater than 300 iu/l. Very high values suggest complicating ingestion of paracetamol (fig. 22.15). The AST : ALT ratio exceeds 2. Serum alkaline phosphatase is usually increased.

The severity is best correlated with the serum bilirubin level and prothrombin time after vitamin K administration [49]. Serum IgA is markedly increased with IgG and IgM raised to a much lesser extent, and serum IgG falls with improvement. The serum albumin level is decreased, increasing as the patient improves. Serum cholesterol levels are usually increased.

The serum potassium value is low, largely due to the low dietary protein intake, diarrhoea and secondary hyperaldosteronism if fluid retention is present. Albumin-bound serum zinc is decreased, and this is related to a low liver zinc concentration, not found in patients with non-alcoholic liver disease. The blood urea and creatinine values increase and these reflect severity. They predict the development of the hepato-renal syndrome.

A polymorph leucocytosis of about 15–20×10⁹/l is in proportion to severity.

Platelet function is depressed even in the absence of thrombocytopenia or of alcohol in the blood.

Hepatic cirrhosis

Established cirrhosis can present without a stage of acute alcoholic hepatitis having been recognized clinically or histologically, and the picture can resemble any end-stage liver disease. Points suggesting an alcoholic aetiology include the history of alcohol abuse (which may be forgotten), the hepatomegaly and the associated features of alcoholism. Splenomegaly is a late feature.

Liver biopsy findings supporting an alcoholic aetiology include a micronodular cirrhosis, peri-venular sclerosis and paucity of hepatic veins. It may be impossible on histological grounds to determine an alcoholic cause.

Cholestatic syndromes

Occasionally, the patient presents with deep jaundice, hepatomegaly and an increase in serum alkaline phosphatase, transaminases, triglycerides and cholesterol [84]. Functional renal failure is usual. This is usually the first episode of decompensation.

Liver biopsy shows massive accumulation of microvesicular fat (see fig. 22.6) with zone 3 cholestasis. Inflammation is inconspicuous and there is little or no hyaline [57]. Electron microscopy shows extensive disorganization of the organelles in affected hepatocytes. The condition has been termed *alcoholic foamy degeneration* [84]. Prognosis is very variable and foamy degeneration can be found in the asymptomatic.

Cholestasis may also be due to compression of the intra-pancreatic portion of the common bile duct by chronic pancreatitis (fig. 22.16). ERCP confirms the diagnosis (fig. 22.17).

Relationship to hepatitis B and C

Markers of past or current hepatitis B or C are commoner in patients with alcoholic disease than in the general population. It may be difficult to distinguish the viral from the alcoholic aetiology. The identification of risk factors is helpful. The effect of abstinence in the alcoholic

Histological cholestasis is a bad prognostic indicator in alcoholic hepatitis [60].

In one study, 50% of patients with alcoholic hepatitis developed cirrhosis after 10–13 years [80]. In another study 23% of patients without cirrhosis developed cirrhosis after an average of 8.1 years [50].

'Pure' fatty liver can be serious. In a study of 86 patients followed for 10.5 years, nine developed cirrhosis and another seven developed fibrosis. Micro- and macrovesicular fat, giant mitochondria and continued alcoholism predicted these serious developments [83].

Features with independent but bad prognostic significance are encephalopathy, low serum albumin, increased prothrombin time, low haemoglobin level and large oesophageal varices [29]. Patients with pre-coma, persistent jaundice and azotaemia are very liable to develop the hepato-renal syndrome.

The patient with decompensated disease improves slowly. Overt jaundice and ascites after 3 months carry a grave prognosis. In the very late, irreversible stage, abstinence cannot be expected to affect the prognosis. The damage has been done and there is no turning back. The highest mortality for patients with either cirrhosis or alcoholic hepatitis or both is in the first year of follow-up [62].

Patients with acute alcoholic hepatitis often deteriorate during the first few weeks in hospital. It may take 1–6 months for resolution, and 20–50% die. Those with a markedly prolonged prothrombin time, unresponsive to intramuscular vitamin K, and with a serum bilirubin level greater than 20 mg, have a particularly bad outlook [49]. Alcoholic hepatitis is slow to resolve even in those who abstain.

In a multi-centre Veterans Hospital study, predictors of survival were age, grams of alcohol consumed, AST : ALT ratio and the histological and clinical severity of disease [17]. Those with poor nutrition, particularly if they had been starving, were liable to die [53].

Prothrombin time and bilirubin can be used to determine a *discriminant function* to estimate prognosis in alcoholic hepatitis (fig. 22.20) [13].

Computer neural networks which can include prothrombin time, bilirubin and encephalopathy have a high prognostic accuracy for mortality in severe alcoholic liver disease [41].

Treatment

The most important measure is to ensure total and immediate abstinence from alcohol. Patients with severe physical ailments are more likely to abstain than those who present with psychological problems. In a long-term follow-up of men attending a liver clinic, severe medical illness was critical in the decision to stop drinking [67]. Continued medical care is also essential. Follow-up of patients with alcoholic liver disease treated at the Royal Free Hospital between 1975 and 1990 showed 50% remained abstinent, 25% took alcohol but were not abusing it and 25% continued alcohol abuse regardless of therapy. The less severely affected can receive *'brief interventional counselling'* from a doctor, nurse or similar person. This results in a 38% treatment benefit albeit often temporary [10]. The more severely affected will need psychiatric referral.

The development of a withdrawal syndrome (*delirium tremens*) should be anticipated by the administration of chlordiazepoxide.

Striking improvement following abstinence and nutritional support is virtually diagnostic of previous alcoholism.

During 'drying out' or recovery from hepatic decompensation, dietary protein should increase to 1 g/kg body weight, as soon as possible. Supplements of potassium chloride, together with magnesium and zinc, are given. Vitamins, especially the B complex, C and K are given in large doses, if necessary intravenously.

Alcoholics should be advised to abstain completely. Nutritional support is essential with 1.2–1.5 g protein/kg body weight [48, 61]. Intake should increase with intercurrent illness. Modest vitamin supplements are advised [77].

Acute alcoholic hepatitis

Ascites is treated cautiously as the hepato-renal syndrome is a likely development (table 22.8).

Table 22.8. Treatment of acute alcoholic hepatitis

Stop alcohol
Investigate precipitant (infections, bleeding, etc.)
Anticipate acute alcohol withdrawal
Intramuscular multivitamins
Treat ascites and encephalopathy
Potassium and zinc supplements
Maintain nitrogen intake—oral or enteral
Consider corticosteroids in severe disease with encephalopathy, without gastrointestinal bleeding

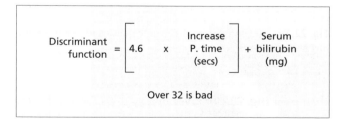

Fig. 22.20. Discriminant function for prognosis in alcoholic hepatitis [13]. P, prothrombin. Serum bilirubin in μmol/l is divided by 17.1 to convert to mg/dl.

Corticosteroids reduce cytokine production and acetaldehyde adduct formation. Results have been extremely conflicting. Seven clinical trials in mild or moderately ill patients showed no effect on clinical recovery, biochemical tests or rate of histological progression. However, more favourable results were reported from a randomized, multi-centre trial [13]. Patients were included with either spontaneous hepatic encephalopathy or a discriminant function value exceeding 32 (see fig. 22.20). Methyl-prednisolone (30 mg daily) or placebo was given within 7 days of admission and continued for 28 days when it was tapered over 2 weeks and discontinued. The mortality rate was 35% of 31 patients receiving placebo, compared with 6% of 35 patients given prednisolone (*P* = 0.006). Prednisolone seemed particularly valuable in those with encephalopathy. The fall in serum bilirubin and pro-thrombin time was greater in the treated group.

A randomized trial [73] and meta-analysis of all trials [36] confirmed initial survival benefit. These positive results are difficult to reconcile with previous negative ones. The numbers may have been too small in the earlier trials and a type 1 error is possible, the control and treated patients not being comparable. The patients may have been less sick, and at risk of death in the later trials. It is now recommended that corticosteroids should be given to those with encephalopathy, but without bleeding, systemic infections or renal failure. Discriminant function values should exceed 32. Only about 25% of hospitalized patients will fulfil all the above criteria. The mortality remains 44% even in those receiving corticosteroids.

Testosterone is of little benefit.

Oxandrolone (an anabolic steroid) is useful in those with moderate disease, but has no effect in those with severe malnutrition and inadequate calorie intake [53].

Protein malnutrition must be corrected. Nutrition is particularly important during the first few days. Most patients can take adequate, natural protein by mouth. An improvement may follow the use of casein-based naso-duodenal tube feeding supplements (1.5 g protein/kg body weight/day) [39]. Oral or intravenous amino acid supplementation should be reserved for the very few jaundiced and severely malnourished patients [48].

Colchicine has failed to improve short-time survival in patients with alcoholic hepatitis [1].

Propylthiouracil. Alcohol induces a hypermetabolic state which potentiates zone 3 anoxic liver injury. This is reduced by propylthiouracil in experimental animals. A long-term beneficial effect has been shown in patients with alcoholic cirrhosis who continue to drink, but at lower levels [63]. This therapy has never gained general acceptance.

S-adenosyl-methionine (SAME) in less advanced disease and phosphatidyl choline [43] have shown benefit in animal disease but cannot be recommended for clinical use at the present time.

Cirrhosis

Cirrhosis is irreversible and therapy has to be directed at the complications. These include portal hypertension, encephalopathy and ascites. Drug metabolism is impaired and particular care must be taken, especially with sedatives. Diazepam seems to be the safest.

Oral supplementation with a purified soya bean, polyunsaturated, lecithin extract containing 94–98% phosphatidyl choline prevents the development of septal fibrosis and cirrhosis in baboons fed alcohol long term [43]. The mechanism is unknown, but is possibly by stimulating lipocyte collagenase.

Porta-caval shunting, including TIPS, is associated with a reduction of bleeding from varices but a 30% incidence of hepatic encephalopathy and only a marginal increase in survival. Results with the selective spleno-renal shunt are less good in alcoholic than in non-alcoholic patients. In general, alcoholics are not good candidates for any surgical procedure, especially if they continue to imbibe.

Hepatic transplantation

Alcoholic liver disease now accounts for 20% of all indications for liver transplant in the USA [5]. Early results are similar to those for other forms of cirrhosis. Initial graft and patient survival is similar to that found in other transplant recipients. The 5-year survival is increased, the benefit being greatest in those with severe disease [71]. After the first 2 years, survival curves decline more rapidly in the alcoholic compared with the non-alcoholic recipient [82]. This could be related to a greater reluctance to re-transplant alcoholics. After the operation, quality of life and return to work are similar.

The selection for transplant is difficult (table 22.9). The cirrhosis is self-inflicted. The patient may return to alcoholism and compliance with immunosuppression may be poor. Should alcoholics compete with other patients when donor livers are in short supply [8]? Those selected should have a stable psychiatric and socioeconomic

Table 22.9. Selection of patients with alcoholic liver disease for liver transplantation

Abstinent for 6 months
Child's grade C
Socioeconomically stable
Job to return to after operation
No extra-hepatic organ alcoholic damage

the protein to the crypt cells of the upper small intestine [69]. Further studies showed that the HFE protein is expressed on the surface of cells [89] and that it interacts with the TfR, reducing the affinity of the TfR for transferrin [37]. The transferrin/TfR interaction is the major mechanism for uptake of iron into many cells. The expression of TfR is inversely related to intra-cellular iron levels.

The association of HFE with TfR may therefore be important for the normal entry of iron into the crypt cell of the villus and hence the regulation of iron absorption. Binding of HFE to TfR may reduce the affinity of TfR for transferrin, allowing the release of iron into the cell from the endosomal compartment. The model that follows this assumption proposes that in iron deficiency crypt cell iron levels are low and villous cell DMT-1 is upregulated leading to iron absorption, while in iron replete or overloaded states the opposite occurs. This control mechanism would be disrupted in genetic haemochromatosis (see below).

Less is known of the regulation of iron absorption in relationship to haemopoiesis and reticulo-endothelial cell iron. A link is possible since macrophage iron handling has been found to be abnormal in genetic haemochromatosis. Transfection of normal *HFE* into these cells corrects transferrin–iron uptake and retention [65]. Thus whether the HFE-related control of iron absorption resides primarily in the intestinal crypt cell, or secondarily through a change in reticulo-endothelial cell iron metabolism, is unclear. Hepcidin may effect iron absorption [40]. Knock-out mice develop iron overload, but the mechanism is not known.

Basolateral transfer

After transport of iron from the intestinal lumen into the mucosal cell of the villus, the iron enters a cytosolic pool. Some passes to be stored in ferritin, and is then either mobilized as necessary, or is lost with exfoliation of mucosal cells. At the basolateral membrane, IREG-1 (also called ferroportin-1) [30, 60] transports iron from the cell to the circulation. Hephaestin, a ferroxidase, appears to promote the transfer of iron from IREG-1 to transferrin [88].

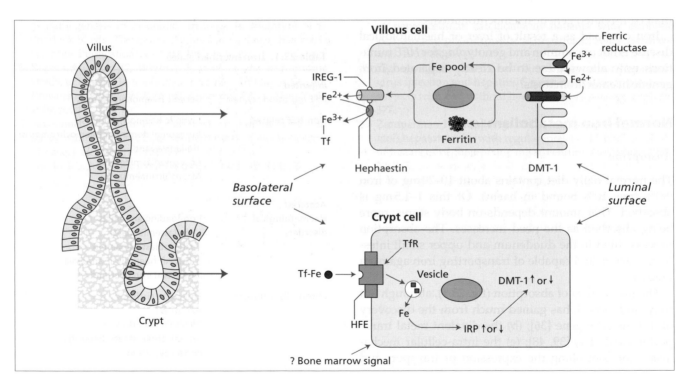

Fig. 23.1. Hypothetical model of regulation of iron absorption. Ferrous iron is transported from the gut lumen into the villous cell by the divalent metal transporter, DMT-1. Iron enters the cellular pool or is stored in ferritin. IREG-1 (ferroportin) transports iron out of the cell across the basolateral surface. Hephaestin converts ferrous to ferric iron which is bound to transferrin (Tf).

Activity of DMT-1 is regulated by intra-cellular iron level. This depends upon entry of iron into the crypt cell. It has been suggested that binding of transferrin receptor (TfR) to HFE protein at the basolateral surface of the crypt cell determines the entry of iron.

In iron deficiency little enters the crypt cell, DMT-1 is upregulated and more iron absorbed. When body stores are normal, DMT-1 is downregulated and iron absorption is reduced. In HFE-related haemochromatosis, it is hypothesized that the C282Y mutation disrupts association between HFE and transferrin receptor, iron does not enter the crypt cell, and DMT-1 is not downregulated as would normally occur with iron overload. Iron absorption continues.

Distribution to tissues

Transferrin (mol. wt 77 000 Da) is a glycoprotein largely synthesized in the liver. It can bind two ferric iron molecules, and is responsible for the 'total iron-binding capacity' of serum of 250–370 μg/dl. This is normally about one-third saturated with iron. Physiological entry of iron into reticulocytes and hepatocytes depends upon transferrin receptors (TfRs) at the cell surface which preferentially bind transferrin-carrying iron. The role of HFE in these tissues is not clear. Receptor/iron complex is internalized and the iron released. This process is saturable. TfRs are downregulated as the cell becomes replete with iron. When serum transferrin is fully saturated, as in overt haemochromatosis, iron circulates in 'non-transferrin-bound' forms, associated with low molecular weight chelators. Iron in this form readily enters cells by a non-saturable process. A stimulator of iron transport (SFT) may also be important for iron uptake when there is iron overload and downregulation of cell surface TfRs [98].

Storage

Iron is stored in cells as ferritin (mol. wt 480 000 Da), the combination of the protein apoferritin (H and L subunits) and iron, which appears under electron microscopy as particles 50 Å in diameter lying free in the cytoplasm. Up to 4500 atoms of iron can be stored within a single ferritin molecule. High concentrations of iron stimulate apoferritin synthesis.

Aggregates of degraded ferritin molecules make up haemosiderin which stains as blue granules with ferrocyanide. Approximately one-third of iron is stored in this form, increasing in iron storage disorders.

Lipofuscin, or wear and tear pigment, accumulates in association with iron overload. It is yellow–brown in colour and does not contain iron.

Iron contained in depots as ferritin or haemosiderin is available for mobilization and haemoglobin formation should the demand arise.

The normal total body content of iron is about 4 g, of which 3 g are present in haemoglobin, myoglobin, catalase and other respiratory pigments or enzymes. Storage iron comprises 0.5 g; of this 0.3 g is in the liver but is not revealed by the usual histological stains for iron. The liver is the predominant site for storage of iron absorbed from the gut. When its capacity is exceeded, iron is deposited in other parenchymal tissues, including the acinar cells of the pancreas, and the cells of the anterior pituitary gland. The reticulo-endothelial system plays only a limited part in iron storage unless the iron is given intravenously, when it becomes the preferential site for deposition. Iron from erythrocyte breakdown is concentrated in the spleen.

Iron overload and liver damage

Fibrosis and hepato-cellular damage are directly related to the iron content of the liver cell [54]. The pattern of damage is similar irrespective of whether the overload is due to genetic haemochromatosis or to multiple transfusions. The severity of fibrosis is maximal in peri-portal areas where iron is particularly deposited.

When iron deposition is low it is stored as ferritin. As the load increases more is present as haemosiderin.

Removal of iron by venesection or chelation leads to clinical and biochemical improvement with reduction or prevention of hepatic fibrosis [13].

There are several processes by which iron can damage the liver. There is enhanced oxidative stress in patients with iron overload and this is associated with increased TGF-β1 expression [53]. Oxidative stress causes lipid peroxidation of membranes of organelles leading to functional defects of lysosomes, mitochondria and microsomes. Mitochondrial cytochrome C oxidase activity is reduced [8]. There is lysosomal membrane fragility and release of hydrolytic enzymes into the cytosol.

Hepatic stellate cells (lipocytes) are activated in genetic haemochromatosis and activation is reversed by iron removal [76]. Stellate cell activation appears related to the release of cytokines and other substances from neighbouring cells rather than oxidant stress within stellate cells [64]. Anti-oxidant treatment protects against hepatic fibrosis in an animal model of iron overload [71]. Although excess iron increases hepatic collagen type I mRNA expression [70], altered matrix degradation also plays a part in the hepatic fibrogenesis due to iron overload (Chapter 21). There are increased levels of tissue inhibitor of metalloproteinase 1 (TIMP-1) and reduced matrix metalloproteinase (MMP) levels [45]. Serum type IV collagen correlates with the degree of hepatic fibrosis due to iron overload [46].

Genetic haemochromatosis

In 1865, Trousseau described the clinical syndrome of skin pigmentation, cirrhosis and diabetes now recognized as characteristic of late stage genetic haemochromatosis. This is an autosomal recessive metabolic disorder in which there is increased iron absorption over many years. The tissues contain enormous quantities of iron, of the order of 20–60 g. If 5 mg of dietary iron were retained by the tissues daily it would take about 28 years for 50 g to accumulate.

Molecular genetics

Sheldon [81] in his classical monograph described idiopathic haemochromatosis as an inborn error of metabolism. The discovery of genetic linkage of

centage of parenchymal cells with positive staining (0–100%). Chemical measurement of iron should be made although it is recognized that the concentration varies between different samples from the same patient [87]. Iron can be measured on tissue extracted from the paraffin block if fresh tissue was not provided. If mutation analysis does not show homozygosity for C282Y then liver biopsy is usually necessary to show whether or not there is iron overload and also the pattern of iron deposition which may give an indication of the cause.

Liver biopsy is not necessary to follow de-ironing during treatment. Serum iron indices are sufficient.

Imaging

Using single-energy *CT scanning*, hepatic attenuation correlates with serum ferritin, but it is unable to detect hepatic iron overload less than five times the normal limit (40% of patients) [15].

The accuracy is greatly improved if dual-energy CT scanning is available.

MRI detects iron which is a naturally occurring paramagnetic contrast agent. In overload states, marked decreases in T2 relaxation time are shown (see fig. 5.20).

Although both CT and MRI detect heavy iron overload, they are not yet sufficiently precise to predict hepatic iron concentrations with accuracy.

Differential diagnosis

Differentiation between classical genetic haemochromatosis and other causes of iron overload has been simplified by the introduction of genotyping for the C282Y mutation in the *HFE* gene. The differential diagnosis is usually with other chronic liver diseases associated with iron accumulation, haematological disease (not related to transfusion overload) and, more rarely, inherited but non-HFE-related iron overload. Acaeruloplasminaemia is exceptionally rare. African iron overload and neonatal haemochromatosis are specific to particular groups.

Serum iron and transferrin saturation, as well as serum ferritin, are sometimes increased in cirrhosis due to causes other than genetic haemochromatosis. These include alcohol and hepatitis C. The clinical picture may confuse, since the association of diabetes mellitus and cirrhosis is not uncommon, and patients with cirrhosis may become impotent, hairless and develop skin pigmentation. Hepato-cellular failure, however, is unusual in haemochromatosis. The degree of iron overload with end-stage liver disease and juvenile haemochromatosis can be within the range of that seen in *HFE*-related haemochromatosis. Both are unrelated to mutations in *HFE*. A family history and clinical picture should make differentiation straightforward.

Prognosis

Much depends upon the amount and duration of iron overload. Early diagnosis and treatment is central to improving prognosis. Those treated in the pre-cirrhotic stage and before diabetes mellitus has developed, and who subsequently have normal iron levels maintained by phlebotomy, have a normal life expectancy [67]. This is important for patients applying for life insurance [73].

Cardiac failure worsens the outlook and such patients rarely survive longer than 1 year without treatment. Hepatic failure or bleeding oesophageal varices are rare terminal features.

The outlook is better than for cirrhosis in alcoholics who stop drinking. However, the patient with haemochromatosis who also abuses alcohol does worse than the abstinent patient.

The risk of developing hepato-cellular carcinoma in haemochromatotic patients with cirrhosis is increased about 200 times [67] and is not reduced by de-ironing [13]. A minority (approx. 15%) of hepato-cellular carcinomas develop in non-cirrhotic haemochromatotic liver [28] — as is found for hepato-cellular carcinoma related to other aetiologies.

Treatment [32, 83]

Iron can be removed by venesection and can be mobilized from tissue stores at rates as high as 130 mg/day [25]. Blood regeneration is extraordinarily rapid, haemoglobin production increasing to six or seven times normal. Large quantities of blood must be removed, for 500 ml removes only 250 mg of iron, whereas the tissues contain up to 200 times this amount. Depending on the initial iron stores, the amount necessary to reduce them to normal varies from 7 to 45 g. Venesections of 500 ml are carried out weekly, or even twice weekly in particularly co-operative patients, and are continued until serum iron, transferrin saturation and ferritin levels fall into the low normal range. Comparison of a venesection-treated with an untreated group showed a survival of 8.2 years compared with 4.9 years and a 5-year mortality of 11% compared with 67% [92]. Venesection treatment results in increased well-being and gain in weight. Pigmentation and hepato-splenomegaly decrease. Liver function tests improve. Control of diabetes improves in some patients [13, 67]. The arthropathy is usually unaffected. Hypogonadism may lessen in men aged less than 40 years at diagnosis [26]. Cardiac function improves depending upon the severity of cardiac damage before venesection.

Hepatic fibrosis can improve following venesection [67], but hepatic cirrhosis is generally regarded to be irreversible.

After de-ironing, venesection of 500 ml of blood every 3–6 months should prevent iron re-accumulation. A low iron diet is difficult to achieve and most patients remain on a normal diet with intermittent venesection.

Gonadal atrophy may be treated by replacement therapy with an intramuscular, depot testosterone. Human chorionic gonadotrophin (HCG) injections will increase testicular volume and sperm counts.

Diabetes should be treated by diet and, if necessary, insulin. Resistant cases may be encountered.

Transplantation

The survival of patients with genetic haemochromatosis after liver transplant is less than for other recipients (53% vs. 81% survival at 25 months) [35]. The lower survival is related to cardiac complications and sepsis, emphasizing the need for early diagnosis and treatment.

Approximately one-third of patients undergoing liver transplantation unrelated to genetic haemochromatosis have hepatic iron deposition. Ten per cent have hepatic siderosis in the range of that seen in genetic haemochromatosis. *HFE* gene mutations are rare in this group. Patient survival after transplantation is significantly lower in those with hepatic iron overload [17]. Transplantation of the liver from a C282Y heterozygote is safe [5].

Whereas previous reports of the transplantation of a haemochromatotic liver into a normal recipient have not shown evidence of subsequent iron accumulation, this has been reported where the donor intestine as well as liver were derived from a C282Y homozygote [3].

Screening for early haemochromatosis in relatives

There are two ways of screening: biochemical tests for iron overload, and mutation analysis (genotyping). Ideally both are done since the results are complementary. If biochemical screening (transferrin saturation and serum ferritin) shows evidence for iron overload then genotyping for the C282Y mutation is done to show whether the individual is homozygous or heterozygous. If heterozygosity for C282Y is shown, H63D analysis is needed to detect the compound heterozygote (C282Y/H63D).

If the transferrin saturation and ferritin levels are very high, then it is likely that the individual is homozygous for C282Y.

If there is only a mild elevation of transferrin saturation and ferritin, not unusual in the younger patient, it is not possible clinically to differentiate the C282Y homozygote from a heterozygote.

If genotyping is done as the first screening step or in the individual with normal iron studies, patients need to give consent. If they are found to be homozygous for C282Y there may be insurance or mortgage issues despite the absence of iron overload. There is a concern that the insurance companies may increase premiums for C282Y homozygotes despite the fact that subsequent monitoring will prevent iron overload and disease.

It is not possible at present to advise a C282Y homozygote who has no evidence of iron overload of the risk of developing iron overload (phenotypic penetrance) or disease (disease penetrance). Studies have shown that there is phenotypic penetrance in 20–80% of homozygotes. There is no information on disease penetrance although it is recognized that there is a discrepancy between the frequency of homozygosity for C282Y in populations of northern European descent (1 in 200–300) and the frequency of clinically overt genetic haemochromatosis.

Children of a patient with genetic haemochromatosis should also be screened because of the 1 in 10 chance in northern European populations of the spouse being a carrier for the C282Y mutation. This would give a 1 in 20 chance of the child being affected. Screening (as for siblings given above) could be done but for young children below the age of consent this is not practical. An alternative approach is to perform mutation analysis in the spouse (C282Y and H63D). This would then give an indication of the possible genotypes in children and the need for later screening.

It is usually recommended that parents are also screened because of the possibility of unrecognized genetic haemochromatosis.

Population screening [32]

Genetic haemochromatosis is a preventable condition and with early diagnosis and de-ironing life expectancy is normal. This is a powerful argument for population screening of appropriate groups. Transferrin saturation for initial screening followed by DNA testing is a cost-effective strategy [10]. Automated measurement of the unbound iron binding capacity (UIBC) is as effective and less expensive [51]. Population screening has not been adopted by public health bodies because of the lack of information on the disease penetrance of genetic haemochromatosis [1].

Other iron storage diseases

Non-*HFE*-related inherited iron overload

Not all patients with haemochromatosis have mutations in the *HFE* gene. The most well-defined group is *juvenile haemochromatosis* [20]. Patients present at an earlier age (second to fourth decade) with iron overload and cardiac and endocrine problems in particular. The male to female ratio is equal. The condition is not linked to chromosome 6 and the disease locus has been mapped

mutated in a new type of haemochromatosis mapping to 7q22. *Nature Genet.* 2000; **25**: 14.

22 Cecchetti G, Binda A, Piperno A *et al.* Cardiac alterations in 36 consecutive patients with idiopathic haemochromatosis: polygraphic and echocardiographic evaluation. *Eur. Heart J.* 1991; **12**: 223.

23 Cotler SJ, Bronner MP, Press RD *et al.* End-stage liver disease without haemochromatosis associated with elevated hepatic iron index. *J. Hepatol.* 1998; **29**: 257.

24 Crawford DHG, Jazwinska EC, Cullen LM *et al.* Expression of HLA-linked haemochromatosis in subjects homozygous or heterozygous for the C282Y mutation. *Gastroenterology* 1998; **114**: 1003.

25 Crosby WH. Treatment of haemochromatosis by energetic phlebotomy. One patient's response to the letting of 55 l of blood in 11 months. *Br. J. Haematol.* 1958; **4**: 82.

26 Cundy T, Butler J, Bomford A *et al.* Reversibility of hypogonadotrophic hypogonadism associated with genetic haemochromatosis. *Clin. Endocrinol.* 1993; **38**: 617.

27 Deugnier Y, Charalambous P, Quilleuc D *et al.* Preneoplastic significance of hepatic iron-free foci in genetic haemochromatosis: a study of 185 patients. *Hepatology* 1993; **18**: 1363.

28 Deugnier Y, Guyader D, Crantock L *et al.* Primary liver cancer in genetic haemochromatosis: a clinical, pathological, and pathogenetic study of 54 cases. *Gastroenterology* 1993; **104**: 228.

29 Diamond T, Stiel D, Posen S *et al.* Osteoporosis in haemochromatosis: iron excess, gonadal deficiency, or other factors? *Ann. Intern. Med.* 1989; **110**: 430.

30 Donovan A, Brownlie A, Zhou Y *et al.* Positional cloning of zebrafish ferroportin 1 identifies a conserved vertebrate iron exporter. *Nature* 2000; **403**: 776.

31 Duane P, Raja KB, Simpson RJ *et al.* Intestinal iron absorption in chronic alcoholics. *Alcohol* 1992; **27**: 539.

32 EASL International Consensus Conference. Genetic haemochromatosis. *J. Hepatol.* 2000; **33**: 485.

33 Faraawi R, Harth M, Kertesz A *et al.* Arthritis in haemochromatosis. *J. Rheumatol.* 1993; **20**: 448.

34 Fargion S, Valenti L, Fracanzani AL *et al.* Hereditary hemochromatosis in a patient with congenital dyserythropoietic anaemia. *Blood* 2000; **96**: 3653.

35 Farrell FJ, Nguyen M, Woodley S *et al.* Outcome of liver transplantation in patients with haemochromatosis. *Hepatology* 1994; **20**: 404.

36 Feder JN, Gnirke A, Thomas W *et al.* A novel MHC class I-like gene is mutated in patients with hereditary haemochromatosis. *Nature Genet.* 1996; **13**: 399.

37 Feder JN, Penny DM, Irrinki A *et al.* The haemochromatosis gene product complexes with the transferrin receptor and lowers its affinity for ligand binding. *Proc. Natl. Acad. Sci. USA* 1998; **95**: 1472.

38 Fellman V, Rapola J, Pihko H *et al.* Iron-overload disease in infants involving fetal growth retardation, lactic acidosis, liver haemosiderosis, and aminoaciduria. *Lancet* 1998; **351**: 490.

39 Fleming MD, Trenor CC, Su MA *et al.* Microcytic anaemia mice have a mutation in Nramp2, a candidate iron transporter gene. *Nature Genet.* 1997; **16**: 383.

40 Fleming RE, Sly WS. Hepcidin: a putative iron-regulatory hormone relevant to hereditary hemochromatosis and the anemia of chronic disease. *Proc. Natl. Acad. Sci. USA.* 2001; **98**: 8160.

41 Fontana RJ, Israel J, LeClair P *et al.* Iron reduction before and during interferon therapy of chronic hepatitis C: results of a multicentre, randomized, controlled trial. *Hepatology* 2000; **31**: 730.

42 Gangaidzo IT, Moyo VM, Saungweme T *et al.* Iron overload in urban Africans in the 1990s. *Gut* 1999; **45**: 278.

43 Ganne-Carrié N, Christidis C, Chastang C *et al.* Liver iron is predictive of death in alcoholic cirrhosis: a multivariate study of 229 consecutive patients with alcoholic and/or hepatitis C virus cirrhosis: a prospective follow up study. *Gut* 2000; **46**: 277.

44 George DK, Goldwurm S, Macdonald GA *et al.* Increased hepatic iron concentration in nonalcoholic steatohepatitis is associated with increased fibrosis. *Gastroenterology* 1998; **114**: 311.

45 George DK, Ramm GA, Powell LW *et al.* Evidence for altered hepatic matrix degradation in genetic haemochromatosis. *Gut* 1998; **42**: 715.

46 George DK, Ramm GA, Walker NI *et al.* Elevated serum type IV collagen: a sensitive indicator for the presence of cirrhosis in haemochromatosis. *J. Hepatol.* 1999; **31**: 47.

47 Gordon HM, Wallace DF, Walker AP *et al.* The role of HFE mutation in determining predisposition to alcohol-related cirrhosis in a Celtic population. *Hepatology* 1998; **28**: 199A.

48 Gunshin H, Mackenzie B, Berger UV *et al.* Cloning and characterization of a mammalian proton-coupled metal-ion transporter. *Nature* 1997; **388**: 482.

49 Guyader D, Jacquelinet C, Moirand R *et al.* Noninvasive prediction of fibrosis in C282Y homozygous haemochromatosis. *Gastroenterology* 1998; **115**: 929.

50 Heilmeyer L, Keller W, Vivell O *et al.* Congenital transferrin deficiency in a seven-year-old girl. *Germ. Med. Mth.* 1961; **6**: 385.

51 Hickman PE, Hourigan LF, Powell LW *et al.* Automated measurement of unsaturated iron binding capacity is an effective screening strategy for C282Y homozygous haemochromatosis. *Gut* 2000; **46**: 405.

52 Hoffbrand AV, Gorman A, Laulicht M *et al.* Improvement in iron status and liver function in patients with transfusional iron overload with long-term subcutaneous desferrioxamine. *Lancet* 1979; **i**: 947.

53 Houglum K, Ramm GA, Crawford DHG *et al.* Excess iron induces hepatic oxidative stress and transforming growth factor β1 in genetic haemochromatosis. *Hepatology* 1997; **26**: 605.

54 Iancu TC, Deugnier Y, Halliday JW *et al.* Ultrastructural sequences during liver iron overload in genetic haemochromatosis. *J. Hepatol.* 1997; **27**: 628.

55 Kato J, Fujikawa K, Kanda M *et al.* A mutation, in the iron-responsive element of H ferritin mRNA, causing autosomal dominant iron overload. *Am. J. Hum. Genet.* 2001; **69**: 191.

56 Lebrón JA, Bjorkman, PJ. The transferrin receptor binding site on HFE, the class I MHC-related protein mutated in hereditary haemochromatosis. *J. Mol. Biol.* 1999; **294**: 1109.

57 Lombard M, Bomford A, Polson RJ *et al.* Differential expression of transferrin receptor in duodenal mucosa in iron overload. *Gastroenterology* 1990; **98**: 976.

58 Martinez PA, Biron C, Blanc F *et al.* Compound heterozygotes for haemochromatosis gene mutations: may they help to understand the pathophysiology of the disease? *Blood Cell. Mol. Dis.* 1997; **23**: 269.

59 McDonnell SM, Hover A, Gloe D *et al.* Population-based screening for haemochromatosis using phenotypic and

DNA testing among employees of health maintenance organizations in Springfield, Missouri. *Am. J. Med.* 1999; **107**: 30.

60 McKie AT, Marciani P, Rolfs A *et al.* A novel duodenal iron-regulated transporter, IREG1, implicated in the basolateral transfer of iron to the circulation. *Mol. Cell.* 2000; **5**: 299.

61 Mendler MH, Turlin B, Moirand R *et al.* Insulin resistance-associated hepatic iron overload. *Gastroenterology* 1999; **117**: 1155.

62 Merryweather-Clarke AT, Pointon JJ, Shearman JD *et al.* Global prevalence of putative haemochromatosis mutations. *J. Med. Genet.* 1997; **34**: 275.

63 Montosi G, Donovan A, Totaro A *et al.* Autosomal-dominant hemochromatosis is associated with a mutation in the ferroportin (SLC11A3) gene. *J. Clin. Invest.* 2001; **108**: 619.

64 Montosi G, Garuti C, Martinelli S *et al.* Hepatic stellate cells are not subjected to oxidant stress during iron-induced fibrogenesis in rodents. *Hepatology* 1998; **27**: 1611.

65 Montosi G, Paglia P, Garuti C *et al.* Wild type HFE protein normalizes transferrin iron accumutation in macrophages from subjects with hereditary hemochromatosis. *Blood* 2000; **96**: 1125.

66 Njajou OT, Vaessen N, Joosse M *et al.* A mutation in *SLC11A3* is associated with autosomal dominant hemochromatosis. *Nature Genet.* 2001; **28**: 213.

67 Niederau C, Fischer R, Purschel A *et al.* Long-term survival in patients with hereditary haemochromatosis. *Gastroenterology* 1996; **110**: 1107.

68 Olynyk JK, Cullen DJ, Aquilia S *et al.* A population-based study of the clinical expression of the haemochromatosis gene. *N. Engl. J. Med.* 1999; **341**: 718.

69 Parkkila S, Waheed A, Britton RS *et al.* Immunohistochemistry of HLA-H, the protein defective in patients with hereditary haemochromatosis, reveals unique pattern of expression in gastrointestinal tract. *Proc. Natl. Acad. Sci. USA* 1997; **94**: 2534.

70 Pietrangelo A, Gualdi R, Casalgrandi G *et al.* Enhanced hepatic collagen type I mRNA expression in fat-storing cells in a rodent model of haemochromatosis. *Hepatology* 1994; **19**: 714.

71 Pietrangelo A, Gualdi R, Casalgrandi G *et al.* Molecular and cellular aspects of iron-induced hepatic cirrhosis in rodents. *J. Clin. Invest.* 1995; **95**: 1823.

72 Piperno A, Sampietro M, Pietrangelo A *et al.* Heterogeneity of haemochromatosis in Italy. *Gastroenterology* 1998; **114**: 996.

73 Powell LW. Hemochromatosis: the impact of early diagnosis and therapy. *Gastroenterology* 1996; **110**: 1304.

74 Powell LW, Halliday JW, Cowlishaw JL. Relationship between serum ferritin and total body iron stores in idiopathic haemochromatosis. *Gut* 1978; **19**: 538.

75 Prieto J, Barry M, Sherlock S. Serum-ferritin in patients with iron overload and with acute and chronic liver diseases. *Gastroenterology* 1975; **68**: 525.

76 Ramm GA, Crawford DHG, Powell LW *et al.* Hepatic stellate cell activation in genetic haemochromatosis. *J. Hepatol.* 1997; **26**: 584.

77 Roberts AG, Whatley SD, Morgan RR *et al.* Increased frequency of the haemochromatosis Cys282Tyr mutation in sporadic porphyria cutanea tarda. *Lancet* 1997; **349**: 321.

78 Roest M, van der Schouw YT, de Valk B *et al.* Heterozygosity for a hereditary haemochromatosis gene is associated with cardiovascular death in women. *Circulation* 1999; **100**: 1268.

79 Roetto A, Totaro A, Cazzola M *et al.* Juvenile haemochromatosis locus maps to chromosone 1q. *Am. J. Hum. Genet.* 1999; **64**: 1388.

80 Sampietro M, Piperno A, Lupica L *et al.* High prevalence of the His63Asp HFE mutation in Italian patients with porphyria cutanea tarda. *Hepatology* 1998; **27**: 181.

81 Sheldon JH. *Haemochromatosis.* Oxford University Press, Oxford, 1935.

82 Sigurdsson L, Reyes J, Kocoshis SA *et al.* Neonatal haemochromatosis: outcome of pharmacologic and surgical therapies. *J. Pediatr. Gastroenterol. Nutr.* 1998; **26**: 85.

83 Tavill AS. AASLD Practice Guidelines. Diagnosis and management of hemochromatosis. *Hepatology* 2001; **33**: 1321.

84 Tsukamoto H, Horne W, Kamimura S *et al.* Experimental liver cirrhosis induced by alcohol and iron. *J. Clin. Invest.* 1995; **96**: 620.

85 Tuomainen P, Kontula K, Nyssnen K *et al.* Increased risk of acute myocardial infarction in carriers of the haemochromatosis gene Cys282Tyr mutation: a prospective cohort study in men in Eastern Finland. *Circulation* 1999; **100**: 1274.

86 Tweed MJ, Roland JM. Haemochromatosis as an endocrine cause of subfertility. *Br. Med. J.* 1998; **316**: 915.

87 Villeneuve J-P, Bilodeau M, Lepage R *et al.* Variability in hepatic iron concentration measurement from needle-biopsy specimens. *J. Hepatol.* 1996; **25**: 172.

88 Vulpe CD, Kuo YM, Murphy TL *et al.* Hephaestin, a ceruloplasmin homologue implicated in intestinal iron transport, is defective in the *sla* mouse. *Nature Genet.* 1999; **21**: 195.

89 Waheed A, Parkkila S, Zhou XY *et al.* Hereditary haemochromatosis: effects of C282Y and H63D mutations on association with β2-microglobulin, intracellular processing, and cell surface expression of the HFE protein in COS-7 cells. *Proc. Natl. Acad. Sci. USA* 1997; **94**: 12384.

90 Wallace DF, Dooley JS, Walker AP. A novel mutation of HFE explains the classical phenotype of genetic haemochromatosis in a C282Y heterozygote. *Gastroenterology* 1999; **116**: 1409.

91 Webster GJM, Saeb-Parsy K, Davies SE *et al.* The effect of heterozygosity for C282Y mutation on fibrosis and liver iron status in chronic hepatitis C. *Hepatology* 1998; **28**: 526A.

92 Williams R, Smith PM, Spicer EJF *et al.* Venesection therapy in idiopathic haemochromatosis. *Q. J. Med.* 1969; **38**: 1.

93 Williams R, Williams HS, Scheuer PJ *et al.* Iron absorption and siderosis in chronic liver disease. *Q. J. Med.* 1967; **36**: 151.

94 Willis G, Wimperis JZ, Lonsdale R *et al.* Incidence of liver disease in people with HFE mutations. *Gut* 2000; **46**: 401.

95 Yang Q, McDonnell SM, Khoury MJ *et al.* Hemochromatosis-associated mortality in the United States from 1979 to 1992: an analysis of multiple-cause mortality data. *Ann. Intern. Med.* 1998; **129**: 946.

96 Yoshida K, Furihata K, Takeda S *et al.* A mutation in the ceruloplasmin gene is associated with systemic haemosiderosis in humans. *Nature Genet.* 1995; **9**: 267.

97 Younossi ZM, Gramlich T, Bacon BR *et al.* Hepatic iron and nonalcoholic fatty liver disease. *Hepatology* 1999; **30**: 847.

98 Yu J, Wessling-Resnick M. Influence of copper depletion on iron uptake mediated by SFT, a stimulator of iron transport. *J. Biol. Chem.* 1998; **273**: 6909.

99 Zoller H, Koch RO, Theurl I *et al.* Expression of the duodenal iron transporters divalent-metal transporter 1 and ferroportin 1 in iron deficiency and iron overload. *Gastroenterology* 2001; **120**: 1412.

34 Scott J, Gollan JL, Samourian S *et al.* Wilson's disease, presenting as chronic active hepatitis. *Gastroenterology* 1978; **74**: 645.

35 Shaver WA, Bhartt H, Combes B. Low serum alkaline phosphatase activity in Wilson's disease. *Hepatology* 1986; **6**: 859.

36 Smallwood RA, Williams HA, Rosenoer VM *et al.* Liver-copper levels in liver disease. Studies using neutron activation analysis. *Lancet* 1968; **ii**: 1310.

37 Sokol RJ, McKim JM, Devereaux MW. α-Tocopherol ameliorates oxidant injury in isolated copper-overloaded rat hepatocytes. *Paediatr. Res.* 1996; **39**: 259.

38 Sokol RJ, Twedt D, McKim JM *et al.* Oxidant injury to hepatic mitochondria in patients with Wilson's disease and Bedlington terriers with copper toxicosis. *Gastroenterology* 1994; **107**: 1788.

39 Srai SKS, Burroughs AK, Wood B *et al.* The ontogeny of liver copper metabolism in the guinea pig: clues to the aetiology of Wilson's disease. *Hepatology* 1986; **6**: 427.

40 Steindl P, Ferenci P, Dienes HP *et al.* Wilson's disease in patients presenting with liver disease: a diagnostic challenge. *Gastroenterology* 1997; **113**: 212.

41 Sternlieb I. Wilson's disease and pregnancy. *Hepatology* 2000; **31**: 531.

42 Stracciari A, Tempestini A, Borghi A *et al.* Effect of liver transplantation on neurological manifestations in Wilson disease. *Arch. Neurol.* 2000; **57**: 384.

43 Strickland GT, Frommer D, Leu M-L *et al.* Wilson's disease in the United Kingdom and Taiwan. I. General characteristics of 142 cases and prognosis. II. A genetic analysis of 88 cases. *Q. J. Med.* 1973; **42**: 619.

44 Togashi Y, Li Y, Kang J-H *et al.* D-Penicillamine prevents the development of hepatitis in Long–Evans Cinnamon rats with abnormal copper metabolism. *Hepatology* 1992; **15**: 82.

45 Walshe JM. Treatment of Wilson's disease with trientine (triethylene tetramine) dihydrochloride. *Lancet* 1982; **ii**: 643.

46 Walshe JM. Penicillamine: the treatment of first choice for patients with Wilson's disease. *Mov. Disord.* 1999; **14**: 545.

47 Walshe JM, Dixon AK. Dangers of noncompliance in Wilson's disease. *Lancet* 1986; **i**: 845.

48 Walshe JM, Yealland M. Wilson's disease: the problem of delayed diagnosis. *J. Neurol. Neurosurg. Psych.* 1992; **55**: 692.

49 Walshe JM, Yealland M. Chelation treatment of neurological Wilson's disease. *Q. J. Med.* 1993; **86**; 197.

50 Wilson AK. Progressive lenticular degeneration: a familial nervous disease associated with cirrhosis of the liver. *Brain* 1912; **34**: 295.

51 Wu M, Cooper JM, Butler P *et al.* Oxidative phosphorylation defects in Wilson's disease liver. *Lancet* 2000; **356**: 469.

Chapter 25
Nutritional and Metabolic Liver Diseases

Malnutrition

Worldwide, protein malnutrition is extremely common. The clinical spectrum includes *kwashiorkor*, historically thought due to protein malnutrition, a view that has been challenged [17], and *marasmus* in which there is decreased energy intake relative to need, through starvation and/or medical illness. The liver suffers in common with other organs.

Kwashiorkor is classically associated with accumulation of fat in the liver (up to 50% of wet weight in severe cases), although the reason remains unclear (see below). It appears that fat can also occur with marasmus, although it is less frequent and less extensive than in kwashiorkor [13], perhaps because of the wide range of causes. Liver biopsies from malnourished children show a reduction in liver protein.

The liver is involved in wasting diseases, especially with chronic diarrhoea such as ulcerative colitis, and the hepatic changes in the alcoholic may be partly nutritional. Hepatic necrosis and fibrosis can be produced in experimental animals by certain diets, particularly those low in protein and essential amino acids [20]. Previous malnutrition may 'condition' the liver to toxic and infective agents, but this has not been proved. Oxidant injury rather than protein deficiency is being proposed as a possible cause of some of the changes in malnutrition [17].

Liver enzymes are usually normal in patients with *anorexia nervosa*. Histological findings have been described in individual patients only.

Fatty liver

This is defined as fat, largely triglyceride, exceeding 5% of the liver weight. It is caused by failure of normal hepatic fat metabolism either due to a defect within the hepatocyte or to delivery of excess fat, fatty acid or carbohydrate beyond the secretory capacity for lipid of the liver cell. Liver biopsy and imaging procedures, such as ultrasound and CT, are increasing the number of patients being identified with excess fat in the liver.

Theoretically fatty liver could accumulate through at least four mechanisms.

1 *Increased delivery of dietary fat or fatty acids to the liver.* Dietary fat is transported in the circulation mainly as chylomicrons (fig. 25.1). Lipolysis in adipose tissue liberates the fatty acids. These are incorporated into trigly-

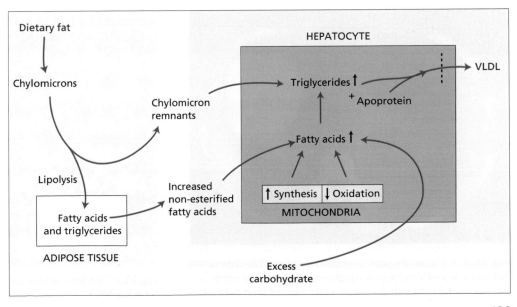

Fig. 25.1. Factors in fatty liver.

Non-alcoholic steato-hepatitis (NASH) is less frequent than pure fatty change but may lead to fibrosis and cirrhosis.

At autospy cirrhosis is seen twice as commonly in 'diabetics' as in the general population, but this excess incidence may be flawed because the hyperglycaemia recorded in life might be secondary to unrecognized cirrhosis.

Clinical features

Type 1 diabetes

There are usually no clinical features referable to the liver. Occasionally, however, the liver is greatly enlarged, firm and with a smooth, tender edge. Some of the nausea, abdominal pain and vomiting of diabetic ketosis may be due to hepatomegaly. Hepatic enlargement is found particularly in young people and children with severe, uncontrolled diabetes. Hepatomegaly is present in around 10% of well-controlled diabetics, in 60% of uncontrolled diabetics and in 10% of patients in ketosis. The liver returns to a normal size when the diabetes is brought under complete control. The enlargement is due to increased glycogen. Insulin therapy in the presence of a very high blood sugar level augments still further the glycogen content of the liver and, in the initial stages of treatment, hepatomegaly may increase.

Type 2 diabetes

The liver may be enlarged with a firm, smooth, non-tender edge. Enlargement is due to increased deposition of hepatic fat largely related to the obesity.

Diabetes in childhood

The liver may be enlarged and this enlargement has been attributed both to fatty infiltration and to increased amounts of glycogen. Aspiration biopsy studies show that the fatty change is slight but that the liver does contain an excess of glycogen. The hepatic changes are similar to those already described in the type 1, insulin-sensitive diabetic.

Liver function tests

In well-controlled diabetics, routine tests are usually normal and any change is due to a cause other than diabetes. Acidosis may produce mild changes including hyperglobulinaemia and a slightly raised serum bilirubin level. These return to normal with diabetic control.

Eighty per cent of diabetics with a fatty liver have abnormal results for one or more serum biochemical test such as transaminases, alkaline phosphatase and γ-glutamyl-transpeptidase.

Hepatomegaly, whether due to increased amounts of glycogen in type 1 diabetes, or to fatty change in type 2, does not correlate with the results of the liver function tests.

Hepato-biliary disease and diabetes

Any real increase of cirrhosis in diabetics seems unlikely. In most instances, the cirrhosis is diagnosed first before impaired glucose tolerance is recognized.

Advanced genetic haemochromatosis causes diabetes mellitus. Diabetes is also associated with chronic hepatitis C virus infection [5], and may occur in patients with autoimmune chronic hepatitis, probably due to the shared immunogenetic predisposition (HLA-B8 and -DR3).

Gallstones are frequent in non-insulin-dependent diabetics. This is probably more related to the biliary changes of obesity than a direct effect of diabetes. The same applies to the finding of a reduced gallbladder contractility in these patients.

Elective surgery for gallbladder disease is not dangerous but emergency biliary surgery in diabetics is associated with an increased mortality and a high risk of wound infections.

Sulphonylurea therapy can be complicated by cholestatic or granulomatous liver disease.

Glucose intolerance of cirrhosis

About 80% of patients with cirrhosis are glucose intolerant, with hyperglycaemia after an oral glucose load (fig. 25.11) [6]. Around 25% become frankly diabetic. The underlying mechanism is complex and not fully understood [2]. There is peripheral insulin resistance [11] and reduced insulin clearance in most cirrhotics. Adipocytes show defects in insulin sensitivity [11]. The first-pass hepatic extraction of insulin is reduced compared with controls [4]. Most patients compensate for the peripheral insulin resistance with increased pancreatic insulin secretion. The result is high circulating insulin levels, a normal fasting blood glucose and minimal glucose intolerance.

In some patients there is a blunted or subnormal pancreatic secretion of insulin after oral glucose, shown by the delayed appearance of C-peptide (fig. 25.11) [4]. This leads to delayed peripheral utilization of glucose. The fasting glucose remains normal.

With more severe hyposecretion of insulin [3], there is also continued hepatic glucose production due to lack of inhibition by insulin [10]. The net result of these changes is fasting hyperglycaemia and marked hyperglycaemia after oral glucose. The patient is diabetic.

The glucose intolerance of cirrhotic patients can be distinguished from genuine diabetes mellitus as the

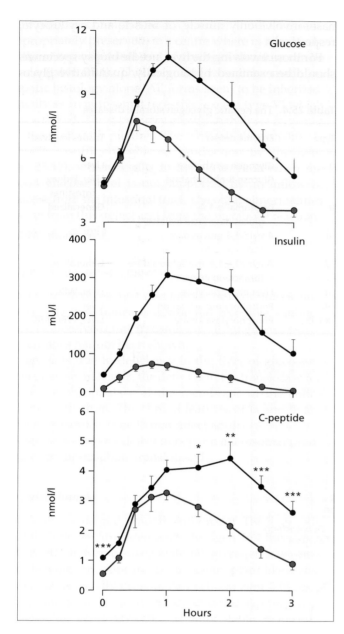

Fig. 25.11. Blood glucose, serum insulin and C-peptide responses to 75 g of oral glucose in cirrhotics ($n=10$) (●) and normal controls ($n=9$) (●). Note the normal fasting glucose followed by hyperglycaemia in the cirrhotics, despite greater insulin levels. The C-peptide response is blunted and only becomes significantly greater than controls at 90 min (*$P<0.05$; **$P<0.01$; ***$P<0.001$) [4].

fasting blood glucose is usually normal. Clinical features of diabetes are not seen.

If the hyperinsulinaemia is reduced in cirrhotics for 96 h by the infusion of the somatostatin analogue octreotide, insulin-mediated glucose uptake returns to normal. This suggests that chronic hyperinsulinaemia in cirrhosis causes insulin resistance [9].

Liver transplantation reverses glucose intolerance and insulin resistance in cirrhotics. Both hepatic glucose uptake and peripheral glucose metabolism improve [7].

Diagnosis of cirrhosis in the presence of diabetes is usually easy from the clinical features. If necessary liver biopsy is diagnostic.

High carbohydrate feeding may be necessary in the management of cirrhosis, especially if there is encephalopathy. This always takes precedence over any impairment of glucose tolerance whether from genuine diabetes or secondary to the liver disease.

Treatment of diabetes in cirrhotic patients

There are few data on the treatment of diabetes in patients with cirrhosis [2]. Decisions depend upon the degree of hyperglycaemia and the severity and prognosis of the liver disease. Diet is appropriate for mild hyperglycaemia. Sulphonylureas can be used if diet is unsuccessful or the blood glucose is higher, but because these agents are metabolized by the liver, the shorter acting agents such as tolbutamide are preferred to reduce the risk of hypoglycaemia [2]. Because of the risk of lactic acidosis, biguanides such as metformin should be avoided. Insulin may be necessary but, as with other diabetics, regular self-monitoring of blood glucose is necessary. Short-acting insulin before meals, and intermediate-acting insulin in the evening, may be used. Strict guidelines do not exist and good control in this group of patients is often difficult and unsatisfactory. Steroid administration, necessary for example in autoimmune chronic liver disease, further complicates diabetic control.

References

1 Blendis L, Brill S, Oren R. Hepatogenous diabetes: reduced insulin sensitivity and increased awareness. *Gastroenterology* 2000; **119**: 1800.
2 Kruszynska YT. Glucose control in liver disease. *Curr. Med. Lit. Gastroenterol.* 1992; **11**: 9.
3 Kruszynska YT, Goulas S, Wollen N *et al.* Insulin secretory capacity and the regulation of glucagon secretion in diabetic and nondiabetic alcoholic cirrhotic patients. *J. Hepatol.* 1998; **28**: 280–91.
4 Kruszynska YT, Home PD, McIntyre N. Relationship between insulin sensitivity, insulin secretion and glucose tolerance in cirrhosis. *Hepatology* 1991; **14**: 103.
5 Mason AL, Lau JYN, Hoang N *et al.* Association of diabetes mellitus and chronic hepatitis C virus infection. *Hepatology* 1999; **29**: 328.
6 Megyesi C, Samols E, Marks V. Glucose tolerance and diabetes in chronic liver disease. *Lancet* 1967; **ii**: 1051.
7 Merli M, Leonetti F, Riggio O *et al.* Glucose intolerance and insulin resistance in cirrhosis are normalized after liver transplantation. *Hepatology* 1999; **30**: 649.
8 Perseghin G, Mazzafero V, Sereni LP *et al.* Contribution of reduced insulin sensitivity and secretion to the pathogenesis of hepatogenous diabetes: effect of liver transplantation. *Hepatology* 2000; **31**: 694.

Biopsy of the subcutaneous abdominal fat pad, rectal mucosa and labial salivary gland are safe and give a positive result in up to 75–80% of cases depending on expertise in the procedure [8, 12]. Liver biopsy is more invasive and carries a reported risk of bleeding of 4–5% and is best avoided in favour of the less invasive routes.

^{123}I-SAP scintigraphy is a specific and sensitive method for detecting and monitoring amyloidosis during treatment of the underlying cause [14]. This method is, however, at present a specialized tool with restricted availability.

Prognosis

This varies according to the type of amyloidosis, the degree of organ involvement and the response to therapy of the underlying condition.

Patients with AL amyloidosis have a mean survival of 1–2 years [12]. There may be longer survival with intensive chemotherapy compared to low-dose oral regimens [4]. Survival is not effected by liver involvement by amyloid [7, 14]. Survival is less when patients have symptomatic heart disease (median survival 6 months).

The prognosis for AA amyloidosis is affected by the underlying chronic disease. The 5-year survival in those with liver deposits is reduced compared with those without liver involvement (43 vs. 72%) (fig. 25.15) [14]. Surviral is significantly better in those with a serum amyloid A value maintained in the reference range (< 10 mg/l) [9].

Patients with FAP may survive for up to 15 years. Patients with transthyretin mutations associated with a younger age of disease onset have a more rapid progression of neurological and cardiac disease and a shorter survival [6]. The 5-year survival after liver transplantation is 75% [17].

Treatment

AA amyloid is treated by controlling the underlying disease. If tuberculosis is cured then amyloid may disappear. Similarly, clinical improvement in rheumatoid arthritis may be paralleled by disappearance of clinical signs of amyloidosis. There is no specific treatment.

Prophylactic colchicine prevents the development of amyloidosis in all cases of FMF.

The treatment of AL amyloid remains difficult because melphalan combined with prednisone only has a 30% response rate with a mean survival of 18 months [13]. Although the response to higher doses of melphalan with peripheral blood stem cell support is greater (60%) [4], the patients have to be fit enough to tolerate the treatment.

Liver transplantation is the definitive treatment for FAP with a 75% 5-year survival [17]. Liver transplanta-

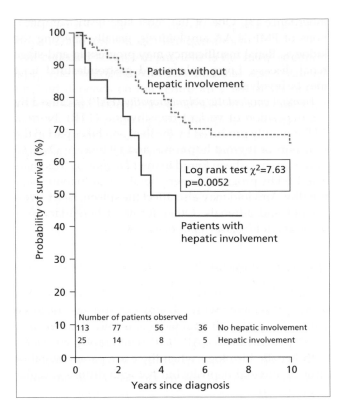

Fig. 25.15. Kaplan–Meier estimate of survival in patients with systemic AA amyloidosis with and without hepatic involvement on ^{123}I-serum amyloid P component. (From [14] with permission.)

tion results in disappearance of the variant TTR from plasma, and regression of some disease. Recovery from autonomic neuropathy is greater than from peripheral neuropathy. The explanted liver from patients with FAP has been transplanted into selected recipients, on the basis that these livers may be normal apart from the production of variant transthyretin, having only been removed to arrest the build-up of further amyloid and clinical progression of polyneuropathy [16]. This has been termed domino liver transplantation. Follow-up of recipients of a FAP liver was uncomplicated over 18 months, and allowed study of the variant transthyretin protein in donors and recipients.

References

1 Ben-Chetrit E, Levy M. Familial mediterranean fever. *Lancet* 1998; **351**: 659.

2 Bion E, Brenard R, Pariente EA *et al.* Sinusoidal portal hypertension in hepatic amyloidosis. *Gut* 1991; **32**: 227.

3 Booth DR, Gillmore JD, Lachmann HJ *et al.* The genetic basis of autosomal dominant familial Mediterranean fever. *Q. J. Med.* 2000; **93**: 217.

4 Comenzo RL, Vosburgh E, Falk RH *et al.* Dose-intensive melphalan with blood stem-cell support for the treatment of AL (amyloid light-chain) amyloidosis: survival and responses in 25 patients. *Blood* 1998; **91**: 3662.

5 Faa G, Van Eyken P, De Vos R *et al.* Light chain deposition

disease of the liver associated with AL-type amyloidosis and severe cholestasis. *J. Hepatol.* 1991; **12**: 75.

6 Falk RH, Comenzo RL, Skinner M. The systemic amyloidoses. *N. Engl. J. Med.* 1997; **337**: 898.

7 Gertz MA, Kyle RA. Hepatic amyloidosis: clinical appraisal in 77 patients. *Hepatology* 1997; **25**: 118.

8 Gillmore JD, Lovat LB, Hawkins PN. Amyloidosis and the liver. *J. Hepatol.* 1999; **30**: 17.

9 Gillmore JD, Lovat LB, Persey MR *et al*. Amyloid load and clinical outcome in AA amyloidosis in relation to circulating concentration of serum amyloid A protein. *Lancet* 2001; **358**: 24.

10 Grateau G, Pêcheux C, Cazeneuve C *et al*. Clinical vs. genetic diagnosis of familial Mediterranean fever. *Q. J. Med.* 2000; **93**: 223.

11 Harrison RF, Hawkins PN, Roche WR *et al*. 'Fragile' liver and massive hepatic haemorrhage due to hereditary amyloidosis. *Gut* 1996; **38**: 151.

12 Kyle RA, Gertz MA. Primary systemic amyloidosis: clinical and laboratory features in 474 cases. *Semin. Haematol.* 1995; **32**: 45.

13 Kyle RA, Gertz MA, Greipp PR *et al*. A trial of three regimens for primary amyloidosis: colchicine alone, melphalan and prednisone, and melphalan, prednisone, and colchicine. *N. Engl. J. Med.* 1997; **336**: 1202.

14 Lovat LB, Persey MR, Madhoo S *et al*. The liver in systemic amyloidosis: insights from ^{123}I serum amyloid P component scintigraphy in 484 patients. *Gut* 1998; **42**: 727.

15 Peters RA, Koukoulis G, Gimson A *et al*. Primary amyloidosis and severe intrahepatic cholestatic jaundice. *Gut* 1994; **35**: 1322.

16 Schmidt HH-J, Nashan B, Pröpsting MJ *et al*. Familial amyloidotic polyneuropathy: domino liver transplantation. *J. Hepatol.* 1999; **30**: 293.

17 Suhr OB, Herlenius G, Friman S *et al*. Liver transplantation for hereditary transthyretin amyloidosis. *Liver Transplant.* 2000; **6**: 263.

α_1-Antitrypsin deficiency [2, 9]

α_1-Antitrypsin is synthesized in the rough endoplasmic reticulum of the liver. It comprises 80–90% of the serum α_1-globulin and is an inhibitor of trypsin and other proteases. Deficiency results in the unopposed action of these enzymes, in particular neutrophil elastase. The lungs are the major target, with damage to alveoli and resulting emphysema.

The gene for α_1-antitrypsin is on chromosome 14. There are about 75 different alleles at this locus which can be distinguished by isoelectric focusing or agarose gel electrophoresis at acid pH, or by PCR analysis. M is the common, normal allele. Z and S are the most frequent abnormal alleles which put the individual at risk of disease. One gene is derived from each parent. The combination results in normal, intermediate, low or zero serum α_1-antitrypsin levels. Protease inhibitor (Pi) MM gives a serum α_1-antitrypsin value of 20–53 µmol/l—the normal state. PiZZ results in a low concentration of 2.5–7 µmol/l and PiNull-Null gives zero levels. Both give a high risk of emphysema. PiSS and PiMZ give levels 50–60% of normal with no increased risk of lung disease. PiSZ gives α_1-antitrypsin levels of 8–19 µmol/l with a mildly increased risk.

Mutation of the gene can give deficiency of circulating α_1-antitrypsin by a number of mechanisms. Liver disease, however, only occurs with mutations where α_1-antitrypsin accumulates in hepatocytes. The classical type is PiZZ but the M_{malton} and M_{duarte} variants may do the same.

Pathogenesis of liver disease [9, 14]

Only the PiZZ phenotype has been clearly associated with liver disease. This is not due to the low circulating levels of α_1-antitrypsin arriving at the liver since other phenotypes with a low circulating level do not develop hepatic damage. Intra-hepatic accumulation of α_1-antitrypsin seems to be responsible. Studies of the molecular structure have shown that with the ZZ mutation there is polymerization of protein units. Normally the reactive loop (fig. 25.16) swings in between the β-helices of the so-called A-sheet of the protein, where it interacts with elastase and other enzymes. In the ZZ mutant protein the

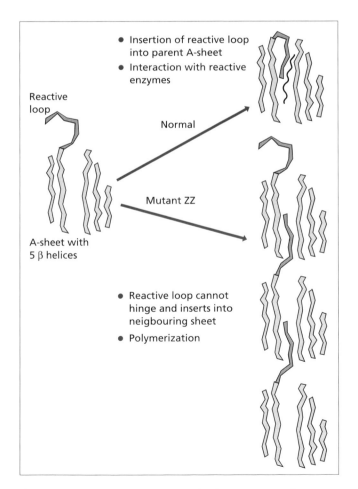

- Insertion of reactive loop into parent A-sheet
- Interaction with reactive enzymes

Reactive loop

Normal

Mutant ZZ

A-sheet with 5 β helices

- Reactive loop cannot hinge and inserts into neigbouring sheet
- Polymerization

Fig. 25.16. Proposed mechanism of polymerization of ZZ α_1-antitrypsin.

Table 26.2. Unconjugated hyperbilirubinaemia in neonates related to time of onset

Birth to 2 days
Haemolytic disease
3–7 days
Physiological ± prematurity
hypoxia
acidosis
1–8 weeks
Congenital haemolytic disorders
Breast milk jaundice
Hypopituitarism
Crigler–Najjar syndrome
Hypothyroidism
Perinatal complications: haemorrhage, sepsis
Upper gastrointestinal obstruction

Table 26.3. Investigations of the jaundiced newborn

Total and direct serum bilirubin
Blood group
Rhesus status
Coombs' test
Haematocrit
Blood smear for morphology
Blood culture
Urine culture

(*physiological jaundice*). It is a benign self-limited process although it is more serious in low birth weight infants where it may persist for as long as 2 weeks. The urine contains both urobilin and bilirubin and the stools are paler than normal.

Hepatic conjugating and transport systems for bilirubin are delayed in the neonate. Absorption of bilirubin from the intestine is increased. Bilirubin binding to albumin is reduced, particularly in premature infants. The jaundice is enhanced by factors which depress liver function, such as hypoxia and hypoglycaemia. Drugs such as water-soluble vitamin K analogues add to the jaundice.

Serum bilirubin levels may be *lower* in infants with circulatory failure, asphyxia and sepsis. Bilirubin may be a physiological anti-oxidant providing protection against perinatal ischaemia–reperfusion tissue injury [8].

The bilirubinaemia is *not* physiological if the level exceeds 5 mg/dl (86 µmol/l) on the first day, 10 mg (171 µmol/l) on the second day, or 12–13 mg (206–223 µmol/l) at any time.

Unconjugated hyperbilirubinaemia in the neonatal period is complicated by bilirubin encephalopathy (*kernicterus*).

Management

Phototherapy. Hyperbilirubinaemia may be prevented or controlled by exposure of the infant to light with a wavelength near 450 nm. The light converts bilirubin IXα photochemically to a relatively stable geometric isomer. Phototherapy is used if the total serum bilirubin exceeds or is equal to 17 mg/dl (289 mmol/l) during the first 48 h of life. It is discontinued after the serum bilirubin has decreased by more than 2 mg or has fallen to 13 mg or less. *Exchange transfusion* is rarely necessary with the advent of phototherapy. It is indicated if the total serum bilirubin exceeds 20 mg by direct spectrophotometry, or a bilirubin rising at a rate greater than 1 mg/dl/h despite phototherapy.

Enzyme induction using phenobarbital is effective when given to the mother.

Tin mesoporphyrin (Sn mesoporphyrin) inhibits haemoxygenase and haem analogues [58]. It may be useful in controlling hyperbilirubinaemia if given in one dose intramuscularly to healthy term or pre-term infants. Its use is still experimental.

Haemolytic disease of the newborn

Fetal–maternal incompatibility usually concerns the Rh blood factors and rarely the ABO or other blood groups. The prevalence is falling, now that anti-D immune globulin is given prophylatically to mothers.

Characteristically, the first-born escapes the disease unless the mother's blood has been sensitized by a previous transfusion of Rh-positive blood.

The infant is jaundiced during the first 2 days of life. Serum unconjugated bilirubin is increased. The critical period is in the first few days when the more deeply jaundiced infants may develop *kernicterus*.

Diagnosis may be suspected by antenatal examination of the mother's blood for specific antibodies and confirmed by a positive Coombs' test in the infant and by blood typing on mother and child.

The risk of mental or physical impairment is low until the serum bilirubin increases well above 20 mg/dl (342 µmol/l).

Kernicterus

This grave condition complicates prematurity jaundice, haemolytic disease and neonatal hepatitis. Management with phototherapy, exchange transfusion and phenobarbital has reduced its occurence. However, diagnosis is increasing as neonates are discharged from hospital earlier and recognition is delayed.

It is prevented by early detection of full-term infants at risk. It is rare in pre-term neonates. Very low birth weight infants with a serum bilirubin level of 10 mg/dl, lower than in full-term babies, may be at risk. Daily transcutaneous serum bilirubin estimations are valuable in management.

Within the first 5 days, the jaundiced infant becomes restless or lethargic and febrile, developing a stiff neck and head retraction which proceeds to opisthotonos. There is stiffness of the limbs with pronated arms, eye squinting, lid retraction, twitching or convulsions and a high-pitched cry

Death may supervene rapidly in 12h and 70% of affected infants die within 7 days of onset. The remaining 30% may survive, but are affected by mental defects, cerebral palsy or athetosis, until they eventually die from intercurrent infections.

MRI T$_2$-weighted images show bilateral high intensity areas in the globus pallidus [87].

Autopsy reveals yellow staining of the basal ganglia and other areas of the brain and spinal cord with unconjugated bilirubin which, being lipid soluble, has an affinity for nervous tissue.

Kernicterus is related to circulating free bilirubin crossing the blood–brain barrier. Reduction of serum bilirubin–albumin binding may play a part and indeed albumin infusions have been used therapeutically.

Mechanisms of bilirubin toxicity and neuron damage are unknown. Bilirubin, however, does inhibit neuronal function [34].

Kernicterus is potentiated by hypoxia, metabolic acidosis and septicaemia [34]. Organic anions which compete for bilirubin binding sites on albumin increase kernicterus although the serum bilirubin level falls. Such anions include salicylates, sulphonamides, free fatty acids and haematin.

Congenital haemolytic disorders

These can all lead to unconjugated hyperbilirubinaemia in the first 2 days of life. They include the red cell enzyme deficiencies (glucose-6-phosphate dehydrogenase and pyruvate kinase) congenital spherocytosis and pyknocytosis.

Glucose-6-phosphate dehydrogenase deficiency. Infants develop jaundice, usually on the second or third day of life. The precipitating haemolytic agent may be a drug such as salicylate, phenacetin or sulphonamides transmitted in the maternal breast milk. This condition is frequent in the Mediterranean area, in the Far East and in Nigeria.

Breast milk jaundice

Hyperbilirubinaemia (serum bilirubin more than 12 mg/dl) affects 34% of newborn breast-fed babies compared with only 15% of those who are formula fed. The aetiology of this breast milk jaundice is unknown. It is diagnosed by exclusion and by showing a fall in serum bilirubin if breast feeding is stopped for 48 h.

The jaundice lasts from 2 weeks to more than 2 months.

Crigler–Najjar hyperbilirubinaemia (Chapter 12)

This may present in the first few days of life. Type I is treated by phototherapy and type II by phenobarbital.

Pituitary or adrenal dysfunction

This is associated with neonatal jaundice in 30%. It is marked by hypoglycaemia, midline facial abnormalities, a low thyroid-stimulating hormone and a free thyroxine level with a low 9.00 a.m. cortisol value. It resolves with hormone replacement, thyroxine and hydrocortisone.

Hypothyroidism

This is more common in girls than boys. Mild anaemia is common and the infant is sluggish. The diagnosis is confirmed by finding low serum thyroxine and tri-iodothyronine levels with high thyroid-stimulating hormone, and by observing the effects of therapy. The mechanism of the jaundice is unknown.

Perinatal complications

Haemorrhage with release of blood into the tissues provides a bilirubin load which may exacerbate jaundice, particularly in the premature. Anaemia depresses hepato-cellular function. Cephalohaematoma is a common association. The prothrombin time should be measured and vitamin K given.

Sepsis, whether umbilical or elsewhere, leads to unconjugated hyperbilirubinaemia in the first few days of life. Blood, urine and, if necessary, cerebrospinal fluid are cultured and appropriate antibodies given.

Upper gastrointestinal obstruction

About 10% of infants with congenital pyloric stenosis are jaundiced due to unconjugated bilirubin. The mechanism may be similar to that postulated for the increase in jaundice when patients with Gilbert's syndrome are fasted.

Hepatitis and cholestatic syndromes (conjugated hyperbilirubinaemia)

The reaction of the neonatal liver to different insults is similar. Proliferation of giant cells is always a part and this reflects increased regenerative ability. In some instances the condition may be the so-called 'idiopathic'

Hepatitis A

Asymptomatic hepatitis A can spread in nurseries for neonates. The source may be infected blood or a nurse carrier. The babies spread the hepatitis A to adults in the nursery and to the community.

Hepatitis C

Babies born to anti-HCV positive mothers show passively transmitted antibody for the first 6 months.

Mothers who are HCV RNA positive can transmit HCV RNA positive disease to their infants [70], but this is infrequent [56, 86]. There is probably no difference between transmission from HIV-positive or HIV-negative mothers. Those with a high serum HCV RNA are more likely to transmit the disease (fig. 26.2) [65]. Breast feeding seems safe [53].

In childhood the usual source of HCV infection is perinatal blood transfusion, multiple transfusions in thalassaemics or renal dialysis patients.

Liver biopsy histology is similar to that seen in adults [4]. Necro-inflammatory activity is low, but fibrosis is often severe suggesting possible progression to chronic disease.

Serum transaminases and HCV viral load are low [31].

Cirrhosis and hepato-cellular carcinoma are possibilities [31]. The response to interferon therapy is one-third, similar to that seen in adults [74].

Cytomegalovirus

This is very common (Chapter 16). The incidence in small children is 5–10% in those living in good hygienic conditions, rising to 80% in the underprivileged.

It is usually acquired placentally from an asymptomatic mother. It can also be transmitted in breast milk and from blood products. Many congenital infections are asymptomatic.

The disease may be fulminant with intense jaundice, purpura, hepatosplenomegaly, chorioretinitis, cataracts and pulmonary defects. Survivors may run a long course with persistent jaundice, hepatomegaly and disappearing bile ducts. The prognosis is good although 30% will develop cirrhosis requiring treatment by liver transplantation.

Intra-nuclear viral inclusions are seen in bile duct epithelium and rarely in hepatocytes. Diagnosis is made on urine or tissue *in situ* using PCR [18].

Herpes simplex

The liver may be involved in the course of a fulminating viraemia, contracted at birth from maternal genital herpes. Jaundice is due to viral involvement of the liver. Histologically, necrosis is seen with little or no inflammatory reaction. Giant cells are absent, but inclusion bodies may be found.

Gancyclovir is often given too late, when massive hepatic necrosis and chronic cholestasis have developed and the mortality is 70% [57].

Congenital rubella syndrome

This disease, if contracted in the first trimester of pregnancy, may cause fetal malformations. It may also persist through the neonatal period and into later life. The liver with the brain, lung, heart and other organs are involved in the generalized virus infection.

Jaundice commences within the first 1 or 2 days with hepatosplenomegaly. The picture is sometimes cholestatic. Serum transaminase levels are slightly elevated.

Hepatic histology shows bile in swollen Kupffer cells and ductules with a focal hepato-cellular necrosis and portal fibrosis. Erythroid haemopoietic tissue is relatively increased. A typical giant cell hepatitis can be seen. The virus can be identified from the liver at necropsy or biopsy.

Usually the hepatitis resolves completely.

Intra-uterine *parvovirus* B19 can cause severe giant cell hepatic disease in the neonate, also fulminant liver failure and aplastic anaemia [49].

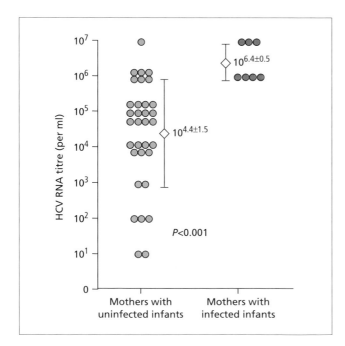

Fig. 26.2. Mean (±SD) serum HCV RNA titres in seven mothers with HCV-infected infants and the 33 mothers with uninfected infants. (From [65] with permission.)

Adenoviruses

These may disseminate in babies with decreased resistance due to thymic alymphoplasia and agammaglobulinaemia. A marked coagulative necrosis with inclusion-bearing cells may be seen. Under similar circumstances this lesion can also complicate *varicella*.

AIDS

Babies and children with AIDS have a very similar picture to that seen in the adult with the same spectrum of infections, primary lymphoma and Kaposi's sarcoma. Hepatic histology shows more giant cell transformation and fewer granulomas [41]. Diffuse, lymphoplasmocytic infiltration is associated with lymphoid interstitial pneumonia.

Non-viral causes of hepatitis

Congenital syphilis

This is very rare. Visceral involvement is late in acquired syphilis but common in fetal infection. Tremendous numbers of treponemes can be found in the liver. Such involvement leads to a fine peri-cellular cirrhosis with a marked connective tissue reaction. Jaundice is usual. The diagnosis is made serologically.

Congenital toxoplasmosis

Infection is intra-uterine. Jaundice develops within a few hours of birth with hepatomegaly, encephalomyelitis, choroidoretinitis and intra-cerebral calcification. Toxoplasmosis may develop later in the neonatal period. It is diagnosed by finding *Toxoplasma* IgM antibodies.

The liver shows infiltration of portal zones with mononuclear cells. Extra-medullary haemopoiesis with increased stainable iron is conspicuous. Histiocytes containing *Toxoplasma* may be present. The jaundice is difficult to relate to the extent of liver damage and haemolysis may be contributory. The liver disease is generally mild.

Bacterial infection

In the neonate, an immature reticulo-endothelial system with decreased complement and opsonins impairs the ability of the liver and spleen to phagocytose bacteria.

The upsurgence of Gram-negative infections, particularly *Escherichia coli*, in nurseries, has led to an increase in cholestatic jaundice due to this cause.

The origins include umbilical sepsis, pneumonia, otitis media or even gastroenteritis. Diagnosis may be difficult as focal signs are minimal or absent. Jaundice appears suddenly in a baby who does not look ill.

Hepatomegaly need not be present and splenomegaly is never great. The leucocyte count exceeds 12 000. A blood culture is usually positive. The umbilical stump should be cultured. Liver function tests are of little value.

Hepatic histology is non-contributory. Culture of liver biopsies is usually negative. The jaundice seems to be due to a combination of haemolysis, hepato-cellular dysfunction and even cholestasis, presumably due to endotoxaemia.

Prognosis depends on early treatment and age of onset, the mortality being 80% below the age of 1 week and 25% later. Antibiotics are appropriate.

Portal vein occlusion may be diagnosed years later.

Liver abscesses in older children are associated with blood-spread organisms. A third have acute blastic leukaemia.

Urinary tract infections

Jaundice may be associated both in infants and children. Infants are usually affected in the first week of life. They are often male, but have no underlying renal tract abnormality. Endotoxaemia contributes to the hepatic dysfunction.

The infants fail to thrive, show fever, jaundice, moderate hepatomegaly and bilirubinuria. Liver biopsy is non-specific. Urine culture is essential in any jaundiced child or infant.

Neonatal hepatitis syndrome

This may be due to intra-uterine infections, endocrine causes such as hypothyroidism, or inherited diseases such as chromosomal abnormalities.

Idiopathic neonatal hepatitis

This is diagnosed after exclusion of known causes. The number of cases being diagnosed has diminished. Inheritance is familial and autosomal recessive. Some instances may reflect disturbances in bile acid metabolism (see p. 463).

Clinical features include small gestational age and dysmorphia. The infant may be stillborn or die soon after or before jaundice has time to develop. More usually, a fluctuating jaundice appears during the first 2 weeks or up to 4 months. Hepatosplenomegaly is usual. The stools contain pigment and the urine bilirubin.

Biochemical changes are not diagnostic but transaminases are usually above 800 iu/l. Hypoglycaemia is common.

Liver biopsy histology is non-specific with giant cells, extra-medullary haematopoiesis and zone 3 inflammation. Bile duct proliferation is minimal and there may be canalicular cholestasis.

Table 27.2. Clinical and laboratory features of 12 patients with acute fatty liver of pregnancy (data from [7])

	No.
Nausea/vomiting	12
Severe heartburn	4
Abdominal pain	7
Jaundice	11
Leucocytosis	12
Thrombocytopenia	9
Proteinuria	7
Oedema	7
Hypertension	8
Serum urea increased	9

in more patients being diagnosed. The incidence is estimated at 1 per 13328 deliveries [30]. It is much rarer than pre-eclampsia.

Clinical features

The onset is between the 30th and 38th week and is marked by nausea, repeated vomiting and abdominal pain followed by jaundice (table 27.2). It is commoner with twins and male births and in primiparae.

In those severely affected, the course is marked by encephalopathy, renal failure, pancreatitis, haemorrhages and disseminated intravascular coagulation.

Ascites is found in 50%, perhaps related to portal hypertension.

Polydipsia and polyuria with transient diabetes insipidus have been reported [33].

Serum biochemical changes

Serum ammonia and amino acid levels are increased, reflecting mitochondrial failure. This is also suggested by lactic acidosis. High serum uric acid levels are usual and may be related to the tissue destruction and lactic acidosis [7].

Hypoglycaemia can be profound.

Hyperbilirubinaemia is found without haemolysis in contradistinction to pregnancy toxaemia where jaundice is rare except when there is haemolysis. Serum transaminase values are variable, usually less than 1000 iu/l, and may be normal.

Haematological findings

Leucocytosis and thrombocytopenia are common but the blood film may be leucoerythroblastic [7].

Prothrombin time and partial prothrombin time are increased. Fibrinogen levels are decreased. Severe bleeding is frequent, but disseminated intravascular coagulation is found in only 10%.

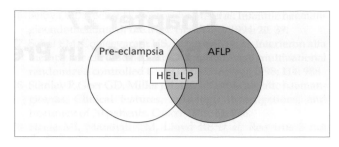

Fig. 27.1. Venn diagram showing the overlap between pre-eclampsia, acute fatty liver of pregnancy (AFLP) and the HELLP syndrome.

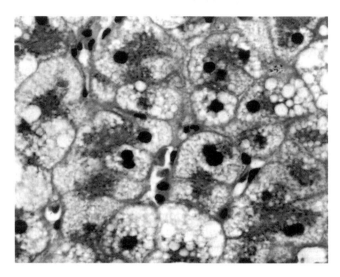

Fig. 27.2. Acute fatty liver of pregnancy. Hepatocytes have a foamy appearance with a central dense nucleus. (H & E, ×120.)

Liver histology

Liver biopsy is not usually necessary but can be performed by the transjugular route. The histological picture is of microvesicular and macrovesicular fat droplets with ballooned hepatocytes containing dense, central nuclei (fig. 27.2). Zone 1 (peri-portal) is relatively spared. The microvacuoles may be clearly recognized only on fresh sections stained for fat with such methods as oil red O (fig. 27.3) [6, 40].

Foci of inflammation and necrosis may be seen; also cholestasis with bile canalicular plugs and bile-stained Kupffer cells. Liver architecture is normal.

Electron microscopy confirms vacuoles and may show a honeycomb appearance in the smooth endoplasmic reticulum. Mitochondria are large and pleomorphic with paracrystalline inclusions [33].

Multi-organ involvement is shown by fatty infiltration of the renal tubules and renal lesions typical of pre-eclampsia. Fatty infiltration of the pancreas and the heart have been reported [40].

Ultrasonography of the liver may show a diffuse increased echogenicity which is very suggestive of acute

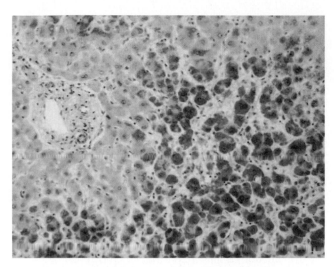

Fig. 27.3. Acute fatty liver of pregnancy: zone 3 hepatocytes are full of microvesicular fat droplets. Portal zones are normal and inflammation is minimal. (Oil red, ×40.)

fatty liver of pregnancy. A normal sonogram does not exclude the diagnosis. CT shows a low attenuation value in 30% [21].

Course and prognosis

Early recognition with prompt treatment has allowed diagnosis of milder cases and the current maternal mortality is 0–15%. The fetal mortality (40–50%) remains high.

Death is usually due to extra-hepatic causes such as disseminated intravascular coagulation with massive haemorrhage, and to renal failure. These features are not seen in the less severe cases.

Recurrences are extremely rare but have been reported. In one such case, a black woman presented with the disease in her fourth and fifth pregnancies [5]. From Australia, a woman had acute fatty liver of pregnancy in her first and second pregnancies [43]. A Chilean report describes the condition in two consecutive pregnancies [33, 34].

Management

The management of the average mild case is careful observation of the mother and fetus in hospital. If the mother's status deteriorates (intractable vomiting, increased jaundice and features of a coagulopathy), the pregnancy should be delivered.

Coagulopathy, renal failure, hypoglycaemia and infections are treated. The prognosis is relatively favourable if intensive care is adequate [29]. Intra-abdominal haemorrhage may necessitate laparotomy for clot evacuation. The intensive care must continue post-partum and intra-abdominal haemorrhage may follow

Table 27.3. The mitochondrial cytopathies

Causes
Acute fatty liver of pregnancy
Reye's syndrome
Genetic defects in mitochondrial function
Drug-related

Features
Vomiting and apathy
Lactic acidosis
Hypoglycaemia
Hyperammonaemia
Microvesicular fat in organs

caesarean section. Hepatic transplantation is sometimes necessary [26, 29].

The baby may need corticosteroids to treat lung immaturity.

Oesophagitis with bleeding is a frequent complication and omeprazole or a similar drug should be given.

Aetiology

Acute fatty liver of pregnancy can be regarded as a member of the *mitochondrial cytopathy family* (table 27.3) [45]. Members include Reye's syndrome, genetic defects in mitochondrial enzymes and drug reactions, especially to sodium valproate and nucleoside analogues (e.g. FIAU).

Apart from the breakdown of carbohydrate, nearly all the reactions involved in energy production take place in mitochondria. Some oxidative phosphorylation includes the oxidation of fuel molecules by oxygen and simultaneous energy transduction into ATP. Fatty acids are broken down in the mitochondria into shorter derivative fatty acids and acyl-CoA. This cycle of repeated fatty acid cleavage requires a series of specific enzymes.

The mitochondrial cytopathies are marked by vomiting and weakness. Lactic acidosis and metabolic acidosis are related to defective mitochondrial energy supply and defects in oxidative phosphorylation. Hypoglycaemia may be related to failure of mitochondrial citric acid cycle function. Raised blood ammonia relates to defects in mitochondrial Krebs' cycle enzymes. Microvesicular fat is seen in the organs.

Young people are predominantly affected in Reye's disease and in genetic defects of mitochondrial enzymes. Patients with acute fatty liver of pregnancy are usually reasonably young. Adverse hepatic effects of sodium valproate are roughly twice as frequent in children than in adults. This has led to the hypothesis that these diseases primarily affect patients having an underlying defect in mitochondrial function. A proportion of women with acute fatty liver of pregnancy are heterozygous for long-chain 3-hydroxy-CoA dehydrogenase deficiency which leads to impaired fatty acid oxidation [51]. Their infants may show hypoglycaemic coma and hepatic steatosis, and have a similar but homozygous defect in fatty acid oxidation. As this defect is autosomal recessive and the mothers are heterozygotes, some of the spouses must be heterozygous. In another report, 11 pregnancies, complicated by features of fatty liver and, HELLP syndrome, were followed by six babies with long-chain 3-hydroxy acyl coenzyme dehydrogenase deficiency [54]. The mothers might be heterozygous for this deficiency because they have had subsequent uneventful pregnancies when the fetus was unaffected.

Pregnancy *per se* may affect mitochondrial function. In mice, late pregnancy is associated with failure of mitochondrial oxidation of fatty acids as a consequence of both decreased mitochondrial β-oxidation of medium-chain fatty acids and decreased activity of the tricarboxylic acid cycle [12].

The mode of initiation of the mitochondrial cytopathies, apart from the genetic enzyme defects, is uncertain. It might be viral, as speculated in Reye's syndrome. It might be toxic and acute fatty liver of pregnancy has followed exposure to toluene [27]. Nutritional factors have also been suggested.

Acute fatty liver of pregnancy should be regarded as part of a systemic mitochondrial dysfunction affecting particularly liver, muscle, nervous system, pancreas and kidneys.

Pregnancy toxaemias

These conditions are characterized by hypertension, proteinuria and fluid retention. The term 'pregnancy toxaemia' includes a spectrum of conditions (table 27.4). The target organs are the uterus, kidney and brain. Hepatic damage is only seen in patients with severe pre-eclampsia and eclampsia.

The aetiology of pre-eclampsia is unknown. It is marked by generalized vasospasm with increased systemic vascular resistance and enhanced pressor responses to endogenous vaso-constrictors. Endothelial cell injury may decrease endothelial-dependent vasodilators and increase production of vaso-constrictors coming from both endothelial cells and platelets. Serum from pre-eclamptic patients contains

factors that increase endothelial cell permeability [13]. The vascular endothelium may be a target for blood-borne products of reduced placental perfusion [39].

Vascular endothelial damage leads to platelet deposition, thrombocytopenia and fibrin deposition in sinusoids. The resultant ischaemia accounts for the focal and diffuse hepato-cellular necrosis and haemorrhages in zone 1 (fig. 27.4).

In mild cases increases in serum alkaline phosphatase and transaminase values are frequent. Minor signs of disseminated intravascular coagulation, such as a reduction in platelets, are also common.

Jaundice is infrequent and often terminal. It is usually haemolytic with disseminated intravascular coagulation. Failure of renal bilirubin excretion may contribute. Serum bilirubin is less than 6 mg/dl (100 μmol/l).

Severe toxaemia may present with epigastric pain, nausea, vomiting, right upper quadrant tenderness and hypertension.

Hepatic histology. Peri-portal (zone 1) fibrin deposits [37] and haemorrhage progress to small necrotic foci, infarcts and haematomas. Zone 3 necrosis and haemorrhage represent shock. An inflammatory reaction is characteristically absent (fig. 27.5). Capillary and hepatic arterial thrombi and, rarely, intra-hepatic portal venous thrombi may be noted. *Serum transaminases* are usually more than 10 times elevated.

Rupture of the liver is associated with shock.

Ultrasound and CT show focal filling defects.

The *treatment* of severe toxaemia is by delivering the pregnancy and by supportive care.

The HELLP syndrome

This is a rare variant of pre-eclampsia [42]. It consists of haemolysis, elevated liver enzymes and low platelet

Table 27.4. Spectrum of pregnancy toxaemias

Pre-eclampsia
HELLP syndrome
Infarction
Bleeding and rupture

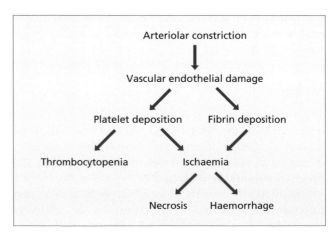

Fig. 27.4. The liver in eclampsia. Hepato-cellular necrosis and haemorrhage follow ischaemia related to vascular endothelial damage.

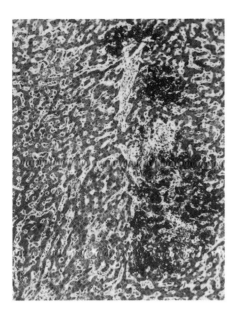

Fig. 27.5. The liver in eclampsia. Focal peri-portal necrosis of liver cells; the lesion contains fibrin. (Mallory's phosphotungstic acid, ×80.)

Table 27.5. Acute fatty liver of pregnancy and toxaemias contrasted: overlaps exist

	Acute fatty liver	Toxaemia
Abdominal pain	50%	100%
Jaundice	100%	40%
Serum transaminases (×normal)	<10	>10
Scans	Diffuse change	Focal abnormalities
Liver biopsy	Microvesicular fat	Fibrin (peri-sinusoidal)
Liver failure	Present	Absent

count [52]. It often affects multipara. The blood pressure may be normal and proteinuria may be absent.

Liver histology shows fibrin deposition [4]. This suggests severe pre-eclamptic liver disease and calls for immediate delivery. The laboratory results do not reflect hepatic histology [4]. Perinatal mortality is 10–60% and the maternal mortality 1.5–5% [46].

Management is supportive, as for eclampsia [49].

Toxaemia and the HELLP syndrome

There is considerable overlap between acute fatty liver of pregnancy, the pregnancy toxaemias and the HELLP syndrome (fig. 27.1, table 27.5). The features include proteinuria and even some peri-sinusoidal fibrin deposition, but hypertension is unusual. The patient with clear pregnancy toxaemia may lack proteinuria and hypertension and yet the liver biopsy, in addition to fibrin deposition, shows some microvesicular fat. Multiparous

patients with acute fatty liver of pregnancy often have a history of pre-eclampsia.

Hepatic haemorrhage

This usually complicates pre-eclampsia or eclampsia and the HELLP syndrome with accompanying disseminated intravascular coagulation and intra-hepatic vascular lesions [11]. The picture includes infarction [19], subcapsular haemorrhage and ruptured liver. Clinically this catastrophe is suspected by sudden constant right upper quadrant or epigastric pain with vomiting and circulatory collapse. The diagnosis is confirmed by ultrasound, CT and angiography. Treatment varies with the severity. Subcapsular haemorrhage is usually treated conservatively. Surgery may be required or even transplant [29]. Hepatic arterial embolization with gelfoam can be used to control haemorrhage.

Hepatic adenomas, often with peliosis hepatis, and often associated with oral contraceptives, may rupture during pregnancy (see Chapters 20 and 30).

Cholestasis of pregnancy

This intra-hepatic cholestasis appears in the last trimester of pregnancy [31].

In its mildest form, pruritus is the only abnormality. It usually commences in the last trimester, but can start as early as the second or third month. Jaundice is rarely deep. The urine is dark and the stools pale. General health is preserved and there is no pain. Weight loss may be great. The liver and spleen are impalpable. After delivery, jaundice disappears and within 1–2 weeks the pruritus has ceased. The condition usually recurs with subsequent pregnancies. Consecutive pregnancies in multiparous patients are associated with variability in the severity and in the time of onset.

Laboratory changes

Serum shows an increase in conjugated bilirubin and alkaline phosphatase values. Serum transaminases are normal or slightly increased, although occasionally very high values are found. These changes return to normal after delivery. Serum bile acids are increased and the primary bile acids (cholic and chenodeoxycholic acids) predominate [1].

Steatorrhoea is usual. It correlates with the severity of the cholestasis.

The prothrombin time is prolonged due to vitamin K deficiency. Cholestyramine enhances the hypoprothrombinaemia.

Hepatic histology shows mild focal and irregular cholestasis. Electron microscopy shows the changes in the

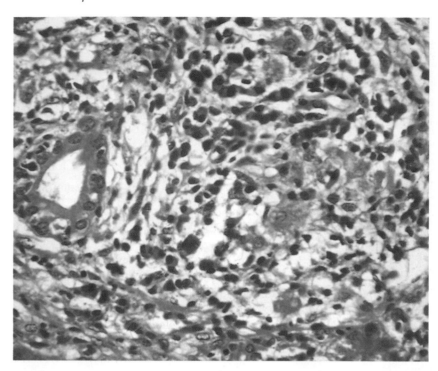

Fig. 28.7. Chronic cholestasis in sarcoidosis. A damaged bile duct is surrounded by an inflammatory infiltrate including lymphocytes. (H & E,×160.)

the fibrosis which may be massive. Sequential liver biopsies show relentless progression of the fibrosis and bile duct loss.

ERCP shows tortuous stretched ducts due to the disturbed liver architecture. Rarely the common hepatic duct is involved [16].

The prognosis is poor. The patients usually die within 2–18 years from the onset.

Corticosteroids are not helpful. Ursodeoxycholic acid may be used to control pruritus [2]. Liver transplantation may be necessary [5]. However, post-transplant multiple hepatic granulomas can recur, but without clinical deterioration [9].

The condition may resemble, and even be indistinguishable from, PBC (see table 14.2).

Granulomatous drug reactions

Drugs are rare causes of hepatic granulomas. However, the identification of a granuloma in a liver biopsy always raises the possibility that it is drug-related. The granuloma may be a reaction to the therapy and not due to the underlying disease. Typically the granuloma is part of a general hypersensitivity reaction. It develops 10 days to 4 months after starting the drug. It may be associated with rash, lymphadenopathy and arthritis. Fever may be related to cytokines from activated macrophages and lymphocytes.

Serum biochemistry shows increases in alkaline phosphatase and γ-glutamyl transpeptidase. Transaminases may be modestly increased. A rise in serum bilirubin is unusual with a simple granulomatous reaction.

Liver biopsy histology shows predominant granulomas. Caseation is absent. Tissue eosinophilia is found in about 70%. Fatty change, portal zone inflammation and bile duct injury are occasionally present. The lesion heals without concentric fibrosis.

Nevertheless, a liver biopsy showing the appearance of granulomas, eosinophils, fatty change, bile duct injury and cholestasis always suggests a granulomatous drug reaction.

Prognosis is usually excellent with recovery within 6 weeks of withdrawing the drug. Rarely, severe reactions may lead to consideration of corticosteroid therapy.

Drug associations

An enormous number of drugs have been linked with a granulomatous hepatic reaction. In most instances the granulomas are not the predominant lesion. In some, the evidence of a causal association is anecdotal and dechallenge has not been recorded. Re-challenge is usually unjustifiable on ethical grounds.

Drugs which can cause a predominantly granulomatous reaction are listed in table 28.3. Allopurinol, carbamazepine, glibenclamide and sulphonamides are the most common culprits. They are all rare, but the reactions can be fatal. In all, the clinicopathological picture is a mixed one with granulomatous, hepato-cellular, cholangitic and vasculitic elements. Carbamazepine and allopurinol are associated with fibrin-ring granulomas

Table 28.3. Important causes of granulomatous drug reactions

Allopurinol
Carbamazepine
Diltiazem
Glibenclamide
Hydralazine
Quinidine/quinine
Sulphonamides

Table 28.4. Hepatic granulomas associated with infections

Mycobacteria	*M. tuberculosis*
	M. avium-intracellulare
	Leprosy
Bacteria	*Brucella*
Spirochaetes	*T. pallidum*
Fungi	Histoplasmosis
	Coccidioidomycosis
	Blastomycosis
Protozoa	Toxoplasmosis
Helminths	Schistosomiasis
	Toxocara canis
	Fasciola hepatica
	Ascaris lumbricades
Rickettsiae	Q fever
Viruses	Hepatitis A
	Hepatitis C
	Cytomegalovirus

Table 28.5. Hepatic granulomas in tuberculosis and sarcoidosis*

	Tuberculosis	Sarcoidosis
Caseation	Present	Absent
Acid-fast bacilli	Present in 10%	Absent
Reticulin framework	Destroyed	Intact
Numbers	Few	Many
Coalescence	Frequent	Rare

*The granulomas may be indistinguishable.

tuberculous meningitis when other methods have failed, and also in miliary tuberculosis at the stage of an indeterminate pyrexia. In such cases, Ziehl–Neelsen stains should be performed, and an unfixed portion of the biopsy cultured for tubercle bacilli.

The distinction between these granulomas and those of sarcoidosis may be impossible to make. Distinctive features of tuberculosis are the presence of acid-fast bacilli and caseation with destruction of the reticulin framework. There is irregularity of the contour with a particularly dense cuff of lymphocytes. Less numerous lesions with a tendency to coalesce also suggest tuberculosis (table 28.5).

Capillary granulomas are found after BCG vaccination, especially in the immunosuppressed.

Rarely, fulminant liver failure can result from tuberculosis [10].

Lepromatous leprosy

Hepatic granulomas indistinguishable from those of sarcoidosis may be found in 62% of patients compared with the tuberculoid form when only 21% are positive. *Mycobacterium leprae* bacilli are sometimes present.

Bacteria

Brucella abortus infection may be complicated by hepatic granulomas. Hepatic tenderness and mild elevations of transaminases and alkaline phosphatase may be found in the acute stage. Hepatic histology shows a nonspecific reactive hepatitis. Granulomas cannot be distinguished from those of sarcoidosis although they tend to be smaller and less clearly demarcated (fig. 28.8). Healing results in scarring. Necrotizing microgranulomas may be found in the bone marrow.

The presence of circulating autoantibodies indicate that the *Brucella* antigen can be responsible for a β-lymphocyte activation of the immune system [3].

Spirochaetes

In the secondary septicaemic stage of *syphilis*,

[30]. Corticosteroids may be considered in severe granulomatous drug reactions.

Granulomas associated with infections

Granulomas can be found with almost all types of infection. The most frequent are tuberculosis, brucellosis, toxoplasmosis, atypical mycobacteriosis, fungal diseases, syphilis, leishmaniasis and the infestations, schistosomiasis and toxocariasis (table 28.4). In many instances, the granulomas are ill-formed and histologically can be distinguished with ease from the classical epithelioid granulomas of sarcoidosis.

Mycobacteria

Tuberculosis

Miliary dissemination accompanies the primary complex, and is also common with chronic adult tuberculosis. Aspiration liver biopsies in patients with tuberculosis have shown positive results in about 25%.

Aspiration biopsy has been used in the diagnosis of

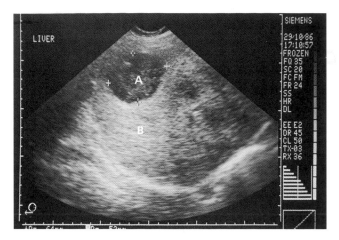

Fig. 29.2. US of a pyogenic liver abscess shows a low-density lesion (A) containing echogenic material which is pus and necrotic tissue. Acoustic enhancement (B) beyond the lesion is characteristic.

About one half of abscesses are *cryptogenic*. This is especially so in the elderly.

Infecting agents

The commonest are Gram-negative *Escherichia coli*, *Streptococcus faecalis*, *Klebsiella* and *Proteus vulgaris*. Recurrent pyogenic cholangitis may be due to *Salmonella typhi*.

Streptococcus milleri, which is neither a true anaerobe nor a micro-anaerobe is a very common cause [13]. Anaerobes are particularly important. Infections are liable to be mixed and often antibiotic resistant. Super-infection is common.

Liver abscesses associated with biliary stents are often due to resistant *Klebsiella*, enterobacter and *Pseudomonas*, *Candida* may be found in the bile. Fungal infections may be associated with underlying malignancy. Staphylococci, usually resistant, are found especially in those who have received chemotherapy. *Klebsiella pneumoniae*, *Pseudomonas* and *Clostridium welchii* may also be found.

Rare causes include *Yersinia enterocolitica* [9] and septicaemic melioidosis. The abscess may be sterile, but this is usually due to lack of adequate, particularly anaerobic, culture techniques or to previous antibiotics.

Pathology

The enlarged liver may contain multiple yellow abscesses, 1 cm in diameter or a single abscess encased in fibrous tissue and usually found in the right lobe. With pylephlebitis, the portal vein and its branches contain pus and blood clots. There may be peri-hepatitis or adhesion formation. A chronic liver abscess may persist for as long as 2 years before death or diagnosis. In biliary-associated cases, multiple foci correspond to the bile duct system.

Small pyaemic abscesses may be found in lung, kidney, brain or spleen. Direct extension may lead to sub-phrenic or pleuro-pulmonary suppuration. Extension to the peritoneum or rupture of a sinus pointing under the skin are rare. A small amount of ascites may be present.

Histologically, areas remote from the abscess show portal zone infection and surrounding disintegrating hepatocytes being infiltrated by polymorphs.

Clinical features

Features such as diabetes, biliary disease, malignancy or immunosuppressive states are recorded.

Presentation is with abdominal pain and fever with features of a space-occupying lesion in the liver.

The onset may be insidious and diagnosis delayed for at least 1 month. A single abscess is often insidious and cryptogenic especially in the elderly. Multiple abscesses are more acute and the cause is more often identified. Sub-diaphragmatic irritation or pleuro-pulmonary spread leads to right shoulder pain and to an irritable cough. The liver is enlarged and tender and the pain is accentuated by percussion over the lower ribs.

Jaundice is late unless there is biliary disease. It is more common than with amoebic abscess.

Recovery may be followed by portal hypertension due to thrombosis of the portal vein.

Serum alkaline phosphatase is usually raised. Polymorph leukocytosis is usual.

Blood cultures may show the causative organism or organisms [2].

Localization of the abscess

Ultrasound (US) distinguishes a solid from a fluid-filled lesion (fig. 29.2). *CT scanning* is particularly valuable although false negatives can be due to lesions near the dome of the liver and to micro-abscesses (figs 29.3–29.5). Multiple small abscesses aggregate, suggesting the beginning of coalescence into single larger abscesses (*cluster sign*) [8].

Endoscopic or *percutaneous cholangiography* may be used to diagnose cholangitic abscesses.

MRI shows a raised lesion with sharp borders, hypo-intense on T_1-weighting, and hyper-intense on a T_2-weighted image. Appearances are not specific or diagnostic of biliary or haematogenous origin [11].

Aspirated material is positive in 90% [2]. It should be cultured aerobically, anaerobically and in carbon dioxide-enriched media for *Streptococcus milleri*.

Treatment

Management has been revolutionized by the wide-

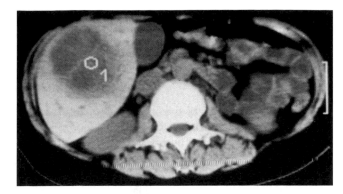

Fig. 29.3. Thalassaemic Greek patient post-splenectomy. CT scan shows a filling defect in the right lobe of the liver with marker over it (labelled 1).

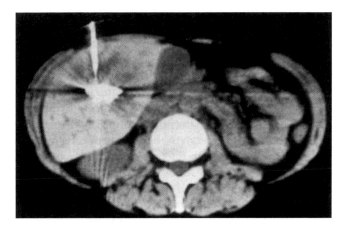

Fig. 29.4. Same patient as in fig. 29.3 with directed puncture of the abscess which resolved without surgery.

spread use of imaging, especially US, allowing localization and easy aspiration for both diagnostic and therapeutic purposes (fig. 29.4). The majority of abscesses can be managed by systemic antibiotics and aspiration, which may need to be repeated [4]. Intravenous antibiotics are rarely effective alone. Drainage is indicated if signs of sepsis persist. Open surgical drainage is rarely indicated. However, solitary left-sided abscess may require surgical drainage, especially in children [12].

With multiple abscesses, the largest is aspirated and the smaller lesions usually resolve with antibiotics. Occasionally, percutaneous drainage of each is necessary.

If amoebiasis is suspected, metronidazole should be given before aspiration [6].

Biliary obstruction must be relieved, usually by ERCP, papillotomy and stone removal. If necessary, a biliary stent is inserted (Chapter 32). Even with eventual cure, fever may continue for 1–2 weeks [2].

Prognosis

Needle aspiration and antibiotic therapy have lowered the mortality [3]. The prognosis is better for a unilocular abscess in the right lobe where survival is 90%. The outcome for multiple abscesses, especially if biliary, is very poor. The prognosis is worsened by delay in diagnosis, associated disease, particularly malignant [17], hyperbilirubinaemia, hypo-albuminaemia, pleural effusion and old age [10].

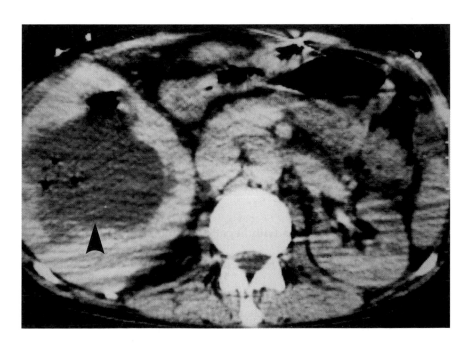

Fig. 29.5. CT shows a large pyogenic abscess with thick shaggy walls in the inferior part of the right lobe of the liver (arrowhead). The abscess contains gas.

acterized by a normal temperature but without clinical improvement. This is the stage of deepening jaundice, with increasing renal and myocardial failure. Albuminuria persists, there is a rising blood urea, and oliguria may proceed to anuria. Death may be due to renal failure. A markedly elevated creatinine phosphokinase level reflects myositis.

Severe prostration is accompanied by a low blood pressure and a dilated heart. There may be transient cardiac dysrhythmias and electrocardiograms may show a prolonged P–R or Q–T interval, with T-wave changes. Death may be due to circulatory failure.

During this stage, the *Leptospira* can be found in the urine, and rising antibody titres demonstrated in the serum.

The third or convalescent stage starts at the beginning of the third week. Clinical improvement is shown by a brightening of the mental state, fading of the jaundice, a rise in blood pressure and an increased urinary volume, with a drop in the blood urea concentration. Albuminuria is slow to disappear.

Temperature may rise during the third week (fig. 29.11), associated with muscle pains. Such relapses occur in 20% of cases.

There is great variation in the clinical course ranging from a mild illness, clinically indistinguishable from influenza, to a prostrating, fatal disease with anuria.

Diagnosis

Before the appearance of antibodies, PCR demonstration of *Leptospira* is the best method of diagnosis [3].

Rising titres of antibodies are sought by Dot-ELISA [4] or immunofluoroscence [1]. The microscopic agglutination test is too complex for routine use.

Leptospira may be cultured from blood during the first 10 days. Urine cultures are positive during the second week and persist for several months.

Liver function tests are non-contributory.

Differential diagnosis

In the early stages, Weil's disease is confused with septicaemic bacterial infections or typhus fever. When jaundice is evident acute viral hepatitis must be excluded (table 29.1). Important distinguishing points are the sudden-onset increased polymorph count and albuminuria of Weil's disease.

Spirochaetal jaundice would be diagnosed more often if blood samples for antibodies were taken from patients with obscure icterus and fever.

Prognosis

Mortality is about 5%. This depends on the depth of

Table 29.1. The differential diagnosis of Weil's disease from viral hepatitis during the first week of illness

	Weil's disease	Viral hepatitis
Onset	Sudden	Gradual
Headache	Constant	Occasional
Muscle pains	Severe	Mild
Conjunctival injection	Present	Absent
Prostration	Great	Mild
Disorientation	Common	Rare
Haemorrhagic diathesis	Common	Rare
Nausea and vomiting	Present	Present
Abdominal discomfort	Common	Common
Bronchitis	Common	Rare
Albuminuria	Present	Absent
Leucocyte count	Polymorph leucocytosis	Leucopenia with lymphocytosis

jaundice, renal and myocardial involvement, and the extent of haemorrhages. Death is usually due to renal failure. The mortality is negligible in non-icteric patients, and is lower in those under 30 years old. Since many mild infections are probably unrecognized, the overall mortality may be considerably less.

Although transient relapses in the third and fourth weeks are common, final recovery is complete.

Prevention

Protective clothing should be provided for workers in industries with a high incidence of Weil's disease, and adequate measures taken to control rodents. Bathing in stagnant water should be avoided.

Treatment

Early, mild leptospirosis is treated by doxycycline (100 mg by mouth) twice daily for 1 week. More seriously ill patients, particularly with vomiting, are given intravenous penicillin G 6 million units/day for 1 week [7].

Prognosis is improving with earlier diagnosis, attention to fluid and electrolyte balance, renal dialysis, antibiotics and circulatory support.

Other types of leptospirosis

In general these infections are less severe than those due to *L. icterohaemorrhagiae*. *L. canicola* infection, for instance, is characterized by headache, meningitis and conjunctival infection. Albuminuria is only found in 40%, and jaundice in only 18% of patients. The frequent presentation is that of 'benign aseptic meningitis'. The disease affects young adults who have usually been in close contact with an infected dog. Fatalities in man are virtually unknown.

Diagnosis is confirmed in a similar way to Weil's disease. A convenient method is rising antibody titres. The spinal fluid shows a lymphocytic picture in most cases.

References

1 Appassakij H, Silpapojakul K, Wansit R *et al.* Evaluation of the immunofluorescent antibody test for the diagnosis of human leptospirosis. *Am. J. Trop. Med. Hyg.* 1995; **52**; 340.
2 Arean VM. The pathologic anatomy and pathogenesis of fatal human leptospirosis (Weil's disease). *Am. J. Pathol.* 1962; **40**: 393.
3 Brown PD, Gravekamp C, Carrington DG *et al.* Evaluation of the polymerase chain reaction for early diagnosis of leptospirosis. *J. Med. Microbiol.* 1995; **43**: 110.
4 Ribeiro MA, Souza CC, Almeida SH *et al.* Dot-ELISA for human leptospirosis employing immunodominant antigen. *J. Trop. Med. Hyg.* 1995; **98**: 452.
5 Tajiki H, Salomao R. Association of plasma levels of tumour necrosis factor alpha—with severity of disease and mortality among patients with leptospirosis. *Clin. Infect. Dis.* 1996; **23**: 1177.
6 Vinetz JM, Glass GE, Flexner CE *et al.* Sporadic urban leptospirosis. *Ann. Intern. Med.* 1996; **125**: 794.
7 Watt G, Padre LP, Tuazon ML *et al.* Placebo-controlled trial of intravenous penicillin for severe and late leptospirosis. *Lancet* 1988; **i**: 433.
8 Weil A. Über eine eigenthumliche mit Milztumour, Icterus and Nephritis einhergehene, acute Infektionskrankheit. *Dtsch. Arch. Klin. Med.* 1886; **39**: 209.
9 Zuerner RL, Alt D, Bolin CA. IS1533-based PCR assay for identification of *Leptospira interrogans* sensu lato serovars. *J. Clin. Microbiol.* 1995; **33**: 3284.

Relapsing fever

This arthropod-borne infection is caused by spirochaetes of the species *Borrelia recurrentis*. It is encountered throughout the world except in New Zealand, Australia and some parts of the west Pacific.

The *Borrelia* multiply in the liver, invading liver cells and causing focal necrosis. Just before the crisis the *Borrelia* roll up and are ingested by reticulo-endothelial cells. This effect is related to immunologically competent lymphocytes. Surviving *Borrelia* remain in the liver, spleen, brain and bone marrow until the next relapse [2].

Clinical features [1]

The incubation period is 3–15 days. The onset is acute with chills, a continuous high temperature, headache, muscle pains and profound prostration. The patient is flushed, sometimes with injected conjunctivae, and epistaxes. In severe attacks, tender hepatosplenomegaly and jaundice develop. The jaundice is similar to that of Weil's disease. Sometimes a rash develops on the trunk. There may be bronchitis.

These symptoms continue for 4–9 days and then the temperature falls, often with collapse of the patient. This peripheral collapse may be fatal, but more usually the symptoms and signs then rapidly abate, the patient remains afebrile for about 1 week, when there is a relapse. There may be a second or even a third milder relapse before the disease ends.

Diagnosis

Spirochaetes can rarely be found in thick blood films. Agglutination and complement fixation tests are available [2]. Organisms may be identified by lymph node aspiration, or from the insect bite site.

Treatment

Tetracyclines and streptomycin are more effective than penicillin. Mortality is 5%.

References

1 Bryceson ADM, Parry EHO, Perine PL *et al.* Louse-born relapsing fever: a clinical and laboratory study of 62 cases in Ethiopia and a reconsideration of the literature. *Q. J. Med.* 1970; **39**: 129.
2 Felsenfeld O, Wolf RH. Immunoglobulins and antibodies in *Borrelia turicetae* infections. *Acta Trop.* 1969; **26**: 156.

Lyme disease

This is due to a tick-borne spirochaete *Borrelia burgdorferi*. It has caused hepatitis with numerous liver cell mitoses [1]. Mild liver function test abnormalities are frequent in the early erythema migrans stage, but these resolve with antibiotic treatment [2]. Lyme disease does not seem to cause permanent hepatic sequelae.

References

1 Goellner MH, Agger WA, Burgess JH *et al.* Hepatitis due to recurrent Lyme disease. *Ann. Intern. Med.* 1988; **108**: 707.
2 Horowitz HW, Dworkin B, Forseter G *et al.* Liver function in early Lyme disease. *Hepatology* 1996; **23**: 1412.

Q fever

This rickettsial disease has predominantly pulmonary manifestations. Occasionally hepatitis may be prominent and clinical features may mimic anicteric viral hepatitis [2, 3].

The liver shows a granulomatous hepatitis. Portal areas contain abundant lymphocytes and the limiting plate is destroyed. Kupffer cells are hypertrophied. The

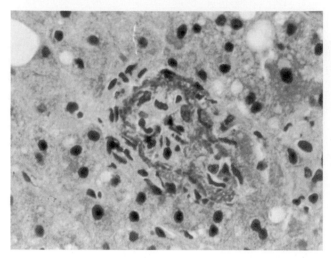

Fig. 29.12. Liver biopsy in Q fever showing a granuloma with fibrin rings having a clear centre. (Martius scarlet blue, ×350.)

granulomas have a characteristic ring of fibrinoid necrosis surrounded by lymphocytes and histiocytes. In the centre of the granuloma is a clear space giving a 'doughnut' appearance (fig. 29.12). The diagnosis is made by showing a rising titre of complement-fixing antibodies to *Coxiella burnetii* 2–3 weeks after the infection.

Rocky mountain spotted fever

Jaundice and rises in serum enzymes sometimes occur. Liver histology shows portal zone inflammation with large mononuclear cells. Hepato-cellular necrosis is inconspicuous but erythrophagocytosis is marked. Rickettsiae may be demonstrated in the portal zones by immunofluorescence microscopy [1].

References

1 Adams JS, Walker DH. The liver in rocky mountain spotted fever. *Am. J. Clin. Pathol.* 1981; **75**: 156.
2 Dupont HL, Hornick RB, Levin HS *et al.* Q fever hepatitis. *Ann. Intern. Med.* 1971; **74**: 198.
3 Tissot-Dupont H, Raoult D, Brouquil P *et al.* Epidemiologic features and clinical presentation of acute Q fever in hospitalized patients: 323 French cases. *Am. J. Med.* 1992; **93**: 427.

Schistosomiasis (bilharziasis)

Hepatic schistosomiasis is usually a complication of the intestinal disease, since emboli of *Schistosoma* ova reach the liver from the intestines via the mesenteric veins. *S. mansoni* and *S. japonicum* affect the liver. *S. haematobium* can sometimes involve the liver.

Schistosomiasis affects more than 200 million people in 74 countries. *S. japonicum* is prevalent in Japan, China, Indonesia and the Philippines. *S. mansoni* is found in Africa, the Middle East, the Caribbean and Brazil [4].

Pathogenesis

Eggs, excreted in the faeces, hatch out in water to release free-swimming embryos which enter appropriate snails and develop into fork-tailed cercariae. These re-enter human skin in contact with infected water. They burrow down to the capillary bed, whence there is widespread haematogenous dissemination. Those reaching the mesenteric capillaries enter the intra-hepatic portal system, where they grow rapidly.

The extent and severity of chronic liver disease correlates with the intensity and duration of egg production and hence with the number of eggs excreted. Adult male and female worms can exist for about 5 years producing 300–3000 eggs daily in portal venules. If liver disease is advanced, faecal egg counts may fall because of senescence of adult worms or previous therapy.

S. japonicum is more pathogenic than *S. mansoni* and produces hepatosplenic schistosomiasis more often and faster.

In the liver, the ova penetrate and obstruct the portal branches and are deposited either in the large radicles, producing the coarser type of bilharzial hepatic fibrosis, or in the small portal tracts, producing the fine diffuse form.

The granulomatous reaction to the *Schistosoma* ovum is of delayed hypersensitivity type, related to antigen released by the egg. TH0- and TH2-type helper lymphocytes play an important role in granuloma formation [10].

Portal fibrosis is related to the adult worm load. The classic, clay-pipestem cirrhosis is due to fibrotic bands originating from the granulomas.

Early on, cytokines, formed from granulomas around ova, may play a central role in fibrogenesis [7]. Fibrosis may be slowly reversible with treatment.

Wide, irregular, thin-walled arteriolar spaces are found in 85% of cases in the thickened portal tracts. These angiomatoids are useful in distinguishing the bilharzial liver from other forms of hepatic fibrosis. Remnants of ova are also diagnostic. There is little or no bile duct proliferation. Nodular regeneration and disturbance of the hepatic architecture is not sufficient to justify the term 'cirrhosis'.

In areas where schistosomiasis, hepatitis virus B and C coexist, a mixed picture of schistosomal fibrosis with cirrhosis may be seen.

Splenic enlargement is mainly due to portal venous hypertension and reticulo-endothelial hyperplasia. Very few ova are found in the spleen. Portal-systemic collateral channels are numerous.

There are associated bilharzial lesions in the intestines

and elsewhere. Fifty per cent of patients with rectal schistosomiasis have granulomas in the liver.

Clinical features

Schistosomiasis shows three stages. Itching follows the entry of the cercariae through the skin. This is followed by a stage of fever, urticaria and eosinophilia. Finally, the third stage of deposition of ova results in intestinal, urinary and hepatic involvement.

Initially, the liver and spleen are firm, smooth and easily palpable. This is followed by hepatic fibrosis and eventually portal hypertension which may appear years after the original infection.

Oesophageal varices develop. Bleeding episodes are recurrent but rarely fatal.

The liver shrinks in size and the spleen becomes much larger. Dilated abdominal wall veins and a venous hum over the liver are indications of the portal venous obstruction. Ascites and oedema may develop. The blood shows leucopenia and anaemia. The faeces at this stage contain few, if any, parasites.

Patients tolerate blood loss well and hepatic encephalopathy is unusual. Hepato-cellular function remains good although there is a large porto-systemic collateral circulation.

Aspiration liver biopsy (fig. 29.13). Eggs or their remnants are seen in 94% of livers from those with faecal eggs.

Remnants of ova may be seen but appearances are not usually diagnostic and the liver biopsy mainly excludes other types of liver disease.

Diagnostic tests

Detection of ova in urine, stool or rectal mucosal biopsy

(rectal 'snip') is still the accepted method of diagnosing active infection (fig. 29.14). Bleeding may be a complication of rectal biopsy in those with portal hypertension. *Serological antibody tests* indicate past exposure without specifying the time.

Detection of circulating schistosomal antigen indicates active disease. An ELISA for detecting circulating soluble egg antigens in serum correlates with egg output. A reagent strip assay is based on glycoconjugates for adult schistosomes [9].

CT shows dense bands following the portal vein to the liver edge; these enhance with contrast [5].

US shows greatly thickened portal veins (fig. 29.15). It may be used to grade fibrosis [1]. Liver, spleen, peri-portal and pancreatic lymph nodes are diffusely enlarged without evidence of portal hypertension.

Colour Doppler shows an increase in blood flow

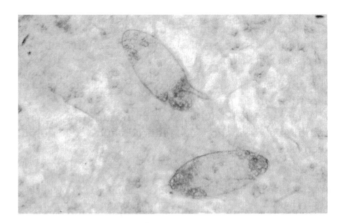

Fig. 29.14. Rectal ('snip') biopsy in schistosomiasis mansoni. A 'squash' preparation in glycerol reveals the ova of *S. mansoni*.

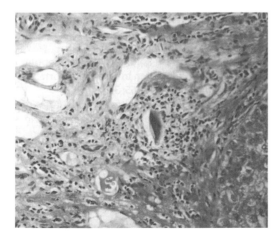

Fig. 29.13. Bilharzial liver. An ovum of *S. mansoni* has lodged in a portal tract which shows a granulomatous reaction. (H & E, ×64.)

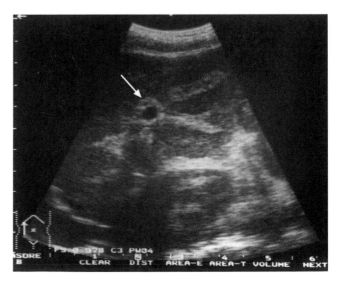

Fig. 29.15. Schistosomiasis: US shows bright portal tracts and a portal vein with greatly thickened walls (arrow).

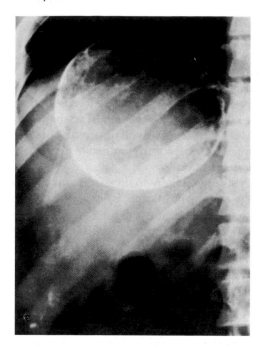

Fig. 29.19. X-ray of the abdomen shows a calcified hydatid cyst in the liver.

Floating bodies indicate the presence of free-moving daughter cysts. Infected gas-containing cysts may show a fluid level.

Hepatic cysts may displace the stomach or hepatic flexure of the colon. Characteristic radiological changes may be seen in the lungs, spleen, kidney or bone.

US or *CT scanning* demonstrates single or multiple cysts which may be uni- or multiloculated, and thin or thick walled (figs 29.20, 29.21, 29.22). US and CT are highly sensitive for diagnosis: 97.7% for US and 100% for CT.

US changes provide the basis for classification (table 29.2) [6]. WHO classification is into active, transitional and inactive cysts. Infected cysts are poorly defined [17].

MRI may show a characteristic intense rim, daughter cysts and detachment of the membranes [12]. Intra-hepatic and extra-hepatic rupture can be defined.

ERCP may show cysts in the bile ducts (figs 29.23, 29.24).

Prognosis

The uncomplicated hepatic hydatid cyst carries a reasonably good prognosis. The risk of complications is, however, always present. Intra-peritoneal or intra-pleural rupture is grave, but rupture into the biliary tree is not so serious because spontaneous cure may follow the biliary colic. Infection is controlled by antibiotics.

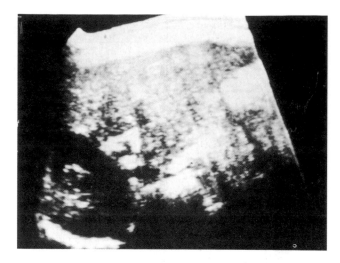

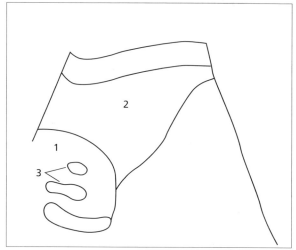

Fig. 29.20. US shows a hydatid cyst (1) in the right lobe of the liver (2). Daughter cysts (3) can be seen inside the larger cyst.

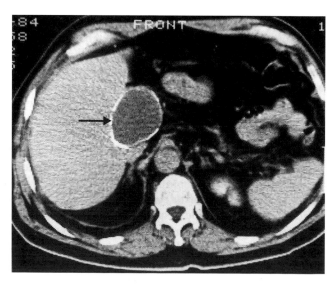

Fig. 29.21. CT scan shows calcified hydatid cyst (arrowed) in a quadrate lobe of the liver (contrast-enhanced scan).

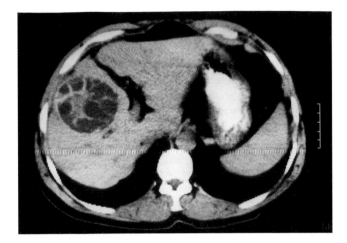

Fig. 29.22. CT scan. Hydatid cyst in right lobe of liver showing patchy calcification of the wall and containing multiple septae produced by daughter cysts (contrast-enhanced scan).

Table 29.2. Classification of ultrasound appearances in hydatid disease [6]

Type	Description
I	Purely cystic
II	Detached membrane
III	Undulating in cyst cavity
	Multiseptate cyst
IV	Heterogenous complex mass (dead parasite)
	Calcified mass (eggshell) (dead parasite)

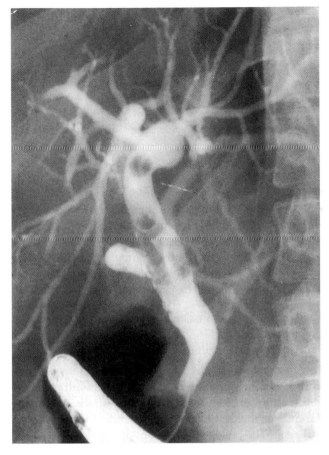

Fig. 29.23. Endoscopic cholangiography showing hydatid cysts in the common bile duct.

Treatment

Dogs are denied access to infected offal and hands are washed after handling dogs [5]. Dogs in affected areas must be regularly de-wormed.

Medical treatment

Mebendazole perfuses through the cyst membrane and interferes with microtubular function. It is poorly absorbed.

Albendazole is better absorbed and cyst levels equal that achieved in plasma. It is more satisfactory than mebendazole.

Medical therapy cannot be regarded as definitive. Albendazole can be given in a 6 to 24-month course for those unsuitable for surgery, with disseminated disease or with rupture. About 30% of cysts disappear, 30–50% degenerate or become smaller and 20–40% of cysts are unchanged [13].

Mebendazole is particularly useful if given 10–14 days

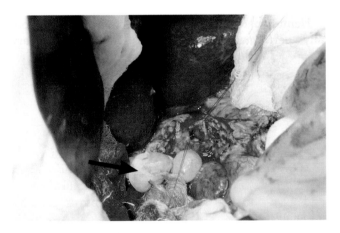

Fig. 29.24. Four glistening hydatid cysts (arrow) were removed surgically from the common bile duct of the patient shown in fig. 29.23.

References

1 Kamath PS, Joseph DC, Chandran R *et al*. Biliary ascariasis: ultrasonography, endoscopic retrograde cholangiopancreatography, and biliary drainage. *Gastroenterology* 1986; **91**: 730.
2 Khuroo MS, Zargar SA, Mahajan R. Hepatobiliary and pancreatic ascariasis in India. *Lancet* 1990; **335**: 1503.
3 Manialawi MS, Khattar NY, Helmy MM *et al*. Endoscopic diagnosis and extraction of biliary *Ascaris*. *Endoscopy* 1986; **18**: 204.
4 Shulman A. Non-Western patterns of biliary stones and the role of ascariasis. *Radiology* 1987; **162**: 425.

Strongyloides stercoralis

This soil-transmitted intestinal nematode is common in tropical countries. It is usually asymptomatic but can cause biliary obstruction due to biliary stenosis [1]. Thiabendazole is effective treatment.

Reference

1 Delarocque Astagneau E, Hadengue A, Degottc C *et al*. Biliary obstruction resulting from *Strongyloides stercoralis* infection: report of a case. *Gut* 1994; **35**: 705.

Trichiniasis

This disease is caused by eating raw, infected pork with subsequent dissemination of *Trichinella* larvae throughout the body.

Hepatic histology may show invasion of hepatic sinusoids by *Trichinella* larvae and fatty change [1].

Diagnosis is difficult unless in an epidemic. Eosinophilia is suggestive. Muscle pain and tenderness may warrant muscle biopsy.

Treatment. ERCP is indicated if the biliary tract is obstructed. Treatment is unsatisfactory. Mebendazole may be effective in the migratory stage but is of doubtful value later.

Reference

1 Guattery JM, Milne J, House RK. Observations on hepatic and renal dysfunction in trichinosis. Anatomic changes in these organs occurring in cases of trichinosis. *Am. J. Med.* 1956; **21**: 567.

Toxocara canis (visceral larva migrans)

This parasite is spread by cats and dogs. The second stage can infect the liver of man, forming granulomas [1]. Hepatomegaly, recurrent pneumonia, eosinophilia and hypergammaglobulinaemia are associated findings. The serum fluorescent antibody test is positive.

Treatment may be tried with diethyl carbamazine or thiabendazole.

Reference

1 Zinkham WH. Visceral larva migrans. *Am. J. Dis. Child.* 1978; **132**: 627.

Liver flukes

Cysts are consumed and larvae develop in the duodenum and eventually reach the bile ducts. The flukes probably invade the liver through its peritoneal coat and are carried via the parenchyma to the bile ducts. During the migratory phase they cause fever and eosinophilia. When they reach the biliary passages they may cause obstruction with complicating suppurative cholangitis.

Clonorchis sinensis

The Chinese liver fluke is found mainly in eastern Asia. It can present years after the patient has left their country of origin as the biliary flukes persist for decades. Cysts are ingested with improperly cooked or raw, fresh-water fish. The cyst wall is destroyed by trypsin in the duodenum and the larvae migrate from the duodenum into the peripheral intra-hepatic bile ducts where they mature to adult worms. In uncomplicated cases, the changes are confined to the bile duct walls with abundant adenomatous formation; fibrosis increases with time [4]. Cholangiocarcinoma is a serious complication [8].

Clinical manifestations depend on the number of flukes, the period of infestation and the complications. With heavy infestation, the patient suffers weakness, epigastric discomfort, weight loss and diarrhoea. Jaundice is due to obstruction to the intra-hepatic biliary tree by worms or inflammation. Infection leads to fever, chills and abdominal pain. Cholangiocarcinoma is marked by progressive jaundice and pruritus.

Diagnosis is based on finding ova in the stool or aspirated bile. Laboratory findings include eosinophilia and an increased serum alkaline phosphatase.

ERCP shows filamentous filling defects in the bile ducts which have blunted tips [7]. The defects are of uniform size and change in position.

US and *CT* changes are based on flukes within dilated ducts and peri-ductal changes without evidence of extra-hepatic biliary obstruction [1, 7].

The *therapeutic response* to praziquantel is poor and relapses may follow bithionol.

The bile ducts must be cleared of stones by endoscopic or percutaneous cholangiography or surgery [5, 6].

Fasciola hepatica

The common sheep fluke is found mostly in mid- and western Europe and in the Caribbean. The animal infestation rate in Britain is high: 30–90% of all sheep and cattle excrete the ova. This increases in wet summers when the intermediate host, the snail *Lymnaea trunculata*, is also more numerous. The encysted cercariae from these snails survive on herbage and patients are usually infected by eating contaminated watercress.

The clinical picture in the acute stage is of cholangitis with fever, right upper quadrant pain and hepatomegaly. Eosinophilia and a raised serum alkaline phosphatase are noted. The picture may simulate choledocholithiasis.

ERCP shows several irregular linear or rounded filling defects in the bile ducts or segmental stenosis, with an inflammatory pattern. Worms can be aspirated.

Liver biopsy shows infiltration of the portal zones with histiocytes, eosinophils and polymorphs. Hepatic granulomas and ova in the liver may occasionally be seen.

Diagnosis is suspected by finding the clinical picture of biliary tract disease with eosinophilia. It is confirmed by finding ova in the faeces. These, however, may not be detected until 12 weeks after the infection when parasites have attained sexual maturity. They disappear later.

The diagnosis may be confirmed by ELISA testing of circulating antibodies to *Fasciola hepatica* excretory-secretory antigens [2, 3].

CT shows peripheral filling defects, sometimes crescentic, in the liver due to the migrating fluke (fig. 29.27) [9].

Treatment of all liver flukes is by praziquantel, bithionol or albendazole.

Recurrent pyogenic cholangitis

This is a common disease in south-east Asia. The initial cause is uncertain, but may be *Clonorchis* or enteric micro-organisms. Biliary stone and stricture formation follow recurrent bacterial infections. Treatment is by antibiotics following biliary drainage either endoscopic or surgical.

References

1 Choi BI, Kim HJ, Han MC *et al.* CT findings of clonorchiasis. *Am. J. Roentgenol.* 1989; **152**: 281.
2 Cordova M, Herrera P, Nopo L *et al. Fasciola hepatica* cysteine proteinases: immunodominant antigens in human fascioliasis. *Am. J. Trop. Med. Hyg.* 1997; **57**: 660.
3 Espino AM, Marcet R, Finlay CM. Detection of circulating excretory secretory antigens in human fascioliasis by sandwich enzyme-linked immunosorbent assay. *J. Clin. Microbiol.* 1990; **28**: 2637.
4 Hou PC, Pang LSC. *Clonorchis sinensis* infestation in man in Hong Kong. *J. Pathol. Bact.* 1964; **87**: 245.
5 Jan YY, Chen MF. Percutaneous trans-hepatic cholangioscopic lithotomy for hepatolithiasis: long-term results. *Gastrointest. Endosc.* 1995; **42**: 1.
6 Jan YY, Chen MF, Wang CS *et al.* Surgical treatment of hepatolithiasis: long-term result. *Surgery* 1996; **120**: 509.
7 Lim JH. Radiologic findings of clonorchiasis. *Am. J. Roentgenol.* 1990; **155**: 1001.
8 Ona FV, Dytoc JNT. Clonorchis-associated cholangiocarcinoma: a report of two cases with unusual manifestations. *Gastroenterology* 1991; **101**: 831.
9 Pagola Serrano MA, Vega A, Ortega E *et al.* Computed tomography of hepatic fascioliasis. *J. Comp. Assist. Tomogr.* 1987; **11**: 269.

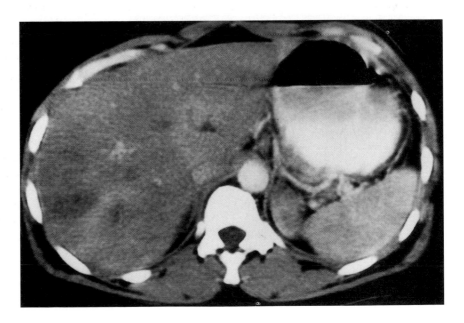

Fig. 29.27. *Fasciola hepatica.* CT in the migratory stage shows multiple, sometimes linear, filling defects at the periphery of the liver. (Courtesy of P.A. McCormick.)

Peri-hepatitis

This upper abdominal peritonitis is associated with genital infections, particularly *Chlamydia trachomatis* and less often with *Neisseria gonorrhoeae* [2]. It affects young, sexually active women and simulates biliary tract disease. Diagnosis is by laparoscopy. The liver surface shows white plaques, tiny haemorrhagic spots and 'violin string' adhesions.

CT may also show 'violin string' adhesions (fig. 29.28) [1]. Treatment is with tetracycline.

References

1 Haight JB, Ockner SA. *Chlamydia trachomatis* perihepatitis with ascites. *Am. J. Gastroenterol.* 1988; **83**: 323.
2 Simson JNL. Chlamydial perihepatitis (Curtis–Fitz Hugh syndrome) after hydrotubation. *Br. Med. J.* 1984; **289**: 1146.

Hepato-biliary disease in HIV infection

HIV does not seem to exert any direct effect on the liver. Many diseases, however, affect the immunodeficient and provide a confusing picture [23, 31]. All parts of the hepato-biliary system can show changes and may be involved in more than one process (table 29.4). Hepatomegaly is seen in at least two-thirds and 50% of patients show abnormal liver function tests. A blood culture is usually more helpful than a liver biopsy.

Hepatic histology is seldom normal, showing macrovesicular fat and mild zone 1 lymphocytes [18].

The causes of hepato-biliary disease differ depending on the extent of immunocompromise [32]. In earlier stages where the CD4 cell count exceeds $500 \times 10^9/l$, hepatic complications are largely liver-specific, such as drug-related, primary neoplasm or infection with hepato-trophic viruses such as hepatitis B and C. With progression of immunodeficiency to CD4 cell counts of less than 200, the liver is generally involved as part of systemic opportunistic infections due to *Mycobacterium avium intracellulare* (MAI), fungi or cytomegalovirus (CMV). The liver is only one site involved in AIDS; liver disease is rarely the primary cause of death.

A high serum alkaline phosphatase level is an indication for US or CT (fig. 29.29). Those with dilated bile ducts should proceed to ERCP to confirm biliary obstruction. Those with a focal lesion should have a guided liver biopsy. In the absence of a focal or bile duct

Table 29.4. Hepato-biliary changes in AIDS

Non-specific
Hepatomegaly
Abnormal biochemistry
Histology
　fatty change
　portal inflammation
　Kupffer cell iron
　diminished lymphocytes

Infections
Mycobacterium avium intracellulare
Mycobacterium tuberculosis
Cytomegalovirus*
Herpes simplex virus
Epstein–Barr virus
*Cryptococcus neoformans**
Histoplasmosis
*Candida albicans**
Coccidiomycosis
Microsporidia*
Toxoplasmosis
Bacillary peliosis
Hepatitis B virus
Impaired response to vaccine and antiviral therapy
Fulminant (rare)
Hepatitis C virus

Tumours
Hodgkin's and non-Hodgkin's lymphoma
Kaposi's sarcoma (rare)

Hepato-toxic drugs
Sulphonamides
Antibiotics
Isoniazid
Antifungals
Tranquillizers
Zidovudine

* Associated biliary tract disease.

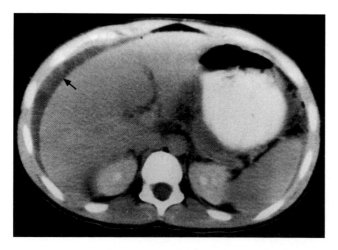

Fig. 29.28. CT in chlamydial peri-hepatitis shows 'violin string' adhesions between liver and anterior abdominal wall (arrowed) and ascites.

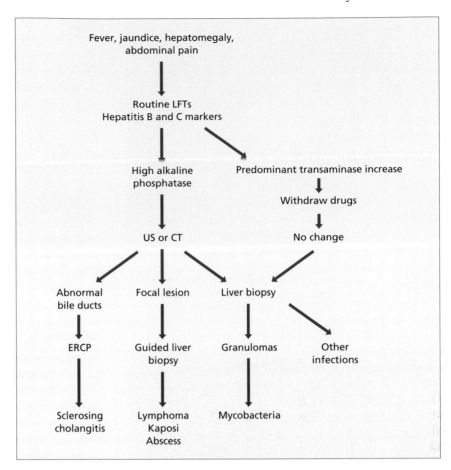

Fig. 29.29. The management of the patient with hepato-biliary AIDS.

lesion a liver biopsy should be performed to exclude mycobacteria (fig. 29.29).

Infections

These are largely opportunistic and part of generalized infection. Liver biopsy in patients with hepatomegaly, fever and abnormal biochemical tests gives the cause in about 25%.

MAI infection is a late complication. It presents with fever, night sweats, weight loss and diarrhoea. Hepatic histology shows poorly formed granulomas without lymphocyte cuffing, giant cells or central caseation. Acid-fast bacilli are present in large numbers in clusters of foamy histiocytes or within Kupffer cells (figs 29.30, 29.31). If MAC is seen in liver biopsies, the mean survival is only 69 days.

Mycobacterium tuberculosis can occur at an earlier stage and is more prevalent in injection drug users than in other categories. When the CD4 count exceeds 200, infection is pulmonary whereas atypical presentations, including hepatic involvement, are seen in patients with more severe immunodeficiency.

CMV is late and part of generalized disease. It is

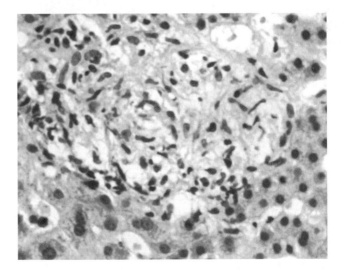

Fig. 29.30. An ill-defined poorly cellular granuloma in the liver of a patient with AIDS. (H & E, ×220.)

associated with fever and weight loss. Diagnosis is made by demonstrating nuclear and cytoplasmic inclusions in Kupffer cells, bile duct epithelium and occasionally hepatocytes.

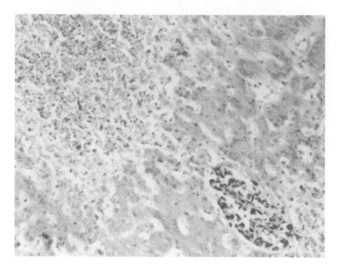

Fig. 29.31. Same patient as in fig. 29.30. Liver stained for acid-fast bacilli shows two granulomas containing many red-staining bacilli (*Mycobacterium avium intracellulare*).

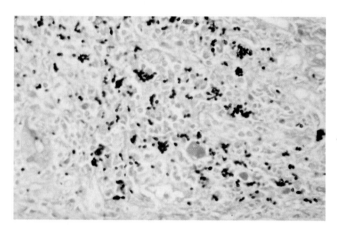

Fig. 29.32. Cryptococcal hepatitis in a patient with AIDS. Many yeast forms of *Cryptococcus neoformans* are stained black. (Methenamine silver, ×350.)

Bacillary peliosis hepatitis. The angioproliferative lesions in the liver resemble Kaposi's sarcoma. It is due to *Bartonella henselae*, a tiny Gram-negative organism which is difficult to cultivate [16, 29]. Systemic features include fever, lymphadenopathy, hepatosplenomegaly and cutaneous and bony lesions. It is treated by erythromycin.

Fungal infections are usually part of late disseminated disease. They include *Cryptococcus neoformans* where yeast can be shown in the liver (fig. 29.32) [4]. Similarly, histoplasmosis (fig. 29.33), coccidiomycosis [27] and *Candida albicans* may involve the liver. Those with low CD4 counts exposed to *Cryptosporidium* are at risk of biliary disease and death within 1 year [30]. *Pneumocystis carinii* can rarely cause hepatitis [20].

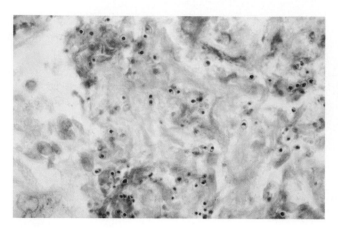

Fig. 29.33. Histoplasmosis hepatitis in a patient with AIDS. Many intracellular forms of *Histoplasma capsulatum* are stained red. (PAS diastase, ×500.)

Hepatitis B, C and D co-infection

Markers of past or present HBV infection are found in approximately 90% of homosexual men or drug abusers with AIDS. In late stage disease, the HBV may activate with conversion to HBe antigen positivity and an increase in HBV polymerase [15]. However, the HBV seems to have little effect on liver histology or survival [24]. Patients respond poorly to HBV vaccination, and to interferon therapy [19, 33]. Hepatitis delta virus (HDV) is present, depending on the location [25].

In contrast, HIV accelerates the course and reduces the survival of HCV-infected patients. The co-infection is particularly frequent in drug absuers and in haemophiliacs where the liver disease is particularly severe [12, 21, 28]. Antibodies to HCV can disappear despite persistent HCV viraemia [26]. Interferon therapy may be tried, but will have the greatest benefit only in those with higher CD4 counts. With the modern therapy of HIV, the number of doubly infected patients with good immune function will increase and combined ribavirin/interferon therapy can be tried.

Neoplasms

Non-Hodgkin's lymphoma is usually metastatic, but can be primary (fig. 29.34). It usually appears late, but may appear at any stage of the disease and can be a primary presentation. It presents as fever, weight loss, night sweats and abdominal pain, with a rise in serum transaminases and especially serum alkaline phosphatase. Large hepatic lesions present with jaundice and pruritus.

US and *CT* show large, usually multifocal solid space-occupying lesions. Guided liver biopsy is diagnostic.

Survival is short and response to chemotherapy poor.

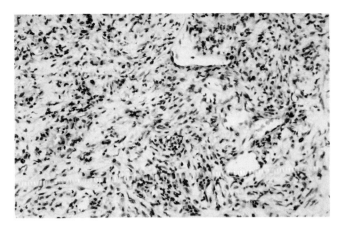

Fig. 29.34. B-cell lymphoma in a patient with AIDS. Sinusoids are infiltrated with large pleomorphic lymphoid cells. (H & E, ×350.)

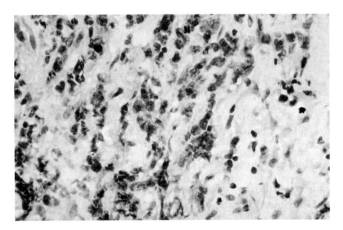

Fig. 29.35. Kaposi's sarcoma in a patient with AIDS. Portal zones show expansion with spindle cell tumour cells which are forming vascular clefts. (H & E, ×150.)

The prognosis depends on the degree of immunocompromise.

Kaposi's sarcoma largely affects homosexual men and is decreasing in prevalence. The patient is usually asymptomatic. It frequently involves the liver as purple–brown, soft nodules. Histology shows multifocal areas of vascular endothelial proliferation with pleomorphic spindle cells and extravasated erythrocytes (fig. 29.35). US shows small hyperechoic nodules and dense peripheral bands. CT shows hypoattenuated lesions enhancing after contrast.

Drug-induced HIV-infected patients are exposed to many potential hepato-toxins. Any agent should be considered at fault. Drug interactions must always be considered. Drug reactions are the commonest cause of jaundice in AIDS [8]. Anti-mycobacterials are most commonly at fault, especially isoniazid and rifampicin.

Trimethoprim-sulfamethoxasole is a common offender, causing granulomatous hepatitis and jaundice [17].

Hepatomegaly and steatosis may be related to nucleoside-analogue retroviral therapy [14]. Zidovudine and dideoxyinosine can cause severe, sometimes fatal, liver failure. The picture is of mitochondrial failure [3].

Hepato-biliary disease

This includes intra- and extra-hepatic sclerosing cholangitis [6], papillary stenosis and acalculous cholecystitis [31]. It is termed *AIDS cholangiopathy*. It is associated with severe immunodeficiency with CD4 lymphocytes counts of less than 200.

Cryptosporidia are the single most common pathogens identified. *Cryptosporidium parvum* is cytopathic for cultured human biliary epithelia via an apoptotic mechanism (fig. 29.36) [9].

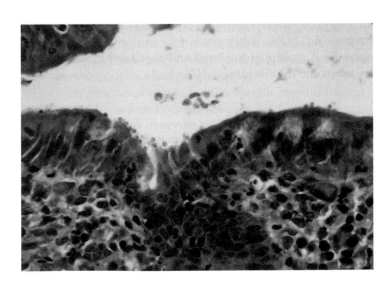

Fig. 29.36. Cryptosporidiosis of the gallbladder in a patient with AIDS. (H & E, ×160.)

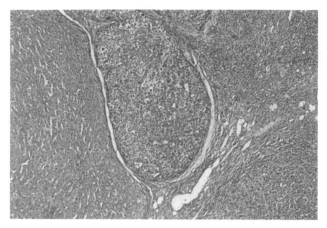

Fig. 30.3. Cirrhosis and a very small hepato-cellular carcinoma.

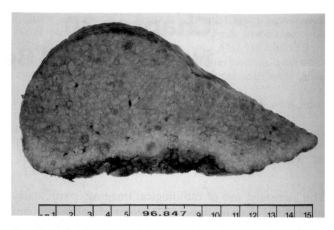

Fig. 30.4. Explant liver of chronic hepatitis C virus cirrhosis: note nodularity. Larger nodules with green/tan appearance are dysplastic.

tocyte nuclei compared with surrounding tissue, clear cell change, small cell dysplasia and fatty change [18]. Features in a dysplastic nodule favouring HCC include nuclear atypia, high nuclear/cytoplasm density, absence of portal tracts, unaccompanied arteries and reduction of reticulin and mitoses [7].

Conclusions. Any focal lesion in a cirrhotic liver must be regarded as suspicious of HCC or of its impending development [14]. Macro-regenerative nodules which are at least 1 cm in diameter and are hypoechoic, are particularly precancerous [5,19]. Screening of focal lesions by ultrasound and α-fetoprotein at 6-monthly intervals at least is mandatory.

Nodules in the absence of underlying liver disease (fig. 30.2)

Discovery of the lesion is followed by the usual detailed history and clinical examination, routine biochemical tests, hepatitis B and C viral markers and an α-fetoprotein level. A family history is taken for cystic disease.

Simple cysts (Chapter 33)

The hepatic cyst may be simple or multiple and may be accompanied by renal or other cysts.

On ultrasound, simple cysts have smooth walls and echo-free contents with through transmission of the sound waves. The CT scan shows a low attenuation value of the centre equivalent to water. There is no enhancement with contrast. MRI with T_2-weighted images shows the cysts as fluid.

Haemangioma

This is the commonest benign tumour of the liver, being found in about 5% of autopsies. Diagnosis is increasing with the greater use of scanning. It is usually single and

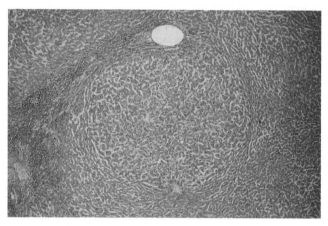

Fig. 30.5. Same patient as in fig. 30.4. Part of a dysplastic nodule: the central nodule (nodule-in-nodule) shows thick trabeculae and focal cholestasis. It is probably a minute hepato-cellular carcinoma. (H & E, × 10.) (Courtesy of Professor A.P. Dhillon.)

small, but occasionally may be multiple or very large. The tumour is commonly subcapsular, on the convexity of the right lobe and is occasionally pedunculated. On section it appears round or wedge shaped, dark red in colour and has a honeycomb pattern, with a fibrous capsule which may be calcified. Histologically, a communicating network of spaces contains red corpuscles. Factor VIII may be expressed. The tumour is lined by flat endothelial cells and contains scanty fibrous tissue. Occasionally, there is a marked fibrous component.

Clinical features. The majority are asymptomatic and discovered incidentally. Symptoms from giant tumours (>4 cm diamater) include abdominal mass and pain due to thrombosis. Symptoms may be due to pressure on adjacent organs. Rarely, a vascular hum is heard over the lesion.

Radiology. A plain X-ray may show a calcified capsule.

Ultrasound shows a solitary echogenic spot with

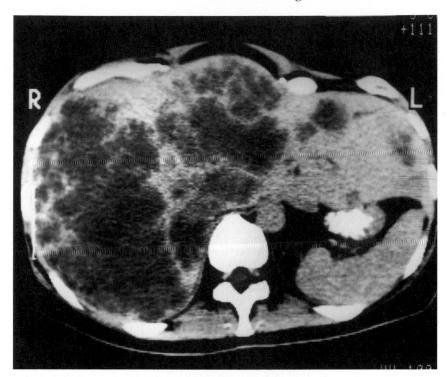

Fig. 30.6. Haemangioma. CT shows a giant benign haemangioma in the right lobe. A few small lesions are seen in the left lobe. The lesions filled in completely after intravenous contrast.

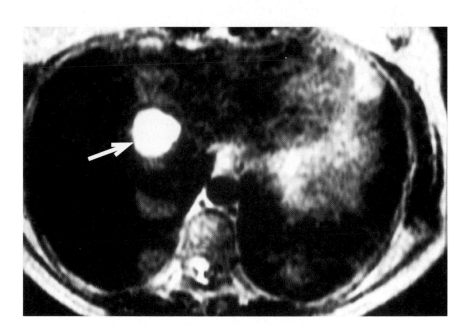

Fig. 30.7. Haemangioma. MRI using long T_2-weighting shows a very bright lesion (arrow). This reflects a profuse and very sluggish circulation usually due to a haemangioma.

smooth well-defined borders. Posterior acoustic enhancement, due to increased sound transmission through the blood of cavernous sinuses, is characteristic.

CT scan enhanced by contrast shows distinctive puddling of contrast in venous channels (fig. 30.6). The contrast fills in the lesion from the periphery to the centre, until opacification is homogeneous after 30–60 min. Foci of globular enhancement are seen after dynamic bolus CT. Calcification may be seen due to previous bleeding or thrombus formation.

MRI shows the tumour as a markedly high intensity area. T_2 is prolonged over 8 ms (fig. 30.7). MRI is of special value in diagnosing small haemangiomas.

SPECT with ^{99m}Tc-labelled red blood cells shows persistent blood pool activity within the lesion.

Arteriography is rarely necessary. Large arterial branches are displaced. The hepatic arteries divide to form small vessels before filling the vascular space. Prolonged, up to 18 s, opacification of the lesion may be shown.

Needle liver biopsy. Using a fine needle this is safe, but unnecessary in view of the diagnostic imaging.

Treatment is usually unnecessary as the lesions do not increase in size [11] or in clinical manifestations. The possibility of rupture is not an indication for surgery. Resection (usually lobectomy or segmentectomy) is safe if pain is severe or expansion rapid [1, 17].

Focal nodular hyperplasia

Focal nodular hyperplasia (FNH) is defined as a nodule composed of benign-appearing hepatocytes in a liver which is otherwise histologically normal or nearly normal (fig. 30.8). It is commonly subcapsular, but can be pedunculated and in either lobe. The lesions vary in size between 1 and 15 cm and may be multiple. The lesion is supported by large arteries accompanied by fibrous stroma containing ductules. The stroma is usually prominent, forming a stellate scar [7]. A central stellate scar (stalk) contains a large artery from which blood flows to the periphery of the lesion. The scar is dense and contains bile ductules, but no portal vein radical. It may represent a vascular anomaly as it is associated with haemangiomas elsewhere. Studies using X-chromosome inactivation showed a random pattern consistent with a polyclonal lesion, thus confirming a reactive disorder related to pre-existing vascular malformation [13]. It does not have an association with sex hormones [10]. It affects both sexes, but especially women in their reproductive years, some of whom have never taken sex hormones. It may present with pain or an abdominal mass. Serum biochemical tests are normal in the uncomplicated case.

The diagnosis is made by imaging with demonstration of the central scar (figs 30.9, 30.10) [14]. Ultrasound shows a nodule of varying echogenicity from patient to patient. The central scar is rarely seen. Colour Doppler shows arterial signals peripherally and centrally.

Contrast-enhanced CT shows a hypervascular mass with a central hypodense stellate scar (fig. 30.9) [2].

MRI shows a mass iso-intense or hypo-intense on T_1-weighted images and slightly intense on T_2-weighted images. The central scar is not usually seen. MRI with

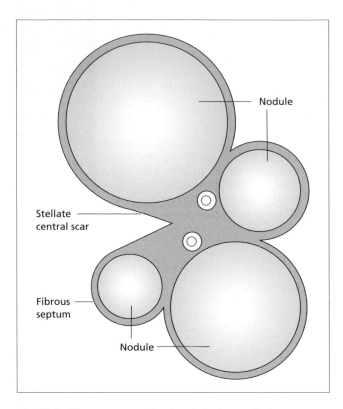

Fig. 30.8. The structure of focal nodular hyperplasia.

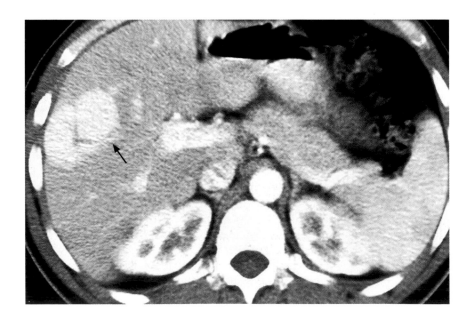

Fig. 30.9. Focal nodular hyperplasia. CT scan, enhanced with intravenous contrast, shows a focal hepatic lesion 5.8 cm in diameter with a central scar (arrow) in the right lobe.

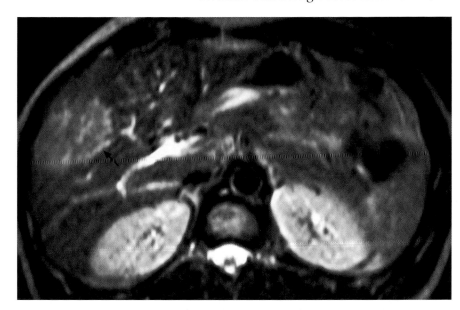

Fig. 30.10. Focal nodular hyperplasia. MRI shows a liver mass in the right lobe (arrow), homogeneously hypervascular after intravenous gadolinium and with a hypo-intense central area.

intravenous gadolinium at the early stages shows a central hypodense area, whereas 4 min later, high signal intensity is present showing that the central scar is vascularized. MRI with gadolinium is the best diagnostic procedure for FNH, having a sensitivity of 70% and a specificity of 98% [3]. Angiography confirms the supply is directed centrally to the scar and is then distributed to the periphery of the lesion like the spokes of a wheel. In most instances, angiography is not considered necessary as CT and MRI are usually diagnostic.

Histologically, the lesion consists of normal hepatocytes and Kupffer cells. The central core is composed of fibrous tissue and proliferating bile ducts (fig. 30.11). Liver biopsy is not usually necessary for diagnosis.

Interpretation may be difficult on the small specimen provided.

FNH is a static lesion, increasing only slowly, if at all, with time. It should be treated conservatively without surgery. Pregnancy may be allowed and any oral hormone therapy continued safely [10, 21].

Hepatic adenoma

Hepato-cellular adenoma is defined as a benign neoplasm composed of hepatocytes in a liver that is otherwise histologically normal or nearly normal (figs 30.12, 30.13). There are no portal tracts or central veins. Bile ducts are conspicuously absent. There is no central scar or predominant arterial supply. Kupffer cells are scarce. Signs of necrosis and infarction may be present and fatty change can be seen in some sections. Large arteries and veins are present in excess, sinusoids may be focally dilated and peliosis may be present (Chapter 20).

There is an association with oral contraceptive use, particularly over many years and in older women. A

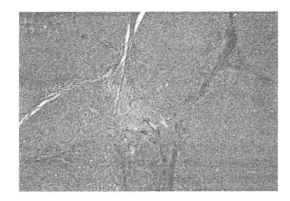

Fig. 30.11. Focal nodular hyperplasia. The central core is composed of fibrous tissue containing a thick-walled artery and proliferating bile ducts. (H & E, ×160.)

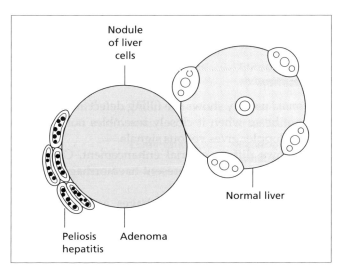

Fig. 30.12. Structure of hepatic adenoma and peliosis hepatis compared with normal liver.

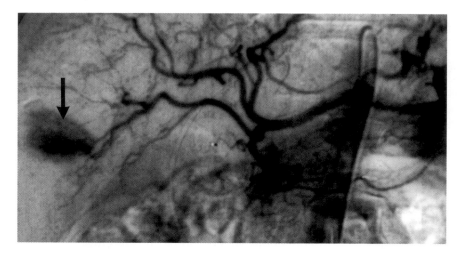

Fig. 31.12. Same patient as in fig. 31.11. Selective hepatic arterial angiography confirms tumour in right lobe (arrow).

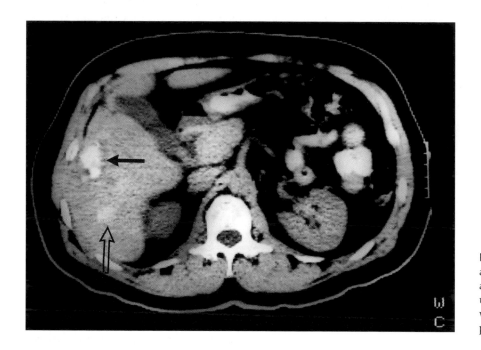

Fig. 31.13. Same patient as in figs 31.11 and 31.12. Oral contrast CT scan 9 days after intra-hepatic arterial lipiodol shows uptake into the right lobe tumour (arrow) with another possible lesion more posteriorly (open arrow).

Needle liver biopsy

Histological confirmation is important if small space-occupying lesions have been detected by ultrasound or CT (fig. 31.6). The biopsy should be done under imaging control. The possibility that biopsy will facilitate spread along the needle tract exists.

Fine-needle aspiration, using a 22-gauge needle, yields cytological specimens which will diagnose moderately and poorly differentiated tumours (fig. 31.14), but the cytological diagnosis of well-differentiated tumours is difficult.

Screening

Small, asymptomatic HCC in a cirrhotic liver may be diagnosed during screening of high-risk patients, by chance during imaging or found in a liver removed at the time of transplantation. Early recognition is important. The 1-year survival of untreated patients with well-compensated liver disease (Child's grade A) and having asymptomatic HCC is 90% at 1 year, whereas the 1-year survival of symptomatic patients is only 40%

Screening is indicated for high-risk patients. These are men, HBsAg or anti-HCV positive, more than 40 years old, and with chronic liver disease especially with cirrhosis and large macro-regenerative nodules. Ultrasound is more sensitive than CT. This is usually followed by directed fine-needle biopsy. Specimens must also be taken from non-tumorous tissue to determine the presence or absence of a concomitant cirrhosis and its activity.

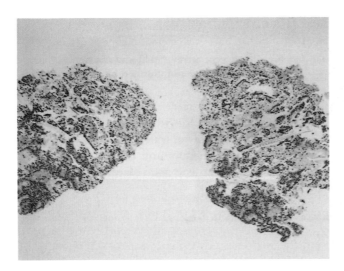

Fig. 31.14. Fine-needle aspiration under ultrasound guidance yielded a clump of HCC cells.

Table 31.2. Okuda staging system [75]

Criterion	Cut-off
Tumour size*	>50% = +; <50% = −
Ascites	Detectable = +; absent = −
Albumin	<3 g/dl = +; >3 g/dl = −
Bilirubin	>3 mg/dl = +; <3 mg/dl = −
Stage	**Survival (months)†**
I: no positives	8.3
II: one or two positives	2.0
III: three or four positives	0.7

*Largest cross-sectional area of tumour to largest cross-sectional area of liver.
†Without treatment.

Serum AFP estimation should be performed at 4–6-monthly intervals, particularly in those who have an initially increased concentration or where macro-regenerative nodules have been detected. Normal serum AFP does not exclude a tumour.

The reported value of screening is high in areas such as Japan where tumours are small and often encapsulated. In South Africa, tumours are rapidly growing and aggressive and screening is of little value. Europe seems to be in an intermediate position. Economics play a part. In Japan, such procedures as ultrasound and AFP estimations are routinely available at no cost to the patient. This is clearly not so in most other parts of the world. The prognosis of HCC is so poor that where cost is an important consideration there is probably a reluctance to screen especially as there is no firm consensus that the death rate will be reduced [15, 18].

Prognosis and risk factors

The outlook is usually hopeless. The time between exposure to hepatitis B or C and tumour development can vary from a few years to many decades [16].

The growth rate of the tumour varies greatly and correlates with survival. Asymptomatic Italian patients had a tumour volume doubling time varying from 1 to 19 months with a mean of 6 months. HCC in Africans is much more rapidly growing. Reasons are speculative, perhaps genetic, perhaps related to malnutrition, to cofactors such as aflatoxin or perhaps to late diagnosis in an itinerant African mine worker.

Small tumours (less than 3 cm in diameter) are associated with a 1-year survival of 90.7%, a 2-year survival of 55% and a 3-year survival of 12.8%. Infiltrating tumours have a worse prognosis than expanding ones. The presence of an intact capsule is a good sign. Although cirrhosis is the main risk factor, macro-regenerative nodules (at least 1 cm in diameter) and hypoechoic ones are particularly precancerous [27, 94].

Severity of liver disease correlates with the chances of developing HCC. Patients less than 45 years old survive longer than older ones. A tumour size exceeding 50% of the liver, a serum albumin less than 3 g/dl and a raised serum bilirubin level are ominous features.

The risk increases if the patient is HBsAg or anti-HCV positive.

In high endemic areas, progression to chronic hepatitis and cirrhosis is increased by infection with hepatitis B and C. Pulmonary metastases adversely affect survival.

Prognostic indices are particularly valuable in clinical trials and in selecting those who would benefit from more aggressive therapy [8]. The Okuda staging system uses tumour size, presence or absence of ascites and the serum bilirubin level (table 31.2).

The Cancer of the Liver Italian Program (CLIP) score [13] is based on the Child's stage, tumour morphology and extension, AFP level and portal vein thrombosis. It may give more accurate prognostic information than the Okuda method.

Surgical treatment (fig. 31.6)

There are various therapeutic options, but the only procedures that offer possibility of cure are resection or transplantation.

Doppler imaging, and particularly enhanced MRI, has revealed more small tumours than those shown by CT or ultrasound. The number of candidates suitable for resection has therefore fallen. Laparoscopic ultrasonography before planned surgery can avoid unnecessary operation [60].

Resection

After partial resection, DNA synthesis increases and the remaining liver cells become larger (*hypertrophy*) and

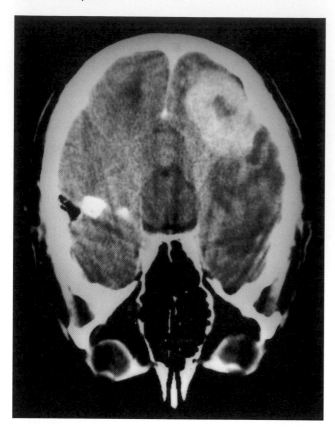

Fig. 31.15. Brain MRI shows large occipital metastasis in a patient with HCC.

Table 31.3. Factors in resection for HCC

Size <5 cm
One lobe
Capsule
Vascular invasion
Cirrhosis grade
Age and general condition

undergo increased mitosis (*hyperplasia*). Up to 90% of a non-cirrhotic liver may be removed with eventual survival.

The resectability rate for HCC is only about 3–30%. Success depends on size (less than 5 cm in diameter), position, particularly in relation to large vessels, presence of vascular invasion, presence of a capsule, absence of satellite lesions and the number of lesions (table 31.3). Multiple lesions have a high recurrence rate and a low survival time.

Cirrhosis is not a definite contraindication but is associated with a higher intra-operative and peri-operative morbidity and mortality. The operative mortality in the non-cirrhotic is less than 3%, but 23% in the cirrhotic. The cirrhosis should be Child's grade A. Over-aggressive resection can lead to hepatic decompensation. The patient's age and general condition must be taken into account.

Metastases must be sought by chest X-ray, CT scan or MRI, and isotope bone scan. Symptoms or signs of metastasis elsewhere should be investigated (fig. 31.15).

Improved results for resection have followed better knowledge of the segmental anatomy of the liver. The left lobe is resected with relative ease. The right lobe is

more difficult. Small tumours may be removed by segmentectomy; in others, lobectomy or trisegmentectomy may be necessary and this demands adequate liver function. The post-resection prognosis is related to the resection of a wide margin around the tumour, the absence of tumour thrombosis in hepatic vein or portal vein and no obvious intra-hepatic metastases.

The chances of 3-year survival are 30–40%; 25% of patients per year will develop recurrence in the residual liver.

Hepatic transplantation

This is used in patients with advanced cirrhosis (Child's grade B and C) who could not survive tumour resection. However, results are particularly poor if the candidate has a large tumour and is considered unsuitable for resection. Tumours greater than 5 cm are unacceptable for transplantation because of the high recurrence rate. Liver transplant is effective for single small (5 cm or less) tumours and no more than three tumour nodules (3 cm or less).

Five-year survival rates are about 20%. The liver is the common site of recurrence, which develops in up to 65% of patients. Those who are HBsAg or HCV positive do considerably worse, as the virus infection recurs in the new liver (Chapter 38). Results are better when tumour is discovered at screening or when a transplant is performed for another indication.

The choice between resection and transplant for a patient with a tumour of less than 5 cm can be extremely difficult. Poor liver function would favour transplant. The decision also depends on the expertise of available physicians and surgeons and the availability of a donor liver.

When the waiting list for transplant is long, resection has been followed by salvage transplant when the tumour recurs or liver function deteriorates [62].

Non-surgical treatment (fig. 31.16)

Systemic therapy

Mitozantrone may be given intravenously in courses

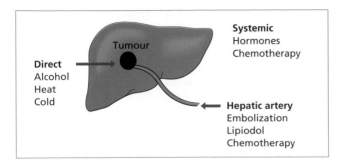

Fig. 31.16. Non-surgical therapeutic options in HCC.

every 21 days. Results are disappointing with a response rate of only 27.3% [21].

Tamoxifen treatment does not prolong survival [14].

Interferon therapy in HCV-positive patients may reduce the risk of later HCC, particularly if the patient has been a sustained responder [98]. Interferon treatment of advanced HCC is not beneficial in terms of tumour progression rate or survival [59].

Trans-arterial embolization

Catheterization of the hepatic artery via the femoral artery and coeliac axis allows embolization of the blood supply to the tumour. Chemotherapeutic agents may be delivered in high concentration. The procedures have limited success due to the development of arterial collaterals which ultimately supply the tumour.

Embolization is used for unresectable tumours. It may be used as an emergency to control intra-peritoneal haemorrhage from a ruptured HCC.

The procedure is performed under local or general anaesthesia and with antibiotic cover. The portal vein must be patent. The hepatic artery branch feeding the tumour is then embolized using gel foam, sometimes with an added agent such as doxorubicin or cysplatin (figs 31.17, 31.18). The tumour undergoes complete or partial necrosis.

Side-effects include pain, which can be severe, fever, nausea, encephalopathy, ascites and massive rises in transaminases. The AFP falls. Abscess formation and misplaced embolization are other complications.

HCCs are not sensitive to radiotherapy.

The results of embolization are variable from failure to prolongation of survival. Prognosis depends on the tumour type and extension, size, portal vein involvement, presence of ascites and jaundice. All lesions without a capsule are resistant to embolization. The technique is more useful in the treatment of *hepatic carcinoid tumours* where there is marked reduction in symptoms and tumour size (figs 31.19, 31.20).

Lipiodol, an iodized poppy seed oil, is retained in the

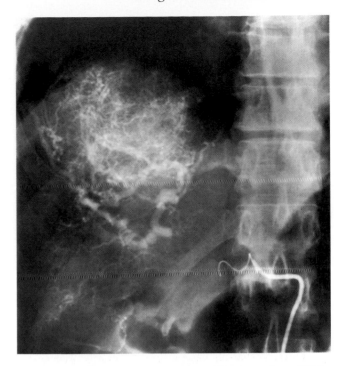

Fig. 31.17. Selective hepatic angiography shows a large HCC in the right lobe of the liver.

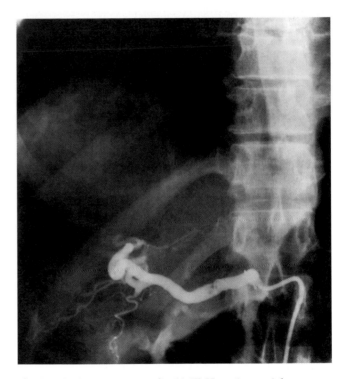

Fig. 31.18. Same patient as fig. 31.17. Hepatic arterial embolization with gel foam occlusion of blood supply to the tumour.

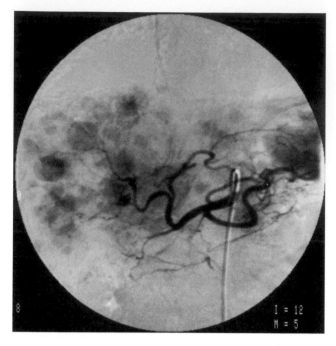

Fig. 31.19. Coeliac angiography in a patient with primary carcinoid tumour of the ileum and multiple, symptomatic liver metastases.

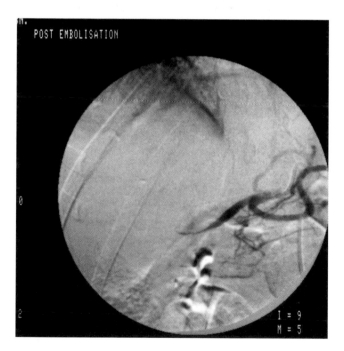

Fig. 31.20. Same patient as fig. 31.19 after selective hepatic arterial embolization to ablate tumour effects.

tumour for 7 or more days after hepatic arterial infusion but disappears from non-tumorous liver (see fig. 31.13). This is valuable in showing very small tumours. It is used to target lipophilic anticancer drugs such as epiru-

Table 31.4. Percutaneous alcohol injection for HCC

Less than 5 cm
Not more than three lesions
Local anaesthesia
Ultrasound or CT control
2–12 ml absolute alcohol
Side-effects

bicin or lipiodol I[131] to the tumour. These drugs all seem to prolong survival. The treatment can be repeated at 3–6-month intervals.

Pre-operative trans-arterial chemo-embolization using lipiodol reduces tumour size and may improve survival after resection or transplant [61]. After resection, adjuvant intra-arterial I[131]-labelled lipiodol decreases the rate of recurrence and increases overall survival [51].

Unfortunately, viable tumour cells often remain in and around the tumour and a complete cure cannot be expected.

Percutaneous ethanol injection

This was originally used for advanced disease in patients who were excluded from any other therapy [57]. It is now used for small (less than 5 cm) tumours, usually not more than three in number. Absolute alcohol is injected percutaneously under ultrasound or CT guidance (table 31.4).

The patient can be treated as an outpatient twice a week with 2–12 ml absolute alcohol for 3–15 sessions. Alternatively, a single session under general anaesthesia using a larger volume may be used for larger lesions [57]. The treatment results in intra-tumoural arterial thrombosis and coagulative necrosis followed by ischaemia of the tumour. It is only used for encapsulated tumours. Necrosis of the tumour is rarely complete. MRI may be useful for showing the effectiveness of therapy.

The injection may be a preliminary to resection and can be repeated if the tumour recurs. Multiple tumours can be treated. Injection is used to control bleeding following rupture of the tumour. The side-effects are similar to those of embolization. Three-year survival for Child's grade A is 71%, and for Child's grade B is 41% [58].

Overall recurrence is related to tumour size and the peri-tumoral capsule. This is 15.6% at 12 months and 45.1% at 24 months [46]. Percutaneous acetic acid injection may be associated with less recurrence and longer survival than alcohol [71].

Percutaneous microwave coagulation may be useful in small, well-differentiated tumours [82].

Radiofrequency obliteration has also been used [31].

Targeted gene transfer

This is used to deliver therapeutic genes specifically to malignant cells without damaging normal tissue.

Viral vectors, such as adenovirus, are efficient, but may exert a host immune response limiting repetitive administration [78]. A tumour-reactive monoclonal antibody coupled with a DNA binding cationic amphiphile, cholesteryl-spermine, has been used for gene delivery to HCC cells [67].

Conclusions

Hepato-cellular cancer remains a fatal disease. In a large trial of 123 patients with stage I HCC, usually with cirrhosis, all treatments increased the probability of survival (fig. 31.21) [3]. Results, however, did not differ between resection, liver transplantation and transarterial oily embolization. The various procedures have rarely been subjected to prospective clinical trials. Results are compared with historical controls or no treatment. The management of the small encapsulated HCC in a patient with well-compensated cirrhosis has improved. However, more often the tumour is large and the patient has decompensated liver disease so that little can be offered.

Fibro-lamellar carcinoma of the liver

This tumour is found in young people (aged 5–35) of both sexes [17]. It presents as an abdominal mass, sometimes with pain. It is unrelated to sex hormones. The liver is non-cirrhotic.

Histologically, clumps of large, polygonal deeply eosinophilic tumour cells are interspersed with bands of mature fibrous tissue (fig. 31.22). The cells have cyto-plasmic pale bodies representing intra-cellular fibrinogen storage. Occasionally the fibrous stroma is lacking.

Electron microscopy shows the cytoplasm packed with mitochondria and thick compact bands of collagen in parallel arrays. The tumour cells are believed to be oncocytes. The hepatocytes contain an excess of copper-associated protein, produced by the cancer cell.

Serum AFP is normal. Serum calcium levels may be raised with pseudo-hyperparathyroidism. Serum vitamin B_{12} binding protein [76] and neurotensin may also be increased.

CT shows a typical stellate scar with radial septa which show persistent enhancement on 10–20-min enhanced CT and MRI [38].

Prognosis is better than for other forms of liver cancer (survival 32–62 months), although the tumour may metastasize to regional lymph nodes.

Treatment is by surgical resection or transplantation [79].

Hepatoblastoma

This rare tumour affects children of both sexes less than 4 years old and very rarely older children and adults. It presents as progressive enlargement of the abdomen with anorexia, failure to thrive, fever and, rarely, jaundice. Associated features include sexual precocity due to secretion of an ectopic gonadotrophin by the tumour, cystathioninuria, hemihypertrophy and renal adenomas. Serum AFP levels are markedly increased. Imaging shows a space-occupying lesion in the liver with displacement of adjacent organs. There may be focal calcification. Angiography shows the features of primary liver cancer with a diffuse parenchymal blush persisting into the venous phase, encasement of vessels, pooling of contrast and an ill-defined margin.

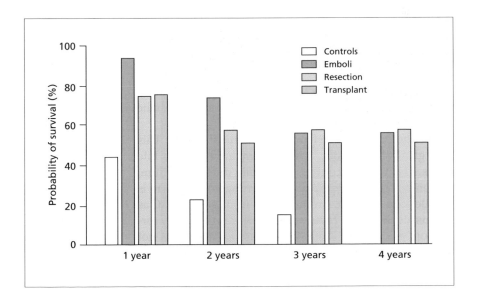

Fig. 31.21. Results of treating early (stage I) HCC on survival [3].

show a raised serum bilirbuin due to chemical sclerosing cholangitis.

Ablative treatment

Cryosurgery destroys tumour by freeze-thawing, using probes cooled by liquid nitrogen to sub-zero temperatures [1]. It is being evaluated in increased numbers of patients suitable for resection and also for unresectable tumours.

Other *local approaches* under investigation include microwave, radio-frequency, focused high intensity ultrasound and interstitial laser photocoagulation [9]. Their therapeutic role is not clearly defined yet.

Colorectal metastases

The liver is most commonly involved. Approximately 20% of patients will have liver metastases at the time of primary diagnosis. Of those without apparent metastases at surgery, 50% will develop metastatic liver disease. Of those treated, only about 20% will survive for about 2 years.

Resection may be possible as the metastases grow slowly, can be single and are mostly found in the subcapsular region. Resection may be possible in about 10% of patients. The peri-operative mortality is less than 5% in experienced hands. The overall 5-year survival is 25–46% [9]. Resection is possible if there are less than four metastases with no extra-hepatic recurrence or disease. Intra-operative ultrasound is essential to diagnose metastases and may alter the management. The surgeon must be prepared at the time of operation to modify the resection planned and to abandon a cure in 10–15% of patients. Lobectomy or a segmentectomy is usually performed.

In a multicentre report of 607 patients having metastases resected, 53% showed a recurrence in the liver and 53% in the lungs [37]. 66% recurred in the first year and 25% were alive and disease-free at 5 years. Patients with a CEA of less than 200 mg/ml with 1-cm surgical margins and less than 1000 g liver removed have a greater than 40% estimated 5-year disease-free survival [5]. In another series of 150 patients, curative resection (46% of patients) gave a median survival of 37 months, non-curative resection (12%), a survival 20.2 months and in the unresectable (52%), the survival was 16.5 months [90].

60% will develop recurrent disease after resection and a second operation must be considered, of similar type to that of the first resection.

Hepatic arterial (HA) infusion chemotherapy can be given continuously by an implantable pump for six 14-day courses, with 1 week rest in between. Starting 4 weeks post-resection, arterial and systemic chemotherapy improves the outlook at 2 years [44]. Survival is 86% for combined HA–5-FU and dexamethasone and 72% for monotherapy.

Metastatic carcinoid tumours

Small bowel carcinoids present with liver or lymph node metastases. Neuroendocrine tumours of the stomach and pancreas are also liable to metastasize to the liver.

Surgical resection has resulted in long-term relief of symptoms and prolonged survival [6, 48]. Surgery can be considered as the tumours shell out easily.

Hepatic artery occlusion and embolization can be palliative (see figs 31.19, 31.20). Transplantation in highly selected patients with metastatic carcinoid has resulted in a 69% 5-year survival.

Octeotride, a somastatin analogue, inhibits 5-HT release and reduces flushing and diarrhoea. Indium-labelled octreotide has been used for scintigraphy (see fig. 5.1) [6].

Indium-III labelled octeotride is under investigation for receptor-targeted therapy.

References

1 Adam R, Akpinar E, Johann M *et al*. Place of cryosurgery in the treatment of malignant liver tumours. *Ann. Surg*. 1997; **225**: 39.

2 Anthony PB. Liver cell dysplasia: what is its significance? *Hepatology* 1987; **7**: 394.

3 Bronowicki J-P, Nisand G, Altieri M *et al*. Compared results of resection (RX), orthotopic liver transplantation (OLT) and transcatheter oily chemoembolization (TOCE) in the treatment of Okuda's stage 1 hepatocellular carcinoma (HCC). *Gastroenterology* 1993; **104**: A881.

4 Buys CHCM. Telomeres, telomerase and cancer. *N. Engl. J. Med*. 2000; **342**: 1282.

5 Cady B, Stone MD, McDermott WV Jr *et al*. Technical and biological factors in disease-free survival after hepatic resection for colorectal cancer metastases. *Arch. Surg*. 1992; **127**: 561.

6 Caplin ME, Buscombe JR, Hilson AJ *et al*. Carcinoid tumour. *Lancet* 1998; **352**: 799.

7 Chen M-F, Jan Y-Y, Jeng L-B *et al*. Obstructive jaundice secondary to ruptured hepatocellular carcinoma into the common bile duct. *Cancer* 1994; **73**: 1335.

8 Chevret S, Trinchet J-C, Mathieu D *et al*. A new prognostic classification for predicting survival in patients with hepatocellular carcinoma. *J. Hepatol*. 1999; **31**: 133.

9 Choti MA, Bulkely GB. Management of hepatic metastases. *Liver Transplant Surg*. 1999; **5**: 65.

10 Chowdhury AR, Black M, Lorber SH *et al*. Hemangioendotheliomatosis of the liver: a 12 year follow-up. *Gastroenterology* 1977; **72**: 157.

11 Clain D, Wartnaby K, Sherlock S. Abdominal arterial murmurs in liver disease. *Lancet* 1966; **ii**: 516.

12 CLIP Group (Cancer of the Liver Italian Program). Tamoxifen in treatment of hepatocellular carcinoma: a randomized controlled trial. *Lancet* 1998; **352**: 17.

13 CLIP Investigators: Prospective validation of the CLIP score: a new prognostic system for patients with cirrhosis and hepatocellular carcinoma. *Hepatology* 2000; **31**: 840.

14 Collier JD, Carpenter M, Burt AD *et al.* Expression of mutant p53 protein in hepatocellular carcinoma. *Gut* 1994; **35**: 98.

15 Collier J, Sherman M. Screening for hepatocellular carcinoma. *Hepatology* 1998; **27**: 273.

16 Colombo M. Hepatocellullar carcinoma. *J. Hepatol.* 1992; **15**: 225.

17 Craig JR, Peters RL, Edmondson HA *et al.* Fibrolamellar carcinoma of the liver: a tumour of adolescents and young adults with distinctive clinico-pathologic features. *Cancer* 1980; **46**: 372.

18 Di Bisceglie AM, Carithers L Jr, Gores GJ. Hepatocellular carcinoma. *Hepatology* 1998; **28**: 1161.

19 Ding S-F, Michail NE, Habib NA. Genetic changes in hepatoblastoma. *J. Hepatol.* 1994; **20**: 672.

20 Dooley JS, Li AKC, Scheuer PJ *et al.* A giant cystic mesenchymal hamartoma of the liver: diagnosis, management, and study of cyst fluid. *Gastroenterology* 1983; **85**: 958.

21 Dunk AA, Scott SC, Johnson PJ *et al.* Mitoxantrone as a single agent therapy in hepatocellular carcinoma. A phase II study. *J. Hepatol.* 1985; **1**: 395.

22 El-Serag HB, Mason AC. Rising incidence of hepatocellular carcinoma in the United States. *N. Engl. J. Med.* 1999; **340**: 745.

23 Erlitzki R, Minuk GY. Telomeres, telomerase and HCC; the long and the short of it. *J. Hepatol.* 1999; **31**: 939.

24 Falk H, Thomas LB, Popper H *et al.* Hepatic angiosarcoma associated with androgenic-anabolic steroids. *Lancet* 1979; **ii**: 1120.

25 Fausto N. Mouse liver tumorigenesis: models, mechanisms and relevance to human disease. *Sem. Liver Dis.* 1999; **19**: 243.

26 Fernandez M, Del P, Redvanly RD. Primary hepatic malignant neoplasms. *Radiol. Clin. North Am.* 1998; **36**: 333.

27 Ferrell L, Wright T, Lake J *et al.* Incidence and diagnostic features of macroregenerative nodules vs. small hepatocellular carcinoma in cirrhotic livers. *Hepatology* 1992; **16**: 1372.

28 Forbes A, Portmann B, Johnson P *et al.* Hepatic sarcomas in adults: a review of 25 cases. *Gut* 1987; **31**: 668.

29 Gerber MA, Shieh YSC, Shim K-S *et al.* Detection of replicative hepatitis C virus sequences in hepatocellular carcinoma. *Am. J. Pathol.* 1992; **141**: 1271.

30 Gerber MA, Thung SN, Bodenheimer HC Jr *et al.* Characteristic histological triad in liver adjacent to metastatic neoplasm. *Liver* 1986; **6**: 85.

31 Goldberg SN, Gazelle GS, Solbiati L *et al.* Ablation of liver tumours using percutaneous RF therapy. *Am. J. Roentgenol.* 1998; **170**: 1023.

32 Harrison HB, Middleton HM III, Crosby JH *et al.* Fulminant hepatic failure: an unusual presentation of metastatic liver disease. *Gastroenterology* 1981; **80**: 820.

33 Harvey CJ, Blomley MJK, Eckersley RJ *et al.* Pulse-inversion mode imaging of liver specific microbubbles: improved detection of subcentimetre metastases. *Lancet* 2000; **355**: 807.

34 Hood DL, Bauer TW, Leibel SA *et al.* Hepatic giant cell carcinoma: an ultrastructural and immunohistochemical study. *Am. J. Clin. Pathol.* 1990; **93**: 111.

35 Hsia CC, Axiotis CA, Di Bisceglie AM *et al.* Transforming growth factor alpha in human hepatocellular carcinoma and coexpression with hepatitis B surface antigen in adjacent liver. *Cancer* 1992; **70**: 1049.

36 Hsu H-C, Huang A-M, Lai P-L *et al.* Genetic alterations at the splice junction of p53 gene in human hepatocellular carcinoma. *Hepatology* 1994; **19**: 122.

37 Hughes KS, Simon R, Songhorabodi S *et al.* Resection of the liver for colorectal carcinoma metastases: a multiinstitutional study of patterns of recurrence. *Surgery* 1986; **100**: 278.

38 Ichikawa T, Federle MP, Grazioli L *et al.* Fibrolamellar hepatocellular carcinoma: imaging and pathologic findings in 31 recent cases. *Radiology* 1999; **213**: 352.

39 Ishak KG, Sesterhenn IA, Goodman MZD *et al.* Epithelioid haemangioendothelioma of the liver: a clinicopathologic and follow-up study of 32 cases. *Hum. Pathol.* 1984; **15**: 839.

40 Johnson DH, Hainsworth JD, Greco FA. Extrahepatic biliary obstruction caused by small-cell lung cancer. *Ann. Intern. Med.* 1985; **102**: 487.

41 Kamby C, Kirksen H, Vejborg I *et al.* Incidence and methodologic aspects of the occurrence of liver metastases in recurrent breast cancer. *Cancer* 1987; **59**: 1524.

42 Keeley AF, Iseri OA, Gottlieb LS. Ultrastructure of hyaline cytoplasmic inclusions in a human hepatoma: relationship to Mallory's alcoholic hyalin. *Gastroenterology* 1972; **62**: 280.

43 Kelleher MB, Iwatsuki S, Sheahan DG. Epithelioid hemangioendothelioma of the liver. Clinicopathological correlations in 10 cases treated by orthotopic liver transplantation. *Am. J. Surg. Pathol.* 1989; **13**: 999.

44 Kemeny N, Huang Y, Cohen AM *et al.* Hepatic arterial infusion of chemotherapy after resection of hepatic metastases from colorectal cancer. *N. Engl. J. Med.* 1999; **341**: 2039.

45 Kew MC. Virchow–Troisier's lymph node in hepatocellular carcinoma. *J. Clin. Gastroenterol.* 1991; **13**: 217.

46 Khan KN, Yatsuhashi H, Yamasaki K *et al.* Prospective analysis of risk factors for early intrahepatic recurrence of hepatocellular carcinoma following ethanol injection. *J. Hepatol.* 2000; **32**: 269.

47 Kojima H, Yokosuka O, Kato N *et al.* Quantitative evaluation of telomerase activity in small liver tumours: analysis of ultrasonography-guided liver biopsy specimens. *J. Hepatol.* 1999; **31**: 514.

48 Kulke MH, Mayer RJ. Carcinoid tumours. *N. Engl. J. Med.* 1999; **340**: 858.

49 Kusano N, Shiraishi K, Kubo K *et al.* Genetic aberrations detected by comparative genomic hybridization in hepatocellular carcinomas: their relationship to clinicopathological features. *Hepatology* 1999; **29**: 1858.

50 Lack EE. Mesenchymal hamartoma of the liver. A clinical and pathological study of nine cases. *Am. J. Pediatr. Hematol. Oncol.* 1986; **8**: 91.

51 Lau WY, Leung TFT, Ho SKW *et al.* Adjuvant intra-arterial iodine-131-labelled lipiodol for resectable hepatocellular carcinoma: a prospective randomized trial. *Lancet* 1999; **353**: 797.

52 Lauffer JG, Zimmerman A, Krahenbuhl L *et al.* Epithelioid haemangioendothelioma of the liver. A rare hepatic tumour. *Cancer* 1996; **78**: 2318.

53 Lederman SM, Martin EC, Laffey KT *et al.* Hepatic neurofibromatosis, malignant shwannoma and angiosarcoma in von Recklinghausen's disease. *Gastroenterology* 1987; **92**: 234.

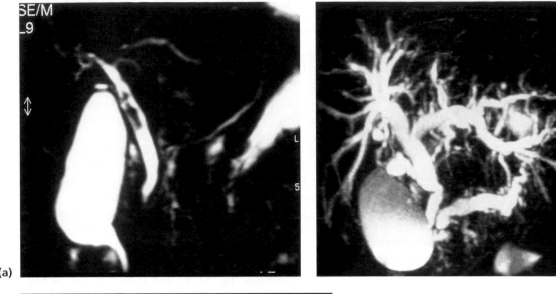

(a)

(b)

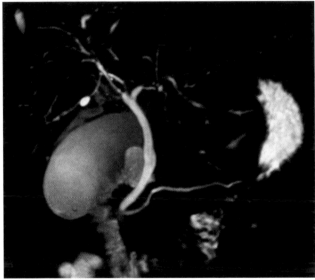

(c)

Fig. 32.7. (a) MRCP in a 39-year-old woman with right upper quadrant discomfort. Ultrasound showed a bile duct of 1 cm but no stones were seen. Gallbladder was normal. Liver function tests were normal apart from marginally abnormal γ-GT. The MRCP shows filling defects in the mid bile duct and stones were removed after endoscopic sphincterotomy. (b) MRCP in a patient presenting with cholestasis and change in bowel habit. Both the common bile duct and pancreatic duct are dilated. ERCP showed carcinoma of the ampulla. (c) MRCP in a 40-year-old woman with chronic cholestasis of unknown aetiology. There are dilatations and strictures of the intra-hepatic and peri-hilar bile ducts. Diagnosis: sclerosing cholangitis.

Endoscopic ultrasound (EUS)

This is done using an endoscope which has a miniature ultrasound transducer mounted on its tip. An endoscopic view is possible but is limited in comparison with normal diagnostic endoscopes.

Most endoscopes used for ultrasonography have a mechanical rotating scanner at the tip and are side or oblique viewing. The transducer rotates at approximately 10 cycles per second providing a 360-degree image. Because of the transducer the endoscope has a long rigid nose over several centimetres at the tip which makes introduction more difficult than a regular endoscope. Another design of endoscope uses a linear transducer which gives a 100-degree ultrasound image.

Recognizing the structures seen at endoscopic ultrasonography requires a sufficient period of training and this has limited its general availability to specialist centres.

EUS has a major application in the evaluation of oesophageal strictures but in the hepato-biliary system its prominent role is in the detection and evaluation of pancreatic tumours (fig. 32.8). It also detects common bile duct stones and can be used for image-directed biopsy.

EUS is at least as sensitive as ERCP in detecting stones and strictures [57]. The sensitivity and accuracy of endoscopic ultrasound for choledocholithiasis is greater than 90% [55] and it is more accurate than transabdominal ultrasound [15].

EUS has a greater sensitivity for detecting pancreatic

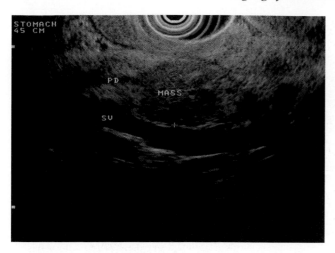

Fig. 32.8. Endoscopic ultrasound in a patient with suspected neuroendocrine tumour in whom CT scan had shown no abnormality. 2.5 cm diameter mass shown in head of pancreas PD, pancreatic duct; SV, superior mesenteric vein. (Courtesy of Dr Steve Pereira.)

tumour (93%) than CT (53%) [52]. Endoscopic ultrasound may also be used to stage pancreatic cancer but its accuracy needs further evaluation [2]. This technique is also highly accurate for localizing pancreatic neuroendocrine tumours which are often not well seen by other methods (fig. 32.8) [6].

Endoscopic ultrasound-guided fine-needle aspiration biopsy is possible from lymph nodes and pancreatic lesions and in experienced hands is safe [75].

With the increased availability of this technique it is being used more frequently for the evaluation of patients with pancreatic tumours, in particular for biopsy and assessing resectability. It may also be valuable for patients with problematic biliary tract pain where MRCP and other scanning has been negative and ERCP unhelpful. Endoscopic ultrasound to look for tiny bile duct stones and for pancreatic disease may be clinically indicated in combination with endoscopic biliary manometry.

Biliary scintigraphy

The technetium-labelled iminodiacetic acid derivative (IDA) is cleared from the plasma by hepato-cellular organic anion transport and excreted in the bile (fig. 32.9a). Biliary radiopharmaceuticals have so improved that one of the newest, Iodida, is easily prepared and is taken up by the liver and excreted into bile efficiently with only 5% of the injected dose excreted in the urine. Effective concentration in the bile duct is achieved in patients with total serum bilirubin levels exceeding 340 μmol/l (20 mg/dl). Resolution is much less than with

other forms of bile duct visualization and the role of cholescintigraphy is therefore limited.

The method may be used to determine patency of the cystic duct in suspected *acute cholecystitis* (fig. 32.9b). The radio-activity is followed until it reaches the duodenum. If the gallbladder fails to visualize, despite common bile duct patency and intestinal visualization, the probability of acute cholecystitis is 99%.

The gallbladder ejection fraction can be calculated from the loss of isotope from the gallbladder after a standard infusion of sincalide (the C-terminal octapeptide of CCK) [78]. This technique can help to identify gallbladder disease in some patients who have gallbladder-like pain but a normal ultrasound.

Cholescintigraphy can show whether the bile duct is obstructed, but in most units US serves this role.

In the more complicated patient, analysis of the pattern of uptake and hepatic clearance of radio-activity, or the combination of scintigraphy with US, can differentiate intra-hepatic cholestasis from bile duct obstruction—useful, for example, in the patient with a biliary stricture, who remains cholestatic despite insertion of a biliary endoprosthesis. Scintigraphy is also useful in assessing the patency of biliary-enteric anastomoses, and may show biliary leaks after cholecystectomy (fig. 32.9c) or liver transplantation [44].

Choledochal cysts can be diagnosed although ultrasound CT and MRI scanning are just as satisfactory (see fig. 33.13).

In the *neonate*, IDA scanning is used to differentiate between biliary atresia and neonatal hepatitis (fig. 32.9d). It may be combined with ultrasound.

Functional obstruction of the sphincter of Oddi after cholecystectomy may be suggested by delayed and reduced excretion of activity with slower emptying of the biliary tree.

Oral cholecystography

Although oral cholecystography shows gallbladder stones with an accuracy of 85–90%, it is now rarely used because of the greater sensitivity and wide availability of transabdominal ultrasonography. In recent years it had a limited role in the evaluation of the gallbladder before oral bile acid therapy but this treatment has also become much less frequent with the development of laparoscopic cholecystectomy.

The contrast agents used were iodine containing, conjugated with glucuronic acid by the liver, and excreted in bile. In the fasting patient contrast enters the gallbladder if the cystic duct is patent. There is reabsorption of water by the lining mucosa, concentration of contrast and gallbladder opacification (fig. 32.10). Complications including hypersensitivity are extremely rare.

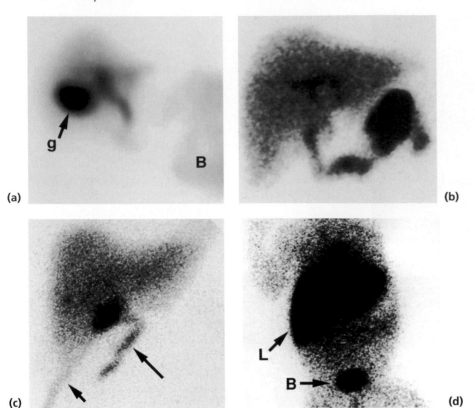

Fig. 32.9. Cholescintigraphy (^{99m}Tc Iodida). (a) Normal scan. At 30 min the gallbladder (g) has filled. Isotope has already entered the bowel (B). (b) Acute cholecystitis. Gallbladder has not filled by 60 min (c) Post-cholecystectomy bile leak. Isotope tracks laterally from gallbladder bed (short arrow) and T-tube track (long arrow). (d) Two-week-old infant with severe jaundice. Radio-activity is concentrated in the liver (L) and did not enter the bowel. Biliary atresia was confirmed. B, bladder.

When this method is used three X-ray films are necessary; control, fasting after oral contrast, and after gallbladder contraction by fat stimulation or CCK. The gallbladder is seen in 85% of patients. Films are taken erect and prone. Normal visualization without stones gives a 95% probability that the gallbladder is normal. The technique is not valuable if the bilirubin is greater than twice the upper limit of normal because of failure of efficient secretion of contrast by the liver.

Oral cholecystography is of value in showing lesions of the gallbladder wall, for example *adenomyomatosis* [47]. This is seen as small fundal outpouchings. *Rokitan-sky–Aschoff sinuses* are seen as a dotted second contour around the gallbladder lumen. Anomalies of the gallbladder may be visualized by oral cholecystography.

Intravenous cholangiography

The contrast (meglumine iotroxate; biliscopin) is concentrated by the liver so that hepatic and common bile ducts are demonstrated. Tomography is used.

However, intravenous cholangiography had become obsolete because of its poor diagnostic accuracy, its morbidity and the advent of MRCP.

Endoscopic retrograde cholangiopancreatography [18]

The ampulla of Vater is visualized endoscopically, the common bile duct or pancreatic duct is cannulated and contrast material injected (fig. 32.11).

Patients with suspected biliary obstruction, a history of cholangitis or a pancreatic pseudocyst are at risk of procedure-related sepsis, and require antibiotic premedication [66]. The elderly are also at greater risk. Micro-organisms responsible include colonic flora (*Escherichia coli*, *Klebsiella*, *Proteus*, *Pseudomonas*, *Streptococcus faecalis*) and the antibiotic choice should reflect this and the hospital antimicrobial policy. Oral ciprofloxacin is as effective as intravenous cefuroxime, and more cost-effective [66].

The patient is starved for 6 h. The procedure is done under sedation with a benzodiazepine (diazepam, midazolam) with an opiate as necessary.

At ERCP, diseases of the oesophagus, stomach, duodenum, pancreas and biliary tract including duodenal diverticula and fistulae may be diagnosed. Manometry of the sphincter area is possible. Immediate treatment may be instituted, for example sphincterotomy for common duct stones. However, endoscopes are costly and the technique demands an experienced team. Usually the patient must be under observation for 24 h

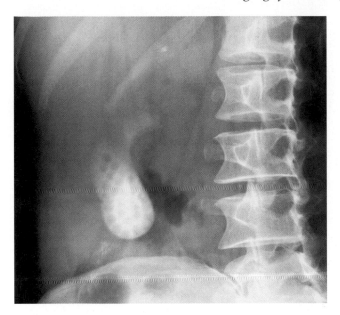

Fig. 32.10. Oral cholecystogram showing gallbladder packed with stones.

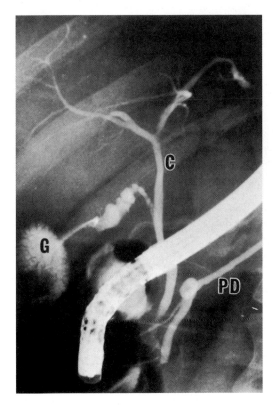

Fig. 32.11. ERCP, normal appearances. C, common bile duct; G, gallbladder; PD, pancreatic duct.

after the procedure. However, outpatient ERCP may be done for selected patients, although around 25% may need admission for complications or observation after a therapeutic procedure [36]. After sphincterotomy observation for 6h or overnight may reduce the need for readmission [30].

The side-viewing duodenoscope is passed. The stomach and duodenum are inspected and biopsy and cytology specimens taken if indicated. The papilla is identified. Duodenal ileus is maintained by intermittent intravenous hyoscine N-butylbromide (Buscopan) or glucagon. The cannula is then introduced under direct vision into the papilla and contrast (e.g. iopromide) injected under fluoroscopic control. Preferential catheterization of bile duct and pancreatic duct is helped by directing the catheter towards 11 and 12 o'clock, respectively, with the ampullary area *en face* seen as a clock face. Use of a dual channel sphincterotome allows selective bile duct cannulation or cannulation after failure with a standard catheter.

The intra-hepatic biliary tree, cystic and common bile ducts and gallbladder are filled (fig. 32.11). Changes in the position of the patient and tilting of the screening table after injection encourage distribution of contrast material throughout the duct system. In difficult cases, such as after sphincterotomy, a balloon catheter in the duct may be used to prevent reflux of contrast into the duodenum and so obtain better bile duct filling. The pancreatic duct is similarly cannulated and X-ray films taken.

An aseptic technique is maintained throughout. Endoscopes are thoroughly cleansed with soap and water and disinfected with activated glutaraldehyde. The danger of introducing infection is shown by a single endoscope which, although cleaned in an automatic machine, remained contaminated with *Pseudomonas aeruginosa* so resulting in biliary infection in 10 patients, with one fatality [3].

A history of minor reactions to intravenous contrast is not important but those who have had a major allergic reaction to iodinated contrast should be premedicated with corticosteroids and antihistamines [25].

The success rate for ERCP is 80–90% but depends on experience. Anatomical causes of failure include a peri-ampullary diverticulum or an ampullary tumour or stricture. Billroth II gastrectomy poses difficulties which may be overcome by an experienced endoscopist if necessary using a forward-viewing endoscope.

Interpretation of the cholangiogram is not always easy. Contrast may obscure small stones. Air bubbles may cause confusion. Failure to fully fill the biliary tree, particularly in non-dependent parts, may add to the difficulty.

Complications

The complication rate is 2–3% and mortality 0.1–0.2%. Complications are directly related to the skill and experience of the operator and to the presence of underlying pancreatic or biliary disease.

Serum amylase levels rise considerably after ERCP and acute pancreatitis is the commonest complication. It almost always follows successful pancreatic cannulation and injection. The volume of contrast injected should be kept to a minimum. Non-ionic lower osmolarity contrast media have not been proven to carry a lower risk of acute pancreatitis. In most cases pancreatitis is clinically mild with recovery over a few days. For this and other reasons (duration of infusion required, cost-effectiveness) somatostatin or gabexate, both shown in randomized studies to reduce post-ERCP pancreatic injury, are not routinely used [4]. Pancreatic pseudocyst is a relative contraindication to ERCP.

Cholangitis is the second most common complication but the commonest cause of death. Bacteraemia is reported in 0–14% [66]. Pre-existing biliary infection and obstruction are important risk factors. Prophylactic antibiotics are important in prevention, together with early decompression of any biliary obstruction.

In patients with primary sclerosing cholangitis and advanced disease, there may be deterioration after ERCP [10].

Indications

ERCP adds to the speed of diagnosis of the jaundiced patient as it can be performed irrespective of depth of jaundice or state of liver function. It outlines the site of any biliary obstruction and in many instances indicates the cause.

It can be used to show duct strictures, and gallbladder and common bile duct stones (figs 32.12, 32.13). It is of particular value in those with biliary disease and undilated intra-hepatic ducts. Diagnoses include primary sclerosing cholangitis, Caroli's disease and other congenital anomalies.

ERCP may be performed after biliary surgery in the investigation of benign post-cholecystectomy symptoms or to define and treat more serious sequelae such as residual calculi, leaks and biliary strictures [22].

ERCP may be used to diagnose pancreatic disease, particularly in those with coincident hepato-biliary problems such as carcinoma of the pancreas and alcoholic pancreatitis with biliary obstruction.

ERCP is occasionally used in the investigation of the patient with obscure epigastric pain. It allows visualization of stomach and duodenum as well as pancreatic and biliary ducts, all at one sitting.

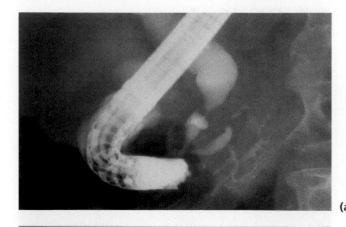

(a)

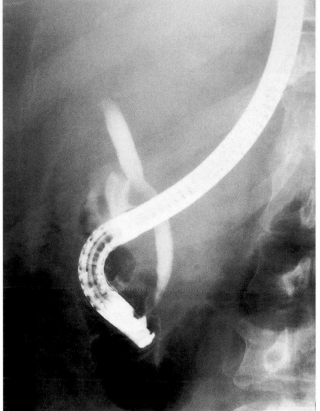

(b)

Fig. 32.12. ERCP showing: (a) dilated bile duct above a stricture. The pancreatic duct comes to an abrupt halt in the head of the pancreas. Appearances are characteristic of carcinoma of the pancreas; (b) common bile duct filling as far as a hilar stricture due to a cholangiocarcinoma.

Pure bile or pancreatic juice may be obtained for culture, aspiration cytology or chemical analysis.

Strictures may be brushed for cytology or biopsied [43].

Endoscopic sphincterotomy [18]

Normal coagulation is a prerequisite for endoscopic

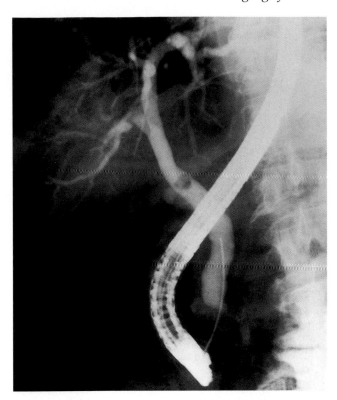

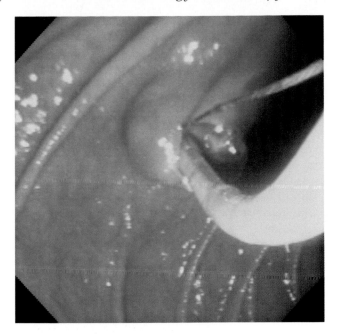

Fig. 32.14. Sphincterotome inserted into ampulla of Vater. The wire has been bowed and the sphincterotomy cut has begun.

Fig. 32.13. ERCP showing common bile duct stone. A sphincterotome has been passed into the lower end of the bile duct.

sphincterotomy and the result of platelet count and pro-thrombin time as well as haemoglobin should be known. Serum is taken for blood group analysis and saved in case transfusion is necessary. Premedication with anti-biotic is routine in most units. A skilled team is required with adequate equipment, in a hospital with facilities to treat any complication.

After the diagnostic ERCP has shown a stone, the ampulla is catheterized with a dual-channel sphinctero-tome appropriate in length and design to the anatomy found. Fluoroscopy is used to establish that this has entered the bile duct. A guide-wire is usually passed into the bile duct to stabilise the sphincterotome position during sphincterotomy. The sphincterotome is with-drawn leaving approximately 1 cm of the wire within the ampulla, the wire is bowed and, under direct vision, a cut is made using a blend or cutting current from the cautery unit (fig. 32.14). The length of cut depends upon the anatomy of the ampulla and the supra-ampullary area, and the size of the stone. If sphincterotomy is being done as a preliminary to endoprosthesis insertion only a small cut is needed. For stones, the aim is to make a cut of sufficient length to allow removal. It may be necessary to cut through the biliary sphincter, shown by the release of bile. Air refluxes up the bile duct. For larger stones

it is necessary to decide when to use a mechanical lithotripter and a moderate cut, rather than risk a larger, possibly complicated sphincterotomy.

The success rate is above 90% [37], reaching 97% in an expert unit [70]. Causes of failure include a large peri-ampullary diverticulum, a Billroth II partial gastrectomy and an impacted stone at the ampulla.

Related techniques which may be helpful include needle knife papillotomy [29], but this should only be used by experienced endoscopists.

Complications [20, 31]

These occur in about 10% and include haemorrhage, cholangitis, pancreatitis, duodenal perforation, Dormia basket impaction and Gram-negative shock. They are life threatening in 2–3%. Mortality is 0.4–0.6%.

Prospective studies show pancreatitis in 8–10% of patients having an endoscopic sphincterotomy. The rate will be influenced by the technique used including selective catheterization of the biliary system using a sphinctertome. Pure cut electrocautery may reduce the risk [27]. Post-sphincterotomy pancreatitis is usually mild.

Bleeding, usually from the retro-duodenal artery, is the most serious potential problem. It usually settles but, if not, surgery can be difficult. Treatment by arterial embolization may be successful. Bleeding is not always immediate and may be delayed several days after the procedure [30].

Cholangitis occurs if biliary decompression (stone removal) is unsuccessful. Prevention is by insertion of a naso-biliary tube or endoprosthesis.

Late results of sphincterotomy show that two-thirds of patients have air in the biliary tract and free reflux of duodenal juice. Bacterial colonization of the bile is present whether or not there are symptoms; the significance of this is unknown. Late complications (5–10% over 5 years) include sphincter stenosis [13] and recurrent stones. The long-term effects of loss of sphincter function are unresolved.

In cirrhotic patients with choledocholithiasis endoscopic sphincterotomy is effective and safe although coagulopathy must be corrected beforehand [58].

Indications

Choledocholithiasis is the commonest indication. Emergency ERCP with endoscopic sphincterotomy is the treatment of choice for patients with *acute suppurative obstructive cholangitis* [45] which is almost always caused by a stone. Where there is *acute cholangitis* of lesser severity elective ERCP is done after a period of antibiotic treatment. Whether or not the gallbladder is in place, sphincterotomy is the treatment of choice.

In patients with *common duct stones without cholangitis* the choice depends on the clinical situation. For *post-*

cholecystectomy retained bile duct stones sphincterotomy is clearly the best treatment in elderly frail patients and those with other medical problems. In this group of patients it is also the accepted treatment even when the gallbladder is still *in situ*. After removal of the common duct stone(s), the decision whether to proceed to cholecystectomy depends upon clinical data, although when the patient is unfit for surgery conservative therapy without cholecystectomy is an option (Chapter 34).

In younger, fit patients with retained stones after cholecystectomy, sphincterotomy is preferred to surgical bile duct exploration. With the gallbladder in place, however, it is not clear whether cholecystectomy should be preceded by endoscopic sphincterotomy or accompanied by duct exploration and stone removal at the time of surgery.

The evolution of laparoscopic cholecystectomy and duct exploration adds to the therapeutic choice.

Acute gallstone pancreatitis, particularly if severe and unresolving, is an indication for emergency ERCP and sphincterotomy if a stone is found (Chapter 34).

Stone extraction is done with wire baskets or balloon catheters (fig. 32.15a,b). In 90% the common bile duct is successfully cleared of stones. If all the stones cannot be extracted from a patient with cholangitis a naso-biliary catheter or endoprosthesis must be left to drain the duct (fig. 32.15c). Stones larger than 15 mm may be difficult to

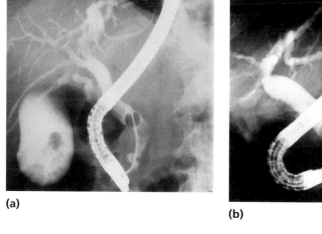

(a)

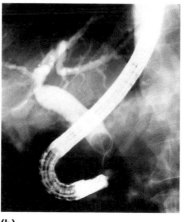

(b)

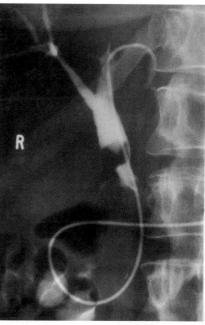

(c)

Fig. 32.15. (a) ERCP showing trawling of bile duct with balloon catheter to remove stones. (b) Removal of duct stone with basket. (c) Naso-biliary tube with stones in the common bile duct.

extract. Mechanical lithotripsy may be used to crush stones with success in 92% of patients [63]. Alternatively, an endoprosthesis may be inserted [50]. This prevents the stone obstructing the bile duct, and is a quicker procedure than lithotripsy. Endoprosthesis insertion may be temporary until another attempt at stone removal, or used for long-term drainage. Administration of oral ursodeoxycholic acid while the endoprosthesis is in place appears to make later clearance of stones from the duct more successful [41].

Extracorporeal shock wave lithotripsy of common bile duct stones fragments them and allows them to pass through the sphincterotomy [26]. Laser lithotripsy is available in some specialist centres.

Sphincterotomy is often done before *endoscopic endoprosthesis* insertion. This was originally recommended to reduce the risk of pancreatic duct obstruction and pancreatitis, but carries the risk of bleeding and is not essential unless the os is particularly small or tight.

Sphincterotomy at the main papilla may be used to treat the rare *sump syndrome* following choledochoduodenostomy [14]. *Papillary stenosis* (Chapter 34) can also be treated by sphincterotomy.

Stone removal without sphincterotomy

Small stones (<8 mm) may be removed through an intact ampulla, with or without balloon dilatation [51]. Larger stones have been removed using the combination of mechanical lithotripsy and balloon dilatation of the sphincter of Oddi. Pancreatitis is a complication in about 7%, but in a randomized trial was as frequent as with endoscopic sphincterotomy [9].

Naso-biliary drainage

A sphincterotomy is not usually necessary. After ERCP, the common bile duct is cannulated and a guide-wire passed deep into an intra-hepatic duct. The cannula is removed and a 300-cm 5 French (Fr) pigtail catheter with multiple side holes is threaded over the wire which is then removed (fig. 32.15c). The catheter is re-routed through the nose. This technique allows decompression of the biliary tree.

There are fewer complications than with percutaneous biliary drainage in terms of infection, bile leak and bleeding.

Naso-biliary drainage can be used as a preliminary to later sphincterotomy in poor risk patients with choledocholithiasis and acute suppurative cholangitis, especially if coagulation is abnormal.

A naso-biliary drain may be left in position when, after sphincterotomy, it has been impossible to clear all the stones from the common bile duct. Later cholangiogra-

phy through the tube shows whether the stones have passed. Naso-biliary drainage may also be used to treat bile leaks after cholecystectomy or liver transplantation, although stent insertion is the first method of choice for both leaks and residual duct stones.

Endoscopic biliary endoprostheses

After catheterization of the ampulla and demonstration of the stricture by contrast, a guide-wire is passed through the catheter and an attempt is made to pass it through the stricture. At the first session this is possible in 60–70% of patients. Using a combination of an inner tube and pushing tube, an endoprosthesis is railroaded into position across the stricture. A 3.3-mm diameter (10Fr) tube requires an endoscope with a 4.2-mm channel and provides effective decompression (fig. 32.16) Barbs on the endoprosthesis prevent it passing all the way up into the bile duct or subsequently back into the duodenum. Two endoprostheses may be used if necessary, for example to left and right hepatic ducts when there is a hilar stricture. Overall success rate of endoprosthesis insertion is 85–90% in skilled hands.

Early complications include cholangitis and pancreatitis. Sphincterotomy is not necessary before 10Fr stent insertion and may cause haemorrhage [48]. Sphinc-

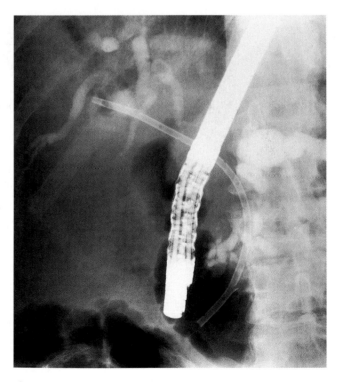

Fig. 32.16. ERCP: polyethylene stent inserted to relieve obstruction due to peri-ampullary tumour.

terotomy may be needed if the ampulla is too tight to admit the stent or if catherization of the biliary system has been difficult so as to allow easy access on a subsequent ERCP.

Late complications include cholangitis and recurrent jaundice due to blockage of the tube, which can easily be removed and replaced endoscopically. Mesh metal endoprostheses are now available which, after insertion in compressed form, expand when released to a diameter of up to 1 cm and remain patent for a longer period than conventional plastic stents (figs 32.17, 32.18). However, blockage still eventually occurs. Coated metal shunts may delay this [39].

Results and indications

Endoscopic plastic endoprostheses successfully decompress the bile duct and relieve symptoms in about 70–80% of patients. The method carries fewer complications than the percutaneous route [65], and has a lower morbidity and mortality than surgical palliative bypass in patients with peri-ampullary carcinoma [64]. Blockage of polyethylene endoprostheses occurs in 25–30% at 3–6 months due to biliary sludge, containing bacteria. Antibiotic and ursodeoxycholic acid adminis-

tration do not prevent this [33]. Tannenbaum stents made of Teflon do not have longer patency rates [28]. When expandable metal mesh endoprostheses block, obstruction is relieved by insertion of a plastic stent or another metal stent within the occluded endoprosthesis [67]. However, the patency of expandable metal mesh endoprostheses is significantly longer than plastic types (fig. 32.18) [19, 42], but the metal type is more expensive. Present experience suggests that a plastic type be placed first, and when it blocks, a metal endoprosthesis is inserted in those patients who are progressing more slowly and are expected to survive longer [53].

Inoperable malignant biliary obstruction from carcinoma of pancreas, ampulla and hilum can be relieved. For a malignant hilar obstruction, drainage of only one lobe provides good palliation. A second endoprosthesis is only needed if cholestasis is not relieved sufficiently or there is sepsis in the undrained side [56].

Benign strictures, whether due to primary sclerosing cholangitis or post-cholecystectomy, can be treated in this way, although balloon dilatation is an alternative.

Failed endoscopic removal of common duct stones. A stent may be introduced into the common bile duct where it

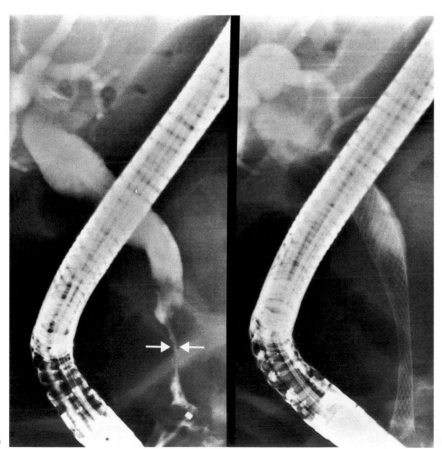

(a)   **(b)**

Fig. 32.17. (a) ERCP showing malignant stricture (arrows) at lower end of bile duct. (b) Mesh metal stent (Wallstent) placed across the stricture. (Courtesy of Dr Kees Huibregtse.)

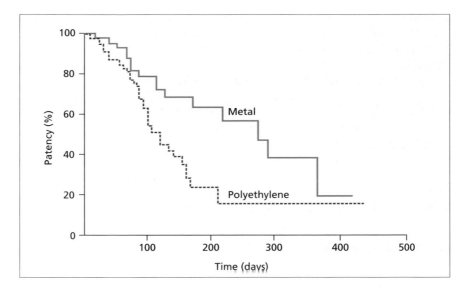

Fig. 32.18. Kaplan–Meier life table analysis of stent patency: randomized trial of metal vs. polyethylene stents. (From [10] with permission.)

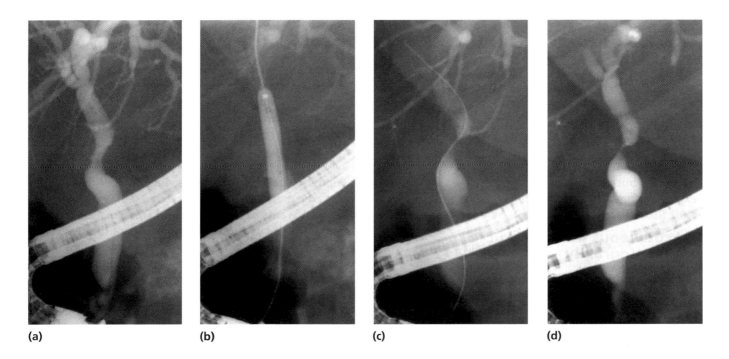

(a)　　　　　(b)　　　　　(c)　　　　　(d)

Fig. 32.19. Endoscopic balloon dilatation of bile duct stricture following liver transplantation. (a) Cholangiogram showing stricture. (b) Wire passed into intra-hepatic ducts. (c) Balloon dilatation to 8 mm diameter. (d) Final cholangiogram with good result.

has been impossible to remove all stones and when the patient is unfit for surgery.

External biliary fistulas. Post-operative leaks from the cystic duct or gallbladder bed may be treated by introduction of a biliary stent. The leak usually seals making re-operation unnecessary. The stent is removed after a few weeks.

Balloon dilatation

Following endoscopic cholangiography, a balloon catheter may be introduced into the common bile duct and inflated. This may be used to dilate a benign stricture (fig. 32.19), whether traumatic or secondary to primary sclerosing cholangitis. It may be a useful preliminary step before insertion of an endoprosthesis.

Per-oral cholangioscopy

The bile duct interior can be inspected using a 'baby' endoscope introduced via a large channel ('mother')

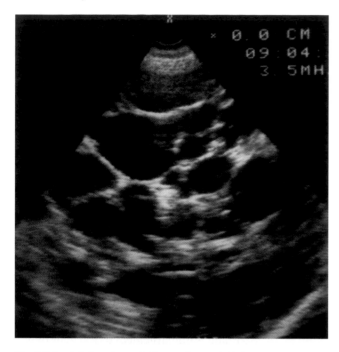

Fig. 33.4. Adult polycystic liver: ultrasound shows numerous echo-free space-occupying lesions.

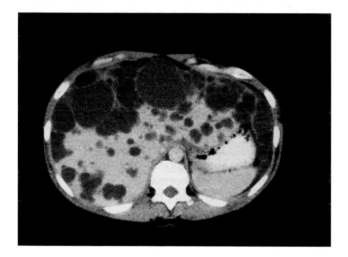

Fig. 33.5. CT scan (contrast enhanced) showing a polycystic liver.

Metastases are accompanied by malaise, weight loss, rapid increase in size of the liver, and, possibly, evidence of a primary neoplasm.

Cirrhosis may be accompanied by signs of hepatocellular disease and the spleen is usually enlarged.

Prognosis and treatment

Polycystic disease of the liver is compatible with long life.

The prognosis is determined by the extent of associ-ated renal cystic disease. Carcinoma is very rare. Surgery is rarely necessary and aspiration under ultrasound control is easy and effective in controlling acute symptoms. However, the fluid returns.

There are several surgical techniques, the choice depending upon the extent of disease [18]. Patients with a limited number of large cysts may be treated by fenestration which can be performed laparoscopically [23]. Where there is localized involvement of the liver parenchyma by multiple medium-sized cysts but with adjacent large areas of normal parenchyma shown by CT, operative fenestration with or without hepatic resection produces symptomatic improvement in the majority [14, 33]. In patients with massive diffuse involvement of the majority of liver parenchyma by all sizes of liver cysts with only a small amount of normal parenchyma between them, fenestration may be useful but carries a high morbidity and mortality. In patients with severe limitation of daily activity and failed previous treatment, liver transplantation can be done (combined with kidney transplantation if necessary) and has a 1-year survival of 89% [41].

Successful liver transplantation has been reported using a donor liver with polycystic change [4].

Congenital hepatic fibrosis

This condition consists, histologically, of broad, densely collagenous fibrous bands surrounding otherwise normal hepatic lobules (fig. 33.6). The bands contain large numbers of microscopic, well-formed bile ducts (fig. 33.7), some containing bile. Arterial branches are normal or hypoplastic, while the veins appear reduced in size. Inflammatory infiltration is not seen. Caroli's syndrome may be associated, also choledochal cyst.

The disease appears both sporadically and in a familial form. It is inherited as autosomal recessive. A ductal plate malformation of interlobular bile ducts has been suggested as the pathogenetic mechanism [11].

Portal hypertension is common. Occasionally this may be due to defects in the main portal veins. More often it is caused by hypoplasia or fibrous compression of portal vein radicles in the fibrous bands surrounding the nodules.

Associated renal conditions include renal dysplasia, adult-type polycystic kidneys [6] and nephronophthisis (medullary cystic disease).

Clinical features

The condition is often misdiagnosed as cirrhosis. The patient is usually diagnosed between the ages of 3 and 10 years but recognition may be delayed until adult life. Sexes are equal. The patient presents with haemorrhage

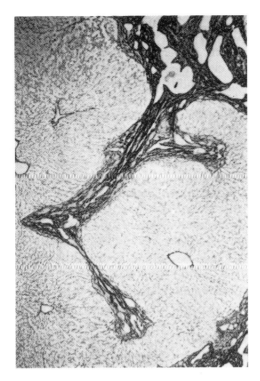

Fig. 33.6. Congenital hepatic fibrosis. Broad bands of fibrous tissue containing bile ducts separate and surround liver lobules. (Silver impregnation, × 36).

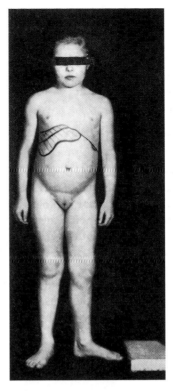

Fig. 33.8. Girl of 8 years with hepatosplenomegaly discovered at routine examination. Liver biopsy showed congenital hepatic fibrosis. Note normal development.

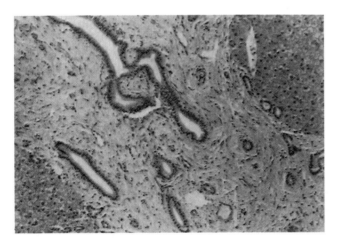

Fig. 33.7. Congenital hepatic fibrosis. Portal area shows dense mature fibrous tissue with a number of abnormal bile ducts. (H & E, × 40.)

from oesophageal varices, a symptomless, large, very hard liver or splenomegaly (fig. 33.8).

There may be other congenital anomalies, especially of the biliary system, with cholangitis [10].

Carcinoma, both hepato-cellular and cholangiocarcinoma, may be a complication [2, 49] as may adenomatous hyperplasia [3].

Congenital hepatic fibrosis is part of the rare disorder

reported with phosphomannose isomerase deficiency [15].

Investigations

Serum protein, bilirubin and transaminase levels are usually normal, but serum alkaline phosphatase values are sometimes increased.

Liver biopsy is essential for diagnosis. Because of the tough consistency of the liver this may be difficult.

Ultrasound shows very bright areas of echogenicity due to the dense bands of fibrous tissue. Direct cholangiography in patients with congenital hepatic fibrosis alone shows tapered intra-hepatic radicals suggesting fibrosis. MR cholangiography shows duct abnormalities including biliary cysts in some patients and this association with congenital hepatic fibrosis has been termed Caroli's syndrome. Choledochal cysts may also be seen [12].

Portal venography reveals the collateral circulation and a normal or distorted intra-hepatic portal tree.

Ultrasound, CT, MRI and *intravenous pyelography* may show cystic renal changes or medullary sponge kidney.

Prognosis and treatment

Congenital hepatic fibrosis must be distinguished from

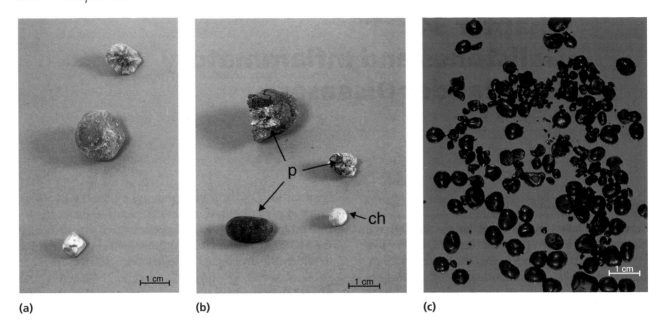

(a)   (b)   (c)

Fig. 34.1. (a) Two faceted cholesterol gallstones. The fragment above shows the concentric structure formed as layer upon layer of cholesterol crystals aggregate. (b) Stones removed from the common bile duct (ch, cholesterol gallstone; p, brown pigment stone). (c) Black pigment gallstones.

Factors in cholesterol gallstone formation [47, 49]

Three major factors determine the formation of cholesterol gallstones. These are: altered composition of hepatic bile, nucleation of cholesterol crystals and impaired gallbladder function (fig. 34.2). Hepatic bile supersaturated with cholesterol and with an increased proportion of deoxycholic acid favours stone formation.

Altered hepatic bile composition

Bile is 85–95% water. Cholesterol, which is insoluble in water and must be maintained in solution, is secreted from the canalicular membrane in unilamellar phospholipid *vesicles* (fig. 34.3). Whether cholesterol remains in solution depends upon the concentration of phospholipids and bile acids in bile, and also the type of phospholipid and bile acid present.

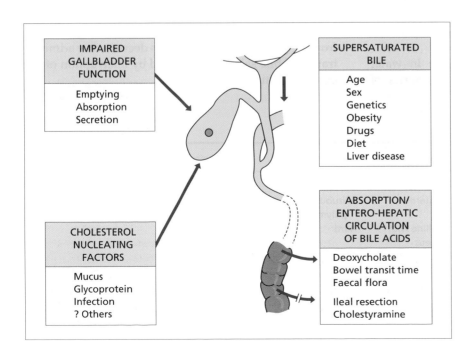

Fig. 34.2. Major factors in cholesterol gallstone formation are supersaturation of the bile with cholesterol, increased deoxycholate formation and absorption, cholesterol crystal nucleation and impaired gallbladder function.

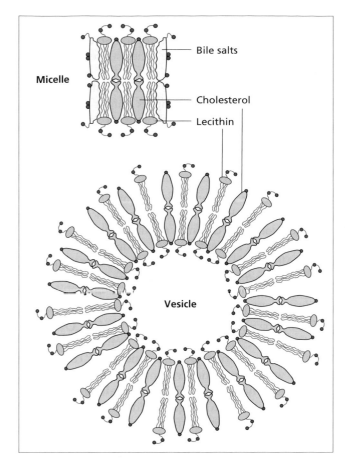

Fig. 34.3. Structure of mixed micelles and cholesterol/phospholipid vesicles.

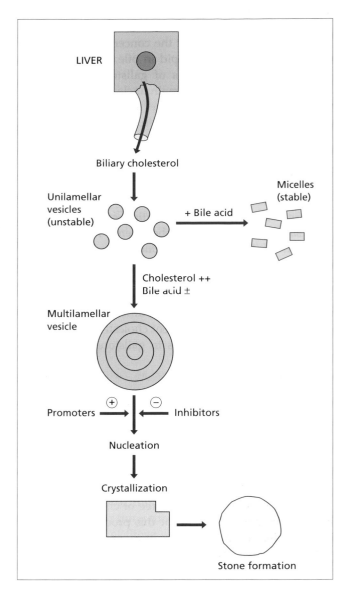

Fig. 34.4. Pathway for cholesterol crystallization in bile.

In hepatic bile unsaturated with cholesterol and containing sufficient bile acid, the vesicles are solubilized into mixed lipid *micelles*. These have a hydrophilic external surface and a hydrophobic interior. Cholesterol is incorporated into the hydrophobic interior. Phospholipids are inserted into the walls of the micelles so that they grow. These 'mixed micelles' are thus able to hold cholesterol in a stable thermodynamic state. This is the situation with a low cholesterol saturation index (derived from the molar ratio of cholesterol, bile acid and phospholipids).

When bile is supersaturated with cholesterol, or bile acid concentrations are low (a high cholesterol saturation index), the excess cholesterol cannot be transported in mixed micelles and unilamellar phospholipid vesicles remain (fig. 34.4). These are not stable and can aggregate. Large multilamellar vesicles form from which cholesterol crystals may *nucleate*. This process involves a sequence of complex events involving several different types of vesicle, micelle and disc [96]. Cholesterol precipitates in many forms including filaments, helices and tubules of non-hydrated cholesterol as well as characteristic plates of monohydrate cholesterol [145].

The type of bile acid present in bile influences gall-

stone formation. A higher proportion of deoxycholate is found in gallstone patients. This is a more hydrophobic bile salt and when secreted into bile extracts more cholesterol from the canalicular membrane increasing cholesterol saturation. It also accelerates cholesterol crystallization.

Deoxycholate is derived from dehydroxylation of cholic acid in the colon by faecal bacteria. There is an entero-hepatic circulation. The amount of deoxycholate present in the bile acid pool depends upon the large bowel transit time, which when increased (as in patients with acromegaly treated with octreotide) correlates with increased serum deoxycholic acid [196]. Other factors affect the amount of deoxycholate formed. Gallstone patients have significantly prolonged small bowel transit times [6] and increased bacterial dehydroxylating activity in faeces [203].

diet to maintain gallbladder emptying may reduce the risk of gallstone formation [63].

Gallstone formation during weight loss following gastric bypass surgery for obesity is prevented by giving ursodeoxycholic acid [180].

Dietary factors

In Western countries, gallstones have been linked to dietary fibre deficiency and a longer intestinal transit time [71]. This increases deoxycholic acid in bile, and renders it more lithogenic [196]. A diet low in carbohydrate and a shorter overnight fasting period protects against gallstones, as does a moderate alcohol intake in males [5]. Vegetarians get fewer gallstones irrespective of their tendency to be slim [141].

Increasing dietary cholesterol increases biliary cholesterol but there is no epidemiological or dietary data to link cholesterol intake with gallstones. Indeed, newly synthesized cholesterol is probably a more important source of biliary cholesterol.

Serum factors

The highest risk of gallstones (both cholesterol and pigment) is associated with low HDL levels and high triglyceride levels which may be more important than body mass [4, 185]. High serum cholesterol is not a determinant of gallstone risk.

Epidemiology (table 34.2)

In the Western world the prevalence of gallbladder stones is about 10%. In the United States more than 20 million people are estimated to have gallbladder disease. The prevalence in non-Hispanic white men is greater than in non-Hispanic black men (8.6 vs. 5.3%) [56]. The prevalence in women is twice that in men. Black Africans and the Eastern world are largely free of stones. The prevalence, however, is rising as lifestyles change. In Japan, the change from traditional to Western diets has been associated with a change from bilirubin to cholesterol gallstones.

American Indians have the highest known prevalence. This is related to supersaturation of the bile with cholesterol [199]. In Chile, the prevalence of gallstones is greatest (35%) in Mapuches. This relates to their strong Amerindian ancestry [126].

Cirrhosis of the liver

About 30% of patients with cirrhosis have gallstones. The risk of developing stones is most strongly associated with Child's grade C and alcoholic cirrhosis with a yearly incidence of about 5% [58]. The mechanisms

Table 34.2. Comparison of gallstone prevalence between countries and races [10]

Very high	High	Moderate	Low
North American Indians	USA whites	USA blacks	Greece
Chile	Great Britain	Japan	Egypt
Sweden	Norway		Zambia
Czechoslovakia	Australia		
	Italy		

are uncertain. All patients with hepato-cellular disease show a variable degree of haemolysis. Although bile acid secretion is reduced, the stones are usually of the black pigment type. Phospholipid and cholesterol secretion are also lowered so that the bile is not supersaturated.

Cholecystectomy and bile duct exploration are poorly tolerated, liver failure being frequently precipitated. Such operations should be done only for life-threatening complications of biliary tract disease, such as empyema or perforation. Endoscopic sphincterotomy is indicated for bile duct stones.

Other factors

Diabetes mellitus is more frequent in individuals with gallstone disease [41]. Diabetics have a higher prevalence of gallstones (or a history of cholecystectomy) than non-diabetics [27]. Hyperinsulinaemia may play a role in gallstone formation [127, 157].

Ileal resection breaks the entero-hepatic circulation of bile salts, reduces the total bile salt pool and is followed by gallstone formation. The same is found in subtotal or total colectomy [117].

Gastrectomy increases the incidence of gallstones [82].

Long-term cholestyramine therapy increases bile salt loss with a reduced bile acid pool size and gallstone formation.

Cholesterol-lowering diets high in unsaturated fat and plant sterols but low in saturated fats and cholesterol result in increased gallstone formation.

Clofibrate enhances biliary cholesterol excretion and makes the bile more lithogenic.

Parenteral nutrition leads to a dilated, sluggish gallbladder containing stones.

Long-term *octreotide* treatment induces cholesterol-rich gallbladder stones in 13–60% of acromegalic patients. The bile is supersaturated with cholesterol, the nucleation time is abnormally rapid and gallbladder emptying is impaired. Serum deoxycholic acid is increased, due to a prolonged large bowel transit time [196].

Endoscopic sphincterotomy improves gallbladder emptying and decreases the lithogenicity of bile in patients with gallstone disease [43]. Patients with gallbladder stones have significantly higher sphincter of Oddi tone [31]. Physical activity is associated with a decreased risk of cholecystectomy [102]. The mechanism is unclear.

Summary

The formation of cholesterol gallstones depends on the production of bile in which cholesterol cannot be maintained in solution. This is due to increased biliary secretion of cholesterol. Increased biliary deoxycholate, in part due to changes in intestinal transit, favours cholesterol crystallization. There are nucleation promoting and inhibiting factors in bile. Imbalance between these generates an environment favouring cholesterol crystallization and stone formation. The gallbladder acts as a reservoir allowing growth of the stone. Changes in motor and other functions of the gallbladder increase the risk of stone formation.

Pigment gallstones

This term is used for stones containing less than 30% cholesterol. There are two types: black and brown (table 34.1) [106].

Black pigment stones are largely composed of an insoluble bilirubin pigment polymer mixed with calcium phosphate and carbonate. There is no cholesterol. The mechanism of formation is not well understood, but supersaturation of bile with unconjugated bilirubin, changes in pH and calcium, and overproduction of an organic matrix (glycoprotein) play a role [106]. Overall, 20–30% of gallbladder stones are black. The incidence rises with age. They may pass into the bile duct. Black stones accompany chronic haemolysis, usually hereditary spherocytosis or sickle cell disease, and mechanical prostheses, for example heart valves, in the circulation. They show an increased prevalence with all forms of cirrhosis, particularly alcoholic [58]. Chemical dissolution therapy of pigment stones remains experimental [106]. Patients with ileal Crohn's disease may form pigment stones because of increased colonic absorption of bilirubin due to failure of ileal absorption of bile acid [23].

Brown pigment stones contain calcium bilirubinate, calcium palmitate, and stearate, as well as cholesterol. The bilirubinate is polymerized to a lesser extent than in black stones.

Brown stones are rare in the gallbladder. They form in the bile duct and are related to bile stasis and infected bile. They are usually radiolucent. Bacteria are present in more than 90%. Stone formation is related to the deconjugation of bilirubin diglucuronide by bacterial β-glucuronidase [106]. Insoluble unconjugated bilirubinate precipitates.

Brown pigment stones form above biliary strictures in sclerosing cholangitis and in the dilated segments of Caroli's disease. There is an association with juxtapapillary duodenal diverticula [161]. In Oriental countries, these stones are associated with parasitic infestations of the biliary tract such as *Clonorchis sinensis* and *Ascaris lumbricoides*. These stones are frequently intrahepatic. Removal from the common bile duct is by endoscopy sphincterotomy and from intra-hepatic ducts by lithotripsy techniques, percutaneous extraction or surgery

Experimentally, stone and sludge formation is prevented by melatonin, a free radical scavenger [169]. Oxidative stress may lead to stones through promoting mucin–glycoprotein formation.

Radiology of gallstones (Chapter 32)

Only about 10% of gallstones are radio-opaque, compared with 90% of renal calculi (fig. 34.5). Visualization is due to the calcium content of the stone. Mixed stones may or may not have sufficient calcium to be rendered visible.

Gallstones are usually multiple and faceted, although a single, round stone may fill the whole gallbladder.

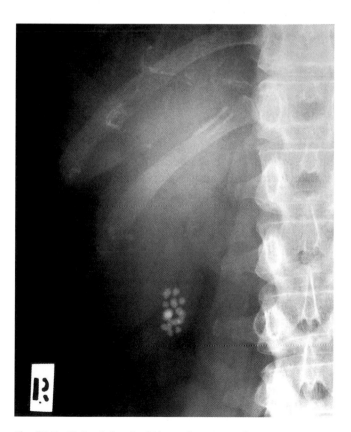

Fig. 34.5. Plain abdominal X-ray showing radio-opaque gallstones. Oral bile acid therapy is contraindicated.

cholecystectomy is planned and common duct stones are suspected. Operative cholangiography, exploration of the bile duct and stone removal is the alternative, with insertion of a T-tube.

The T-tube is in position in the common bile duct for about 2 weeks. Culture of the bile is done, for postoperative complications are often due to sepsis. Cholangiography precedes removal of the T-tube.

Slight and transient increases in serum bilirubin and transaminase levels can be expected in the normal postoperative cholecystectomy course [69]. Greater increases indicate such complications as a retained duct stone or injury to the bile ducts.

Acalculous cholecystitis

Acute

About 5–10% of acute cholecystitis in adults and about 30% in children occurs in the absence of stones. The most frequent predisposing cause is an associated critical condition such as after major non-biliary surgery, multiple injuries, major burns, recent childbirth, severe sepsis, mechanical ventilation and parenteral nutrition.

The pathogenesis is unclear and probably multifactorial, but bile stasis (lack of gallbladder contraction), increased bile viscosity and lithogenicity, and gallbladder ischaemia are thought to play a role. Administration of opiates which increase sphincter of Oddi tone may also reduce gallbladder emptying. Shock impairs cystic arterial blood flow.

Clinical features should be those of acute calculous cholecystitis with fever, leucocytosis and right upper quadrant pain but diagnosis is often difficult because of the overall clinical state of the patient who may be intubated, ventilated and receiving narcotic analgesics.

There may be laboratory evidence of cholestasis with a raised bilirubin and alkaline phosphatase. Cholescintigraphy is reported to have a sensitivity of 60–90% for acalculous cholecystitis [88, 118]. Ultrasound and CT are complementary and useful in showing a thickened gallbladder wall (>4 mm), pericholecystic fluid or subserosal oedema without ascites, intramural gas, or a sloughed mucosal membrane. Because of the difficulties of diagnosis a high index of suspicion is needed, particularly in patients at risk. Gangrene and perforation of the gallbladder are common. The mortality is high, 41% in a recent series [88], often due to delayed diagnosis.

Treatment is emergency cholecystectomy. In the critically ill patient percutaneous cholecystostomy under ultrasound guidance may be life saving.

Chronic

This is a difficult diagnosis as the clinical condition resembles others, particularly the irritable bowel syndrome and the functional dyspepsias. Ultrasound scans and oral cholecystograms are normal. Nevertheless, chronic inflammation can be present in the gallbladder without gallstones and relief will follow cholecystectomy.

Cholescintigraphy with measurement of the gallbladder ejection factor 15 min after CCK infusion has been used to try and identify patients who would benefit from cholecystectomy. Normal individuals have an ejection fraction of 70% [34]. In those with a low ejection fraction (less than 40%) or who develop pain during the infusion, symptom relief after cholecystectomy is reported in between 70 and 90% of patients [103, 172, 174, 205]. However, decisions on management based on this test alone appear inappropriate and the result should be taken in the context of the other clinical features of the patient. In patients with acalculous gallbladder disease undergoing cholecystectomy, chronic cholecystitis, muscle hypertrophy and/or a narrowed cystic duct have been shown in patients in whom symptoms were relieved [205]. Management of this group of patients remains a clinical challenge.

Typhoid cholecystitis

Circulating typhoid bacilli are filtered by the liver and excreted in the bile. The biliary tract, however, is infected in only about 0.2% of patients with typhoid fever.

Acute typhoid cholecystitis is becoming very rare. Signs of acute cholecystitis appear at the end of the second week or even during convalescence, and are sometimes followed by perforation of the gallbladder.

Chronic typhoid fever cholecystitis and the typhoid carrier state. The typhoid carrier passes organisms in the faeces derived from a focus of infection in the gallbladder or biliary tract. Chronic typhoid cholecystitis is symptomless.

The carrier state is not cured by antibiotic therapy. Cholecystectomy is successful if there is not an associated infection of the biliary ducts. Chronic typhoid cholecystitis is not an important cause of gallstones, but carries an increased risk of gallbladder carcinoma [24].

Biliary carriers of other salmonellae have been reported and treated with ampicillin and cholecystectomy.

Acute cholecystitis in AIDS [25]

Four per cent of 904 patients with AIDS needed an abdominal operation over a 4-year period [147]. One-third of these cases had cholecystectomy for acute acalculous cholecystitis. This is thought to occur because of gallbladder stasis and increased bile lithogenicity in the critically ill patient, opportunistic pathogens, such as cytomegalovirus (CMV) and cryptosporidium, or vascular insufficiency due to oedema or infection.

Patients present with fever, right upper quadrant pain and tenderness. The white cell count is often normal but with a left shift of neutrophils. Ultrasound shows features of acute cholecystitis (without stones).

Treatment is by cholecystectomy with a mortality of around 30% due to sepsis.

Other infections

Actinomycosis can very rarely involve the gallbladder, as may *Vibrio cholerae* [68] and *Leptospirosis* [197] which have been associated with acalculous cholecystitis. The pathological significance of *Helicobacter* spp. in the biliary tree is uncertain [59, 123].

Other associations

A *chemical cholecystitis* may follow long-term infusion of cytotoxic drugs, such as FUDR, into the hepatic artery.

Diseases involving the *cystic artery*, such as polyarteritis nodosa, may lead to cholecystitis [138].

The gallbladder may be involved in *Crohn's disease*.

Other gallbladder pathology

Cholesterolosis of the gallbladder

There is accumulation of cholesterol and triglyceride in the gallbladder wall. It is present in 50% of patients with gallstones, and 35% of symptomatic patients without stones having cholecystectomy for polyp or adenomyomatosis [160].

Cholesterol esters and other lipids are deposited in the submucosal and epithelial cells as small, yellow, lipid specks and, together with the intervening red bile-stained mucosa, give the appearance of a ripe strawberry. The deposits are at first found only on the mucosal ridges but later they extend into the troughs. As more lipid is deposited, it projects into the lumen as polyps which may become pedunculated. The change is confined to the gallbladder and never extends to the ducts.

The lipid is seen in reticulo-endothelial xanthoma cells of the mucosa, which is not inflamed. The cholesterolosis is related to the biliary, not blood, cholesterol concentration.

The aetiology is uncertain. The gallbladder mucosa may simply be taking up excess cholesterol from bile. Other possibilities are a defect in submucosal macrophages, impaired transport of cholesterol out of the mucosa [160], or increased cholesterol ester synthesis by the gallbladder mucosa [202].

There is controversy concerning the relation of cholesterolosis to symptoms. However, cholesterolosis may sometimes cause right upper quadrant pain and features causing confusion with the irritable bowel syndrome. Diagnosis is difficult. Oral cholecystography, preferably with CCK, shows filling defects in the gallbladder in only a third, and ultrasonography is usually negative.

Xanthogranulomatous cholecystitis

This is an uncommon inflammatory disease of the gallbladder characterized by a focal or diffuse destructive inflammatory process with lipid-laden macrophages. Macroscopically, areas of xanthogranulomatous cholecystitis appear as yellow masses within the wall of the gallbladder [154]. The gallbladder wall is invariably thickened and cholesterol or mixed gallstones are usually present.

The pathogenesis is uncertain, but an inflammatory response to extravasated bile, possibly from ruptured Rokitansky–Aschoff sinuses, is likely.

Symptoms often begin as an episode of acute cholecystitis and persist for up to 5 years. There is extension of yellow tissue into adjacent organs. Fistulae from gallbladder to skin or duodenum may develop [154]. At operation, carcinoma seems likely and frozen sections are usually required to make the differentiation.

Adenomyomatosis

This may affect the gallbladder wall profusely or locally. There is epithelial proliferation with muscular hypertrophy and mural diverticulae (Rokitansky–Aschoff sinuses), which may be seen as spots of contrast medium outside the lumen of the gallbladder on oral cholecystography after a fatty meal. Adenomyomatosis (*cholecystitis glandularis proliferans*) may cause chronic symptoms which are relieved by cholecystectomy.

Porcelain gallbladder

This rare condition (0.4–0.8% at cholecystectomy) is due to extensive calcification of the gallbladder wall. Circumferential calcification is seen on abdominal X-ray or CT. Ultrasound is helpful in showing the extent of involvement of the gallbladder wall. The condition is associated with a high frequency of cancer (12–61%) [171].

Post-cholecystectomy problems

Poor results after cholecystectomy can be expected in about one-third of patients. These may be due to wrong diagnosis. About 90–95% of those *with gallstones* are freed of symptoms or improved post-operatively. The absence of stones questions the original diagnosis. The

Table 34.3. Sphincter of Oddi dysfunction: classification

Group I (definite)	
Biliary-type pain	
Abnormal liver function tests (AST; alkaline phosphatase > 2 × normal) documented on two or more occasions	
Dilated common bile duct > 12 mm	
Delayed drainage of ERCP contrast > 45 min	Manometry unnecessary
Group II (presumptive)	
Biliary-type pain and one or two of other group I criteria	Manometry essential
Group III (possible)	
Biliary-type pain only. No other abnormalities	Manometry essential if intervention contemplated

patients may have been suffering from a psychosomatic or some other disorder including non-visceral pain [167]. Results of surgery are poor when done for vague symptoms such as abdominal bloating or dyspepsia, or in patients using psychiatric medication [110, 194]. A biliary cause is likely if stones are found at cholecystectomy and if a period of relief follows the operation. The colon and pancreas are common alternative culprits.

Symptoms may be related to technical difficulties at the time of surgery. These include traumatic *biliary stricture* (Chapter 35) and *residual calculi*.

Amputation neuromas can be demonstrated in some patients but removal offers no relief and this seems unlikely to be the cause of the symptoms.

Chronic pancreatitis, a common association of *choledocholithiasis*, may persist post-operatively.

US is the first test to image the bile duct. Depending on the result and the clinical features MRCP may be indicated. Despite all these efforts, ERCP is usually necessary. Residual calculi, stricture, ampullary stenosis, a cystic duct stump or normal appearances are significant findings.

Sphincter of Oddi dysfunction [34]

This has been an area of controversy but now appears to be a cause of post-cholecystectomy pain in some patients. Two forms exist.

Papillary stenosis is defined as narrowing of all or part of the sphincter of Oddi. There is fibrosis. It may follow injury due to stones [74], operative instrumentation, biliary infection or pancreatitis. There may be episodes of pain associated with abnormal liver function tests. On ERCP the bile duct is dilated and drains slowly. The basal sphincter tone is raised on manometry and is not reduced by smooth muscle relaxants. Endoscopic sphincterotomy is helpful [189].

Sphincter of Oddi (biliary) dyskinesia is a more difficult area. Biliary manometry shows a range of abnormalities including sphincter spasm, increased phasic contraction frequency (tachyoddia), paradoxical contraction response to CCK, and abnormal propagation of phasic waves.

There are clinical features (table 34.3) which are valuable in management decisions in patients with sphincter of Oddi dysfunction. Group I benefit from sphincterotomy in 90% of cases. In group II manometry is important. Patients with an elevated basal sphincter pressure have greater benefit from sphincterotomy than those with a normal pressure (91 vs. 42%) [64]. Studies continue in group III. Duodenal distension reproduces the symptoms in most patients [42]. Sphincterotomy in those with abnormal manometry may be beneficial in only 50% of patients [34]. Drug treatment with nitrates, nitroglycerin and calcium channel blockers which relax the sphincter are worth a trial, although the vasodilating side-effects limit their therapeutic use.

Gallstones in the common bile duct (choledocholithiasis)

The majority of stones in the common bile duct have migrated from the gallbladder and are associated with calculous cholecystitis. Migration is related to the size of the stone relative to the cystic and common bile duct. The stones grow in the common bile duct so causing biliary obstruction and facilitating the migration of further stones from the gallbladder.

Secondary stones that are not of gallbladder origin usually follow partial biliary obstruction due to such causes as residual calculus, traumatic stricture, sclerosing cholangitis or congenital biliary abnormalities. Infection may be the initial event. Stones are brown, single or multiple, oval and conforming to the long axis of the duct (fig. 34.1b).

Effects of common bile duct stones

Bile duct obstruction is usually partial and intermittent since the calculus exerts a ball-valve action at the lower

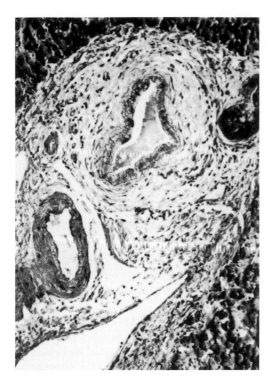

Fig. 34.12. Portal zone from operative liver biopsy of a patient with sclerosing cholangitis secondary to choledocholithiasis. The duct wall shows concentric fibrosis and the whole portal area is fibrosed. (PAS stain, ×126.)

end of the common bile duct. In the anicteric, hepatic histology is virtually normal. In the icteric, it shows cholestasis. In chronic cases, the bile ducts show concentric scarring (fig. 34.12) and eventually secondary sclerosing cholangitis and biliary cirrhosis.

Cholangitis. The stagnant bile is readily infected, probably from the duodenum. The bile becomes opaque and biliary sludge appears. Rarely the infection is more acute and the bile is purulent. The common bile duct is thickened and dilated, with desquamated or ulcerated mucosa, especially in the ampulla of Vater. The cholangitis may spread to the intra-hepatic bile ducts and, in severe and prolonged infections, cholangitic liver abscesses are seen. The cut section of liver shows cavities containing bile-stained pus, communicating with the bile ducts. *Escherichia coli* is the commonest infecting organism. Others include *Klebsiella, Streptococcus, Bacteroides* and *Clostridia*.

Acute or *chronic pancreatitis* may result from stones wedged in or passing through the ampulla of Vater.

Clinical syndromes

Choledocholithiasis may be silent and symptomless, discovered only by imaging at the time of a routine cholecystectomy for chronic calculous cholecystitis. Alternatively, the stones may cause an acute cholangitis with jaundice, pain and fever. In the elderly, they may present simply as mental and physical debility [33]. Residual stones detected early or late after cholecystectomy can be silent or symptomatic.

Acute jaundice and cholangitis

The classical picture is of an elderly, obese woman, with a previous history of flatulent indigestion, fat intolerance and mid-epigastric pain, presenting with jaundice, abdominal pain, chills and fever.

The *cholestatic jaundice* is usually mild, but may be deep or absent. Bile duct obstruction is rarely complete and the amount of pigment fluctuates in the stools.

Pain occurs in about three-quarters of patients, is usually severe, colicky and intermittent and needs analgesics for its relief. Sometimes it is a constant, sharp, severe pain. The site may be right upper quadrant or epigastric. It radiates to the back and to the right scapula. It is associated with vomiting. Palpation of the epigastrium is painful. *Fever* occurs in about a third of the patients, and there may be rigors. *Urine* is dark according to the degree of obstruction.

The *bile* shows a mixed growth of intestinal organisms, predominantly *E. coli*.

The *serum* has the changes of cholestasis with raised alkaline phosphatase, γ-glutamyl transpeptidase and conjugated bilirubin. In acute obstruction the transaminase levels may be briefly very high.

If a stone obstructs the main pancreatic duct, the serum amylase concentration may rise sharply and there may be clinical pancreatitis.

Haematological changes. The polymorph leucocyte count may be raised; the level depends on the acuteness and severity of the cholangitis.

Blood culture should be performed during the febrile period and the antibiotic sensitivity of any organism determined. Although the usual organisms encountered are the colonic ones, such as *E. coli* and anaerobic streptococci, other unusual ones such as *Pseudomonas* must be sought. Bile should be taken at ERCP for culture.

X-rays of the abdomen may show calculi in the gallbladder, or more medially and posteriorly in the common bile duct.

Ultrasound may show dilated intra-hepatic ducts although more often these are undilated. Stones in the lower end of the common bile duct are often missed by ultrasound.

Cholangiography, usually by the endoscopic route, confirms the presence of stones. Where the clinical features are equivocal, and ERCP is considered too invasive as a first test, MRCP is valuable in showing whether or not there is a duct stone.

Diagnosis

This is not difficult if jaundice follows biliary colic and febrile episodes. Too often, however, there is only vague indigestion, no fever, no gallbladder tenderness and an unhelpful white blood count. Alternatively, the patient may present with painless jaundice and sometimes itching. The condition must then be differentiated from other forms of cholestasis, including neoplastic, and acute viral hepatitis (see table 12.2). The bile in total biliary obstruction due to carcinoma is rarely infected and cholangitis is unusual unless there has been previous endoscopic cholangiography or stenting.

Residual common duct stones

Between 5 and 10% of patients having a cholecystectomy with exploration of the common bile duct will have retained stones. Calculi in the intra-hepatic ducts are especially liable to be overlooked. Residual bile duct calculi may be suspected if the patient experiences pain when the T-tube draining the bile duct is temporarily clamped. Cholangiography reveals filling defects. Sepsis and cholangitis occur post-operatively. In many instances, however, the residual bile duct calculi remain silent for many years.

Management of common duct stones

This depends on the clinical situation—emergency or elective—on the age and general condition of the patient and on the facilities and clinical expertise available. Antibiotics will be given for their systemic effect to treat or prevent septicaemia, and this is probably more relevant than their entry into bile. They are only temporarily effective in controlling the septicaemia if the bile duct is completely obstructed. Drainage is needed. Other measures include control of fluid and electrolyte balance and intravenous vitamin K, if the patient is jaundiced.

Acute obstructive suppurative cholangitis

Clinical features that identify this syndrome are fever, jaundice, pain, confusion and hypotension (*Reynold's pentad*) [151]. Renal failure and thrombocytopenia, as part of a disseminated intravascular coagulopathy, develop later. This situation is an emergency.

Laboratory tests should include blood cultures, as well as white cell and platelet count, prothrombin time and renal function tests. *Ultrasound* should show a dilated biliary system with or without stones. Even if ultrasound is negative, *endoscopic cholangiography* should be done if the clinical features suggest bile duct disease. MRCP is valuable if the clinical picture is equivocal.

Treatment is by intensive broad-spectrum antibiotics and emergency decompression of the biliary tract, as well as resuscitation with intravenous fluids. Antibiotics should cover Gram-negative colonic bacteria [179]. There are several alternatives but piperacillin/tazobactam is a good choice, with an aminoglycoside (gentamicin or netilmicin) if the clinical picture is life threatening. Aminoglycoside should only be used for a few days because of the risk of nephrotoxicity. Most cases are caused by common duct stones. ERCP is done with sphincterotomy and stone removal, if coagulation and anatomy permit. If not, then a naso-biliary tube is inserted.

The aim of any procedure is to *guarantee decompression of the biliary system*. The endoscopic approach is now accepted as the first choice, although there is still a mortality of around 5–10% [99, 104]. If this method fails, percutaneous trans-hepatic external bile drainage is the second choice. Surgical operation carries a greater mortality than non-surgical techniques, being between 16 and 40% [104]. After decompression there is usually rapid resolution of septicaemia and toxaemia. If not, drainage of the biliary system should be checked, or another source of sepsis sought, such as empyema of the gallbladder or liver abscess.

Antibiotics should be continued for 1 week, particularly if there are gallbladder stones, since empyema can be a complication of cholangitis.

Such severe cholangitis may also complicate malignant strictures after an interventional procedure, for example cholangiography without drainage, or previous endoprosthesis insertion. The management is the same: antibiotics and biliary decompression.

Acute cholangitis

The same principles govern the treatment of cholangitis of a lesser degree, but endoscopic therapy can be done electively if the patient's condition allows.

Malaise and fever are followed by shivering and sweating (*Charcot's intermittent biliary fever*). Not all features of Charcot's triad (fever, pain, jaundice) may be present. Laboratory tests include white cell count, renal and liver function tests and blood cultures. Ultrasound may show biliary tract disease.

The choice of antibiotic depends upon the state of the patient and local policy. A cephalosporin usually suffices [179]. Quinolones (e.g. ciprofloxacin) are an alternative. Cholangiography is timed according to the state of the patient and the response to antibiotics. Stones are removed after endoscopic sphincterotomy. If the stones cannot be extracted, bile drainage is provided by insertion of a naso-biliary tube or endoprosthesis (fig. 34.13). This management is necessary independent of whether the gallbladder is *in situ* or not. Subsequent decisions on cholecystectomy are discussed below.

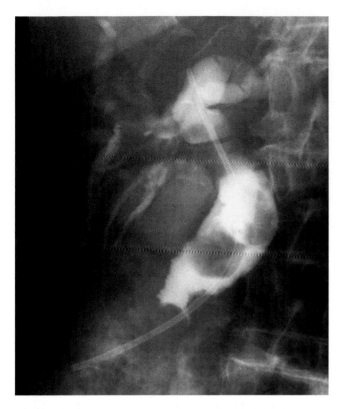

Fig. 34.13. ERCP in a patient with acute cholangitis. The common bile duct contains a large stone which could not be removed. A stent was inserted to provide drainage.

Multivariate analysis has identified seven features associated with a poor outcome in a mixed group of patients with cholangitis treated surgically and by non-surgical techniques. These were acute renal failure, cholangitis associated with liver abscess or liver cirrhosis, cholangitis secondary to high malignant biliary strictures or after percutaneous trans-hepatic cholangiography, female gender and age over 50 years [65].

Common duct stones without cholangitis

These are usually treated by elective endoscopic cholangiography, sphincterotomy and stone removal. Antibiotics are given to cover the procedure. Stone removal without sphincterotomy is possible, in most cases after balloon dilatation of the sphincter [15]. Pancreatitis occurs in 5–10%.

Patients with gallbladder *in situ*

Endoscopic sphincterotomy is definitive for residual post-cholecystectomy stones with only 10% having further biliary problems [70]—a similar outcome to surgical treatment.

If the gallbladder is still *in situ* and contains stones,

subsequent management depends upon the age and clinical state of the patient. In the elderly, several studies have shown that, after endoscopic sphincterotomy, only 5–10% need cholecystectomy for gallbladder disease during 1–9 years follow-up [81]. However, a randomized trial of sphincterotomy alone versus open cholecystectomy with surgical removal of duct stones found that 15% of patients treated by sphincterotomy subsequently required cholecystectomy during a mean follow-up of 17 months [183]. This compared with 4% of the surgical group needing sphincterotomy after the cholecystectomy for a retained duct stone.

In an otherwise fit patient, the choices are endoscopic sphincterotomy (ES) followed by laparoscopic cholecystectomy, cholecystectomy with duct exploration, or ES without cholecystectomy unless gallbladder complications occur. The decision depends upon local expertise. In the patient who is unfit for surgery, ES without cholecystectomy is appropriate.

In younger patients—the age point is as yet undefined—cholecystectomy is generally recommended because of the concern that complications will occur in the long term.

Acute gallstone pancreatitis

Gallstones travelling down the bile duct may produce acute pancreatitis as they pass through the ampulla. The stones are usually small and pass into the faeces. The inflammation then subsides. Sometimes the stone does not pass out of the ampulla and pancreatitis persists and may be severe. Abnormal liver function tests, particularly transaminases, and ultrasound are the most useful tests to identify the patient with pancreatitis due to gallstones [40]. Early ERCP and sphincterotomy to remove the stone(s) has been shown to reduce complications and cholangitis in patients with severe, but not mild, pancreatitis [54, 166]. The optimal timing and selection of patients awaits further study.

Biliary sludge may also cause attacks of acute pancreatitis [101].

Large common duct stones

Stones greater than 15mm in diameter are difficult or impossible to remove with a standard basket or balloon after sphincterotomy. Some may pass spontaneously. There are several options (table 34.4), which will depend upon local expertise and enthusiasm.

Mechanical lithotripsy may crush the stone but is limited by basket design and stone shape and size. With the latest baskets 90% success is possible [168].

The easiest method, particularly in the poor risk patient, is the insertion of an *endoprosthesis* (fig. 34.13), which may be long term, or temporary before surgical or

Table 34.4. Non-surgical treatment options for large common duct stones

---
Mechanical lithotripsy ('crushing basket')
Endoprosthesis
Extracorporeal shock-wave lithotripsy
Contact dissolution therapy
Electrohydraulic lithotripsy
Laser lithotripsy
---

endoscopic duct clearance. Early complications are seen in 12%, with a mortality of 4% [131]. Biliary colic, cholangitis and cholecystitis are late complications [139]. Stones may become smaller after stenting and may then be easier to remove at later ERCP [26].

Extracorporeal shock-wave lithotripsy can fragment 70–90% of large common duct stones with subsequent clearance of fragments through the sphincterotomy in the majority of patients, with less than a 1% 30-day mortality [52, 163].

Endoscopic electrohydraulic and laser lithotripsy remain experimental [133].

Trans T-tube tract removal of stones

Retained stones can be removed percutaneously along the T-tube tract in 77–96% of patients [135] with a complication rate of 2–4% (cholangitis, pancreatitis, tract perforation). The T-tube should have been in place for 4–5 weeks before stone removal to allow a fibrous tract to form. This method is complementary to endoscopic sphincterotomy, which with a T-tube in place is successful in about 75% [135]. The endoscopic approach may be favoured in the older patient, or when there is patient intolerance of the T-tube, or the size or path of the T-tube is not optimal.

Intra-hepatic gallstones

Stones in the intra-hepatic ducts are particularly common in certain parts of the world such as the Far East and Brazil where they are associated with parasitic infestation. Gallstones form in chronically obstructed bile ducts due to such conditions as anastomotic biliary–enteric stricture, primary sclerosing cholangitis or Caroli's disease. They are usually of brown pigment type. Secondary hepatic infection may result in multiple abscesses.

Percutaneous techniques using large-bore transhepatic catheters [132], combined with surgery if necessary, can clear stones in over 90% of patients, leaving the majority symptom-free [140]. The percutaneous transhepatic cholangioscopic approach can clear intra-hepatic stones in over 80% [83]. There is stone recurrence in 50% of patients with duct strictures.

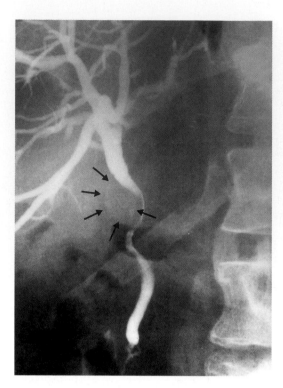

Fig. 34.14. Percutaneous cholangiography in Mirizzi's syndrome shows a large gallstone impacted in the cystic duct (arrowed) which has caused partial obstruction to the common hepatic duct.

Mirizzi's syndrome

Impaction of a gallstone in the cystic duct or neck of the gallbladder can cause partial common hepatic duct obstruction [60]. Recurrent cholangitis follows and the stone may erode into the common hepatic duct creating a single cavity [36].

Ultrasound shows dilated intra-hepatic and common hepatic ducts, but the cause may not been seen or correctly interpreted. Cholangiography shows mid duct obstruction (fig. 34.14). There may be the appearances of a stone, and from the outset it may be obvious that this is in cystic rather than bile duct. However, the appearances may initially suggest a common duct stone and only when attempts have failed to remove it does it become clear that the situation is more complicated. The operator must be alert to the possibility of a cystic duct stone and Mirizzi's syndrome. Endoscopic therapy is possible (stent insertion) to decompress the biliary system before surgery. Endoscopic stone retrieval is occasionally possible [53]. Surgery consists of removing the diseased gallbladder and the impacted stone.

A higher frequency of gallbladder carcinoma has been reported in Mirizzi's syndrome than with long-standing gallstone disease alone [146].

Biliary fistulae

External

These follow procedures such as cholecystotomy, transhepatic biliary drainage or T-tube choledochotomy. Very rarely they follow gallstones, carcinoma of the gallbladder or trauma.

Because of the sodium and bicarbonate content of bile, patients with external biliary fistulae run a risk of severe hyponatraemic acidosis and rise in blood urea levels.

Distal biliary obstruction contributes to the failure of the fistula to heal and the placement of an endoscopic or percutaneous biliary stent is followed by healing without the need for further difficult re-operations.

Internal

In 80% these are due to long-standing calculous cholecystitis. The inflamed gallbladder, containing stones, adheres and ruptures into a segment of the intestine, usually the duodenum and less often the colon (fig. 34.15). The ejected gallstones may be passed or cause intestinal obstruction (*gallstone ileus*), usually in the terminal ileum.

Post-operative biliary strictures, especially after multiple efforts at repair, may be complicated by fistula formation, usually hepatico-duodenal or hepatico-gastric. The fistulae are short, narrow and liable to block.

Biliary fistulae may also follow rupture of a chronic duodenal ulcer into the gallbladder or common bile duct. Fistulae may also develop between the colon and biliary tract in ulcerative colitis or Crohn's disease, especially if the patient is receiving corticosteroid therapy.

Clinical features

There is a long history of biliary disease. The fistula may be symptomless and, when the gallstones have discharged into the intestine successfully, the fistula closes. Such instances are often diagnosed only at the time of a later cholecystectomy.

About one-third give a history of jaundice or are jaundiced on admission. Pain may be absent or as severe as biliary colic. The features of cholangitis may be present. In cholecystocolic fistula the common bile duct may be filled with calculi, putrefying matter and faeces, which cause the severe cholangitis. Bile salts entering the colon produce severe diarrhoea. Weight loss is profound.

Radiological features

These include gas in the biliary tract and the presence of a gallstone in an unusual position. A barium meal, in the case of a cholecysto-duodenal fistula, or a barium

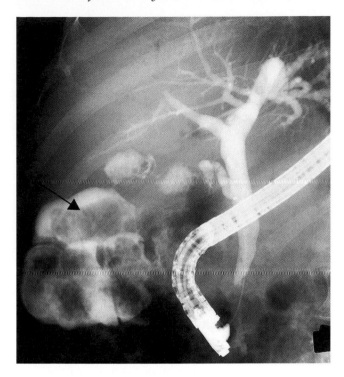

Fig. 34.15. ERCP showing a fistula between the gallbladder and colon (large arrow).

enema, in the case of a cholecystocolic fistula, may fill the biliary tree. Small bowel distension may be noted.

ERCP should be diagnostic (fig. 34.15).

Treatment

Fistulae due to gallbladder disease are treated surgically. Adherent viscera are separated and closed and cholecystectomy and drainage of the common bile duct performed. There is an operative mortality of around 10% [159].

Endoscopic treatment of common duct stones can result in closure of cholecystocolic and bronchobiliary fistulae [22, 121].

Gallstone ileus

A gallstone over 2.5 cm in diameter entering the intestine causes obstruction, usually of the ileum, less often of the duodeno-jejunal junction, duodenal bulb, pylorus or colon [32]. The impacted gallstone may excite an inflammatory reaction in the intestinal wall, or cause intussusception.

Gallstone ileus is very rare but is the cause of a quarter of all cases of non-strangulated intestinal obstruction in patients over 65 [98].

The patient is usually an elderly, afebrile female, possibly with a preceding history suggestive of chronic cholecystitis. The onset is insidious, with nausea, occasional vomiting, colicky abdominal pain and a somewhat distended but flaccid abdomen. Complete intestinal obstruction leads to rapid physical deterioration.

A plain X-ray of the abdomen may reveal loops of distended bowel with fluid levels and possibly the obstructing stone. Gas may be seen in the biliary tract and gallbladder, indicating a biliary fistula.

The plain film on admission is diagnostic in about 50% of patients. Ultrasound, barium studies and CT provide diagnostic information in a further 25%. Leucocytosis is not usual unless there is associated cholangitis with pyrexia.

Pre-operative diagnosis is made in about 70% of cases [32].

Treatment

After the patient's general condition has been restored by intravenous fluids and electrolytes, the intestinal obstruction should be relieved surgically. This may be done by manual propulsion of the stone or by enterotomy. Whether fistula repair and cholecystectomy are also done at the time of the first operation to relieve intestinal obstruction depends upon the operative feasibility and the clinical state of the patient [32]. If not done at the initial operation, subsequent cholecystectomy is not mandatory [109]. Mortality is about 20%.

Haemobilia [19]

Haemorrhage into the biliary tract may follow trauma including surgical and needle liver biopsy, aneurysms of the hepatic artery or one of its branches, extra- or intra-hepatic tumours of the biliary tract, hepatocellular carcinoma, gallstone disease, inflammation of the liver especially helminthic or pyogenic, and rarely varicose veins related to portal hypertension. Iatrogenic disease such as liver biopsy and percutaneous trans-hepatic cholangiography and bile drainage now accounts for 40%.

Clinical features are pain related to the passage of clots, jaundice and haematemesis and melaena. Minor episodes may be shown only by positive occult blood tests in faeces.

Diagnosis is suspected whenever upper gastrointestinal bleeding is associated with biliary colic, jaundice or a right upper quadrant mass or tenderness.

MRCP, ERCP or percutaneous cholangiography may show the clot in the ducts (fig. 34.16).

Treatment

Many resolve spontaneously. If bleeding continues angiography with embolization of a bleeding vessel if seen is indicated [38]. If clot obstructs the bile duct or

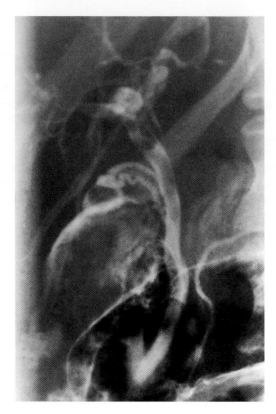

Fig. 34.16. ERCP in haemobilia shows filling defects, representing blood clot in the bile ducts.

gives colic, ERCP and drainage or sphincterotomy may be necessary [97].

Bile peritonitis

Aetiology

Post-cholecystectomy. Bile may leak from small bile channels between the gallbladder and liver or from an imperfectly ligated cystic duct. If the biliary pressure is raised, perhaps by a residual common duct stone or papillary stenosis, leakage is facilitated and the subsequent paraductal bile accumulation favours the development of biliary stricture.

Post-transplantation. Leakage of bile from the bile-duct anastomosis is a recognized complication of liver transplantation.

Rupture of the gallbladder. Empyema or gangrene of the gallbladder may lead to rupture and the formation of an abscess; this is localized by previous inflammatory adhesions.

Trauma. Crushing or gunshot wounds may involve the biliary tree. Needle biopsy of the liver or percutaneous cholangiography may rarely be complicated by puncture of the gallbladder or of a dilated intra-hepatic bile duct in a patient with deep cholestasis. Oozing of bile rarely follows operative liver biopsy.

Spontaneous. Biliary peritonitis may develop in patients

with prolonged, deep obstructive jaundice without demonstrable breach of the biliary tree. This is presumably due to bursting of minute superficial intra-hepatic bile ducts.

Common bile duct perforation is exceedingly rare. The factors concerned are similar to those for perforated gallbladder. They include increases of intra-ductal pressure, calculous erosion and necrosis of the duct wall secondary to thrombosis [89].

Spontaneous perforation of the extra-hepatic bile ducts is a rare cause of jaundice in infancy, the most common site being at the confluence of the cystic and common hepatic duct. Pathogenesis is unknown.

Clinical picture

This depends on whether the bile is localized or free in the peritoneal cavity, sterile or infected. Free rupture of bile into the peritoneal cavity causes severe shock. Due to the irritant effect of bile salts, large quantities of plasma are poured into the ascitic fluid. The onset is with excruciating, generalized, abdominal pain. Examination shows a shocked, pale, motionless patient, with low blood pressure and persistent tachycardia. There is board-like rigidity of the diffusely tender abdomen. Paralytic ileus is a frequent complication. Bile peritonitis should always be considered in any patient with unexplained intestinal obstruction. In a matter of hours secondary infection follows and the temperature rises while abdominal pain and tenderness persist.

Laboratory findings are non-contributory. There may be haemoconcentration. Abdominal paracentesis reveals bile, usually infected. Serum bilirubin rises and this is followed by an increase in alkaline phosphatase levels. Cholescintigraphy or cholangiography will show the leakage of bile. Bile drainage by the endoscopic or percutaneous route has improved the prognosis.

Treatment

Fluid replacement is imperative. Paralytic ileus may demand nasogastric intubation. Antibiotics are given to prevent secondary infection.

Rupture of the gallbladder is treated by cholecystectomy. Biliary leakage from the common bile duct can be treated by endoscopic stenting (with or without sphincterotomy) or naso-biliary drainage. If the leak does not seal over in 7–10 days, surgery may be necessary.

Association of gallstones with other diseases

Colorectal and other cancers

Population surveys show that gallstone sufferers do not seem at increased risk from other malignancies except perhaps that of the gallbladder [120] and extra-hepatic bile ducts [51].

Changes in faecal bile acids and cholesterol metabolites may promote colorectal oncogenesis [165]. Cholecystectomy may allow greater exposure of conjugated primary bile acids to anaerobic intestinal bacteria and so the increased production of carcinogens. Cholecystectomy and gallstones and colorectal cancer have been linked, although the association was not confirmed [2, 61]. The association may be related to increased diagnostic efforts in symptomatic post-cholecystectomy patients incidentally detecting early colorectal cancers.

Diabetes mellitus

About 30% of all diabetics over 20 years old have gallstones, compared with 11.6% of the general population of the same age. The older diabetic tends to be obese, and this may be the important factor in gallstone formation. Chronic pancreatitis and gallstones are associated and chronic pancreatitis can produce mild diabetes.

Patients with diabetes may have large, poorly contracting and poorly filling gallbladders [90]. A 'diabetic neurogenic gallbladder' syndrome has been postulated.

Patients with diabetes mellitus undergoing cholecystectomy, whether emergency or elective, have increased complications. These are probably related to associated cardiovascular or renal disease and to more advanced age.

References

1 Abei M, Nuutinen H, Kawczak P *et al*. Identification of human biliary alpha$_1$-acid glycoprotein as a cholesterol crystallization promoter. *Gastroenterology* 1994; **106**: 234.

2 Adami HO, Meirik O, Gustavsson S *et al*. Colorectal cancer after cholecystectomy: absence of risk increase within 11–14 years. *Gastroenterology* 1983; **85**: 859.

3 Apstein MD, Carey MC. Pathogenesis of cholesterol gallstones: a parsimonious hypothesis. *Eur. J. Clin. Invest.* 1996; **26**: 343.

4 Attili AF, Capocaccia R, Carulli N *et al*. Factors associated with gallstone disease in the MICOL experience. *Hepatology* 1997; **26**: 809.

5 Attili AF, Scafato E, Marchiolo R *et al*. Diet and gallstones in Italy: the cross-sectional MICOL results. *Hepatology* 1998; **27**: 1492.

6 Azzaroli F, Mazzella G, Mazelo P *et al*. Sluggish small bowel motility is involved in determining increased biliary deoxycholic acid in cholesterol gallstone patients. *Am. J. Gastroenterol.* 1999; **94**: 2453.

7 Barkun JS, Barkun AN, Sampalis JS *et al*. Randomised controlled trial of laparoscopic vs. mini cholecystectomy. *Lancet* 1992; **340**: 1116.

8 Barkun JS, Fried GM, Barkun AN *et al*. Cholecystectomy without operative cholangiography: implications for common bile duct injury and retained common bile duct stones. *Ann. Surg.* 1993; **218**: 371.

9   Barton JR, Russell RCG, Hatfield ARW. Management of bile leaks after laparoscopic cholecystectomy. *Br. J. Surg.* 1995; **82**: 980.

10 Bateson MC. Gallstone epidemiology. *Curr. Gastroenterol.* 1986; **5**: 120.

11 Bearcroft PW, Lomas DJ. Cholesterol crystallization in bile. *Gut* 1997; **41**: 138.

12 Behar J, Lee KY, Thompson WR *et al.* Gallbladder contraction in patients with pigment and cholesterol stones. *Gastroenterology* 1989; **97**: 1479.

13 Bennion LJ, Ginsberg RL, Garnick MB *et al.* Effects of oral contraceptives on the gallbladder bile of normal women. *N. Engl. J. Med.* 1976; **294**: 189.

14 Berger MY, van der Velden JJIM, Lijmer JG *et al.* Abdominal symptoms: do they predict gallstones? *Scand. J. Gastroenterol.* 2000; **35**: 70.

15 Bergman JJGHM, Rauws EAJ, Fockens P *et al.* Randomised trial of endoscopic balloon dilation vs. endoscopic sphincterotomy for removal of bileduct stones. *Lancet* 1997; **349**: 1124.

16 Bergman JJGHM, van den Brink JR, Rauws EAJ *et al.* Treatment of bile duct lesions after laparoscopic cholecystectomy. *Gut* 1996; **38**: 141.

17 Berr F, Mayer M, Sackmann MF *et al.* Pathogenic factors in early recurrence of cholesterol gallstones. *Gastroenterology* 1994; **106**: 215.

18 Bertomeu A, Ros E, Zambon D *et al.* Apolipoprotein E polymorphism and gallstones. *Gastroenterology* 1996; **111**: 1603.

19 Blochle C, Izbicki JR, Rashed MYT *et al.* Hemobilia: presentation, diagnosis and management. *Am. J. Gastroenterol.* 1994; **89**: 1537.

20 Boston Collaborative Drug Surveillance Program. Oral contraceptives and venous thromboembolic disease: surgically confirmed gall-bladder disease and breast tumours. *Lancet* 1973; **i**: 1399.

21 Boston Collaborative Drug Surveillance Program. Gallbladder disease, venous disorders, breast tumours: relation to oestrogens. *N. Engl. J. Med.* 1974; **290**: 15.

22 Brem H, Gibbons GD, Cobb G *et al.* The use of endoscopy to treat bronchobiliary fistula caused by choledocholithiasis. *Gastroenterology* 1990; **98**: 490.

23 Brink MA, Slors JFM, Keulemans YCA *et al.* Enterohepatic cycling of bilirubin: a putative mechanism for pigment gallstone formation in ileal Crohn's disease. *Gastroenterology* 1999; **116**: 1420.

24 Caygill CPJ, Hill MJ, Braddick M *et al.* Cancer mortality in chronic typhoid and paratyphoid carriers. *Lancet* 1994; **343**: 83.

25 Cello JP. AIDS-related biliary tract disease. *Gastrointest. Endosc. Clin. North Am.* 1998; **8**: 963.

26 Chan ACW, Ng EKW, Chung SCS *et al.* Common bile duct stones become smaller after endoscopic biliary stenting. *Endoscopy* 1998; **30**: 356.

27 Chapman BA, Wilson IR, Frampton CM *et al.* Prevalence of gallbladder disease in diabetes mellitus. *Dig. Dis. Sci.* 1996; **41**: 2222.

28 Cheslyn-Curtis S, Gillams AR, Russell RCG *et al.* Selection, management, and early outcome of 113 patients with symptomatic gall stones treated by percutaneous cholecystolithotomy. *Gut* 1992; **33**: 1253.

29 Chin PT, Boland S, Percy JP *et al.* 'Gallstone hip' and other sequelae of retained gallstones. *HBP Surg.* 1997; **10**: 165.

30 Chow WC, Ong CL, Png JC *et al.* Gall bladder empyema—another good reason for early cholecystectomy. *J. R. Coll. Surg. Edin.* 1993; **38**: 213.

31 Cicala M, Habib FI, Fiocca F *et al.* Increased sphincter of Oddi basal pressure in patients affected by gall stone disease: a role for biliary stasis and colicy pain? *Gut* 2001; **48**: 414.

32 Clavien P-A, Richon J, Burgan S *et al.* Gallstone ileus. *Br. J. Surg.* 1990; **77**: 737.

33 Cobden I, Lendrum R, Venables CLO *et al.* Gallstones presenting as mental and physical debility in the elderly. *Lancet* 1984; **i**: 1062.

34 Corazziari E, Jensen PF, Hogan WJ *et al.* Functional disorders of the biliary tract. *Gastroenterol. Int.* 1993; **6**: 129.

35 Cox MR, Wilson TG, Luck AJ *et al.* Laparoscopic cholecystectomy for acute inflammation of the gall bladder. *Ann. Surg.* 1993; **218**: 630.

36 Csendes A, Carlos Diaz J, Burdiles P *et al.* Mirizzi syndrome and cholecystobiliary fistula: a unifying classification. *Br. J. Surg.* 1989; **76**: 1139.

37 Cuschieri A, Berci G. *Laparoscopic Biliary Surgery.* Blackwell Scientific Publications, Oxford, 1990.

38 Czerniak A, Thompson JN, Hemingway AP *et al.* Hemobilia: a disease in evolution. *Arch. Surg.* 1988; **123**: 718.

39 Davidson BR, Neoptolemos JP, Carr-Locke DL. Endoscopic sphincterotomy for common bile duct calculi in patients with gallbladder *in situ* considered unfit for surgery. *Gut* 1988; **29**: 114.

40 Davidson BR, Neoptolemos JP, Leese T *et al.* Biochemical prediction of gallstones in acute pancreatitis: a prospective study of three systems. *Br. J. Surg.* 1988; **75**: 213.

41 De Santis A, Attili AF, Corradini SG *et al.* Gallstones and diabetes: a case-control study in a free-living population sample. *Hepatology* 1997; **25**: 787.

42 Desautels SG, Slivka A, Hutson WR *et al.* Postcholecystomy pain syndrome: pathophysiology of abdominal pain in sphincter of Oddi type III. *Gastroenterology* 1999; **116**: 900.

43 Dhiman RK, Phanish MK, Chawla YK *et al.* Gallbladder motility and lithogenicity of bile in patients with choledocholithiasis after endoscopic sphincterotomy. *J. Hepatol.* 1997; **26**: 1300.

44 Diehl AK, Beral V. Cholecystectomy and changing mortality from gallbladder cancer. *Lancet* 1981; **i**: 187.

45 Doctor N, Dooley JS, Dick R *et al.* Multidisciplinary approach to biliary complications of laparoscopic cholecystectomy. *Br. J. Surg.* 1998; **85**: 627.

46 Donald JJ, Cheslyn-Curtis S, Gillams AR *et al.* Percutaneous cholecystolithotomy: is gall stone recurrence inevitable? *Gut* 1994; **35**: 692.

47 Donovan JM. Physical and metabolic factors in gallstone pathogenesis. *Gastroenterol. Clin. North Am.* 1994; **28**: 75.

48 Dowling RH. The enterohepatic circulation. *Gastroenterology* 1972; **62**: 122.

49 Dowling RH. Pathogenesis of gallstones. *Aliment. Pharmacol. Ther.* 2000; **14** (Suppl. 2): 39.

50 Dunn D, Fowler S, Nair R *et al.* Laparoscopic cholecystectomy in England and Wales: results of an audit by the Royal College of Surgeons of England. *Ann. R. Coll. Surg. Engl.* 1994; **76**: 269.

51 Ekborn A, Hsieh C, Yuen J *et al.* Risk of extrahepatic bile duct cancer after cholecystectomy. *Lancet* 1993; **342**: 1262.

52 Ellis RD, Jenkins AP, Thompson RP *et al.* Clearance of

refractory bile duct stones with extracorporeal shockwave lithotripsy. *Gut* 2000; **47**: 728.

53 England RE, Martin DF. Endoscopic management of Mirizzi's syndrome. *Gut* 1997; **40**: 272.

54 Enns R, Baillie J. The treatment of acute biliary pancreatitis. *Aliment. Pharmacol. Ther.* 1999; **11**: 1379.

55 Erlinger S, Go AL, Husson J-M *et al.* Franco-Belgian Co-operative Study of ursodeoxycholic acid in the medical dissolution of gallstones: a double-blind, randomized, dose–response study, and comparison with chenodeoxycholic acid. *Hepatology* 1984; **4**: 308.

56 Everhart JE, Khare M, Hill M *et al.* Prevalence and ethnic differences in gallbladder disease in the United States. *Gastroenterology* 1999; **117**: 632.

57 Festi D, Sottili S, Colecchia A *et al.* Clinical manifestations of gallstone disease: evidence from the multicentre Italian study on cholelithiasis (MICOL). *Hepatology* 1999; **30**: 839.

58 Fornari F, Imberti D, Squillante MM *et al.* Incidence of gallstones in a population of patients with cirrhosis. *J. Hepatol.* 1994; **20**: 797.

59 Fox JG, Dewhirst FE, Shen Z *et al.* Hepatic *Helicobacter* species identified in bile and gallbladder tissue from Chileans with chronic cholecystitis. *Gastroenterology* 1998; **114**: 755.

60 Freeman ME, Rose JL, Forsmark CE *et al.* Mirizzi syndrome: a rare cause of obstructive jaundice. *Dig. Dis.* 1999; **17**: 44.

61 Friedman GD, Goldhaber MK, Queensbury CP Jr. Cholecystectomy and large bowel cancer. *Lancet* 1987; **i**: 906.

62 Gadacz TR. Update on laparoscopic cholecystectomy, including a clinical pathway. *Surg. Clin. North Am.* 2000; **80**: 1127.

63 Gebhard RL, Prigge WF, Ansel HJ *et al.* The role of gallbladder emptying in gallstone formation during diet-induced rapid weight loss. *Hepatology* 1996; **24**: 544.

64 Geenen JE, Hogan WJ, Dodds WJ *et al.* The efficacy of endoscopic sphincterotomy after cholecystectomy in patients with sphincter of Oddi dysfunction. *N. Engl. J. Med.* 1989; **320**: 82.

65 Gigot JF, Leese T, Dereme T *et al.* Acute cholangitis: multivariate analysis of risk factors. *Ann. Surg.* 1989; **209**: 435.

66 Gilat T, Somjen GJ, Leikin-Frenkel A *et al.* Fatty acid bile acid conjugates (FABACs)—new molecules for the prevention of cholesterol crystallization in bile. *Gut* 2001; **48**: 75.

67 Gleeson D, Ruppin DC, Saunders A *et al.* Final outcome of ursodeoxycholic acid treatment in 126 patients with radiolucent gallstones. *Q. J. Med.* 1990; **279**: 711.

68 Gomez NA, Gutierrez J, Leon CJ. Acute acalculous cholecystitis due to *Vibrio cholerae*. *Lancet* 1994; **343**: 1156.

69 Halevy A, Gold-Deutch R, Negri M *et al.* Are elevated liver enzymes and bilirubin levels significant after laparoscopic cholecystectomy in the absence of bile duct injury? *Ann. Surg.* 1994; **219**: 362.

70 Hawes RH, Cotton PB, Vallon AG. Follow-up 6–11 years after duodenoscopic sphincterotomy for stones in patients with prior cholecystectomy. *Gastroenterology* 1990; **98**: 1008.

71 Heaton KW, Emmett PM, Symes CL *et al.* An explanation for gallstones in normal-weight women: slow intestinal transit. *Lancet* 1993; **341**: 8.

72 Hellstern A, Leuschner U, Benjaminov A *et al.* Dissolution of gallbladder stones with methyl tert-butyl ether and stone recurrence: a European study. *Dig. Dis. Sci.* 1998; **43**: 911.

73 Henriksson P, Einarsson K, Eriksson A *et al.* Estrogen-induced gallstone formation in males. *J. Clin. Invest.* 1989; **84**: 811.

74 Hernandez CA, Lerch MM. Sphincter stenosis and gallstone migration through the biliary tract. *Lancet* 1993; **341**: 1371.

75 Hickman MS, Schwesinger WH, Page CP. Acute cholecystitis in the diabetic. A case control study of outcome. *Arch. Surg.* 1988; **123**: 409.

76 Holzbach RT, Marsh M, Olszewski M *et al.* Cholesterol solubility in bile: evidence that supersaturated bile is frequent in healthy man. *J. Clin. Invest.* 1973; **52**: 1467.

77 Hood K, Gleeson D, Ruppin DC *et al.* Prevention of gallstone recurrence by nonsteroidal anti-inflammatory drugs. *Lancet* 1988; **ii**: 1223.

78 Hood KA, Gleeson D, Ruppin DC *et al.* Gall stone recurrence and its prevention: the British/Belgian gall stone study group's postdissolution trial. *Gut* 1993; **34**: 1277.

79 Hopman WPM, Jansen JBMJ, Rosenbusch G *et al.* Role of cholecystokinin and the cholinergic system in intestinal stimulation of gallbladder contraction in man. *J. Hepatol.* 1990; **11**: 261.

80 Howard DE, Fromm H. Nonsurgical management of gallstone disease. *Gastroenterol. Clin. North Am.* 1999; **28**: 133.

81 Ingoldby CJH, El-Saadi J, Hall RI *et al.* Late results of endoscopic sphincterotomy for bile duct stones in elderly patients with gallbladder *in situ*. *Gut* 1989; **30**: 1129.

82 Inoue K, Fuchigami A, Higashide S *et al.* Gallbladder sludge and stone formation in relation to contractile function after gastrectomy. *Ann. Surg.* 1992; **215**: 19.

83 Jan Y-Y, Chen M-F. Percutaneous trans-hepatic cholangioscopic lithotomy for hepatolithiasis: long-term results. *Gastrointest. Endosc.* 1995; **42**: 1.

84 Janowitz J, Kratzer W, Zemmler T *et al.* Gallbladder sludge: spontaneous course and incidence of complications in patients without stones. *Hepatology* 1994; **20**: 291.

85 Jazrawi RP, Pazzi P, Petroni ML *et al.* Postprandial gallbladder motor function: refilling and turnover of bile in health and cholelithiasis. *Gastroenterology* 1995; **109**: 582.

86 Jüngst D, Del Pozo R, Dolu MH *et al.* Rapid formation of cholesterol crystals in gallbladder bile is associated with stone recurrence after laparoscopic cholecystotomy. *Hepatology* 1997; **25**: 509.

87 Jüngst D, Lang T, von Ritter C *et al.* Cholesterol nucleation time in gallbladder bile of patients with solitary or multiple cholesterol gallstones. *Hepatology* 1992; **15**: 804.

88 Kalliafas S, Ziegler DW, Flancbaum L *et al.* Acute acalculous cholecystitis: incidence, risk factors, diagnosis, and outcome. *Am. Surg.* 1998; **64**: 471.

89 Kerstein MD, McSwain NE. Spontaneous rupture of the common bile duct. *Am. J. Gastroenterol.* 1985; **80**: 469.

90 Keshavarzian A, Dunne M, Iber FL. Gallbladder volume and emptying in insulin requiring male diabetics. *Dig. Dis. Sci.* 1987; **32**: 824.

91 Keulemans YCA, Mok KS, de Wit LTH *et al.* Hepatic bile vs. gallbladder bile: a comparison of protein and lipid concentration and composition in cholesterol gallstone patients. *Hepatology* 1998; **28**: 11.

92 Kibe A, Holzbach RT, LaRusso NF *et al.* Inhibition of cho-

tion and chemotherapy following curative resection of the pancreatic head. *Cancer* 1987; **59**: 2006.

21 Hammel P, Couvelard A, O'Toole D *et al*. Regression of liver fibrosis after biliary drainage in patients with chronic pancreatitis and stenosis of the common bile duct. *N. Engl. J. Med.* 2001; **344**: 418.

22 Kawa S, Tokoo M, Hasebe O *et al*. Comparative study of CA 242 and CA 19-9 for the diagnosis of pancreatic cancer. *Br. J. Cancer* 1994; **70**; 481.

23 Kurzawinski TR, Deery A, Dooley JS *et al*. A prospective study of biliary cytology in 100 patients with bile duct strictures. *Hepatology* 1993; **18**: 1399.

24 Legman P, Vignaus O, Dousser B *et al*. Pancreatic tumours: comparison of dual-phase helical CT and endoscopic sonography. *Am. J. Radiol.* 1998; **170**: 1315.

25 Lesur G, Levy P, Flejou J-F *et al*. Factors predictive of liver histopathological appearance in chronic alcoholic pancreatitis with common bile duct stenosis and increased serum alkaline phosphatase. *Hepatology* 1993; **18**: 1078.

26 Lewandrowski K, Lee J, Southern J *et al*. Cyst fluid analysis in the differential diagnosis of pancreatic cysts: a new approach to the preoperative assessment of pancreatic cystic lesions. *Am. J. Roentgenol.* 1995; **164**: 815.

27 Lillemoe KD, Cameron JL, Kaufman HS *et al*. Chemical splanchnicectomy in patients with unresectable pancreatic cancer: a prospective randomized trial. *Ann. Surg.* 1993; **217**: 447.

28 Lowenfels AB, Maisonneuve P, Cavallini G *et al*. Pancreatitis and the risk of pancreatic cancer. *N. Engl. J. Med.* 1993; **328**: 1433.

29 Lowenfels AB, Maisonneuve P, DiMagno EP *et al*. Hereditary pancreatitis and the risk of pancreatic cancer. *J. Natl. Cancer Inst.* 1997; **89**: 442.

30 McDowell RK, Gazelle GS, Murphy BL *et al*. Mucinous ductal ectasia of the pancreas. *J. Comput. Assist. Tomogr.* 1997; **21**: 383.

31 Menges M, Lerch MM, Zeitz M. The double duct sign in patients with malignant and benign pancreatic lesions. *Gastrointest. Endosc.* 2000; **52**: 74.

32 National Institute for Clinical Excellence (NICE) (2001). Guidance on gemcitabine for pancreatic cancer. HTTP://www.nice.org.uk. May 2001.

33 Nevitt AW, Vida F, Kozarek RA *et al*. Expandable metallic prostheses for malignant obstructions of gastric outlet and proximal small bowel. *Gastrointest. Endosc.* 1998; **47**: 271.

34 Norton ID, Geller A, Petersen BT *et al*. Endoscopic surveillance and ablative therapy for periampullary adenomas. *Am. J. Gastroenterol.* 2001; **96**: 101.

35 O'Brien S, Hatfield ARW, Craig PI *et al*. A three-year follow-up of self expanding metal stents in the endoscopic palliation of longterm survivors with malignant biliary obstruction. *Gut* 1995; **36**: 618.

36 Pemert J, Marsson J, Westermark GT *et al*. Islet amyloid polypeptide in patients with pancreatic cancer and diabetes. *N. Engl. J. Med.* 1994; **360**: 313.

37 Polati E, Finco G, Gottin L *et al*. Prospective randomized double-blind trial of neurolytic coeliac plexus block in patients with pancreatic cancer. *Br. J. Surg.* 1998; **85**: 199.

38 Prat F, Chapat O, Ducot B *et al*. A randomized trial of endoscopic drainage methods for inoperable malignant strictures of the common bile duct. *Gastrointest. Endosc.* 1998; **47**: 1.

39 Prat F, Chapat O, Ducot B *et al*. Predictive factors for survival of patients with inoperable malignant distal biliary strictures: a practical management guide. *Gut* 1998; **42**: 76.

40 Queneau P-E, Adessi G-L, Thibault P *et al*. Early detection of pancreatic cancer in patients with chronic pancreatitis: diagnostic utility of a K-*ras* point mutation in the pancreatic juice. *Am. J. Gastroenterol.* 2001: **96**; 700.

41 Rivera JA, Fernandez-del Castillo C, Rall CJN *et al*. Analysis of K-*ras* oncogene mutations in chronic pancreatitis with ductal hyperplasia. *Surgery* 1997; **121**: 42.

42 Smith AC, Dowsett JF, Russell RCG *et al*. Randomised trial of endoscopic stenting vs. surgical bypass in malignant low bileduct obstruction. *Lancet* 1994; **344**: 1655.

43 Soetikno RM, Lichtenstein DR, Vandervoort J *et al*. Palliation of malignant gastric outlet obstruction using an endoscopically placed Wallstent. *Gastrointest. Endosc.* 1998; **47**: 267.

44 Speer AG, Cotton PB, Russell RCG *et al*. Randomized trial of endoscopic vs. percutaneous stent insertion in malignant obstructive jaundice. *Lancet* 1987; **ii**: 57.

45 Stahl TJ, Allen MO'C, Ansel HJ *et al*. Partial biliary obstruction caused by chronic pancreatitis: an appraisal of indications for surgical biliary drainage. *Ann. Surg.* 1988; **207**: 26.

46 Stewart CJR, Mills PR, Carter R *et al*. Brush cytology in the assessment of pancreatico-biliary strictures: a review of 406 cases. *J. Clin. Pathol.* 2001; **54**: 449.

47 Taheri S, Meeran K. Islet cell tumours: diagnosis and medical management. *Hosp. Med.* 2000; **61**: 824.

48 Tersmette AC, Petersen GM, Offerhaus GJA *et al*. Increased risk of incident pancreatic cancer among first-degree relatives of patients with familial pancreatic cancer. *Clin. Cancer Res.* 2001; **7**: 738.

49 Traverso LW, Longmire WP Jr. Preservation of the pylorus in pancreaticoduodenectomy. *Surg. Gynecol. Obstet.* 1978; **146**: 959.

50 Van Laethem J-L, Vertongen P, Deviere J *et al*. Detection of c-K-*ras* gene codon 12 mutations from pancreatic duct brushings in the diagnosis of pancreatic tumours. *Gut* 1995; **36**: 781.

51 Warshaw AL, Zhuo-yun G, Wittenberg J *et al*. Preoperative staging and assessment of resectability of pancreatic cancer. *Arch. Surg.* 1990; **125**: 230.

52 Yamaguchi K, Enjoji M. Carcinoma of the ampulla of Vater. A clinico-pathologic study and pathologic staging of 109 cases of carcinoma and five cases of adenoma. *Cancer* 1987; **59**: 506.

53 Yamaguchi K, Enjoji M. Adenoma of the ampulla of Vater: putative precancerous lesion. *Gut* 1991; **32**: 1558.

54 Zoepf T, Zoepf D-S, Arnold JC *et al*. The relationship between juxtapapillary duodenal diverticula and disorders of the biliopancreatic system: analysis of 350 patients. *Gastrointest. Endosc.* 2001; **54**: 56.

Chapter 37
Tumours of the Gallbladder and Bile Ducts

Benign lesions of the gallbladder

At ultrasound, polypoid lesions of the gallbladder are occasionally seen and there is usually concern as to their nature and how to manage them. The vast majority are benign. They may be true tumours or pseudo-tumours. True tumours comprise adenoma, lipoma and leiomyoma. Pseudo-tumours include cholesterol polyps, inflammatory polyps and adenomyomatosis.

These lesions are seen most often as an echogeneic focus that projects into the gallbladder lumen, does not cast an acoustic shadow, and does not move when the patient is moved (unlike a stone). The diagnostic accuracy of ultrasound for the commonest lesions is 50–90% depending on the pathology [34].

Cholesterol polyps are usually multiple, with a higher echogenicity than liver, a pedicle and a mulberry-like surface [34]. They may contain a hyperechoic spot. Pathologically they consist of hypertrophied villi laden with cholesterol.

Adenoma is seen as a polypoid lesion which on ultrasound has an echogenicity similar to the liver, a smooth surface and usually no pedicle [34].

80%–90% of gallbladder polypoid lesions do not change in size on follow-up scans [41, 57]. However, they cause concern because of the low chance of malignancy in adenomas. Cholecystectomy will be done for the symptomatic patient. This is also appropriate for the lesion greater than 10 mm in diameter, where the risk of malignancy is greater [34]. Other features of malignant tumour are a sessile lesion, isoechoic with the liver, growing rapidly on serial ultrasounds.

Patients with a smaller lesion without these features should undergo a second scan. Some lesions disappear but the majority remain, and these patients may be offered a cholecystectomy for peace of mind. Alternatively, a repeat scan is done at 6-monthly intervals to detect any change in size [39]. In practice ultrasound lesions less than 10 mm in diameter with benign appearances in an asymptomatic patient tend to be treated conservatively but follow-up scanning is important. If the result of trans-abdominal ultrasound is inconclusive, endoscopic ultrasound if available is useful with a diagnostic accuracy for neoplastic lesions of 80% [10].

Carcinoma of the gallbladder [1]

This is an uncommon neoplasm. Gallstones coexist in about 75% of cases and chronic cholecystitis is a frequent association. There is a clear association with large, multiple gallbladder stones [62], but a causal relationship is unproven.

The calcified (porcelain) gallbladder is particularly likely to become cancerous [51]. An anomalous pancreatico-biliary ductal union, greater than 15 mm from the papilla of Vater, is associated with congenital cystic dilatation of the common bile duct and with gallbladder carcinoma [40]. Regurgitation of pancreatic juice may be tumorigenic. The common gallbladder cholesterol polyps are not precancerous.

Chronic typhoid infection of the gallbladder increases the risk of gallbladder carcinoma by 167-fold [6], emphasizing the need for antibiotic treatment to eradicate the chronic typhoid and paratyphoid carrier state, or for elective cholecystectomy.

Papillary adenocarcinoma starts as a wart-like excrescence. It grows slowly into, rather than through, the wall until a fungating mass fills the gallbladder. Mucoid change is associated with more rapid growth, early metastasis and gelatinous peritoneal carcinomatosis. *Squamous cell carcinoma* and *scirrhous* forms are recognized. The *anaplastic type* is particularly malignant. The most common tumour is a differentiated adenocarcinoma [1, 16] which may be papillary.

The tumour usually arises in the fundus or neck, but rapid spread may make the original site difficult to locate. The rich lymphatic and venous drainage of the gallbladder leads to early spread to related lymph nodes, causing cholestatic jaundice and widespread dissemination. The liver bed is invaded and there may also be local spread to the duodenum, stomach and colon resulting in fistulae or external compression.

Clinical. The patient is usually an elderly, white female, complaining of pain in the right upper quadrant, nausea, vomiting, weight loss and jaundice. Sometimes an unsuspected carcinoma is found in a cholecystectomy specimen at histology. These small lesions may not even be recognized at the time of operation [13].

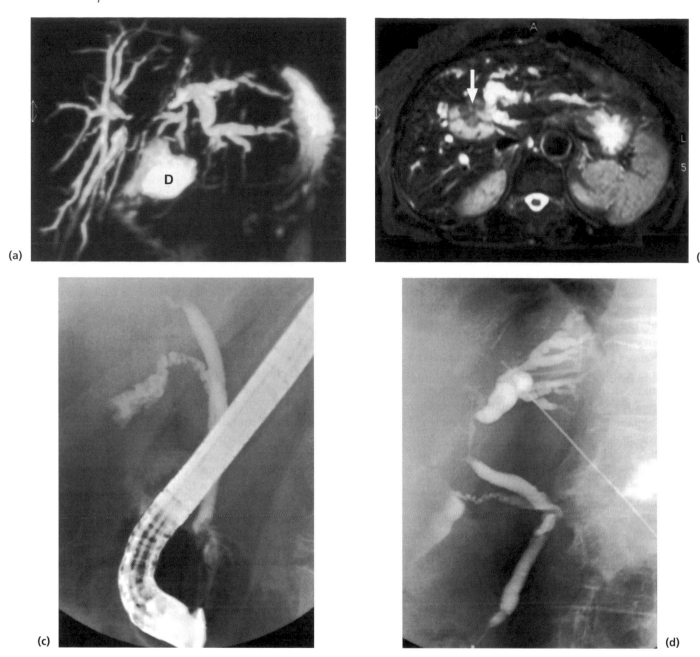

Fig. 37.3. A 75-year-old woman presenting with cholestatic jaundice. Ultrasound showed dilated intra-hepatic ducts, a hilar mass and a normal common bile duct. (a) MRCP shows dilated intra-hepatic ducts with at least three segments obstructed in the right lobe and the left hepatic system obstructed at the hilum. If non-surgical drainage is to be done, these appearances favour drainage of the left- rather than the right-sided system (D, duodenum). (b) MRI scan shows a mass in the liver (arrow) above the hilum. (c) Non-operative drainage was chosen since the patient was considered inoperable. ERCP shows a normal common duct with a hilar structure. A stent could not be placed. (d) Following on the MRCP appearances, the left-sided duct system was chosen for percutaneous cholangiography and a stent inserted.

unusual cause but it should be detected if an orderly work-up is used. History and examination are usually unhelpful.

The first step in the cholestatic patient is ultrasound scanning. Intra-hepatic bile ducts will be dilated in cholangiocarcinoma. The common duct is normal,

equivocal or may be dilated down to an extra-hepatic tumour. If there is a suspicion of hilar cholangiocarcinoma and other clinical features do not indicate inoperability, the choice is MRCP or, if this is not available, referral to a specialist hepato-biliary unit.

If ultrasound does not show dilated bile ducts in the

cholestatic patient, other causes (Chapter 13) need to be considered including drug jaundice (history) and primary biliary cirrhosis (anti-mitochondrial antibody). Liver histology will help. If primary sclerosing cholangitis is possible, cholangiography is diagnostic.

With scanning and cholangiography it should be possible to diagnose the bile duct stricture due to cholangiocarcinoma. At the hilum, the differential diagnosis is a benign stricture [25] or metastatic gland, in the mid-duct carcinoma of the gallbladder, and in the peri-ampullary region carcinoma of the pancreas. Differentiation will depend upon history and other imaging techniques.

Prognosis

Prognosis depends on the site of the tumour. Those distally placed are more likely to be resectable than those at the hilum. The histologically differentiated do better than the undifferentiated. Polypoid cancers have the best prognosis.

If unresected, the 1-year survival for cholangio carcinoma is 50%, with 20% surviving at 2 years and 10% at 3 years [18]. This reflects that some tumours are slow growing and metastasize late. Jaundice can be relieved surgically or by endoscopic or percutaneous stenting. The tumour kills by its site making it inoperable, rather than by its malignancy. Average survival after resection is longer, making proper assessment in patients fit for surgery essential.

Staging [7]

If the clinical state of the patient does not rule out surgery the resectability and extent of tumour is assessed. Metastases, usually late, should be sought.

Low and mid common bile duct lesions are usually resectable although vascular imaging is needed to exclude invasion.

Hilar cholangiocarcinoma is more problematic (table 37.1). If cholangiography shows involvement of the secondary hepatic ducts in both hepatic lobes (fig. 37.4, type

IV) or imaging shows encasement of the main portal vein or hepatic artery, the lesion is irresectable. A palliative procedure is needed.

If the tumour is limited to the hepatic duct bifurcation, affecting one lobe of the liver only, or only obstructs the portal vein or hepatic artery on the same side, the lesion may be resectable. Pre-operative imaging is aimed at establishing whether after surgical removal a viable unit of liver remains [7]. This must contain a biliary radicle large enough to anastomose to bowel, and a normal portal vein and hepatic arterial branch. At surgery, further assessment is done with intra-operative ultrasound and a search for lymph node involvement.

In a department with a high resection rate, pre-operative cholangiography predicted clinical management in 82% of patients, and angiography determined management in 80% [38].

Treatment

Surgery

Tumours of the lower bile duct may be resected with a 1-year survival of about 70%. More proximal tumours may be resected by local or major liver surgery including excision of the whole bifurcation of the common hepatic duct, lobectomy if necessary and bilateral hepatico-jejunostomy.

Table 37.1. Criteria of irresectability for hilar cholangiocarcinoma

Bilateral bile duct involvement or multifocal disease on cholangiography
Main trunk of portal vein encased/occluded
Bilateral involvement of hepatic arterial or portal vein branches or both
Unilateral hepatic artery involvement and extensive contralateral bile duct involvement

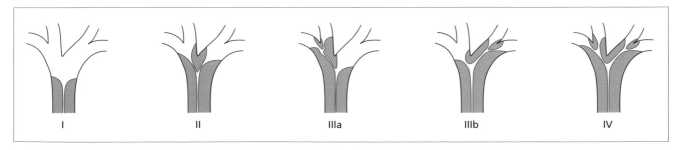

I	II	IIIa	IIIb	IV

Fig. 37.4. Classification of hilar cholangiocarcinoma according to the involvement of bile ducts. Resectability of type I to III depends on angiographic findings. Type IV (bilateral involvement of secondary hepatic ducts) indicates incurable disease. In inoperable patients median survival after stent insertion depends upon the extent of tumour [53].

Some advocate caudate lobectomy, based on the observation that two to three bile ducts from this lobe drain directly into the main bile ducts adjacent to the confluence of the hepatic ducts and thus are likely to be involved by tumour.

The proportion of cholangiocarcinomas being resected has increased from 5–20% of patients in the 1970s to 30% or more in specialist centres in the 1990s. This relates to earlier diagnosis and referral to a tertiary centre, more accurate and complete pre-operative assessment, and a more aggressive surgical approach. The problem is to achieve a resection with tumour-negative margins. Median survival after aggressive resection of hilar cholangiocarcinoma is 18–40 months with good palliation for most of this time [7, 38]. Local resection of Bismuth type I and II tumours (fig. 37.4) carries a peri-operative mortality of 5% or less. Liver resection is needed for type III lesions, and carries a greater morbidity and mortality.

Liver transplantation is not appropriate for cholangiocarcinoma because of early recurrence in the majority [64].

Surgical palliative procedures include anastomosis of jejunum to the segment III duct in the left lobe which is usually accessible despite the hilar tumour (fig. 37.5). Jaundice is relieved for at least 3 months in 75% of patients [26]. If segment III bypass is not possible (atrophy, metastases), a right-sided intra-hepatic anastomosis to the segment V duct can be done.

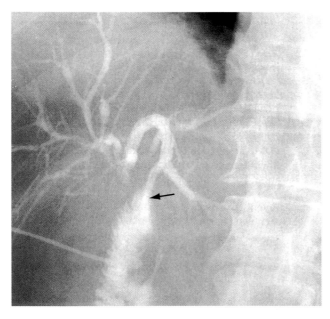

Fig. 37.5. Check cholangiogram after surgical bypass for hilar cholangiocarcinoma. The anastomosis is between the jejunum and the third segment duct of the left lobe (arrow).

Non-surgical palliation

In those patients unfit for surgery or with irresectable tumours, jaundice and itching may be relieved by placing an endoprosthesis across the stricture either by the endoscopic or percutaneous route.

By the endoscopic route, stents can be inserted successfully in about 90% of patients if a combined endoscopic/percutaneous procedure is included after a failed endoscopic attempt. The major early complication is cholangitis (7%). Thirty-day mortality is between 10 and 28% depending upon the extent of the tumour at the hilum and the mean survival is 20 weeks [53]. Stenting of only one lobe is necessary [14].

Percutaneous trans-hepatic endoprosthesis insertion is also successful but carries with it a higher risk of complications such as bleeding and bile leakage (Chapter 32). Metal mesh endoprostheses, which expand to 10 mm diameter in the stricture after insertion of a 5 or 7 French catheter, are more expensive than plastic types, but have longer patency for peri-ampullary strictures [36]. They may be used for hilar strictures. Studies suggest a similar advantage over plastic endoprostheses [63] but their insertion requires an experienced operator.

There are no trials comparing surgical versus non-surgical palliation. There are benefits and disadvantages of both approaches [44]. Generally, non-operative techniques are appropriate for high-risk patients expected to have a shorter survival. Because of recurrent stent blockage requiring replacement [24], surgical bypass should be considered as an alternative palliative approach.

Internal radiotherapy using an iridium-192 wire or radium needles may be combined with biliary drainage [21]. The value of this technique is unproven. Cytotoxic drugs are ineffective. External radiotherapy has appeared to show some benefit in retrospective studies but in a randomized trial showed no benefit [50]. Intra-duct photodynamic therapy combined with stenting has given encouraging results in Bismuth type III and IV cholangiocarcinoma [2]. There is a local tumour response of 30–75% and hilar bile ducts occlusion can be reversed. The treatment is costly and controlled studies are needed to establish survival benefit. Symptomatic treatment is that of chronic cholestasis (Chapter 13).

Cholangiocellular carcinoma

This intra-hepatic bile duct derived tumour is classified as a primary hepatic carcinoma. It becomes symptomatic as it enlarges producing abdominal pain rather than jaundice [8]. It grows rapidly with early metastasis and a particularly poor prognosis. There is an association with Thorotrast (thorium dioxide), an intravenous contrast medium used many years ago. Scanning shows an intra-hepatic mass. Distinction from hepato-cellular carcinoma may be difficult. Hepatic venous and portal vein involvement is rare. Surgery is the only chance for effective treatment. Resection is possible in 30–60% of cases [8]. One-year survival after resection is 50–60%. Transplantation for irresectable tumour gives a median survival of 5 months [49].

Metastases at the hilum

Cholestatic jaundice developing following the diagnosis of carcinoma elsewhere (in particular the colon) may be due to diffuse metastases within the liver or duct obstruction by nodes at the hilum. Differentiation between the two is by ultrasound. If dilated bile ducts are shown and the patient is symptomatic with itching, biliary obstruction can be relieved by insertion of an endoprosthesis by the endoscopic or percutaneous approach [61]. Palliation is achieved depending upon the extent of tumour but the 30-day mortality is greater and the survival significantly shorter compared with endoprosthesis insertion for primary bile duct malignancy [53].

References

1 Bartlett DL. Gallbladder cancer. *Semin. Surg. Oncol.* 2000; **19**: 145.

2 Berr F, Wiedmann M, Tannapfel A *et al*. Photodynamic therapy for advanced bile duct cancer: evidence for improved palliation and extended survival. *Hepatology* 2000; **31**: 291.

3 Björnsson E, Kilander A, Olsson R. CA 19-9 and CEA are unreliable markers for cholangiocarcinoma in patients with primary sclerosing cholangitis. *Liver* 1999; **19**: 501.

4 Broomé U, Löfberg R, Veress B *et al*. Primary sclerosing cholangitis and ulcerative colitis: evidence for increased neoplastic potential. *Hepatology* 1995; **22**: 1404.

5 Butterly LF, Schapiro RH, LaMuraglia GM *et al*. Biliary granular cell tumour: a little-known curable bile duct neoplasm of young people. *Surgery* 1988; **103**: 328.

6 Caygill CPJ, Hill MJ, Braddick M *et al*. Cancer mortality in chronic typhoid and paratyphoid carriers. *Lancet* 1994; **373**: 83.

7 Chamberlain RS, Blumgart LH. Hilar cholangiocarcinoma: a review and commentary. *Ann. Surg. Oncol.* 2000; **7**: 55.

8 Chen M-F. Peripheral cholangiocarcinoma (cholangiocellular carcinoma): clinical features, diagnosis and treatment. *J. Gastroenterol. Hepatol.* 1999; **14**: 1144.

9 Chijiiwa K, Tanaka M. Carcinoma of the gallbladder: an appraisal of surgical resection. *Surgery* 1994; **115**: 751.

10 Choi W-B, Lee S-K, Kim M-H *et al*. A new strategy to predict the neoplastic polyps of the gallbladder based on a scoring system using EUS. *Gastrointest. Endosc.* 2000; **52**: 372.

11 Cook DJ, Salena BJ, Vincic LM. Adenomyoma of the common bile duct. *Am. J. Gastroenterol.* 1988; **83**: 432.

12 Cubertafond P, Gainant A, Cucchiaro G. Surgical treatment of 724 carcinomas of the gallbladder. Results of the French Surgical Association Survey. *Ann. Surg.* 1994; **219**: 275.

13 De Aretxabala X, Roa I, Brugos L *et al*. Gallbladder cancer in Chile: a report on 54 potentially resectable tumours. *Cancer* 1992; **69**: 60.

14 De Palma GD, Galloro G, Siciliano S *et al*. Unilateral vs. bilateral endoscopic hepatic duct drainage in patients with malignant hilar biliary obstruction: results of a prospective, randomized, and controlled study. *Gastrointest. Endosc.* 2001; **53**: 547.

15 Diamantis I, Karamitopoulou E, Perentes E *et al*. p53 protein immunoreactivity in extrahepatic bile duct and gallbladder cancer: correlation with tumour grade and survival. *Hepatology* 1995; **22**: 774.

16 Donohue JH, Nagorney DM, Grant CS *et al*. Carcinoma of the gallbladder: does radical resection improve outcome? *Arch. Surg.* 1990; **125**: 237.

17 Ekbom A, Hsieh C, Yuen J *et al*. Risk of extra hepatic bile duct cancer after cholecystectomy. *Lancet* 1993; **372**: 1262.

18 Farley DR, Weaver AL, Nagorney DM. 'Natural history' of unresected cholangiocarcinoma: patient outcome after non-curative intervention. *Mayo Clin. Proc.* 1995; **70**: 425.

19 Feydy A, Vilgrain V, Denys A *et al*. Helical CT assessment in hilar cholangiocarcinoma: correlation with surgical and pathologic findings. *Am. J. Roentgenol.* 1999; **172**: 73.

20 Fleming KA, Boberg KM, Glaumann H *et al*. Biliary dysplasia as a marker of cholangiocarcinoma in primary sclerosing cholangitis. *J. Hepatol.* 2001; **34**: 360.

21 Fletcher MS, Brinkley D, Dawson JL *et al*. Treatment of hilar carcinoma by bile drainage combined with internal radiotherapy using 192-iridium wire. *Br. J. Surg.* 1983; **70**: 733.

22 Fritscher-Ravens A, Broering DC, Sriram PVJ *et al*. EUS-guided fine-needle aspiration cytodiagnosis of hilar cholangiocarcinoma: a case series. *Gastrointest. Endosc.* 2000; **52**: 534.

23 Fujita N, Noda Y, Kobayashi G *et al*. Diagnosis of the depth of invasion of gallbladder carcinoma by EUS. *Gastrointest. Endosc.* 1999; **50**: 659.

24 Gerhards MF, den Hartog D, Rauws EA *et al*. Palliative treatment in patients with unresectable hilar cholangiocarcinoma: results of endoscopic drainage in patients with type III and IV hilar cholangiocarcinoma. *Eur. J. Surg.* 2001; **167**: 274.

25 Gerhards MF, Vos P, van Gulik TM *et al*. Incidence of benign lesions in patients resected for suspicious hilar obstruction. *Br. J. Surg.* 2001; **88**: 48.

26 Guthrie CM, Banting SW, Garden OJ *et al*. Segment III cholangiojejunostomy for palliation of malignant hilar obstruction. *Br. J. Surg.* 1994; **81**: 1639.

27 Hintze RE, Abou-Rebyeh H, Adler A *et al*. Magnetic resonance cholangiopancreatography-guided unilateral endoscopic stent placement for Klatskin tumours. *Gastrointest. Endosc.* 2001; **53**: 40.

28 Hisatomi K, Haratake J, Horie A *et al*. Relation of histopathological features to prognosis of gallbladder cancer. *Am. J. Gastroenterol.* 1990; **85**: 567.

29 Hochwald SN, Burke EC, Jarnagin WR *et al*. Association of preoperative biliary stenting with increased postoperative infectious complications in proximal cholangiocarcinoma. *Arch. Surg.* 1999; **134**: 261.

30 Keiding S, Hansen SB, Rasmussen HH *et al*. Detection of cholangiocarcinoma in primary sclerosing cholangitis by positron emission tomography. *Hepatology* 1998; **28**: 700.

31 Klatskin G. Adenocarcinoma of the hepatic duct at its bifurcation within the porta hepatis. An unusual tumour with

distinctive clinical and pathological features. *Am. J. Med.* 1965; **38**: 24.

32 Kluge R, Schmidt F, Caca K *et al.* Positron emission tomography with [^{18}F] fluoro-2-deoxy-D-glucose for diagnosis and staging of bile duct cancer. *Hepatology* 2001; **33**: 1029.

33 Kubicka S, Kohnel F, Flemming P *et al.* K-ras mutations in the bile of patients with primary sclerosing cholangitis. *Gut* 2001; **48**: 403.

34 Kubota K, Bandai Y, Noie T *et al.* How should polypoid lesions of the gallbladder be treated in the era of laparoscopic cholecystectomy? *Surgery* 1995; **117**: 481.

35 Kurathong S, Lerdverasirikul P, Wongpaitoon V *et al. Opisthorchis viverrini* infection and cholangiocarcinoma. A prospective, case-controlled study. *Gastroenterology* 1985; **89**: 151.

36 Lammer J, Hausegger KA, Flockiger F *et al.* Common bile duct obstruction due to malignancy: treatment with plastic vs. metal stents. *Radiology* 1996; **201**: 167.

37 Leidenius M, Höckerstedt K, Broomé U *et al.* Hepatobiliary carcinoma in primary sclerosing cholangitis: a case control study. *J. Hepatol.* 2001; **34**: 792

38 Lillemoe KD, Cameron JL. Surgery for hilar cholangiocarcinoma: the Johns Hopkins approach. *J. Hepatobil. Pancreat. Surg.* 2000; **7**: 115.

39 Mainprize KS, Gould SWT, Gilbert JM. Surgical management of polypoid lesions of the gallbladder. *Br. J. Surg.* 2000; **87**: 414.

40 Misra SP, Dwivedi M. Pancreaticobiliary ductal union. *Gut* 1990; **31**: 1144.

41 Moriguchi H, Tazawa J, Hayashi Y *et al.* Natural history of polypoid lesions in the gall bladder. *Gut* 1996; **39**: 860.

42 Nakeeb A, Pitt HA. The role of preoperative biliary decompression in obstructive jaundice. *Hepatogastroenterology* 1995; **42**: 332.

43 Neumaier CE, Bertolotto M, Perrone R *et al.* Staging of hilar cholangiocarcinoma with ultrasound. *J. Clin. Ultrasound* 1995; **23**: 173.

44 Nordback IH, Pitt HA, Coleman J *et al.* Unresectable hilar cholangiocarcinoma: percutaneous vs. operative palliation. *Surgery* 1994; **115**: 597.

45 Oikarinen H, Paivansalo M, Lahde S *et al.* Radiological findings in cases of gallbladder carcinoma. *Eur. J. Radiol.* 1993; **17**: 179.

46 Parkin DM, Ohshima H, Srivatanakul P *et al.* Cholangiocarcinoma: epidemiology, mechanisms of carcinogenesis and prevention. *Cancer Epidemiol. Biomarkers Prev.* 1993; **2**: 537.

47 Patel AH, Harnois DM, Klee GG *et al.* The utility of CA 19–9 in the diagnoses of cholangiocarcinoma in patients without primary sclerosing cholangitis. *Am. J. Gastroenterol.* 2000; **95**: 204.

48 Patel T. Increasing incidence and mortality of primary intrahepatic cholangiocarcinoma in the United States. *Hepatology* 2001; **33**: 1353.

49 Pichlmayr R, Lamesch P, Weimann A *et al.* Surgical treatment of cholangiocellular carcinoma. *World J. Surg.* 1995; **19**: 83.

50 Pitt HA, Nakeeb A, Abrams RA *et al.* Perihilar cholangiocarcinoma. Postoperative radiotherapy does not improve survival. *Ann. Surg.* 1995; **221**: 788.

51 Polk HC. Carcinoma and calcified gallbladder. *Gastroenterology* 1966; **50**: 582.

52 Ponsioen CY, Vrouenraets SME, van Milligen de Wit AWM *et al.* Value of brush cytology for dominant strictures in primary sclerosing cholangitis. *Endoscopy* 1999; **31**: 305.

53 Polydorou AA, Cairns SR, Dowsett JF *et al.* Palliation of proximal malignant biliary obstruction by endoscopic endoprosthesis insertion. *Gut* 1991; **32**: 685.

54 Rosen CB, Nagorney DM, Wiesner RH *et al.* Cholangiocarcinoma complicating primary sclerosing cholangitis. *Ann. Surg.* 1991; **213**: 21.

55 Sato Y, van Gulik TM, Bosma A *et al.* Prognostic significance of tumour DNA content in carcinoma of the hepatic duct confluence. *Surgery* 1994; **115**: 488.

56 Stewart CJR, Mills PR, Carter R *et al.* Brush cytology in the assessment of pancreatico-biliary strictures: a review of 406 cases. *J. Clin. Pathol.* 2001; **54**: 449.

57 Sugiyama M, Atomi Y, Yamato T. Endoscopic ultrasonography for differential diagnosis of polypoid gall bladder lesions: analysis in surgical and follow up series. *Gut* 2000; **46**: 250.

58 Tamada K, Ido K, Ueno N *et al.* Preoperative staging of extrahepatic bile duct cancer with intraductal ultrasonography. *Am. J. Gastroenterol.* 1995; **90**: 239.

59 Taylor-Robinson SD, Toledano MB, Arora S *et al.* Increase in mortality rates from intrahepatic cholangiocarcinoma in England and Wales 1968–98. *Gut* 2001; **48**: 816.

60 Tompkins RK, Saunders KD, Roslyn JJ *et al.* Changing patterns in diagnosis and management of bile duct cancer. *Ann. Surg.* 1990; **211**: 614.

61 Valiozis I, Zekry A, Williams SJ *et al.* Palliation of hilar biliary obstruction from colorectal metastases by endoscopic stent insertion. *Gastrointest. Endosc.* 2000; **51**: 412.

62 Vitetta L, Sali A, Little P *et al.* Gallstones and gall bladder carcinoma. *Aust. NZ J. Surg.* 2000; **70**: 667.

63 Wagner H-J, Knyrim K, Vakil N *et al.* Plastic endoprostheses vs. metal stents in the palliative treatment of malignant hilar biliary obstruction: a prospective randomized trial. *Endoscopy* 1993; **25**: 213.

64 Wall WJ. Liver transplantation for hepatic and biliary malignancy. *Semin. Liver Dis.* 2000; **20**: 425.

65 Watanabe M, Asaka M, Tanaka J *et al.* Point mutation of K-ras gene codon 12 in biliary tract tumours. *Gastroenterology* 1994; **107**: 1147.

66 Zidi SH, Prat F, Le Guen O *et al.* Performance characteristics of magnetic resonance cholangiography in the staging of malignant hilar strictures. *Gut* 2000; **46**: 103.

Chapter 38
Hepatic Transplantation

In 1955, Welch performed the first transplantation of the liver in dogs [118]. In 1963, Starzl and his group carried out the first successful hepatic transplant in man [101].

The number of transplants is escalating and, in 1997, 4099 patients were transplanted in the USA. Elective liver transplantation in low-risk patients has a 90% 1-year survival. Improved results can be related to more careful patient selection, to better surgical techniques and post-operative care, and to greater willingness to re-transplant after rejection. Better immunosuppression has contributed.

Selection of patients

The patient selected for transplant should suffer from irreversible, progressive disease for which there is no acceptable, alternative therapy. The patient and the family must understand the magnitude of the undertaking and be prepared to face the difficult early post-operative period and life-long immunosuppression.

Improved results have led to a greater acceptance of the procedure. Demand has exceeded supply of donor organs (fig. 38.1). The time spent awaiting transplant

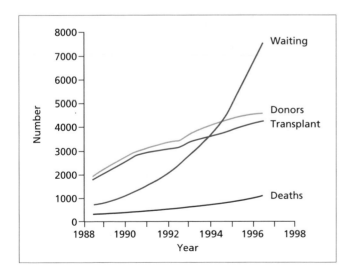

Fig. 38.1. Over the last 8 years availability of donors has not kept up with the demand for transplants. Waiting time and deaths have increased.

and deaths occurring before it can be performed have increased. The waiting time for low-risk patients is approximately 6–12 months. Although in general this may be longer for those of blood group B and AB, group O recipients may have the longest waiting time because group O is the universal donor type. Depending on the system of organ distribution, such livers can be given to recipients having any ABO group. Donor livers suitable for children are particularly rare and this has led to the split-liver technique (see fig. 38.5).

The equitable distribution of the precious donor livers is difficult. Results (and costs) are much better if the patient is low risk (ambulatory) compared with high risk (intensive care). Decisions are usually made by a multi-disciplinary panel including the patient and patient's family. In the USA, the United Network for Organ Sharing (UNOS) guidelines are followed (tables 38.1, 38.2) [63]. A modified Child–Pugh score is used as the basis by which to evaluate the severity of liver disease. The priorities expressed by the general public are not the same as those of clinicians. There has been a perceived lack of fairness in organ allocation [76]. The UNOS website (www.unos.org) allows the public and clinicians access to transplant activities and outcomes. Livers should be allocated for medical need and not on the basis of financial or other considerations. Unacceptable criteria include the patient's contribution to society, inability to comply with treatment (e.g. antisocial behaviour), the patient's contribution to the disorder (e.g. drug or alcohol abuse) and the past use of medical resources [27]. Recipients are broadly defined as having an intolerable quality of life because of liver disease or having an anticipated length of life of less than 1 year because of liver failure. There are few guidelines predicting survival. Patients more than 65 years old have a substantially worse 5-year survival, but age itself is not a contraindication.

Candidates: outcome (table 38.3)

In Europe, the pattern of primary indication for liver transplantation is changing. The main indication is cirrhosis, including primary biliary cirrhosis. More patients with acute and sub-acute hepatic failure are being

revascularization is essential. If not corrected, re-transplant is necessary.

Portal vein thrombosis is often silent, presenting as variceal bleeding weeks to months after the transplant.

Hepatic vein occlusion. This is common in patients who have had liver transplantation for the Budd–Chiari syndrome. Occasionally there is stricturing of the supra-hepatic–caval anastomosis and this can be treated by balloon dilatation.

Biliary tract complications

Bile secretion recovers spontaneously over a 10–12-day period and is strongly dependent upon bile salt secretion. The incidence of complication is 6–34% of all transplants usually during the first 3 months (table 38.10) [67, 109].

Bile leaks may be early (first 30 days) related to the bile duct anastomosis or late (about 4 months) after T-tube removal. Abdominal pain and peritoneal signs may be masked by immunosuppression.

Early leaks are diagnosed by ERCP or percutaneous cholangiography. HIDA scanning may be useful. They are usually treated by the endoscopic insertion of a stent or nasobiliary drain.

Extra-hepatic anastomotic strictures. These present after about 5 months as intermittent fever and fluctuating serum biochemical abnormalities. There is a wide differential diagnosis including rejection and sepsis. They are diagnosed by MRI cholangiography [44], ERCP or percutaneous cholangiopancreatography and treated by balloon dilatation (see fig. 32.19) and/or insertion of a plastic stent [109]. Hepatic arterial patency must be established.

Non-anastomotic or *'ischaemic-type' biliary strictures* develop in 2–19% [43]. They are associated with multifactorial damage to the hepatic arterial plexus around bile ducts. Factors include prolonged cold ischaemia time, hepatic arterial thrombosis, ABO blood group incompatibility, rejection, foam cell arteriopathy and a positive lymphocytotoxic cross-match. Peri-biliary arteriolar endothelial damage contributes to segmental microvascular thrombosis and hence to multiple segmental biliary ischaemic strictures.

Table 38.10. Biliary complications of liver transplantation

Leaks
Early (0–2 weeks)
anastomotic
Late (4 months) after T-tube removal
Strictures
Anastomotic (6–12 months)
Non-anastomotic/intra-hepatic (3 months)

Non-anastomotic strictures usually develop after several months. They develop in the donor common hepatic duct, with variable extension into the main intra-hepatic ducts. On cholangiography the wall of the duct may appear irregular and hazy, presumably reflecting areas of necrosis and oedema. Attempts are made to treat them by balloon dilatation and stenting. Hepatico-jejunostomy is sometimes possible. Re-transplant may be necessary.

Biliary stones, sludge and casts. These can develop any time following transplant. Obstruction, particularly biliary stricture, may be important. Foreign bodies such as T-tubes and stents may serve as a nidus for stone formation. Cyclosporin is lithogenic.

Treatment is by endoscopic sphincterotomy and stone extraction with naso-biliary irrigation if necessary.

Renal failure

Oliguria is virtually constant post-transplant, but in some renal failure is more serious. The causes include pre-existing kidney disease, hypotension and shock, sepsis, nephrotoxic antibiotics and cyclosporin or tacrolimus. Renal failure often accompanies severe graft rejection or overwhelming infection.

Pulmonary complications

In infants, death *during* liver transplantation may be related to platelet aggregates in small lung vessels. Intravascular catheters, platelet infusions and cell debris from the liver may contribute.

In the ICU, pulmonary infiltrates are most frequently due to pulmonary oedema and pneumonia. Other causes are atelectasis and respiratory distress syndrome [99]. In the first 30 days, pneumonia is usually due to methicillin-resistant *Staphylococcus aureus*, *Pseudomonas* and aspergillosis. After 4 weeks pneumonia due to CMV and *Pneumocystis* is seen. Later (more than 1 year), when the patient has developed recurrent HCV or HBV, lymphoproliferative disorder or chronic rejection are seen.

In one report, 87% of patients with pneumonia required ventilation and 40% were bacteraemic. Pyrexia, leucocytosis, poor oxygenation and cultures of the bronchial secretions indicate pneumonia and demand antibiotic therapy. The overall mortality for those having pulmonary infiltrates in the ICU is 28% [99].

Pleural effusion is virtually constant and in about 18% aspiration is necessary.

A post-transplant hyperdynamic syndrome tends to normalize with time.

The hepato-pulmonary syndrome (Chapter 6) is usually corrected by liver transplant but only after a stormy post-transplant course with prolonged hypoxaemia, mechanical ventilation and intensive care [60].

Non-specific cholestasis

This is frequently seen in the first few days, with the serum bilirubin peaking at 14–21 days. Liver biopsy suggests extra-hepatic biliary obstruction but cholangiography is normal. Factors involved include mild preservation injury, sepsis, haemorrhage and renal failure. If infection is controlled, liver and kidney function usually recover but a prolonged stay in the ICU is usually necessary.

Rejection

Immunologically, the liver is a privileged organ with regard to transplantation, having a higher resistance to immunological attack than other organs. The liver cell probably carries fewer surface antigens. Nevertheless, episodes of rejection, of varying severity, are virtually constant.

Cellular rejection is initiated through the presentation of donor HLA antigens by antigen-presenting cells to host helper T-cells in the graft. These helper T-cells secrete IL2 which activates other T-cells. The accumulation of activated T-cells in the graft leads to T-cell-mediated cytotoxicity and a generalized inflammatory response.

Hyper-acute rejection is rare and is due to pre-sensitization to donor antigens. Acute (cellular) rejection is fully reversible, but chronic (ductopenic) is not. The two may merge into one another. The diagnosis of rejection from opportunistic infections is difficult and protocol liver biopsies are essential. Increased immunosuppression to combat rejection favours infection.

Acute cellular rejection

64% of patients will have at least one episode, usually 5–20 days post-transplant and within the first 6 weeks [121]. Acute rejection does not have an adverse effect on patient or graft survival [51, 75]. There is little need to give higher immunosuppression during the first few days. The patient feels ill, there is mild pyrexia and tachycardia. The liver is enlarged and tender. Serum bilirubin, transaminases and prothrombin time increase. The liver enzyme changes lack specificity and a liver biopsy is essential.

Rejection is shown by the classical triad of portal inflammation, bile duct damage (fig. 38.8) and sub-endothelial inflammation of portal and terminal hepatic veins (endothelialitis) (fig. 38.9). Eosinophils may be conspicuous [50], and hepato-cellular necrosis may be seen.

Rejection may be graded into mild, moderate and severe (table 38.11) [32]. Follow-up biopsies may show eosinophils, resembling a drug reaction, and infarct-like

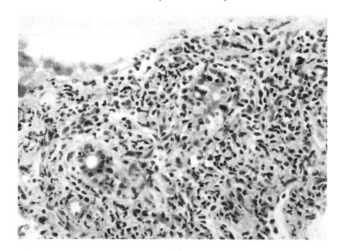

Fig. 38.8. Acute rejection: a damaged bile duct infiltrated with lymphocytes is seen in a densely cellular portal tract. (H & E, ×100.)

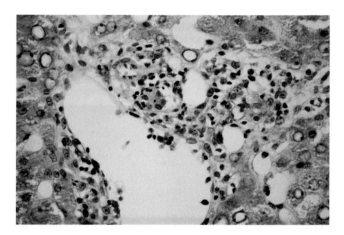

Fig. 38.9. Acute cellular rejection 8 days post-transplant. Liver biopsy shows portal zone infiltration with mononuclear cells and endothelialitis of cells lining the portal vein. (H & E, ×100.)

areas of necrosis, perhaps secondary to portal venous obstruction by lymphocytes. Hepatic arteriography shows separation and narrowing of hepatic arteries (fig. 38.10). Histological severity correlates prognostically with steroid failure, early death or re-transplant [121]. In 85%, treatment is successful by increasing immunosuppression. Boluses of high dose methylprednisolone are given, for example 1 g intravenously daily for 3 days. Those who are steroid-resistant receive IL2 monoclonal antibody for 10–14 days. Tacrolimus rescue may also be tried. Those failing to respond to these measures proceed to ductopenic rejection. Re-transplant may be needed if the rejection continues.

Chronic ductopenic rejection

Bile ducts are progressively damaged and ultimately

infection is associated with cholestatic hepatitis and the vanishing bile duct syndrome.

'Pizza-pie' retinitis and gastroenteritis are other features.

Liver biopsy shows clusters of polymorphs and lymphocytes with CMV intranuclear inclusions (fig. 38.14). Bile duct atypia and endothelialitis are absent. Immunostaining, using a monoclonal antibody against an early CMV antigen, allows early diagnosis (fig. 38.15) [84]. Cell culture techniques, such as DEAFF (Detection of Early Antigen Fluorescent Foci), may be positive within 16 h. PCR techniques are now routine for diagnosis.

Routine prophylaxis for CMV with oral ganciclovir is effective [45] and is used in some centres, but there is concern over the appearance of resistant strains.

If possible, immunosuppression should be reduced. Re-transplant may be necessary.

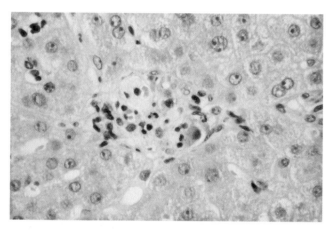

Fig. 38.14. CMV hepatitis 4 weeks post-transplant. A focus of inflammation shows hepatocytes containing inclusion bodies. (H & E, ×160.)

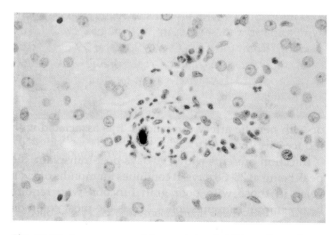

Fig. 38.15. Immunoperoxidase staining (×160) confirms the presence of CMV as a brown intranuclear deposit.

Herpes simplex virus

This infection is usually related to immunosuppression-induced reactivation. Liver biopsy shows confluent areas of necrosis with surrounding viral inclusions. This infection has virtually disappeared with prophylactic acyclovir.

Epstein–Barr virus

This is most frequent in children as a primary infection. It causes a mononucleosis–hepatitis picture (fig. 38.16). It is often asymptomatic. The diagnosis is made serologically (see Chapter 16).

Lymphoproliferative disorders

These complicate all solid organ transplants, the incidence being 1.8–4%. The tumour is usually a non-Hodgkin's B-cell lymphoma. It usually affects children but can also be seen in adults. There is a strong association with Epstein–Barr infection. The tumour presents 3–72 months post-transplant in lymph nodes or in the allograft itself. The prognosis is very poor. Treatment is by reducing immunosuppression and by giving antiviral therapy with acyclovir. Systemic chemotherapy may increase survival but has to be given cautiously as withdrawal may be followed by fulminant liver failure or reactivation of the hepatitis B virus. The outcome is poor [6].

Adenovirus

These infections are seen in children. They are usually

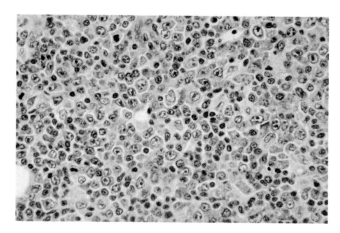

Fig. 38.16. Epstein–Barr-associated lymphoproliferative syndrome in a child aged 3 years, at 6 months post-transplant. A lymph node from the porta hepatis showing sheets of lymphocytes replacing the normal lymph gland architecture. (H & E, ×300.)

mild, but fatal hepatitis can develop. There is no recognized treatment.

Varicella

This can complicate transplants in children. It is treated with intravenous ganciclovir.

Nocardia

This infection usually affects the chest but skin and cerebral lesions may also occur.

Fungal infections

Aspergillosis has a high mortality with increases in serum bilirubin and renal failure. Brain abscess may be a complication. It may be treated by liposomal amphotericin.

Pneumocystis pneumonia

This presents in the first 6 months. It is diagnosed by bronchoscopy and broncho-alveolar lavage. It is prevented by Bactrim (Septrin) prophylaxis, one tablet daily for the first 6 months post-transplant.

Malignancies

Six per cent of organ transplant recipients will develop cancer, usually within 5 years of the transplant [107]. Many are related to immunosuppression. Malignancies include lymphoproliferative diseases, skin cancers and Kaposi's sarcoma [107]. Yearly cancer surveillance is essential for all patients post-transplant.

Drug-related toxicity

This must always be considered in any reaction whether hepatitic or cholestatic. Causative drugs include azathioprine, cyclosporin, tacrolimus, antibiotics, antihypertensives and antidepressants.

Disease recurrence

Hepatitis B appears at 2–12 months and may lead to cirrhosis and liver failure within 1–3 years (see p. 659). Hepatitis C is seen at any time after the first 4 weeks.

Hepato-cellular malignancies recur in the graft or as metastases, usually within the first 2 years.

The possible recurrence of primary biliary cirrhosis is discussed in Chapter 14. Budd–Chiari syndrome may re-appear quite soon after transplantation if anticoagulation is not well controlled.

Central nervous system toxicity

Several central nervous changes can follow liver transplantation [18]. Half the patients show fits, children being more susceptible than adults [26]. Cyclosporin-associated fits are controlled by phenytoin but this induces (accelerates) cyclosporin metabolism.

Central pontine myelinolysis is related to sudden alterations in serum electrolytes, perhaps in combination with cyclosporin. CT scan shows white-matter lucencies.

Cyclosporin is bound to lipoprotein fractions in the blood. Patients with low serum cholesterol values are at particular risk of central nervous system toxicity after the transplant.

Cerebral infarction is related to peri-operative hypotension, or air/micro-thrombus embolism.

Cerebral abscess is seen although rarely.

Headaches in the first few weeks can persist. Cyclosporin has been incriminated but in most instances the cause is obscure [18].

Tremor is a common side-effect of immunosuppressants including corticosteroids, tacrolimus and cyclosporin. It is usually mild, but occasionally requires reduction or cessation of medication.

A second transplant is associated with more and greater mental abnormalities, seizures and focal motor defects.

Bone disease

Patients having liver transplants usually have some previous degree of hepatic osteodystrophy. The bones deteriorate post-transplant with vertebral collapse in 38% during the second 3 months. The cause is multifactorial and includes cholestasis, cyclosporin, corticosteroid therapy and bed rest [91]. Recovery takes place with time.

Ectopic soft-tissue calcification [70]

This can develop diffusely and is associated with respiratory insufficiency and bone fractures. It is secondary to hypocalcaemia due to citrate infused in fresh frozen plasma, and, in addition, renal failure and secondary hyperparathyroidism. Tissue injury and administration of exogenous calcium lead to the soft-tissue calcium deposition.

Conclusion

Hepatic transplantation is a tremendous undertaking that does not begin or end with the surgery. The patient and family need psychiatric and social support. There must be a back-up programme to procure organs.

dine in controlled hepatitis B virus recurrence after liver transplantation. *Transplantation* 1998; **65**: 1615.

74 Neuberger JM, Adams DH. Is HLA matching important for liver transplantation? *J. Hepatol.* 1990; **11**: 1.

75 Neuberger J, Adams DH. What is the significance of acute liver allograft rejection? *J. Hepatol.* 1998; **29**: 143.

76 Neuberger J, James O. Guidelines for selection of patients for liver transplantation in the era of donor-organ shortage. *Lancet* 1999; **354**: 1636.

77 Nghiem HV. Imaging of hepatic transplantation. *Radiol. Clin. North Am.* 1998; **36**: 429.

78 Olivieri NF, Liu PP, Sher GD *et al.* Brief report: combined liver and heart transplantation for end-stage iron-induced organ failure in an adult with homozygous beta-thalassaemia. *N. Engl. J. Med.* 1994; **330**: 1125.

79 Ong JP, Reddy V, Gramlich TL *et al.* Cryptogenic cirrhosis and risk of recurrence of nonalcoholic fatty liver disease after liver transplantation. *Gastroenterology* 2000; **118**: A973.

80 Orons PD, Zajko AB. Angiography and interventional procedures in liver transplantation. *Radiol. Clin. North Am.* 1995; **33**: 541.

81 Otte G, Herfarth C, Senninger N *et al.* Hepatic transplantation in galactosaemia. *Transplantation* 1989; **47**: 902.

82 Otte JB. Recent developments in liver transplantation: lessons from a 5-year experience. *J. Hepatol.* 1991; **12**: 386.

83 Otte JB, de Ville de Goyet J, Sokal E *et al.* Size reduction of the donor liver is a safe way to alleviate the shortage of size-matched organs in paediatric liver transplantation. *Ann. Surg.* 1990; **211**: 146.

84 Paya CV, Holley KE, Wiesner RH *et al.* Early diagnosis of cytomegalovirus hepatitis in liver transplant recipients: role of immunostaining, DNA hybridization and culture of hepatic tissue. *Hepatology* 1990; **12**: 119.

85 Ratziu Y, Samuel D, Sebagh M *et al.* Long-term follow-up after liver transplantation for autoimmune hepatitis: evidence of recurrence of primary disease. *J. Hepatol.* 1999; **30**: 31.

86 Reding R, de Groyet J de V, Delbeke I *et al.* Paediatric liver transplantation with cadaveric or living related donors: comparative results in 90 elective recipients of primary grafts. *J. Pediatr.* 1999; **134**: 280.

87 Rela M, Musien P, Volea-Melendez H *et al.* Auxiliary partial orthotopic liver transplantation for Crigler–Najjar syndrome type 1. *Ann. Surg.* 1999; **239**: 565.

88 Revell SP, Noble-Jamieson G, Johnston P *et al.* Liver transplantation for homozygous familial hypercholesterolaemia. *Arch. Dis. Child.* 1995; **73**: 456.

89 Ringe B, Lang H, Oldhafter KJ *et al.* Which is the best surgery for Budd–Chiari syndrome: venous decompression or liver transplant action? A single-centre experience with 50 patients. *Hepatology* 1995; **21**: 1337.

90 Riordan SM, Williams R. Tolerance after liver transplantation: does it exist and can immunosuppression be withdrawn? *J. Hepatol.* 1999; **31**: 1106.

91 Roding MA, Shane E. Osteoporosis after organ transplantation. *Am. J. Med.* 1998; **104**: 459.

92 Rosenau J, Bahl MJ, Tillmann HL *et al.* Lamivudine and low-dose hepatitis B immune globulin for prophylaxis of hepatitis B reinfection after liver transplantation — possible role of mutations in the YMDD motif prior to transplantation as a risk factor for reinfection. *J. Hepatol.* 2001; **34**: 895.

93 Sanchez-Fuey OA, Rimola A, Grande L *et al.* Hepatitis B immunoglobulin discontinuation followed by hepatitis B virus vaccination: a new strategy in the prophylaxis of hepatitis B virus recurrence after liver transplantation. *Hepatology* 2000; **31**: 496.

94 Schissky ML, Scheinberg IH, Sternlieb I. Liver transplantation for Wilson's disease: indications and outcome. *Hepatology* 1994; **19**: 583.

95 Schluger LK, Sheiner PA, Thung SN *et al.* Severe recurrent cholestatis hepatitis C following orthotopic liver transplantation. *Hepatology* 1996; **23**: 971.

96 Seaberg EC, Belle SH, Beringer KC *et al.* Long-term patient and retransplantation-free survival by selected recipient and donor characteristics: an update from the Pitt-Unos liver transplant registry. *Clin. Transplant.* 1997; **18**: 15.

97 Sheiner PA, Boros P, Klion FM *et al.* The efficacy of prophylactic interferon alfa-2b in preventing recurrent hepatitis C after liver transplantation. *Hepatology* 1998; **28**: 831.

98 Sheiner PA, Schwartz ME, Mor E *et al.* Severe or multiple rejection episodes are associated with early recurrence of hepatitis C after orthotopic liver transplantation. *Hepatology* 1995; **21**: 30.

99 Singh N, Gayowski T, Wagener MM. Pulmonary infiltrates in liver transplant recipients in the intensive care unit. *Transplantation* 1999; **67**: 1138.

100 Singh N, Gayowski T, Wagener MM *et al.* Quality of life, functional status and depression in male liver transplant recipients with recurrent viral hepatitis C. *Transplantation* 1999; **67**: 69.

101 Starzl TE, Marchioro TL, von Kaulla KN *et al.* Homotransplantation of the liver in humans. *Surg. Gynecol. Obstet.* 1963; **117**: 659.

102 Starzl TE, Rao AS, Murase M *et al.* Will xenotransplantation ever be feasible? *J. Am. Coll. Surg.* 1998; **186**: 383.

103 Starzl TE, Todo S, Fung J *et al.* FK 506 for liver, kidney and pancreas transplantation. *Lancet* 1989; **ii**: 1000.

104 Starzl TE, Todo S, Tzakis A *et al.* The many faces of multivisceral transplantation. *Surg. Gynecol. Obstet.* 1991; **172**: 338.

105 Stieber AC, Zetti G, Todo S *et al.* The spectrum of portal vein thrombosis in liver transplantation. *Ann. Surg.* 1991; **213**: 199.

106 Tan KC, Yandza T, de Hemptinne B *et al.* Hepatic artery thrombosis in paediatric liver transplantation. *J. Pediatr. Surg.* 1988; **23**: 927.

107 Tan-Shalaby J, Tempero M. Malignancies after liver transplantation: a comparative review. *Semin. Liver Dis.* 1995; **15**: 156.

108 Todo S, Starzl ET, Tzakis A. Orthotopic liver transplantation for urea cycle enzyme deficiency. *Hepatology* 1992; **15**: 419.

109 Tung BY, Kimmey MB. Biliary complications of orthotopic liver transplantation. *Dig. Dis.* 1999; **17**: 133.

110 US Multicentre FK 506 Liver Study Group. A comparison of tacrolimus (FK 506) and cyclosporin for immunosuppression in liver transplantation. *N. Engl. J. Med.* 1994; **331**: 1110.

111 Van Hoek B, de Boer J, Boudjema K *et al.* Auxiliary vs. orthotopic liver transplantation for acute liver failure. *J. Hepatol.* 1999; **30**: 699.

112 Van Hoek B, Ringers J, Kroes ACM *et al.* Temporary heterotopic auxiliary liver transplantation for fulminant hepatitis B. *J. Hepatol.* 1995; **23**: 109.

113 Van Thiel DH, Gavaler JS, Kam I *et al.* Rapid growth of an intact human liver transplanted into a recipient larger than the donor. *Gastroenterology* 1987; **93**: 1414.

114 Wachs ME, Bak TE, Karrer FM *et al.* Adult living donor liver transplantation using a right hepatic lobe. *Transplantation* 1998; **68**: 1313.

115 Wade JJ, Rolando N, Hayllar K *et al.* Bacterial and fungal infections after liver transplantation: an analysis of 284 patients. *Hepatology* 1995; **21**: 1328.

116 Watson CJ, Friend PJ, Jamieson NY *et al.* Sirolimus: a potent new immunosuppressant for liver transplantation. *Transplantation* 1999; **67**: 505.

117 Watts RWE, Morgan SH, Danpure CJ *et al.* Combined hepatic and renal transplantation in primary hyperoxaluria type I: clinical report of nine cases. *Am. J. Med.* 1991; **90**: 179.

118 Welch CS. A note on transplantation of the whole liver in dogs. *Transpl. Bull.* 1955; **2**: 54.

119 Whitington PF, Balistreri WF. Liver transplantation in paediatrics: indications, contraindications, and pretransplant management. *J. Pediatr.* 1991; **118**: 169.

120 Wiesner RH. A long-term comparison for tacrolimus (FK506) vs. cyclosporin in liver transplantation. *Transplantation* 1998; **66**: 493.

121 Wiesner RH, Demetris AJ, Belle SH *et al.* Acute hepatic allograft rejection: incidence, risk factors, and impact on outcome. *Hepatology* 1998; **28**: 638.

122 Wiesner RH, Ludwig J, Vanhoek B *et al.* Current concepts in cell-mediated hepatic allograft rejection leading to ductopenia and liver failure. *Hepatology* 1991; **14**: 721.

123 Zandi P, Panis Y, Debray D *et al.* Paediatric liver transplantation for Langerhans' cell histiocytosis. *Hepatology* 1995; **21**: 129.

124 Zignego AL, Dubois F, Samuel D *et al.* Serum hepatitis delta virus RNA in patients with delta hepatitis and in liver graft recipients. *J. Hepatol.* 1990; **11**: 102.